The Encyclopedia of Ailments

"This book has helped me in my personal life and also in my practice. I use it a lot with my patients because when someone has a physical blockage, it is generally coming from an emotional blockage that creates the physical symptom. Therefore, if the patient really wants to get the full mind, body, spirit connection, they have to understand where the emotions are coming from. When I explain this to them, it is not clear, but when I use the encyclopedia they tend to understand a lot more. If I compare this book to other books that I ever read on the subject, it contains the easiest and clearest way to really look into the emotional blockage and understand it properly. Using the encyclopedia in my practice has helped me become the best practitioner I can be."

— PAM STILWELL-BOON, D.O., kinesiologist, registered massage therapist, and fitness trainer

"*The Encyclopedia of Ailments and Diseases* is not a book to read. It's a book to treasure and consult when you need guidance and support in deciphering the messages your body is trying to convey to you. All explanations are written in the first person, and the author cleverly encourages us to read in syllables, very slowly. As a result, the act of reading itself can positively affect the third chakra and the third level of the aura (the mental chakra and level). Reading becomes healing. This encyclopedia is a truly comprehensive source of information regarding psychosomatic disorders."

— TJITZE DE JONG, Brennan Healing Science practitioner and author of *Energetic Cellular Healing and Cancer*

"I have been a therapist for 21 years and work with *The Encyclopedia of Ailments and Diseases* in my practice daily. I highly recommend it to my clients because it can help them relieve their physical and emotional ailments. I use the encyclopedia as a complement to the techniques I use. The information it contains is comprehensive, easy to understand, and accessible to all. It provides food for thought to help my clients make positive changes in their lives."

— RICHARD CLOUTIER, naturopath and massage therapist, Centre du Renouveau, Québec

"Global science has developed a holistic view of health as a phenomenon that supports its four parts—physical, mental, social, and spiritual. All of these parts are closely interconnected and in a harmonious unity, constantly interacting with each other. This book is a unique reference tool that reveals the emotional and psychological causes of illnesses. It indicates feelings, thoughts, and emotions at the level of the consciousness and the subconscious present in more than 900 diseases and ailments. It explains the method of heart integration and acceptance of information that initiates the process of healing, and it offers positive affirmations that transform ailments and illnesses. Medical workers can use this book in their practice and for research to help patients in their healing process."

— OLEG SHEKERA, M.D., professor of the National Academy of Sciences of Ukraine

"I have been using this book for a few years. At the beginning, I was only consulting when needed but recently I have read it in its entirety. This book is a real bible on the subject. You will find what emotional state corresponds to each illness or discomfort in the body. A wart? Shoulder pain? There is no coincidence. These ailments always reflect an internal conflict between your body and mind. Any therapist or individual who wishes to be in tune with their body and their emotions should use this as a reference book."

— LUDIVINE STAHL, France

"I'm a firm believer in diving deep into the personal world of emotions and beliefs in order to unravel issues presenting in the physical body. This classic book provides healer wisdom for the reader to explore, which enables potentially unhelpful patterns or repressed emotions to be brought into consciousness, with love, for their resolution. Lots of food for thought and insight to help us understand the power of thought and emotion on our health and well-being. The magic, of course, arises from using this insight for our liberation."

— NIKKI GRESHAM-RECORD, counselling psychologist, healer, and author of *Working with Chakras for Belief Change: The Healing InSight Method*

THE ENCYCLOPEDIA OF

Ailments AND Diseases

How to Heal the
Conflicted Feelings, Emotions,
and Thoughts at the Root of Illness

JACQUES MARTEL
With Lucie Bernier

Translated by Dan Conley

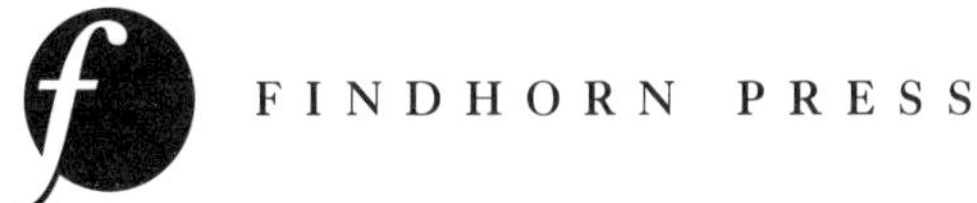

FINDHORN PRESS

Findhorn Press
One Park Street
Rochester, Vermont 05767
www.findhornpress.com

Findhorn Press is a division of Inner Traditions International

Originally published in French in 1998 by Les Éditions ATMA Internationales, Canada, under the title *Le grand dictionnaire des malaises et des maladies*
Second edition published in French in 2007
First English edition published in 2012 by Les Éditions ATMA Internationales, Canada, under the title *The Complete Dictionary of Ailments and Diseases*
First U.S. edition published in 2020 by Findhorn Press

Disclaimer
The information in this book is given in good faith and is neither intended to diagnose any physical or mental condition nor to serve as a substitute for informed medical advice or care. Please contact your health professional for medical advice and treatment. Neither author nor publisher can be held liable by any person for any loss or damage whatsoever which may arise from the use of this book or any of the information therein.

Cataloging-in-Publication Data for this title is available from the Library of Congress

ISBN 978-1-64411-189-5 (print)
ISBN 978-1-64411-190-1 (ebook)

Printed and bound in the United States by P. A. Hutchison

10 9 8 7 6 5 4 3 2 1

Text design and layout by Marie-France Côté
This book was typeset in ITC-Clearface and Frutiger
with Sagona used as a display typeface.

To send correspondence to the author of this book, mail a first-class letter to the author c/o Inner Traditions • Bear & Company, One Park Street, Rochester, VT 05767, USA and we will forward the communication, or contact the author directly at **www.atma.ca**

To All Seekers of Truth

To Peddar Zask, my spiritual father

Acknowledgements

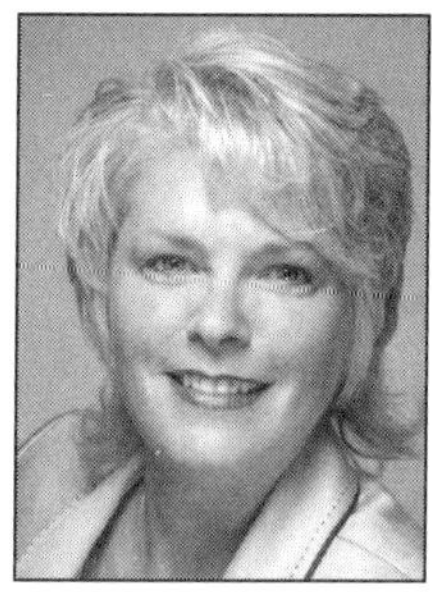

Lucie Bernier
lucie.bernier@atma.ca

I especially want to thank **Ms. Lucie Bernier** for her collaborative work throughout all the years we were engaged in producing this book. Her experience from her personal life and as a psychotherapist, her training in the metaphysical approach of ailments and diseases, her capacity for comprehensive thinking and her intuition have significantly contributed to advancing the work on this book.

I also want to thank the following persons for their participation in producing this book:

Ms. Denise Boucher
Ms. Ginette Caron
Mr. Laurent Chiasson
Ms. Nicole Cloutier
Ms. Fleurette Couture
Mr. Pierre Couture
Ms Heather Dixon
Ms. Louise Drouin
Mr. Paul-Émile Drouin
Mr. Jean Dumas
Ms. Danielle East
Ms. Nicole Gagné
Ms. Catherine Guin
Mr. Robert Lenghan
Ms. Micheline Pascal
Ms. Ginette Plante
Ms. Denise Quintal
Mr. Denis Tremblay

My father: Noé Martel

Contents

Preface

I accept↓♥ my healing

Becoming **aware** of who I am and of what I am becoming is always very exciting when my discoveries about myself and others are beautiful and positive. What happens, however, when the discoveries that result from a personal self-exploration of any sort lead me to see hidden facets of myself and make me become **aware** of ailments and diseases that have happened to me or that probably took place within my body?

This is what happened throughout these past few years, when I realized that diseases had subtly taken hold in me because of poorly managed emotions and that, by learning to re-harmonize this whirlwind of all sorts of emotions that inhabited me, I could acquire a healing power over any ailment or any disease that I had allowed to take over as king and master in my **Temple of Flesh**.

Of course, accepting↓♥ to reclaim the responsibility for my own health has been a long process of introspection involving a questioning of my values and, most especially, has given me **the certainty that I have the power to heal myself.**

In getting there, I have had the privilege, since 1988, of knowing Jacques and working closely with him and learning many things through the numerous conferences and workshops that he gave. By his ability to present simply and accessibly a subject that many people may see as very complex, by his unconditional **love** and his desire to help people achieve greater physical, emotional and spiritual well-being, he has been, and still is, a pillar and a guide who knows how to help me chase away my guilt and replace it, instead, by taking charge of my own life, so that I feel increasingly free, comfortable within myself, and in charge of my life. Jacques has helped me to accept↓♥ illness, of whatever sort, as a positive experience, because now it is an opportunity for me to stop and question myself about what is happening in my life. For many people such as myself, illness has given me an opportunity to ask for help, something that I quite often wish to avoid. I must remind myself that **to fall is human; but to get up again is divine** and that, to start a healing process, it is essential to open up to others, to open up to oneself and, first and foremost, to open up to **love,** for any ailment or any disease can be healed if I am ready to accept↓♥ to drop my blinders and cast a new and positive look upon any situation I may happen to experience, however difficult it may be, for I know that once I have understood the coming of this experience into my life, it will be able to go on its way and I shall recover perfect health.

That is what this book, which I consider to be an exceptional transformational tool, is intended to be. It is a window opened on this still very poorly understood world of emotions. It is an instrument that gives me the opportunity to open myself up to the grain that allowed this microbe, this virus, this tumor or any other physical ailment to germinate in my body and suddenly appear in full daylight. By enabling me to **love** and accept↓♥ myself through all these poorly or hardly experienced emotions, I shall take a step towards more harmony, more peace, more **love**.

By learning to **decode this new dictionary of emotions**, I shall now be able to invest in my own **capital of health**, being now capable of preventing and avoiding many of the ailments that may threaten me.

Throughout these recent years when I collaborated with Jacques in giving birth to this book, I was always surprised to see the sheer amount of time (thousands of hours) that had to be invested in it, not counting all the energy and the openness required for channelling all these poorly managed items of information that, quite often, involved either a period in my personal life or a situation experienced by a person I knew.

We have all been 'sick' at least once in our lives, and the fact of dissecting the causes of an illness that affects us or affects someone close to us enables us to detach and distance ourselves from it (in the sense of seeing an illness in a positive way and disengaging ourselves from the negative hold we have allowed it to have on us), and become the witnesses rather than the victims of all these ailments.

This is what I wish for everyone to discover for themselves, through using this tool. May each and all of us become more and more autonomously independent, more and more capable of recognizing the sources giving rise to the ailments and diseases that affect, or could affect us. This recognition and acknowledgment will serve as a means of prevention and will bring about the necessary changes in our lives in order to reclaim our health. This is an extraordinary complement that is now adding itself to the numerous techniques that already exist, in the traditional as well as the new medicine, and is proving to be essential not only for healing at the physical level, but also at the level of the heart ♥ (of **love**), where true healing takes place...

To your good health!

Lucie Bernier
Therapist and Co-author

Introduction

Health has always been a matter of great concern to me. In fact, from an early age I began to experience health problems, without having any exact notion of what had caused them. My mother was faced with difficult situations that, over many years, required care in the form of operations, various treatments and even years of hospitalization.

In my own case, since nobody seemed able to find out exactly what my illness was, a doubt appeared to constantly hover over the whole issue: I believed that these illnesses could be psychological. I then said to myself: "Either it's 'in my head', or else there must be some reason for what's happening". I decided to go with the second choice, and that is when I began to explore whatever was causing me to experience all those ailments.

In 1978 I began to work in the health field, in food supplements. That is when I began to realize by myself, during the individual consultations I was giving and through my other observations, that there could exist a relation between emotions, thoughts and illnesses. I had begun intuitively to discover the link that existed between certain emotions and certain illnesses. It was in 1988, while registering for some personal growth courses, that I was put in contact with what is described today as **the metaphysical approach to ailments and diseases.** I can still see myself, together with others at that time, perusing the compilation of ailments and diseases that Louise Hay had set out in her book. I also observed people who were beginning their own investigations of themselves or of others in order to verify the validity of her assertions, all passionate about discovering new avenues of research in order to gain a better understanding of what they were experiencing.

From that moment on, my interest in this approach never stopped growing, all the more so that I was reorienting my work to engage in the more specific field of personal growth. Since that day, I have never ceased verifying, through my individual consultations and the courses I teach or the workshops I lead, the relevance of these data on ailments and diseases. Even today, I still find myself, whether in a grocery store or when I go to make photocopies, asking people questions about what they are experiencing in relation to their ailments or diseases.

I still see these people looking at me with a surprised or questioning expression, wondering if I am a clairvoyant or an extraterrestrial to know such things about their personal lives without them having told me anything about themselves. In fact, the answer is simple. When one knows how to decode ailments and diseases and also knows to which emotions or thoughts these are related, it is then easy to tell a person what she, or he, is experiencing. I then tell these people that it is simply my knowledge of the functioning of human beings and my knowledge of the links between thoughts, emotions and illnesses that enable me to give them this information. In a sense, I explain to them that all the relevant data could be entered into a computer database and that one could then give the computer the symptoms of their ailment or disease, or simply name it, and the computer could then output the information on what one is experiencing in one's personal life, consciously or not. **So it is not a matter of clairvoyance but clearly a matter of knowledge.**

Today, with my accumulated experience and knowledge, I can state that it is impossible for someone to suffer from diabetes without feeling a deep sadness or aversion towards a situation that the person has experienced. For me, it is impossible for a person to suffer from arthritis without experiencing self-criticism or dissatisfaction with someone else or with certain situations in that person's life. For me, it is impossible for someone to experience liver problems without feeling anger and frustration towards oneself or towards others, and so on. I have occasionally received the following comment: *"When you decode ailments and diseases, you 'fix' things to make them fit".* Then I am told that everybody experiences anger, frustration, sorrow, rejection, etc. My response to this is that everyone does not react to a given condition in the same manner. For instance, take the fact that I grew up in a family of 12 children with a father who was an alcoholic and a mother who was depressive. My brothers and sisters will have had the same parents as I, but each child, including myself, will be affected or not, or affected differently, because of their different interpretations of their respective experiences with those same parents.

Why? Because we are all different, and we must all become consciously aware of various issues in our personal development. Thus, a manifestation of rejection can set off an illness in one person but not in someone else. **All depends on how I feel myself being affected, consciously or unconsciously.** If my psychological stress is sufficiently high, it will be converted into biological stress in the form of an illness.

During a workshop I was giving on the metaphysical approach to ailments and diseases, in the context of an exhibition on natural health and alternative therapies, the ailments and diseases that were submitted for discussion were decoded quickly and accurately enough, to my great satisfaction. Some time later, a friend who was in the audience during this workshop told me: *"Jacques, you should be more careful when you give your answers directly and quickly to respond to people's questions. Some people around me got the impression that the workshop had been artfully contrived with accomplices to create the impression of a perfect fit."* Of course, nothing of the sort had transpired. What is important to understand here is that first, the person who is concerned by the ailment or disease being discussed knows that the stated answer is true for her or his own case, which may not appear quite so obvious to the other people present who are not personally so concerned.

Secondly, what is new and still freshly revealed for our **conscious awareness** can appear to be unreal. Denying this reality can also be a means of self-protection to avoid feeling responsible for what is happening to oneself.

Here is an anecdote illustrating this observation. The famous inventor Thomas Edison met the members of the U.S. Congress to formally present his newest invention, the phonograph, a speaking machine. It is reported that when he demonstrated the machine in actual operation, certain members of Congress called him an impostor, saying that there had to be some subterfuge afoot because, for them, it was simply impossible for the human voice to issue forth out of a box.

Times have truly changed. That is why it is important to remain open to new ideas that may provide innovative answers to many problems. Many people in the United States and in Europe have developed this approach about the link that exists between conflicted emotions and thoughts and physical illnesses, which helps in making this whole field of investigation better known not only here in Quebec (Canada) but also more widely throughout the world.

I often say, during my conferences, that I have very strong mental powers, but also have very strong intuitive powers, and that the greatest challenge in my life has been, and still is, to reconcile those two powers. My academic training as an electrical engineer has helped me to work through the logical and rational side of things. Physics has taught me that a cause is always linked to very real effects. It was this law of cause and effect that I was later able to apply to the domain of emotions and thoughts, although these are less tangible than physical reality itself. But is this truly the case? Even in a sub-field of physics such as electricity, we are working with something that no human being has ever actually seen: electricity. For in fact we are working with effects such as **light**, heat, electromagnetic induction, and so on. Similarly, thoughts and emotions are not necessarily physical in the proper sense of the term, but they can have physical repercussions in the form of ailments and diseases. That is why one of the goals of this book is to demonstrate that something that is non-visible, such as thoughts and emotions, can induce a reaction that is physical and measurable, very often in the form of ailments and diseases. Can I measure anger? No, but I can take the measure of my fever when that symptom affects me. Can I measure the fact that I often get the impression of having to struggle in life to get what I want? No, but I can measure the diminishing number of red globules in my blood when I present anemia. Can I measure the fact that not enough joy is permeating my life? No, but I can measure my excessive level of blood cholesterol, and so on. Then, if I become aware of the thoughts and emotions that have brought about the onset of an ailment or a disease, could it be that, by changing these thoughts and emotions, I could recover my health? I dare say: Yes.

However, the links involved can be in fact more complex and deeper, involving more than just those facets of which I happen to be consciously **aware.** That is why I may need to call upon people working in the medical field or people using other professional approaches to help me in achieving the necessary changes in my life. If I must undergo a surgical operation while understanding at the same time whatever has led me to experience such a situation, it's quite likely that I'll recover from my operation much more quickly than another person having the same operation but who doesn't want to know what was going on in his or her life or who is simply unaware of it.

Furthermore, if I have not understood the message conveyed by my disease, then the operation or treatment may seem to make the disease disappear, but the illness may shift later on to some other part of my body, in a different form.

It is to be hoped that more and more businesses will become **aware** of the solid reasons for helping their employees in their personal development, on the emotional level. This will make it possible to diminish the number of accidents in the company and the rate of absenteeism, and will increase each individual's effectiveness. If my personal, family and occupational life is such that I don't feel right within myself, I'll become more likely to 'attract', albeit unconsciously, a disease or an accident as a means for taking some leave or for getting other people to take care of me.

It was in 1990 that the idea came to me to write an encyclopedia dealing with the metaphysical causes of ailments and diseases, and it was in 1991 that I started working on it. At that time, I hadn't anticipated the tremendous sum of work that was awaiting me. And fortunately so, for if I had known it then, I believe I would never have engaged in this project. But I said to myself: *"One thing at a time! I'll get there; I'm going to work until I'm satisfied enough with the results to publish this book."*

I am saying this also because making changes in oneself takes a lot of work, energy and willpower. An American writer[1] said one day: ***"Only the brave and the adventurous will personally experience God."*** What I understand from this quotation is that my determination in taking up life's challenges and my courage in tentatively exploring pathways that are new to me will enable me to reach a certain state of achievement and well-being. This state of well-being defines physical, mental and emotional health.

From 1978 to 1988, I worked in the field of nutritional supplementation, also called the **orthomolecular approach,** which means "providing the organism with the necessary nutriments, such as vitamins, minerals and other nutriments, in the form of food or dietary supplements, in order to regain or maintain **optimal health**". At that time I relied mainly on the work of psychiatrists and other physicians, biochemists and various Canadian and American (mostly) researchers who demonstrated, in their experimenting, that by providing the necessary nutriments, one could manage to improve, or even restore in some cases, a person's physical, mental and emotional health. In fact, there exist several approaches to obtaining **optimal health**, all of them important, each of them acting in some way on all the aspects of our beings. In 1996 I saw a report[2] on television about a hospital, the Columbia-Presbyterian Hospital in New York City, mentioning the case of a patient, Mr. Joseph Randazzo, who was to be operated on for three coronary bypass procedures. This patient benefited from sessions of visualization, energy and reflexology treatments before his operation. During the operation he benefited from energizing

---

1. **Twitchell, Paul:** Found in an American periodical, *Mystic World,* for the years 1969-1970.
2. Also reported in LIFE Magazine of september 1996 under the general theme of "The Healing Revolution".

treatments. After his operation, this same patient again took part in visualization sessions and received energizing and reflexology treatments to allow him to recover more quickly. These interventions were fruitful because the patient recuperated much more rapidly after this operation than another patient would have under the usual conditions. The attending physician, Dr. Mehmet Oz, explained that he was conducting such an experiment on 300 of his patients in order to analyze the results of adding these alternative therapies to the conventional medical treatment.

Thus, the aim of this book is to complement any approach, whether medical or linked to alternative forms of medicine. It thus deals comprehensively with the allopathic, more medical approach as well as with the holistic approach, which is more inclusive of the physical, mental, emotional and spiritual dimensions of our beings. I strongly hope that all health professionals, wherever they work, will use this encyclopedia as a complement to their practice, **as a tool for working and investigating,** to help their patients in their healing process. In my case, I have experienced operations, traditional medicine, medications, acupuncture, energy treatments, divination, naturopathy, massage, colour therapy, dietetics, vitamin therapy, Dr. Bach's floral essences, chiropractic, orthotherapy, iridology, psychotherapy, rebirth (conscious breathing), homeopathy, etc. I know that if a technique were valid for everyone, it would be the sole existing technique. But such is not the case, because of all the animals on this planet, human beings are the species with the most possibilities but also the greatest complexity.

That is the reason why I must try to understand by myself what I am experiencing, including, when the need arises, by requesting the help of others in their respective domains of competence. The same writer I mentioned above wrote one day: ***"One must learn from those who know".*** That is how I must seek out the best of what is available in each profession. When I am facing a physician, I tell myself that he knows more than I do about medicine, and that I must pay attention to what he is telling me and suggesting to me, leaving me free to then choose my orientation. Similarly, when I am facing an acupuncturist, I pay attention to what he is telling me or suggesting as a treatment, because he knows more than I do about the functioning of energy balancing amongst my meridians. And the same goes as well for all the other professions.

The other day, a lady told me that she didn't believe in all these stories about thoughts and emotions being related to illnesses. I answered that it was not necessary to believe in them. After someone had read to her some texts related to certain ailments and diseases that she had previously suffered from or still had herself, we noted that her attitude had changed and that she had now become more receptive to this approach. In fact, there is an inner part of me that knows what is going on and that what is being said about me fits with what I am experiencing and that this is not a mere chance occurrence. We must be careful here: I must not feel guilty about what is happening to me and I must not believe that what I'm being told means that it's my own fault if I'm sick.

I am responsible for what happens to me but, in most cases, it is not my fault. **It is our lack of awareness of the laws that regulate the links between our thoughts and emotions and our physical bodies that leads us to experience situations of ailments and diseases. I must therefore become aware of the trajectory of my personal progression or, in the broadest sense, of my spiritual development.** In places where I have found little or no **love**, I must rediscover that love was present there nevertheless. Not obvious, you may reply! But that is the way it is. If I throw myself down from a balcony and break a leg, shall I then say that God punished me? In fact, there does exist a law, called gravity, which tends to 'bring me down to earth'. This law is neither good nor bad, it's the law of gravity. Even if I rail and rage against this law for it's because of it that I broke my leg, this will change nothing in the law, because **the law is the law.** Thus, all illnesses are explained by a lack of love. It is said that love is the only healer. But if this is true, should it not be enough to simply give love to then see healing occur?

This is true, in certain cases. In fact, it is as though **love** has to enter through certain doors for healing to occur, through those very doors that were closed off from **love** when previous injuries were sustained. That is quite a vast field for discovery and for broadening one's **awareness!**

The aim of this book is not to directly provide solutions for my ailments and diseases, but rather to help me become aware of the fact that the ailment or disease I am experiencing originates from my thoughts and my emotions and that, on that basis, I can then choose the means I feel to be the most appropriate to bring about changes in my life.

However, the mere fact of knowing where my ailment or my disease comes from can sometimes suffice to bring about changes in my physical body. In certain cases, the positive change can reach 50% and sometimes even as far as 100%, or complete healing.

As for myself, when I discovered the personal development courses in 1988 and was able to become **aware** of the changes taking place in me, I got the feeling that I was beginning to be born again and I saw hope for better days emerging on the horizon. At last I had found a way to achieve important changes in my life and to see the results for myself. I had to act because I was in reaction against authority. I was experiencing enormous rejection, abandonment and misunderstanding. **I knew all that, but it still remained for me to find a way to change and to heal my inner injuries.** That is why I engaged in this field of activity called personal development. My work allowed me to work on myself while working with others to help them in opening up their **conscious awareness. I sincerely believe that each one of us can take ourselves in hand more or less autonomously and that each one of us can achieve a higher degree of wisdom, love and freedom! We all deserve this.**

This encyclopedia was designed to be a tool for opening up conscious awareness and for inquiry into self-discovery. When something happens to me that affects my health, I read over again what is said about it in this encyclopedia in order to be even more **aware** of what is happening. Indeed, human beings tend to obliterate, to remove from their conscious memory, whatever bothers them. Thus when I read the encyclopedia, I do so with the eyes of someone who wants to learn and to become more consciously aware of what is happening inside. My mental, intellectual side collects the information with which I'll be working. **Because the only true power I have is my power over myself: I am the creator of my own life. The more aware I am, the more able I'll be to achieve the appropriate changes.**

Over the past century, and more especially in the past 50 years, we have experienced an extraordinary leap with respect to our technology, which has made it possible, in many cases, to improve our living conditions. Despite all this progress, we do not realize very well that science does not hold answers for everything and that there exist, on this planet, many men and women suffering from illnesses. Whether we live in industrialized countries or in developing countries, we must take care of ourselves and we must face these questions: Who am I? Where am I going? What is my goal in life?

It is important that I use this book as a tool for understanding, investigation and transformation.

If any new ideas come to me while reading these texts, I must feel comfortable about completing them in my own words. **This tool must become a living instrument to which each and every one of us can add his, or her, own contribution.** This is how certain passages in the book came to be written, at the request of persons who knew that I was working on this project. For instance, when someone asked me: *"Have you dealt in your book with peanut butter allergies?"*, the answer was: *"No, but now I'm going to do it"*. The same thing happened with several other illnesses that I was asked to include.

I wish you, then, 'Good reading!'

Jacques Martel

Author, Professional Speaker and Trainer

General Remarks

This book is a document of inquiry into the metaphysical aspect (thoughts, feelings, emotions) of ailments and diseases. The author apologizes in advance for any errors that may have slipped through and invites the reader to inform him of any such errors directly on the Internet site or in writing.

The author of this book does not claim to provide any medical advice directly or indirectly. He also does not claim to determine any diagnoses directly or indirectly. The ideas contained in this book are there as items of information, as opportunities for investigating an ailment or a disease in order to help the persons themselves, their attending physicians or their therapists in gaining a better understanding of the origin of the ailment or disease.

The statements contained in this book are only intended as information. The author is quite **aware** that the ailments and diseases in this book are dealt with from a metaphysical approach of an ailment or a disease, and that several other health-related aspects may be involved also. The author is **aware** that illnesses can be far more complex than what is explained here.

The simplified approach to certain diseases such as cancer or diabetes is to enable the reader to open a door of inquiry into the metaphysical cause of the ailment or disease with the help of a health professional.

The guiding idea of this dictionary is first to start off with a simple point of view on the ailment or disease in order to make the information as accessible as possible so that the greatest number of people may understand it. **This approach is designed to be complementary to all prevailing allopathic[3] and holistic[4] medical approaches.**

Any person who would want to make any changes to an ongoing treatment should first speak about it with their attending physician or their professional therapist. Anyone experiencing situations of diseases such as diabetes (insulin-dependent) or cardiac diseases (requiring taking pills daily), etc., must obtain medical advice before making any changes to their medication, even if they 'believe' they have found the cause of their illness, and even if they 'believe' that everything is now fixed and under control.

However, persons who use this book for its information do it for themselves, which is strictly their right. The author and the editor decline any responsibility for any acts that might be performed after reading this book, whereby any readers might be led to do things or to make decisions that could be contrary to their well-being.

---

3 **Allopathic:** An approach that uses a medical treatment for the purpose of combating sickness. This term is generally used to designate conventional medecine.

4 **Holistic:** An approach that takes into account the person viewed as a whole, including the physical, mental and emotional aspects and sometimes even the spiritual aspect.

↓♥ : This dual symbol, often used in the text, represents the energy associated with a mental image or associated with an emotion related to a situation, which I figuratively move from my head to my heart♥ ! What happens then is either a healing in **love**, or the reinforcement of a positive attitude.

Most of the following terms or expressions are explained in footnotes when they appear for the first time. However, as people do not usually read a dictionary from cover to cover like a novel, the author wanted to outline the explanations on certain terms or expressions that can be found here and there in the text, in order to clarify the meaning he wanted to give them.

To be O.K.: This means to be and feel in agreement with my personal values, whether or not they are in harmony with the values of the society in which I live and with which I identify.

Integrate: Refers to the fact of assimilating a situation or an idea within myself. When it refers to an emotional injury and I say that I have 'integrated the situation', it means that I have completely healed the inner injury that was attached to this situation and that I have become accordingly **aware** of this experience.

My 'bubble': This expression refers to my own personal space around me, my vital energy space.

Grounded: Refers to the sense of feeling familiarly connected to the earth and to the material, concrete, actual, practical world.

My higher self: Refers to the higher part of ourselves, which we call **Conscience**, **Soul**, etc.

My inner guide: As with the explanation for my 'higher self', this term refers to that inner part of me that can guide me, if this is consistent with my beliefs.

Obliteration: The fact of erasing something from my conscious memory or from my sensitivity.

Pattern: In this context, this refers to a scheme of thought that tends to make me repeat certain events in my life.

Psychic : Refers to what concerns the level of my thoughts, the mental level.

Reincarnation: This is a topic increasingly referred to in the new therapeutic approaches, which is why the author occasionally refers to it. However, the author wants the reader to feel entirely free to adhere or not to this idea, knowing that any mentions made on the subject of reincarnation are included as information only.

Yin and Yang: Yin is the name given in Chinese medicine to designate the negative, feminine or intuitive energy polarity; Yang is the name used to designate the positive, masculine or rational energy polarity. These Yin and Yang terms are encountered in acupuncture in particular. When the terms Yin and Yang are used in this text, they refer to the energy polarity, namely the intuitive or rational aspect within ourselves, rather than to acupuncture.

WARNING

This book provides avenues for investigation as to thoughts, feelings and emotions that could be the source of some discomfort or illness. Anyone who has any discomfort or illness should go to their doctor or health professional. The information contained in this book does not replace traditional medicine that is recognized by the governmental authorities of the country concerned, it is only a complement.

The Reading Integration Technique

I can use the information contained in this book to effect changes at the level of my emotions. For this we use the Reading Integration Technique by Monosyllabic, Rhythmic and Sequential Pronunciation ©. By doing the following exercise, I can activate my emotional memory to make it possible, from my head to my heart ↓♥, for some part of my emotions to be healed in **love**.

It is a matter of taking the text dealing with an ailment or a disease and reading it syllable by syllable, taking at least one second per syllable. For example, let us take the following disease:

> **ARTHRITIS (in general)**
> **Arthritis** is defined as the inflammation of a joint. It can affect each of the parts of the human locomotor system: this includes the bones, the ligaments, the tendons and the muscles. It is characterized by inflammation, muscular stiffness and pain, which **correspond,** on the metaphysical level, to an experience of **closing off, criticism, sorrow, sadness** or **anger.**
>
> Then becomes:
>
> **AR-THRI-TIS (in-ge-ne-ral)**
> Ar-thri-tis is de-fined as the in-flam-ma-tion of a joint. It can af-fect each of the parts of the hu-man lo-co-mo-tor sys-tem: this in-cludes the bones, the li-ga-ments, the ten-dons and the mus-cles. It is cha-rac-te-rized by in-flam-ma-tion, mus-cu-lar stiff-ness and pain, which **cor-res-pond**, on the me-ta-phy-si-cal le-vel, to an ex-pe-ri-ence of **clo-sing off, cri-ti-ci-sm, sor-row, sad-ness** or **an-ger.**

And I continue my reading until I have covered the complete text I am reading in the book. **It is very important to proceed very slowly,** one syllable per second at the most or even more slowly. It is not important that I be concerned about whether or not my intellect understands the words or the sentences I am pronouncing. It is possible that emotions of sorrow or sadness may manifest themselves during the exercise; it is a matter of putting **love** into the situation. I can take the text of a disease I currently have or of a disease I previously had, or of a disease I may fear contracting. If I experience any emotions during the exercise, I can do it over again later in the day, or on another day, until I no longer experience any emotions and I feel comfortable with the text.

I can do this exercise, if I wish, after a meditation, after listening to relaxing music or after a guided relaxation session.

I can also do the exercise by reading the text of the *Preface* or the text of the *Introduction.*

The purpose of the following information is to give further explanations on the use of this technique. I shall start by saying that for me, the term *'integration'* refers to the fact of becoming **conscious** in one's being; which also means *'healing'* to some degree, in the sense that the ailment or the disease is a message that my body is sending me to enable me to become **aware** of what I am currently experiencing.

I first used this technique in the ***'Retrieving our Inner Child'*** workshops that I have led since March 1993. It is used when an adult writes a letter to his, or her, inner child and when the inner child then responds to the adult.

What happens during the application of this technique, which consists in reading a text syllable by syllable and taking at least one second per syllable? The first thing to understand is that the faster I read, then the more my reading takes place in my mental sphere, 'all in my head'. The more slowly I read, then the more my reading will take place in contact with the energy centre of the heart♥, also called the chakra of the heart♥. **All ailments and diseases are conscious or unconscious interpretations that I have made in relation to a situation or a person involving a lack of love.** So it works as if this message, or this injury I might say, was registered at the level of **love**, which, in humans, corresponds to the energy centre of the heart♥.

My injuries related to a lack of **love** are registered in my heart♥ in the form of rejection, abandonment, anger, incomprehension, sadness, disappointment, and so on. In order for me to be able to change this message registered within myself, **I must first activate the information at the starting point;** in other words, I must be in contact with the 'inner folder' in which this injury has registered a piece of information that becomes activated whenever a new similar situation occurs in my life. It is as though the situation allows the emotion to be activated because the event that occurs induces it to resonate.

Thus, when I activate in my heart♥ the situation that caused me to experience sorrow, sadness, anger, etc., I thereby open up the heart's♥ energy centre to let in the energy of **love**, which brings healing with it, along with the **awareness** that accompanies it, or vice-versa (i.e. with **awareness** preceding healing).

To make the pronunciation exercise more effective, I imagine that my words are issuing from me at the level of my heart♥, as though my mouth were at the level of my heart♥. It follows that during the exercise I may experience tingling sensations in different parts of my body; currents of heat may travel through different parts of my body, along with feelings of sorrow, sadness or any other sort of emotion that may emerge. It will be enough to remain calm if any such strong emotions of sorrow or sadness manifest themselves, for things are usually under control and it is as if my body knows what it is capable of taking.

If for any reason I fear experiencing too much emotion, I can do the exercise in the presence of a person who can support me in what I am experiencing, a responsible person in charge or a therapist.

How are the Ailments and Diseases Classified?

They are generally entered in the *Index* at the end of the book, in alphabetical order of ailment or disease as, for example:

ACIDOSIS 33

This disease is in the 'A's.

When you find the following title:

DISEASE (Addison's).................................... 34

You place at the end of the parenthesis the title preceding the parenthesis, which produces: Addison's **DISEASE**.

When you find, after the name of the illness, the reference indication **'SEE'**, as in the following example:

FATNESS / OVERWEIGHT *See: weight [excess]*

You must refer to **WEIGHT** (excess) and find the title of this ailment among the 'W's, in order to get the information on the ailment itself in relation to **FATNESS / OVERWEIGHT.**

You can go and look up a complement of information on the illness itself, or about certain features related to it, by looking up other illnesses. Thus, the extended reference indication **'SEE ALSO'** leads you to a complement of information on the illness, which is presented as follows:

AGORAPHOBIA *See also: anxiety, death, fear.*

For instance, if you find yourself in the **'SEE ALSO'** reference indication following the name of the illness, indicated here with items separated by forward slashes /, as in the following example:

HAIR — TINEA *See also: hair [loss]/baldness/alopecia areata*

This must be read as: See also: Hair – loss,
Hair – Baldness,
Hair – Alopecia areata

Certain illnesses were re-sorted to place them closer to their complements of information. Thus, all the topics related to **BLOOD** were re-sorted by using the appropriate reference indications such as:

ANEMIA *See: blood—anemia*

DIABETES *See: blood — diabetes*

HYPOGLYCEMIA *See: blood — hypoglycemia*

LEUKEMIA *See: blood — leukemia*

Hence, to get the most information possible about **ANEMIA**, you must first read the following articles:

BLOOD (in general)
BLOOD disorders
BLOOD — ANEMIA

In the case where you find yourself in a subsection, for example if you want information about **ANEMIA**, you will find it under **BLOOD — ANEMIA**. Even if it is not indicated in **'SEE ALSO'**, this supposes that you must read the parts about **BLOOD (in general)** and **BLOOD disorders**.

Similarly, while exploring still another subsection, as in **ECZEMA**, found under **SKIN - ECZEMA**, you must also read the information about **SKIN (in general)** and **SKIN diseases**. The same applies to any other sections where the name titles **(in general)** and **(disorders/diseases...)** appear.

Among the ailments, diseases or body parts that include several ailments or diseases, let us mention:

ALLERGIES
ANUS
ARTHRITIS
BACK
BLOOD
BONES
BRAIN
BREASTS
BRONCHI
CANCER
EARS
EYES
FEET
FINGERS
GLANDS
HAIR
HEART♥
INTESTINES
KIDNEYS
LEGS
LIVER
LUNGS
MOUTH
MUSCLES
NAILS
NOSE
RESPIRATION
SKIN
SPINE
STOMACH
TEETH
THROAT
VAGINA

Ailments

AND

Diseases

FROM

A to Z

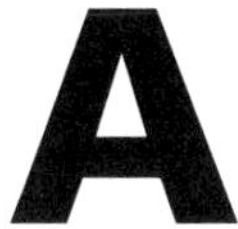

ABASIA

Although my muscles and my whole locomotor system are not causing me any discomfort, I am only partly able to walk, or I am incapable of walking. It is my command system, located in the cerebellum, which can be affected by a lesion, a vascular disorder or a tumor.

This sometimes originates from a great fear related to my thoughts, which has had the effect of **freezing me in place**. This fear or guilt is related to the fact of advancing, of going forward in life. I feel despondent, dejected. Life 'down here' is a constant struggle. I have the impression that I am among the disadvantaged. I feel I am falling between two stools, casting doubt on my values and the basics of my life, and this prevents me from moving forward. I have great difficulty in engaging myself in life.

I accept↓♥ to seek out the cause of this insecurity, or this guilt, and develop more confidence in myself. I can begin to visualize myself walking more and more easily, while amplifying my feeling of self-confidence. I also become more **Aware** that life can provide me with the tools necessary for my advancement.

ABSCESS (anal) *See: ANUS — ANAL ABSCESS*

ABSCESS (brain) *See: BRAIN [ABSCESS IN]*

ABSCESS (liver) *See: LIVER [ABSCESS]*

ABSCESS OR EMPYEMA *See also: INFLAMMATION*

An **abscess** is a type of infection characterized by the formation and accumulation of pus in normally constituted tissues. It generally produces a lump, and I can find it only on body tissue or on an organ. An **abscess** is related to the lymphatic system when it is in overload (filled with toxins), and the organism shows it outwardly by redness, pain, or fever.

An **abscess** indicates that I am showing a response to **anger** or to an emotional injury, a feeling of **irritation**, **confrontation**, **incapacity**, **failure,** or **vengeance** that I have been unable to express concretely (the pus is related to my body fluids and to my emotions). I received an insult that is difficult to accept↓♥. I may have fallen very low, having tried to accomplish too many things at once: my aggressive temperament made me forge ahead, but beneath it all there was a doubt within me, an uncertainty, often related to a past painful and humiliating experience that I wish I could exorcise from my life but is still present. It is often **an excess of irritation or dissatisfaction that I can't succeed in expressing about myself, another person or a situation.** Unhealthy thoughts, which can go as far as vengeance and seethe and 'ferment' within me, will produce the infection and the pus. I may feel dirty. This contained frustration may present itself to make a situation **come to a head**, in a sense **bursting the abscess**. It can produce mental turmoil in me (like a swelling) leading to emptiness and exhaustion. This type of infection (the **abscess**) is only a manifestation (or a creation) of my mental activity, of my thoughts. I wonder if there is a secret I have kept for myself, or some negative thoughts that I have held in so much that they have concentrated in one point of my body, and often tainted with guilt. It is high time for me to go on to other things, to change attitudes, if I want to improve my life… and my body, before some more generalized infection manifests itself. I am tense, physically as well as mentally, and I need to learn to focus my attention on the positive in my life and use my creative energy to externalize my whole inner Universe. Furthermore, an **abscess** corresponds to a deep **sorrow**, even an **inner desperation** that will generate a deep feeling of helplessness or failure. Emptiness and exhaustion may follow. I have the impression of having lost everything, or am afraid that this might happen. It appears at the **source** of the sorrow, which means that the emotion experienced is associated with the function and the body part where the **abscess** manifests itself. For example, if it is located on my **leg**, it is related to my resistances and conflicts, and thereby indicates to me that I must orient my life in certain directions. If it is located at the level of my **eyes**, it has to do with a difficulty in seeing who I am, what I am, where I am going and what is in store for me. If it affects my **feet**, I am experiencing difficulties, doubts or fears related to the future or to how I imagine it. If it affects my **ears**, it concerns something I hear. If it is on my **hips**, I have difficulty in dashing forward in life, and so on. All of that is related to my **ability to stand up**, to express my independence and my freedom. I accept↓♥ in my **heart♥** to bring my fears and my insecurities to a head, and my **abscess** will burst too, along with them. A **superficial abscess**, which can be seen and touched, is related to my **rage** about situations in my life that can be easily identifiable. It also bears a relationship with the affected body part such as the neck, the back, the fingers, and so on. A **deep abscess** can be found inside my body and is related to a **disappointment** involving deeper feelings of my being. Depending upon its location, an **abscess** can have serious consequences. For example, if it is located in the region of the **brain**, it is related to my individuality and to the way I conceive of myself; in the area of the **lungs**, it is related to life; of the **kidneys**, it is related to my fears; of the **liver**, it is related to criticism. I want to find out why this **concentrated anger** is affecting my life, by looking up the corresponding meaning for the affected body part. I can focus more **Love** and understanding this way upon the situation that led me to experience this anger. The **shirt-button abscess** designates one or several **superficial abscesses** that are jointly related to a **deep abscess** or to deeper tissues. It is therefore invisible to the naked eye. Thus, my body is telling me that my **anger** is now affecting my outer and my inner life. It is as though 'this **irritation** is piercing my body' and expressing my pressing need to heal these injuries through **Love**. The **hot abscess** usually induces an inflammatory reaction and can form rapidly. The fact that an **abscess** frequently encloses itself in a membrane clearly indicates that it originates from non-beneficial thoughts that provoke anger. The **cold abscess** presents no inflammatory reaction and its progress is rather slow. It can be due to fungi or to Koch's bacillus[1]. This type of **abscess** indicates that my anger shows itself in the form of **disappointment** or **resignation** toward a situation.

I accept↓♥ the new thoughts of **Love** and I remain with an open **heart♥** toward the people around me, rather than fixate my attention on my old injuries, on my past or on certain forms of vengeance. By becoming **conscious** of this process of acceptance↓♥, the **abscess** is then likely to disappear forever.

ABDOMEN / BELLY / STOMACH *See also: INTESTINAL AILMENTS, SWELLING / BLOATING [OF THE ABDOMEN]*

The **abdomen** or **belly** is the lower anterior part of the human trunk, containing mainly the intestines.

Just as in my everyday life, when I stuff myself with too much food, I have a 'full **belly**', I feel like sleeping and I experience some discomfort. I must learn to take my time, to take in each new situation one by one, to leave myself some time to adapt to the changes taking place in my life, and thereby avoid experiencing impatience and frustration. As it is in the **abdomen** that a child starts to grow and gets ready to move from its initial solitary state to a more social state, the **abdomen** is therefore the region of **relations**. All the difficulties in this region are related to the conflicts or the blockages between me and the world in which I live, these conflicts being expressed through the personal relations that make up my reality. If I am experiencing an ***abominable*** or awful situation, my **stomach** reacts strongly, especially when I feel forced to 'lie down flat on my **stomach** in front of someone' and feel humiliated by this. This region is **tense** when I feel fragile, unsure of myself, and with the impression some people are 'rolling over my **stomach**'. It is **slack** instead, when I feel disabused with life, when I don't care about anything any longer. An upset **stomach** indicates to me that I have a negative perception of life, and I may experience **rancor**, having difficulty in integrating new ideas that could make my life better. This **rancor** can result from my feeling of powerlessness toward the paternal figure that I consider to have been dominant in my life. I have the impression that I have a duty to sacrifice myself or that I am being manipulated.

I accept↓♥ to acknowledge my thoughts and feelings through others and in the world around me. Because it is in my **abdomen** that my deepest intentions and my feeling of what is good or bad reside, then any discomfort

---

1. **Koch** (Robert): A German physician (Clausthal, Hanover, 1843 – Baden-Baden 1910). In 1882 he identified the bacillus (a bacterium in the form of a stick) of tuberculosis. He described the modes of transmission of this disease and invented a method of diagnosis. In 1905, he received the Nobel Prize for medicine for all of his discoveries.

in this area gives me a good indication of what is going on in my inner life and my emotions.

ABORTION *See: CHILDBIRTH – ABORTION*

ACCIDENT *See also: BURNS, CUT*

An **accident**, just as an **injury**, occurs when my emotions are disturbed. It is quite often synonymous with **guilt** or **fear**. It is related to my feelings of **guilt**, to my way of thinking and to how I function in society. It also denotes a certain **reaction toward authority**, and even to several aspects of violence. I may sometimes have difficulty in asserting myself before this authority, speaking of my needs, presenting my points of view. I then '**cause violence to myself**''. An **accident** indicates a direct and immediate need to turn to action. The need for a change of direction is so great that my thought uses an extreme, even a dramatic, situation to make me **Aware** that I must probably change the route I am currently following. It is like a break-off point in one aspect of my life, a point of no return, and not necessarily in my couple. **It is a form of conscious or unconscious self-punishment**. The body part **injured** during the **accident** is usually already ill or weakened, whether by a disease, an ailment, a cut, a burn, or any predisposition to **accidents**. The **accident** enables me to observe this weakness by bringing it to the surface. An **accident** is also my inability to see myself and accept myself↓♥ as I am. **As I am 100% responsible for my acts and my whole life, I can better explain to myself why I have attracted a specific form of accident on myself**. 'Attracted', you say? Yes, for all this originates from my deepest thoughts, from my *patterns* or schemes of childhood thought. It is quite possible that I am attracting punishments on myself <u>if, today, I have the impression</u> of doing something in which **I am not OK** and am feeling vulnerable. Exactly as during my childhood, I was punished when **I was not OK** It is registered in my mental memory and it is time for me to change my attitude. The 'moral' side of a human being leads me to punish myself if I feel guilty, hence the pain, the afflictions and the **accidents**. It is essential for me to know that I may feel guilty in a given situation **if, and only if,** I know that I am doing harm to someone else. **In any other situations, I am responsible but not guilty**. I must remember that I am my own authority (in the individual sense). I need to take my place in the Universe. I must stop doing violence to myself. As I wrote above, an **accident** is related to **guilt**, which in turn is related to my **fear** toward a situation. The fear of not being OK is often perceived from the standpoint of guilt rather than from that of responsibility. An **accident** often forces me to stop or slow down my activities. A certain period of questioning follows. By remaining open and objective toward myself, I will quickly discover the reason or reasons behind this **accident**. Did I lose control over a situation? Is it time for me to change orientations, to change directions? Do I have difficulty in listening to my inner signs or my intuition, to the point that I attract a physically **radical** sign? Or I tend to be fatalistic. I worry constantly and I live more in terms of suppositions than in terms of the facts and reality. Did I observe how the **accident** occurred? What state was I in before and after? It is very important to review the conditions surrounding the **accident**; I analyze the words I use and they make me **Aware** of the fact that they highLight what I was experiencing at the moment of the **accident**. If any **wounds** result from this **accident** or **injury**, I will experience anger and resentment toward a situation that I find extremely **nasty**. I observe all the signs and symbols of this situation (the **accident**) and listen to my inner voice to find a solution that will probably avoid further aggravating all this. The **predisposition to accidents** is a state that occurs during a conflicted relation with reality, the incapacity of being fully present and **Aware** of the world as it presents itself to me. It is as though I wished to be somewhere else. I am disconnected from what is happening around me, maybe because I find my reality unacceptable or difficult to live through.

I accept↓♥ to see that I need to be more **connected** to myself in order to discover my security and my inner confidence. I stop this wild race and take the time to look at my life. I question myself by testing my choices in line with my fundamental values. I accept↓♥ the opening that takes place in order for me to feel more free and happy.

ACHILLES' HEEL TENDON

The **Achilles' heel tendon** connects the muscle of the calf to the heel bone. It is the strongest **tendon** in our body: it can carry up to 880 pounds (400 kilos).

It enables my thoughts and my desires, physical as well as spiritual, to become realities. It also serves to express any blockage in the ankle's movement. For example, I may have a great desire for stability, but this is difficult to achieve because of a precarious financial situation.

The **Achilles' heel tendon** can support a lot: do I have the impression that I too am supporting a heavy load? It can only be strong and carry a heavy load if its inner base is solid, but if I feel empty inside, what can I rely on? Maybe I give too much importance to the 'container', to the external side of things, but what about the 'content'? What are my priorities, my values? What is my life based on? Am I in contact with my divine essence, or am I only at the level of 'appearance'? Is there a break-up in my relations with others, especially with my children or parents? Do I always need to move, to go away, as if I couldn't stand to remain in one single place for too long, a little like a gypsy? I become **Aware** that the **Achilles' heel tendon** works more when I am in the standing position (vertical) than when I am lying down.

It becomes more fragile if I experience it as impossible for me to go higher. It may be the desire for a promotion, a change in social rank, or the desire to belong to a professional sports team, but obstacles prevent this from materializing.

I accept↓♥ to take action and get things moving in order to achieve my dreams and reach the goals I have set for myself. I base my life on solid human values. I increase my inner strength by being myself.

ACIDOSIS / OXYOSIS *See also: GOUT, RHEUMATISM*

Acid is often related to what eats at metal and to what is bitter (psychic bitterness). Thus, **acidosis** indicates that I have **refused to assimilate** a situation that is now unconsciously accumulating, spreading in the body a high level of acidity in the blood or in the fluid in which the cells are bathed. To **assimilate** means to process, resolve and fix any problem, situation or conflict that is disturbing me, that I refuse, that is **poisoning** my existence! For example, I can ask myself what the situation is (often of an emotional nature) that is eating at me inside and is making me **so bitter toward life**. It is possible that I am currently experiencing a situation that is calling up in my dissatisfaction over the relations I had with **my mother**. I can even feel similar dissatisfaction with my children, some friends or some employees toward whom I feel '**like a mother**'. I have difficulty in stopping myself; I don't dare get any rest or take any time for myself. **Metabolic acidosis**, which is related to my body in general, reflects my bitter side toward life in general. **Respiratory acidosis or gaseous acidosis** originates from the fact that I do not eliminate sufficient carbon gas when I breathe. Thus, my bitter side in life has to do with my relations with my environment and the people around me. The usual **acidosis** of diabetics is **acidocetosis**. However, **lactic acidosis** remains exceptional. Both generate a coma and dehydration. In the case of **lactic acidosis**, an excessive amount of lactic acid is found in the blood. Because the blood normally transports joy, the result is that my bitter side in life, involving everything that happens in it, greatly affects me. That is why I can find myself in this state again if I am a diabetic (which corresponds to deep sadness), if I am experiencing kidney failure (which corresponds to great fears toward life), or if I have leukemia, a form of blood cancer (which corresponds to the fact that I always feel I have to struggle in life). In the extreme case, **rheumatism** is a direct and sometimes inevitable result of the excess acidity that is **acidosis**.

I accept↓♥ to see, and deal with, the situations of my life at the level of the **heart♥** even if they irritate me and bother me. By focusing my attention on a conscious process of openness and acceptance↓♥, I can avoid physically enduring this painful disease (as well as its treatment!). I resolve situations to experience more joy, freedom and inner peace.

ACNE *See: SKIN – ACNE*

ACRODERMATITIS *See: SKIN – ACRODERMATITIS*

ACROKERATOSIS *See: SKIN – ACROKERATOSIS*

ACROMEGALIA *See: BONE – ACROMEGALIA*

ADDISON'S DISEASE *See also: GLAND – CAPSULE [SUPRARENAL]*

An insufficient secretion of ***cortisol*** by the surrenal glands[2] is what generates **Addison's disease**[3].

It is a form of disappointment with myself. It is an extreme state of emotional and spiritual under-nourishment. Having this disease can mean that I experienced much submission in my childhood toward one of my parents. I may have felt myself psychically assaulted, or experienced a trauma or an intense irritation where I may have felt my life in danger. I have the impression that somebody is 'out to get me' and that I should run away as fast as I can. This condition has made me experience great insecurity about the future and to have great doubts about my capacities. This disease stands out by an extremely defeatist attitude, an absence of purpose or interest in myself or in anything around me. I was forced to give up, to 'throw in the towel' without saying a word and that broke my **heart♥**. I may compensate my disappointments by becoming dependent upon a substance or a person. I consider myself as an anguished victim. I have the impression that my whole life is made of torture. I feel much anger against myself. I cannot receive any **Love** from others. I experience great anxiety and antipathy.

I accept↓♥ to take my place, go ahead and spend some energy in working out certain personal goals without expecting any approval or permission from others around me, whatever the importance of my undertaking or my goal. I will find a method for better **connecting** myself to my inner self, which has unlimited resources and high self-esteem. I can thus retrieve some control over my life.

ADENITIS *See also: GANGLION – LYMPHATIC NODE, INFLAMMATION*

When I have an inflammation in a ganglion of the lymphatic system, it is because I am experiencing insecurity related to some fear on the affective level. I am irritated in one or several relationships, and I find it difficult to outwardly show my frustrations, which often change into anger. It is like a stick of dynamite on the point of exploding! The part of the body that is affected gives me an indication about the aspect of my life that is involved.

I accept↓♥ to try and find out the source of my sorrow in order to become **Aware** of the fear that inhabits me and develop my self-confidence to get beyond this emotion. I must express it externally in order to free myself from it.

ADENOIDS *See: TONSILS, TUMORS*

---

2. **Surrenal glands**: endocrine glands located above the kidneys in the form of a pyramid, and whose function is to enable me to develop superhuman strength for my survival when my life is in danger.
3. **Addison** (Thomas): An English physician (1793–1860) who in 1855 described this disease as a slow suprarenal (adrenal) failure.

ADENOMA *See also: BREAST DISORDERS, TUMORS*

An **adenoma** is generally a benign tumor on a gland.

As any tumor, it originates from an emotional shock that has become densely focused on the part of the body related to this shock, whether it is the pancreas, a breast, the prostate or even an endocrine gland, such as the liver or a kidney. Instead of drawing upon my own resources, I base my life on the opinions, beliefs or words of others. I have no overall view of things and I have difficulty in making decisions, namely about the direction in which I want to move. I shuffle about in place. I fear certain changes in my life by integrating certain new ideas and I don't know how to apply them. It is difficult for me to say NO to an outside influence and to search within myself instead for the true answers.

I accept↓♥ the events of the past, to enable me to move confidently ahead. I allow my creativity to manifest itself. Above all, I listen to my inner voice, who knows what is good for me.

ADENOPATHY *See also: GANGLION – LYMPHATIC NODE, INFECTIONS (IN GENERAL), INFLAMMATION, TUMORS*

Adenopathy is characterized by an increase in the volume of the lymphatic ganglia and can originate from an inflammation, a tumor or an infection.

As the ganglions of the lymphatic system act as filters for the lymphatic system, it means that I am experiencing an emotional stress or shock related to fears on the affective level. I thus feel blocked, stuck on that level. If I am experiencing a conflict, I keep everything sealed inside myself. I have difficulty in seeing what is good or bad for me. The affected region indicates to me more specifically the aspect of my life that is involved, whether it is the thorax, the abdomen, the neck, the armpits or the groin.

I accept↓♥ to develop my autonomy and my self-confidence, in order to take charge of my life!

ADHESIONS

Adhesions are characterized by a form of joining of two body organs by conjunctive tissue.

If I 'adhere' excessively, or 'stay hooked' to negative, unhealthy or inadequate ideas, to resentment, **hate** or anger toward someone, to **guilt**, to illusory dreams, to a life too focused on the family context or the home (for example, the 'brood mother'), I risk showing **adhesions** in the viscera[4]. Some are **pathological**, which means they occur following an inflammation related to **rage** or to some tumor that originates from repressed emotions or a situation that I have difficulty in digesting. I am experiencing confusion related to some situation. I associate emotions and/or ideas that are in fact unrelated. I feel lost. I am like a stray dog.

4. **Viscera**: The general term to designate each of the organs contained within the cranium, the rib cage or the abdomen.

I accept↓♥ to let go of the past, of the old ideas and negative thoughts that are impeding my happiness. I return to others what is theirs, such as their own responsibilities. I live in the present moment and savor each instant of my life.

AGEUSIA *See: TASTE DISORDERS*

AGGRESSIVENESS *See also: ANGUISH, ANXIETY, BLOOD — HYPOGLYCEMIA, NERVOUSNESS, TANTRUM*

Aggressiveness is a quantity of repressed energy that generally derives from frustration experienced in a situation.

It is often unconscious, and the frustration can poison my existence so much that I use my **aggressiveness** as a means of expression (**aggressiveness** is indeed one), as a valve to let out all this pressure built up within me. It is a way to defend myself because I feel I am under attack, not respected, abused, tense and misunderstood. I want to be understood! **Aggressiveness** diminishes my level of vitality. It can be difficult for me to remain open and let the energy flow. Obviously, if I am in a state of **aggressiveness** I cut myself off temporarily, especially from spiritual energy and the openness of the **heart♥**. It is an **innate, instantaneous** and thoughtless state of defense and protection: I doubt my worth and even tend to silently depreciate myself, telling myself that I am not up to it. I feel vulnerable, with the impression that some danger is threatening me. My powerlessness leads me to want to attack those I consider to be better or stronger than me. I may have the impression that I am being prevented from being myself, but in fact I am the one who is setting up barriers and limitations against myself. If I am aggressive, I often have the **feeling** that I am the strongest because I decide to attack first. I place myself in a state of domination-submission and I am **torn** inside. The person in front of me acts as a **mirror**. I project a part of myself that I have yet to accept↓♥, and this **pushes** my **button**![5] The result? The excitation is amplified, the tension mounts, and now the muscular contraction appears! I am stiff and tense, on guard, ready to leap against any attacks! I am on the defensive and struggling against my anxieties. What to do?

I accept↓♥ to remain open, to work on myself **first**, to listen to my intuition and my inner voice, which protect me and guide my steps. I express my emotions, whatever they may be. I accept↓♥ that my greatest strength resides in the fact of being myself and that the true power I can manifest can only be found in the fact of being true instead of wanting to project the image of a 'hard-boiled' individual.

---

5. **Press my button**: An expression indicating that one can activate a triggering element of a reaction or an emotion.

AGING (ailments of)

In **aging**, my body loses some of its flexibility. I move about with more difficulty, my dexterity deteriorates. What is my body trying to tell me? I probably regret some parts of my past; I may believe I no longer have my place in this world, that the time has come for me to **stop myself**. I also believe that life used to be better before. I refuse to see any of the beautiful things of today. My thoughts are turned toward yesterday and I criticize the present. This rigidity in my way of thinking is transmitted to my whole being. **Aging** is a stage to which I must adjust. But since I have started to age from the very first moment of my birth and so on until the moment of my death, at which point in my life do I start to grow old 'too fast' or 'too poorly'? There really is no yardstick. The process of **aging** risks being accelerated when I live too much in my head and not in my **heart♥**. Or if I leave my power of creation to someone besides myself, or allow society to dictate to me what is good for me. Or if I want to play a role in order to be accepted↓♥ by the people around me, but do not live according to my own personal values (thereby limiting my own freedom myself). If I refuse to see my emotions as allies, if I am closed to **Love**, if I kill my creativity and my deepest impulses, then under these conditions, I may feel bitter and think about my age.

I accept↓♥ to trust myself. I also accept↓♥ to live the present moment in my **heart♥**. I let go of what is not beneficial for me. I keep whatever gives me joy, laughter, energy, the **Love** of self and of others. I accept↓♥ to open myself up to changes and I accept↓♥ to receive and give more with my **heart♥**. My state thus improves day by day. I believe that the youth of **heart♥** and body is eternal. My physical body can only show the positive thoughts of health and youth.

AGING (pathological) *See: SENILITY*

AGITATION *See also: HYPERACTIVITY*

Agitation is a state that can affect me if I am a very nervous person who nevertheless succeeds in channeling her energy as well as she can! It is close to a **state of emergency**, an inner insecurity I can't control, a process of outward expression of my emotions, often a cry of alarm to show others how I am feeling inside: stuck, distrustful, fearful in certain situations, enterprising but often awkward and especially very irritating for the people around me! If I am very **agitated** physically and internally, I can experience a form of instability because I have difficulty in remaining 'centered' (stable and anchored) in myself: I therefore unconsciously use this state because I need to increase my self-confidence, to prove that I can succeed, by attracting attention: *"Watch me go!"*

I accept↓♥ to become **conscious** of the fact that the more I can understand why I have this insecurity inside me,the more I succeed in controlling the agitation. I remain calm, I verbally communicate my feelings and my needs, and everything will be for the best.

AGNOSIA *See also: ALEXIA [CONGENITAL]*

Agnosia is an object recognition disorder, inexplicable by sensory deficit and reflecting (or explaining) a specific intellectual deficit. It exists for all the sense organs: blindness, deafness, verbal.

If it is **visual**, what I see reminds me of some of my injuries that I was unable to overcome when they occurred: if I don't enter into contact with my environment, I avoid reconnecting with my own injuries. When it is **auditory**, it is generally accompanied by a language disorder: I am also protecting myself from others, thereby preventing myself from communicating and creating deep and enduring relations in order to avoid suffering if those relations were ever to break up. **Tactile agnosia** (touch) prevents me from entering into physical contact with my surroundings. It is somewhat like a child who discovers what is outside of her: if I am insecure, I fear whatever I may discover out there, and so I manage to make my body incapable of defining objects. It puts me in contact with my incapacity for building anything with certain elements of my life. **Spatial agnosia** is the impossibility of locating an object in space: it is related to the disorientation or the loss of certain memories that were too painful for me, and I therefore no longer have any points of reference. I thus remain remote from my own nature and I can't locate myself in society because I feel lost.

I accept↓♥ that all my past experiences will become part of a learning process. I accept↓♥ to acknowledge and examine what the lessons to be learned will be. From now on, I will remain in contact with reality, and I realize that it is by healing my inner injuries that I will resume contact with all of what I am. Later on, I will be able to be **Aware** of the Universe around me and feel well and free.

AGORAPHOBIA *See also: ANXIETY, DEATH, FEAR*

Agoraphobia, derived from the Greek words **AGORA** (marketplace, place of assembly) and **PHOBOS** (fear), is the panic of the crowd and also that of fearing it.

It is strongly related to an unconscious fear of death. If I suffer from **agoraphobia**, I am probably a very sensitive person, receptive on several levels (mainly psychic[6]) and possessing a very fertile imagination. I am very dependent affectively, and I never truly cut the maternal tie(s). I have difficulty in discerning my true self amidst what I create on the psychic level, namely thought-forms, which feeds my anxieties. I am like a **sponge**: I absorb the emotions of others (mainly the fears) without discerning, filtering or protecting what belongs to me, so I amplify my fears as well as those of others. I thus tend

6. **Psychic**: At the level of my thoughts, the mental level.

to withdraw into myself, to feel responsible for everything, to communicate very little except with the person whom I **trust enormously**, with whom I feel safe; I thus isolate myself for fear of moving away from this form of **security**. I am like a rat in a cage and I even tend to hang onto this person, feeling my fragility and how far my self-created limits reach and curtail my freedom. I have difficulty taking on my role as an adult. I may even think I am suffering from insanity and I **must stop believing that as soon as possible**. It is easy for me to 'control' everything from a place where I am totally secure. However, as soon as I leave that place, everything falls apart! I fear the look of others upon me, and their judgment. I am anxious about everything, as if my fears were invading me to the point where I have the impression of losing control! As soon as an experience stimulates me too strongly (a birth, an accident, a death, a catastrophe), I risk sinking once again into my anxieties (noises, people, etc.), without ever finding an enduring situation, hence the amplification of my **agoraphobia**. Furthermore, my criticism level is high because I am experiencing much insecurity, I trust people very little, and I believe that things and situations are not going as well as I would like: so I criticize. **Agoraphobia** sometimes underlies a conflict with my mother, whom I constantly criticize. She may have greatly relied upon me, thus enacting a form of dependence. The relationship became based upon expectations instead of **Love**. I may then have felt a great emptiness, which is making itself felt now that I have become an adult. I had such an impression of having to fuse with my mother (or another adult of reference who saw to my education) that I have difficulty in being surrounded by people, for I unconsciously fear I may have to fuse with them, which is too much to ask of me.

I accept↓♥ to change my attitude right now. I choose the directions I will take, **Aware** that I enjoy full freedom of movement and action. I accept↓♥ my fears one by one, such as they are, for I know they are poisoning my life, but they can also serve to make me go ahead! **I learn to Love and accept myself↓♥**, to **Love** my maternal and protective side (mother), to build myself a physical and inner world of happiness, with no criticism or dependence. It is also an advantage for me to express myself in my verbal communication and my creativity. I must go beyond the fear of 'losing my place', and be in harmony with myself. I remain responsible for my happiness, even if I tend to believe that I determine the happiness as well as the unhappiness of others. I accept↓♥ to take risks and to meet my fears, which are impeding my creative power. This will help me better manage my life and my inner impulses. A balanced and active sexuality will help me to free myself from this emotional fixation in my mind.

AHT (Arterial Hypertension) *See: TENSION (ARTERIAL) — HYPERTENSION*

AIDS (Acquired Immune Deficiency Syndrome)

If I am carrying the **AIDS** virus (**HIV**: **H**uman **I**mmunodeficiency **V**irus) and am in good health, it will simply be said that I am **seropositive**, and I may never develop the disease. If my immune system weakens because of the **HIV virus,** then I can say that I have **AIDS**, the disease.

If I am a person afflicted with **AIDS**, I see my immune system becoming deficient in T cells (lymphocytes or varieties of white globules in the **blood** and the lymph) and it thereby becomes incapable of protecting me against certain infections, such as pneumonia and cancer. The **AIDS virus** is transmitted by the blood (blood contaminated during a blood transfusion, an infected syringe, a wound in contact with infected blood, etc.) or sexual fluids. The thymus gland (located in front of the trachea), the site where T cells are formed, is thus affected and, by this very fact, the energy of the **heart♥** is affected also. The diffusion of infected cells into the extracellular fluids, mainly the blood, corresponds to emotional energy. Blood related to the **heart♥** symbolizes **Love**, sorrow and creativity. Thus, my emotional system is unbalanced and incapable of expressing itself freely. **I am experiencing great guilt about Love; I have the impression of not being up to what the situation requires**. My system is weakening and becoming increasingly vulnerable to all forms of invasion. It is as if my immune system can no longer tell the difference between what is good for me and what is not. I need to become **Aware** of the fact that I am repressing emotions such as fear and anger, that I am repudiating the person I am to the point of wishing for my complete destruction. To this repression of my feelings is usually also added a deep guilt that eats away at me from inside. My self-esteem is practically non-existent and I fear the judgment of others. **The result of my incapacity to Love and accept↓♥ myself as I am is that I can no longer protect myself**, I am as defenseless as when I was little. My inner strength, which is normally backed by **Love**, acceptance↓♥ and an intense desire to live, is becoming slowly weakened and undermined. **Even unconsciously, death may appear to me as a solution to my despair**. I am ashamed of myself, I am out of contact with my own emotions, and total emptiness looms. I have had the impression, for a long time now, that I have no authority over my own life. I am unable to ask for **help**[7] from the people I **Love**, in any area of life. It could turn out to be the only way, finally, to get some attention and **Love** from my parents. I consider myself as a shame for my family, and it may be best for me to disappear. I will no longer be a source of suffering for them because I don't fit all their expectations. My integrity is undermined. It is important to **realize** that the **HIV virus** is transmitted either by the **blood** or by **sperm** during a sexual encounter; both are generally synonyms of life (a blood transfusion can save a life, and through the sexual act I can give life, continuing the bloodline). These are unconditional acts of **Love**. Then how is it possible for 'death' to be transmitted through these same acts? Where did the inner break occur with the **Love** that previously inhabited me, which allowed this virus to settle as the king and master in my body? Why have I become my own parasite instead of being my own best friend? I am discovering that going through a sexual experience can prove to be emotionally very revealing. Even spiritually, it can lead me to experience beneficial events

---

7. **AIDS** sounds close to **'aid'**.

as soon as the sexual energy surges from the basic chakra[8] that is the source of my spiritual ascent. On the other hand, if this energy is badly used, merely for self-gratification and self-indulgence, it can turn against me. Without a sincere sign of purity, it can turn into a pathological or bothersome energy. I therefore learn to recognize the forms of energy that are in me and I use them to better further my development.

I accept↓♥ to take myself in hand, I trust myself and I learn to **Love** every part of my person. I must be born to life a second time, but this time, I accept↓♥ to live for myself and to be happy. I accept↓♥ who I am: a divine and magnificent being. In so doing, if I have any children, it will help them at the same time to become sovereign in their own lives and will foster their blooming and the acceptance↓♥ of their whole beings.

AILMENTS (various)

An **ailment** is not a disease, but rather a discomfort that I am feeling, with an intensity that can vary.

It is an '**un-ease'** or an '**un-wellness**' that I am experiencing, and I am in conflict with myself or with a situation in my life. The way to decode an **ailment** is the same as for a disease. However, the clinical symptoms are more vague and may vary from feeling 'out of sorts' to fainting. As in the case of a disease, an **ailment** originates from a conscious or unconscious conflict or trauma. An **ailment** can be temporary, but it can indicate an inner conflict that should be resolved before the message is sent more strongly in the form of a disease.

AIR SICKNESS *See: SEA SICKNESS*

ALCOHOLISM *See also: ALLERGIES, BLOOD — HYPOGLYCEMIA, CANCER OF THE TONGUE, CIGARETTES, DEPENDENCE, DRUGS*

The abuse of **alcoholic** drinks causes a whole set of disorders: physically, the body changes and tenses, the brain's capacities and functioning diminish, the nervous and muscular systems become "**tense and over-tensed**". Similar to all the other forms of dependence, "**alcoholism**" manifests itself mainly at times when I need to fill a deep affective or inner void, an aspect of myself that is truly «poisoning» my existence!

I can drink abusively for various reasons: to **escape my reality**, whatever the situation (conflict or other) because of something that does not suit me; to resist my fears toward authority (especially paternal) and those I **Love** because I am afraid that I may unveil myself one day; to expose who I really am; to give me the **courage** to move forward, to speak, to confront people (note that, if I am a bit tipsy, I am often more open because I am less fixated on my inhibitions); it gives me a feeling of power and strength; it gives me power in an emotional relationship because my state will surely bother the other person.

---

8. **Basic Chakra:** One of the body's seven main energy centers, located in the coccyx, at the base of the spine.

I no longer see situations that may be threatening to me. I live in solitude and isolation, with **guilt**, **misunderstanding, inner anxiety** and some **form of abandonment** (family or other) and I have the feeling that I am **useless**, **worthless**, inept, inferior, and incapable of being and acting for myself or others. I have confined myself in overly-rigid principles. As I believe that I don't deserve any **Love** and happiness, I find myself in a cold environment where nobody understands me. Instead of building solid relationships with people, I do it with **alcohol**, which becomes my 'best friend'. I don't find my place in society. In the past, I used to live intensely: I could experience the **intoxication** of speed, of heights, of nature, and it all disappeared from my life. I therefore needed 'a little boost'. Often I want to escape a conflict or something that is hurting me by drowning my sadness or any other emotion that I have trouble dealing with. I don't feel myself supported in a situation, and **alcohol** becomes my support, my 'crutch'. **Alcoholism** can be related to one or more situations that make me tense. When I drink a glass of **alcohol**, this tension diminishes; and at first, I register that the connection seems to be: tension→ **alcohol**→ well-being, which means that, as soon as I feel tension, I have a glass of **alcohol** and I feel better. The result being that I may thereby develop a sort of **automated** response to tension and every time I feel any tension it is inscribed in my brain that I must have a drink of **alcohol** in order to feel better. One source of **alcoholism** is the difficulty I experienced, as a child, in dealing with a family where one of the members (often the mother or father) was an **alcoholic**: there is generally more strife, sometimes physical and psychological violence or abuse of all sorts. I may even want to disassociate myself from the family in which I am living and which does not suit me. There is then a decline in my moral sense: the frequent scenes of strife provoke in me a devalued parental image and a deficient integration of ethical structures. I would have wanted to reconcile my parents, as I was no longer able to get by in this home that was destroyed, in my view. In some families the addiction to alcohol is fostered by education, the adults having induced me as a child to drink it as a game, or having made the regular consumption of **alcohol** a '**normal** thing to do'. The neurotic disorders and personality alterations that result from this have become powerful factors of **alcoholism** for me since I became an adult. Even nutritional deficiencies can drive one to search for a nutritional complement provided by **alcohol**. **Alcoholism** can even induce hypoglycemic states, as **alcohol** molecules can transform rapidly but temporarily into blood sugar. This explains why, if I am an **alcoholic** and I stop consuming, I may find myself consuming impressive amounts of coffee, a source of stimulation in the form of **caffeine**, and of sugar, pastries or desserts (sources of sugar). Sometimes I may smoke a lot because cigarettes provide a source of stimulation (heightened heartbeat rates) that I need to feel in shape. It is important to discover the source of this sadness that is related to hypoglycemia and to find what causes it in my life, for I have not yet resolved the cause. Another cause of **alcoholism** may be **allergies**, which means I may be allergic only to cognac, gin, rye or scotch, etc. It would seem that only a particular sort of **alcohol** may satisfy me. It is possible that I may be allergic to one or many of the ingredients that make up a particular drink, whether it is wheat, barley or rye, etc. I can then ask myself, what am I allergic to? **Alcoholism** can also come from me not accepting↓♥ a person or a situation from my youth. If I was inappropriately touched in a sexual manner by an **alcoholic** person when I was young, or if I feel guilty whenever I think about it, I may be driven to drink. If I have not accepted↓♥ the anger of my **alcoholic father**, it is possible that by association, I may become angry, **like my father**, and become an **alcoholic** myself. I therefore drink to avoid my anxieties and forget my past and future, but especially the **present**. I constantly escape and create a Universe of illusions and fantasies, a form of artificial exaltation, to escape the physical world and thus to disassociate an often difficult reality from a continually unsatisfied dream. I don't see the real meaning of my life. By living according to the norms of my parents or of society, I become distant from myself. I feel different, out of phase with the rest of the world. What is the use of diplomas or important titles? I perceive the world as very materialistic and I don't know how to belong to this world. I must move away from my creativity and my imagination and 'do as the others do'. In so doing, I have the impression of 'losing my **Soul**'. I momentarily lose contact with my feelings of solitude, of being misunderstood, with the powerlessness of not being like the others and my self-rejection. I can abandon my responsibilities, and I am 'saved' for a moment. This scenario only further worsens my dependence on **alcohol** (or drugs), for I become more and more dissatisfied with my existence. I want to separate myself from reality by going into a world of illusion but, once I become sober, reality appears to be even more difficult and life ever harder to handle, which can then bring on depression. I am faltering, not functioning with a clear **head**, especially when I become **dependent**, **with the same type** of emotional dependence **I may have desired** and that I have the impression **my mother or father** never gave me: to be Loved unconditionally. I may wish to become fused with my mother, whom I miss, or wish, on the contrary, to be rid of her because I haven't been capable of receiving her **Love** and I am resisting her. I also become **Aware** that when I drink, I can express things that are usually impossible to express. **Alcohol** then becomes a way to 'make my unconscious speak'. I express in my moments of crisis what I can't say or do while I am sober.

I accept↓♥ from now on to look at my life face on, to stop destroying myself and to become responsible. It is time to emphasize my good qualities, physical and spiritual, even if the past was painful for me and, in a sense, even if my bottle was often **my best friend**. From now on, I accept↓♥ to get my life in order, to start loving my qualities and the person I am. I am now on the path to success. I will respect myself and find easier ways to deal with my problems (experiences) instead of staying in a temporary or almost permanent state of Light and despair. I accept↓♥ my difference and fully take it on. I allow my unique qualities to express themselves, **Aware** that I no longer have to satisfy society's expectations. By allowing my inner fullness to grow, by drinking the **Love** and the gentleness that people and the Universe want to give me, I no longer need to 'fill' myself to excess with alcoholic drink.

ALEXIA (congenital) / WORD BLINDNESS

Congenital alexia is also called **word blindness**. It is a pathological incapacity for reading. I may either be able to read the letters but not the words, or read the words without making out the letters, or be unable to read all the words together in a sentence, which prevents me from understanding its meaning.

If I am affected by this disease, I may experience great **concern** or exaggerated attention about the thoughts that I have. The more exaggerated the attention I lavish on aspects of my life that don't really need it, the more I risk suffering by thus remaining oblivious, or closed, to thoughts that enhance my development. What is unknown to me makes me experience great insecurity. I thereby have much less power over my life, and I feel a great emptiness.

I accept↓♥ the fact that I need to open up inside to my intuition and my imagination, two marvelous faculties that the **Soul**[9] that I am possesses to express itself. If I want to heal this disease, I need only look for how disturbed my life is, what the disease prevents me from (or allows me to avoid) doing, saying or seeing. By opening up my **heart♥**, I resolve this situation **consciously**. It is easier for me as a child to show inner listening, because I am more 'connected' than adults, **I can read the Love messages from my heart♥ more easily!** So then, I open myself up to my intuition and I manifest my creativity more.

ALLERGIES *See also: ALCOHOLISM, ASTHMA*

To be **allergic** is to be in a state where one is prone to a different and often stronger and more uncontrollable reaction upon a second exposure to a specific antigen. An **allergy** is the overactive response by the immune system to a foreign antigen. The allergenic substance does not usually provoke a reaction with most people, but my immune system identifies it as being dangerous.

This response results from an inner cause and is often the way that my body uses to tell me that I am living in a state of aggressiveness and hostility toward a given person or situation, <u>depending on my mental interpretation of what I am experiencing specifically.</u> An **allergy** is therefore a defense and a sign that my Ego is protecting itself. My great sensitivity wants to give me a signal that something or someone is hostile to me, that some danger is afoot. I no longer feel safe. **Allergies** (including hay fever) are similar to asthma, but the reaction is located in the region of the eyes, nose and throat instead of in the lungs and chest area. What am I **allergic** to? What is making me overreact so much? What is the real cause of this irritation and of my body's strong emotional response (snuffling, teary eyes, feeling the need to cry)? These are all responses from my **emotional system**, the liberation of emotions suppressed by my body's reaction. It is my body's reaction to something, a sort of mental symbol, because my body is trying to reject, obliterate[10] or ignore what is

9. **The Soul**: The divine spark that I am, my **Conscience**.

10. **To obliterate**: To erase from my conscious memory or my sensitivity.

bothering it. I am therefore rejecting the part of myself that is attacking me. This is the means that I use to express my emotions, **to let out the badness.** Nothing can stop this reaction of refusal for the time being, and it is not rational, because it operates at the instinctual and subconscious level. It is as if there is something that has no business being there, an **enemy** that is interfering with my protective barriers. This enemy takes over my **power** to be and act and this impresses me. I am **impressed** by the power that others wield to the detriment of my own power. I feel threatened by a certain unconscious fear that I am refusing to experience. My **allergies** therefore tend to indicate a **deep level of intolerance**, perhaps the fear of having to fully engage in life, to rid myself of all the emotional crutches that support me, and allow myself to live self-sufficiently. By my **allergy**, I **separate** myself from the people around me and I live in a constant state of alertness because I must avoid coming into contact with the antigen, the source of my **allergic** reactions. I remain withdrawn and I communicate very little. I may have difficulty in discerning, choosing and taking my rightful place. I can feel the need to reach the members of my family through verbal and, mainly, physical contact. A key characteristic of persons with **allergies** is often that they don't feel they **are good enough**! I want to attract and get attention, sympathy and support from others. Am I using this **allergy** to get **Love**? It is possible. Whatever the case may be, one thing is certain: I have an **allergy** <u>because I am refusing a part of myself, and my subconscious struggle is great</u>. **It is my resistance, my way of saying 'no'**. The fact that I feel repelled by some part of myself, (often my sexual desires that I repudiate) makes my senses revolt, for they aspire to fully enjoy life. When I learn to say NO to certain situations, I open myself to saying YES to new situations. I have the power to decide what suits me in my own Universe. Individuals can be **allergic** to many things: food, objects, forms, smells. Anything that involves the five senses (particularly the sense of smell, which is the most powerful sense involving memory). My mind registers a multitude of impressions, **good or bad for me**. It is quite possible that if I am **allergic** to something, it is because I have mentally associated it with a certain good or bad memory and my instinct is to suppress it at this time. An **allergy** refers to something from the past that thwarts or irritates me in the present. Sometimes, I no longer want to remember certain events with my memory; my body then takes over, to remind me of what I would prefer to forget. An **allergy** often surfaces when I feel **separated** from a thing, an animal or a person. Whenever I relive a situation that reminds me of this sad, wrenching event, I will have this **allergic** reaction because at some level my body (my senses) remembers everything and registers it somewhere in its cells. When a person I **Love** leaves her physical body and my bereavement is not over, I may become **allergic** to something that reminds me of this person and, therefore, of this definitive separation that I don't accept↓♥. My **skin** then reacts to my sorrow involved in this separation. If the situation experienced is accompanied by great anxiety, my **sinuses** will be affected (**hay fever** and sneezing). In this case, a situation 'doesn't smell good', and I try to avoid it or 'stay away from it'. If it turns into **sinusitis**, I have the impression that I can't get rid of this situation or get out of it, I am stuck. If fear predominates, my **allergy** will more likely express itself through **coughing** (difficulty in breathing), and if the separation itself was what I had a hard time going through, the **allergies** will more likely show up through **skin** diseases (eczema, rash, hives, dermatitis, etc.). **Allergies to food** (for example: sugar and alcohol for the alcoholic) are related to an experience or to having been in a situation where I had to say **NO** to something that was perhaps what I Loved the most, so frustration ensued and I became **allergic to it**. It is often the fear of something new or adventurous, a lack of trust in life. I now feel compelled to deprive myself of this sort of joy by thinking that life is something ordinary and unchallenging. What do I want to avoid facing? What makes me react so strongly? What is frightening me so, from inside? Is there something that I so distrust that it makes me want to push it away from me? What would I like to control or have some power over, but I feel that it escapes me (somewhat as in the case of anorexia, I must now carefully control what I eat, at the risk of dying from it, as in acute cases of **food allergies**)? It seems that, in certain cases, my mind associates situations involving substances by using like-sounding words. So if I don't want to *be*, I become **allergic** to a *bee* sting, an insect bite. Years later, once I have accepted↓♥ and wholly integrated this change, the **allergy** will disappear. Another example: a baby is born and is **allergic** to thyme: why? Months before, when his mother was ready to give birth, she kept saying to her partner: *"Hurry up, it is time to go to the hospital, we're not going to make it"!* Here the word time is the homonym of **thyme.** Therefore at the basis of an **allergy** is an emotion of irritation or frustration that is associated with a product or a situation because of what it represents, to remind me that this ailment is something I must be Aware of and integrate. An **allergy** appears when my life context changes, is unsettled or challenged. My points of reference change, even if it is a happy event that is good for me. A new job or a move, for example, brings on a degree of insecurity and can lead me to protect myself. My self-confidence diminishes, and I 'feel dizzy'. The fact that I don't acknowledge my own worth implies that I put my partner, my child or my best friend on a pedestal. Unconsciously, this irritates me, and I may become **allergic** to that person.

By starting to accept↓♥ in my **heart♥** my life and my fears, the process of integration will be triggered, and the **allergies** that complicate my existence will return to the Universe. I need inner peace and above all, **Love**. I will remain open and everything will be for the best. I accept↓♥ to acknowledge my own worth and to dig to the roots of things. I can discover happiness within myself. By accepting↓♥ my beauty and all my divine qualities, I will be in harmony with the people around me, and the frustration will disappear.

ALLERGIES to ANIMALS (in general)

Animals possess an innate instinct and sexuality and each animal represents a facet of **Love**. An **allergy to an animal** (or to its fur) generally reflects a **resistance** to the instinctual or sexual aspect that the animal represents for me.

I accept↓♥ all the aspects of sexuality. I also accept↓♥ my desires, **conscious** as well as unconscious, for they are integral parts of my being.

ALLERGIES to ANTIBIOTICS

An **antibiotic**[11] (anti = against/bio = life) is a body (of a bacterial or other origin) specialized in fighting microbes.

But microbes also represent life. Therefore there is a contradiction. If the role of an antibiotic is to 'kill' a certain form of life in me, why then am I **allergic to antibiotics**? Probably because I refuse certain forms of life, certain **living** situations in my existence (various and more or less pleasant experiences).

There is something about which I must become more **conscious**, which is to accept↓♥ these experiences because, though they be difficult for me, I have lessons to draw from them. I trust my creative potential.

ALLERGY to CATS

The **cat** is an animal that is much more sensitive to what is **invisible** than most persons are. It embodies sensuality and gentleness. An **allergy to cats** may be more related to the aspect of my personality that can 'feel' things (the 'feminine' side), though I may have no concrete proof of this. I may therefore experience intolerance because I have no rational proof. It is clear, then, that the **cat** (or the **female cat**) symbolizes the **female sexual side**[12] and all the feminine qualities such as gentleness, charm and tenderness. I experience a certain duality between the need to receive gentleness, for instance, and my fear of it. There is an anxiety related to sexuality that can originate from a prohibition, guilt, or even death. I must therefore accept↓♥ these aspects, which I probably refuse either to receive or to manifest.

*NOTE: This **feline sensitivity** is explained by the fact that the **cat's** morphology features a nervous system concentrated mainly in the periphery of the body, whereas in humans the nervous system is more concentrated in the body's core. This special morphology makes the **cat** more **sensitive** to the special vibrations or energies of persons and places or, in a sense, to what a person or a place **'gives off'**.*

ALLERGY to DOGS

The **dog**, they say, is 'Man's best friend' (human's), so I may well wonder, when I experience this type of **allergy**, what person or what situation involving friendship is making anger surge up in me? If I am **allergic to dogs**, I may even experience some aggressiveness and even a degree of violence toward the sexuality that I relate to friendship. I may be experiencing uneasiness, not

---

11. **Antibiotic**: It was to Sir Alexander Fleming, a British physician and bacteriologist (Darve 1881 – London 1955) that we owe the discovery of penicillin in 1928, which was extracted only in 1939 and tried out on humans in 1941, which opened up the era of antibiotics.

12. **Female**: See: FEMALE PRINCIPLE

feeling able to sort out more clearly in my mind the places taken up in my life by sexuality, friendship and **Love**. This malaise makes anger rise in me, showing up in the form of an **allergy**.

I accept↓♥ to mark off the boundaries of friendship, and carefully define it in order to clarify certain situations in my life that may be, for the moment, in a gray area. I respect myself in my needs and in my choices.

ALLERGY to DUST

As **dust** is related to **dirt** and **impurity**, if I am **allergic to dust**, I am feeling some insecurity involving aspects of my life that I may believe to be 'dirty and impure', and this fear quite probably manifests itself in my sexuality. If I am **allergic to dust**, I may have a great need to attend to my self-esteem. Also, the expression used in the Bible: *"For **dust** you are, and to **dust** you will return"* expresses well the sense of futility that I may experience in certain situations. The expression *"Everything is blowing off into **dust**"* also renders the feeling of futility that can inhabit me regarding what I have undertaken or am currently undertaking, whether it involves something psychological, affective (emotional) or material. I tend to do my best to be Loved and accepted↓♥ because I have the impression that I am not good enough. This self-criticism can make people avoid me. Even if I have no physical symptoms related to an **allergy to dust**, I may be a person who is a 'cleanliness maniac', in the sense of being excessively so. I can now examine what part of me seems to find my sexuality 'dirty', or wonder if I am afraid of it being 'dirty'.

I learn to value myself and everything I do. I learn to accept↓♥ each aspect and part of my body. I view it as a whole. By taking the time to go and see the deeply hidden emotions within me, I get to know myself better, and from this I will draw an extraordinary strength that will allow me to live my life joyfully and creatively.

ALLERGY to FEATHERS

Have I become **allergic** to a situation or a person who makes me feel that I am **nailed to the ground** and can't **fly away** to feel freer and happier? Then I am probably experiencing anger over **feeling stuck** inside, between a situation and the **freedom I crave** to be happier. Maybe I was in a situation where I **'lost some feathers'** or was **'plucked clean'** [13], and this irritates me no end.

I accept↓♥ that the world will take care of me and give me everything I need to be happy.

ALLERGY to FISH OR SEAFOOD

If I am always heedlessly unsuspicious when faced with **'fishy'** propositions or statements, it means that I am a person who can be easily misled or 'had'. My

---

13. **To be plucked clean:** To be stripped, dispossessed or robbed of something.

allergy therefore expresses well my feeling of **frustration** over one or several situations where I **happened to be naive**.

I accept↓♥ to take my place and to become **Aware** of the fact that life is a succession of experiences for learning. The more I increase my self-confidence and my sense of responsibility, the more this feeling of frustration will fade away and make this **allergy** disappear.

ALLERGY to HAY FEVER (cold)

This **allergy** is basically a reaction to pollen, a vegetal grain that is the **male element** of the flower.

This male element conveys the symbol of reproduction and fertilization. This **allergy** usually affects the eyes, the nose and the sinuses. The **allergy** is at the basis of a **resistance** to a situation in my life, to a past memory or even to a facet of my own personality. I don't like my life to be programmed in advance. It is therefore possible that often, unconsciously, **I resist a form of sexuality or certain aspects of it**, especially if what I feel about sexuality 'doesn't smell right'. A fear of reproduction may be present. Am I an adult who sees time quickly slipping by and who fears that her dream of having children and raising a family will vanish as time goes by? Am I a teenager struggling with many questions related to the fact of having children? It can also be a resistance and a non-acceptance↓♥ of the passing of time, which is especially noticed with each new season, when the **allergy** reappears. **Hay fever** can also be related to the fact that I was separated from a person, and this greatly affected me. A **pollen allergy** brings me back to my difficulty in going out to encounter life, to go out on an adventure. Novelty scares me and I am anxious when faced with any changes in my life. I can certainly **attract** an **allergy** for several reasons, but one thing is sure: I suffocate or I feel suffocated by a situation. I revolt, something doesn't suit me at all, but I do it all the same to please someone, and I suffocate. I change my mind under the influence of someone else, I am ready to do anything, and I am suffocating. I can feel **suffocated** in things to say or to do, especially if I have difficulty in taking my place and in saying no. I also tend to experience a lot of guilt. I feel inferior and fear the reactions of others. I reject myself and I want to expel whatever disturbs me. I fear I may find myself **straw-poor**. However, I remain imprisoned in old habits. I am rigid, just as the succession of the seasons always unfolds in the same sequence. I manipulate to get what I want. You see the programming? It can be mental (a way of crying) as well as 'seasonal', for the summer period is ideal for manifesting this **allergy**, especially if I need an excuse to be less busy during this beautiful period of the year! Some people have **hay fever** for periods as long as seven years! It is time for me to change that immediately, or at least to become **Aware** of it. I become **conscious** of the fact that **hay fever** can become a means for me to avoid certain situations, because in any case I would not be capable of refusing to do some chore or to go to some place in particular. So now, I have a good reason! It can also be a means for me to feel different, to need to attract attention. This way, people will at least have to notice me during the **allergy** season. By taking and occupying my vital space, my 'bubble' of **Light**[14], I am able to open myself up to others in my true **Light**, without any artifice. I thereby avoid living in a situation of fLight and secrets. The first manifestation of **hay fever** may have been unconsciously related to a striking event where I probably experienced strong emotions. When the same period of the year comes around again, I remember or, rather, my body remembers, and the **hay fever** again reappears. It is therefore important for me to become **conscious** of this event so that I can break the *pattern* of the ailment: I will no longer need it in the future because I took the step to **consciousness** that I had to take. The **hay fever** was just a sign to help me stop and find the deeper cause of my ailment. I will feel more free, more in charge of my life.

I accept↓♥ what is good for me, even if this involves a new and unfamiliar form of sexuality. I know that everything is possible, in **Love** and harmony. I accept↓♥ to come out of my isolation and go toward people, as I no longer need this **allergy** to attract attention, because I know that I am different and unique.

ALLERGY to HORSES

The **horse** is associated with the **instinctual aspect of sexuality**. As an instinct is more related to the first *chakra* (or coccyx)[15], my fear may focus on the issue of 'having base sexual instincts', and may then manifest itself by an **allergy** to this strong and spirited animal. It may be that I find sexuality not 'spiritual' enough for me, if I feel deep inside of me the desire to go through these experiences to help me bring more spirituality into my physical reality.

I accept↓♥ to open myself up to new experiences that will help me know myself better and become more fulfilled.

ALLERGY to MILK PRODUCTS

Milk represents our **contact** with our mothers from the first instants of our arrival in this world. It is a complete food that allows me to have all the nutriments I need for my growth during the first weeks of my life. Because originally, I get this **milk** through my **contact** with my mother, this food also signifies the **Love that I receive from my mother**. Therefore if, amongst the people around me, there is a person I identify, either my mother or someone else acting in her stead, and I experience frustration involving her in the role I have attributed to her, this could explain why I have an **allergy to milk**. I am experiencing frustration with the form of attention and even of criticism that this person directs at me, which makes my contact with her unpleasant. I may also find myself in a situation where I feel trapped, dependent and at the mercy

---

14. **My 'bubble' of Light**: I can imagine and envision myself in a bubble of **Light**, which will increase my protection against my environment and give me more self-confidence.
15. **First chakra**: The first chakra is one of the seven main energy centers in the body; it is located at the level of the coccyx, at the base of the spine.

of someone else. It is as if my life depended on her decision to feed me or not, and that is very frustrating and agonizing. Or is it I who is clinging too much? If this **allergy** developed since my birth, I must find out what fears or frustrations my mother experienced while carrying me, and which I may have made my own, leading me to experience this **allergy**. This attention focused on me could lead me to ask: "Who does she think she is? Does she take herself to be my mother?"

It is important for me to accept↓♥ to put some **Love** in the situation and to harmonize my feelings about this relation that is special and fundamental for the survival of the human species, and which is recorded in me, the link between a mother and her child.

ALLERGY to PEANUTS (butter or oil)

When I eat **peanut oil** or **peanut butter**, it activates in me the memory of an event when I was young, where I had an especially bad time of it and about which I now experience regrets. At that time, I may have had the impression that I was required to do work for which I felt I was not being sufficiently paid (in money, in affection, etc.). I worked then, and even today, I still can do heavy work for very little pay, and I found this situation ***ugly,*** repugnant. Working just 'for **peanuts'** made me seethe with anger inside. By trying to identify the event or the situations where I experienced such a feeling, I will be able to modify my emotional memory and resolve the situation.

I accept↓♥ to become **conscious** of all the areas of my life where I feel I am being helped and where life is relatively easy for me, and I amplify this feeling of well-being to help me balance out the feelings of difficulty that I may have recorded in my childhood memory.

ALLERGY to POLLEN *See: ALLERGY — HAY FEVER*

ALLERGY to STRAWBERRIES

An **allergy to strawberries** is associated with frustration that places in contradiction the feeling of **Love** and that of pleasure**,** the latter being for me a fundamental need, along with food or sleep. This **allergy** can originate from an event that I experienced, or even that I didn't experience, in relation to a person or a situation. A feeling of hate and frustration, combined with guilt, can start up this **allergy** in me. Pleasure is such a part of my life as a human being that strong **strawberry allergy** attacks can induce an incapacity for breathing, which could result in death. The lungs represent life and I thus reveal, by my **allergy** attack, an unsatisfied fundamental need in my life. It is important for me to become **conscious** of my fundamental needs by learning that when I eat food, it is **Love** I am giving to myself; when I feel pleasure, it is also **Love** that I am showing myself. An **allergy to strawberries** can also originate from a feeling I may have experienced toward a person or that a person may have felt toward me. For instance, I may have said to myself: *"I* *don't like this guy's* ***strawberry*** *mark"*, meaning this as emblematic of everything I don't like about his face. It may be related to a member of my family, and I am saddened by the discord that I see.

I must accept↓♥ that each and every one of us has their individuality, with their qualities and their fears, and that in each being, is this spark that shines.

ALLERGY to SUNLIGHT

The **sun** is the representation of the active principle and the Yang energy. It is therefore the symbol of the Father.

When I am **allergic to the sun**, the contact I have with my father (physical as well as symbolic) is a source of suffering or discomfort. The relationship may have been painful, burning or stifling, and in some cases, it suddenly stopped. This contact may have been broken off, altered or became too invasive. In all cases, there was some conflict, disagreement or disappointment with someone or something from whom/which I had to separate, which caused a painful reaction that I was unable to overcome and of which I still carry the repercussions today as an adult. Is there also a refusal to accept↓♥ my own inner Father?

I accept↓♥ to see what is bothering me and to trustfully let myself be touched by the heat of the **sun** (and my Dad!). I free myself of those emotions that were festering deep in my **heart♥**. The **sun** is the source of **Light**, heat and life. I choose to contact my inner **Sun**, and I make peace with the past to become responsible, to feel free, and to shine on the way to reaching my own destiny.

ALLERGY to WASP OR BEE STINGS

I certainly have the impression of being constantly **harassed** or **criticized** by my close entourage. It acts on me as if I was constantly being '**pricked**'. Whenever I am actually **pricked** physically, it sets off all the hate I have accumulated in myself from all those situations where I felt myself being attacked. I tend to curl up within myself, in the hope of thereby avoiding further attacks. I reach the point of feeling inferior. The 'poison' contained in the 'aggressor's stinger' reminds me of how much I can poison my own life by living according to the expectations of society, my family or my spouse. I aspire to become the 'Queen Bee', but instead, I actually live my life as a simple 'worker bee' who resembles all the others. I live like a victim. I am distrustful and fatalistic.

I accept↓♥ to start looking at the good, attractive side of things. By my acceptance↓♥ of no longer being a victim, the insects will go looking for other victims! I learn to take my appropriate place and I examine by what means I can make criticism diminish from the people around me and how I can become more detached from what others may think of me. I look at myself with the eyes of the **heart♥**, and I accept↓♥ my true worth!

ALOPECIA *See: HAIR — BALDNESS*

ALOPECIA AREATA *See: HAIR — ALOPECIA AREATA*

ALTITUDE SICKNESS *See: MOUNTAIN / ALTITUDE SICKNESS*

ALZHEIMER'S[16] DISEASE *See also: AMNESIA, SENILITY*

This disease makes brain cells degenerate, and a progressive loss of intellectual faculties leads to a state of dementia (lunacy).

This modern-day illness, mainly characterized by the unconscious desire to terminate my life, to leave this world once and for all or to **escape my reality,** is due to a chronic incapacity to accept↓♥ or to face, and deal with, this reality and certain situations in life because I am afraid and am finding it painful to live. I therefore make myself insensitive to my surroundings and to my inner emotions. I *'numb myself'*, I *'become **Light**-headed'*, and life then seems easier and death, more acceptable↓♥. I am afraid, or have the impression, that I am no longer Loved, that I am being forgotten. I have suffered so much that I can no longer feel anything. I don't have the impression that I was recognized in life (often by my mother), so I no longer recognize the others today. **Alzheimer's disease** generates in me a form of dementia that associates memory degradation, mental confusion and an inability to express myself clearly, violence, certain forms of unAwareness of my surroundings, and even innocent behavior similar to that of a young child. **Desperation, irritability and melancholy** lead me to become withdrawn and to cut myself off from others. I let myself *'die a slow death'*. I quietly **separate** myself from the rest of the world. This illness tells me that I am not enjoying life and that I am escaping a situation that I fear, that irritates or hurts me, for I feel abandoned. It is a fLight from the adult world by the loss of recent memory and the return to the old memory. At first glance, it is a situation that seems serious, of which I may remain oblivious for a long time. I am seen as a 'normal', balanced person, but others notice that I have withdrawn inward out of desperation, anger or frustration, which makes me insensitive to the world around me. I refuse to feel what is happening around and within me; I prefer to let myself go. I may have a hard time letting go of my old ideas, because my memory is so filled with all of them! And as I am so much more focused on the past than on the **present moment**, my short-term memory becomes deficient and **atrophies,** no longer brings anything new or creative into my life. The consequence is that my memory is being **used up in remembering** old things instead of generating new and fresh ideas. This disease generally affects elderly persons, especially if I have reached retirement age: I go from a condition where I am productive, where I have power and responsibilities, to a life where I feel useless, helpless and dependent, emotionally, physically and financially.

16. **Alzheimer** (Alois): A German neuropathologist who in 1906 described alterations in the brain of a person affected by dementia (lunacy).

How I wish I could wind back up the clock's hands of time! *"When I was a child, I wasn't afraid of dying, of the future, of my responsibilities... how happy I was!"* From a medical point of view, the emotional and mental factors, along with their corresponding body parts (fluids, blood, tissues, and bones), become involved in the onset of this disease. When blood no longer reaches certain parts of the brain, a type of mental trauma occurs. These reactions are very hard on the brain. It is a sort of retreat of blood flow from certain cerebral areas. There may be an extreme fear of many facets of aging or of impending death, which triggers an unconscious return to childlike behavior and an obliteration of the present, the past and the future from conscious memory or sensitivity in order to ignore it all. My body, under attack by the brain's degenerating cells, unconsciously makes me prepare for the time when I must part. This takes the form of childlike behavior where I allow myself to live out and 'achieve' all my fantasies and fancies.

I live in the moment and accept↓♥ to let go of the past and to start off by taking care of myself. **Love** and support from others are necessary in an experience such as this.

AMENORRHEA (absence of menstruations) *See: MENSTRUATION — AMENORRHEA*

AMNESIA *See also: MEMORY [FAILING]*

Amnesia is the partial or total loss of my memory, including information already acquired in the past as well as current information. **Amnesia** is comparable to Alzheimer's disease in several respects. The **amnesic** person suffers terribly from the present moment in their current life.

My **desire to flee** and to 'go away' is so great (whatever the situation experienced) that I curl up into myself out of **pain**, **anger**, **incapacity** or **despair,** and I close in on myself by becoming insensitive to almost everything. By becoming **amnesic**, I am no longer responsible for myself, because I separate myself from my conscious mind. I therefore entrust myself into the hands of others. I have the impression that this way, nobody will be able to judge me or condemn me. I escape, I become numb or I make myself insensitive to a person or a situation. I refuse to go through everyday situations and experiences, whatever their intensity. My inner pain is in proportion to the seriousness of the **amnesia**, whether it is **partial** (partial mental obliteration[17] of very painful childhood images) or **total** (an unconscious attempt to have a new life and a new desire to live, because I no longer can live through this first life!). Shame and guilt can manifest themselves, for whatever reason. I try to ignore several things, including my family and several difficult situations. I am more or less separated from current reality. **Amnesia** manifests itself at a time when I have the impression that I am carrying too much on my shoulders, that I am overloaded with tasks to carry out, that a very great danger is looming. I don't know what direction to take, and I feel like I am going to

17. **Obliteration**: The fact of erasing something from my **conscious** memory or my sensitivity.

'explode' at any moment. I may frequently experience **partial amnesia** when faced with a difficult situation, which I prefer to forget so as not to have to come into contact with painful emotions such as the separation from someone close to me. The process of acceptance↓♥ and integration is very important, because the phenomenon of **obliteration** of certain experiences by the mind can play tricks on me in future experiences. It is possible that I may experience some of them without knowing or understanding why they are happening to me!

I accept↓♥ to become **conscious** every day of who I am and of what still remains for me to resolve in order to regain contact with my true **higher self**.

AMPHETAMINES (consumption of) *See: DRUGS*

AMPUTATION *See also: SELF-MUTILATION*

An **amputation** is a surgical operation that consists in removing a limb, a limb segment or a salient body part (tongue, breast, penis).

The total or partial **amputation** of a limb, whether it is by reason of an accident or for other medical reasons (gangrene, tumor), is very often related to a feeling of **great guilt** about some facet of my life. I want this situation to disappear from my life. I want to 'cut it away once and for all'. But instead of it being this situation that disappears, it is the part of my body that manifests it that will be cut off. All this occurs unconsciously. If my left foot is **amputated**, it is as if my fear or my guilt is such that I prefer to 'die' rather than take the direction or the turn I took in my affective life; the right leg concerns my fear or my guilt regarding my responsibilities, etc. If I have not accepted↓♥ this **amputation**, then an emotional pain will remain attached to it (**phantom limb pain**). As this limb has become like a phantom, I wonder what special fear is preventing me from making contact with reality. Long before the **amputation**, I was experiencing powerlessness and dependence. I may even have felt handicapped in one facet of my body, of my life or in my interpersonal relations. This psychological and emotional handicap has been transferred to my physical body. If I undergo an **amputation**, it is important for me to remember that my body is not **amputated** energetically speaking, so I can remain open to the metaphysical aspect that the **amputated** part represents. Thus, if my right leg was **amputated**, I can invest the **Love**, the understanding and the integration required to achieve the greater degree of **consciousness** I need in order to advance more rapidly in carrying out my responsibilities **as if I still had my leg**.

I accept↓♥ to make all guilt disappear, being **Aware** that I am always acting for the best. I make peace with myself and I learn to appreciate what I am. Whatever the conditions, I choose to advance at my own stride, and I appreciate what is beautiful and good in life.

AMYOTROPHIA, AMYOTROPHY *See: ATROPHY*

ANAL FISSURA *See: ANUS — ANAL FISSURA*

ANDROPAUSE *See also: PROSTATE / (IN GENERAL) / DISEASES*

Andropause, specific to men, corresponds to menopause in women, although it does not involve any equivalent hormonal changes.

All the insecurities related to aging, sexual capacities and feelings of uselessness and weakness manifest themselves mentally and physically by ailments affecting the genital organs (mainly the prostate) and one or several aspects of the male concept. I have reached a stage in my life when I can take a rest, take a pause and change my priorities.

As a man, instead of rejecting myself, I accept↓♥ to take my place in the world, in harmony with each facet of my person, including the female side as well as the male side. I have a right to take more time for myself; I will be all the more effective for it when I am active or at work.

ANEMIA *See: BLOOD — ANEMIA*

ANEURYSM (arterial) *See also: BLOOD — HEMORRHAGE*

An **aneurysm** is a condition that causes a dilation of an arterial wall, thereby creating the risk of a hemorrhage by a rupture of the weakened blood vessel.

It occurs when I experience a conflict with my family or with the persons whom I consider to be like my family. Some want to force me to do something, but I am resisting with all my strength and I must prove my point of view, which puts great **pressure** on my shoulders. I am nervous, I risk 'losing' something that is out of my control. I am afraid of being abandoned and am blocking the circuits because I feel powerless. I find my life difficult, and I see everything that happens to me negatively and pessimistically. I am losing my energy, scattering it in all directions. I am trying to maintain at all costs a situation that is going more or less well and that risks breaking down at any moment: a job, an affective relationship, or something else. My blood vessels are contracting because I don't take into account my biological rhythm, and I put a sort of pressure on myself that risks rupturing. I refuse to advance joyously and allow life to circulate. A head **aneurysm** (cranial) **illuminates** how my ideas are sometimes different, and I have to fight to defend them because there is a lot of misunderstanding around me. I may also experience this misunderstanding following a break-up I have gone through (either I left, or someone else left me), which greatly affected me. An **aneurysm of the aorta** shows me the pressure that is put on me, mainly by a person in authority, to make me let go of something that I believe belongs to me. The **aneurysm** shows me how closed I can be to new ideas or solutions that are available to me.

I accept↓♥ to give myself **Love**. I stop my futile struggling when the time comes to let go of what is tied to the past. I accept↓♥ to let go, in order to free myself from it. I learn to let the movement of life circulate. I thus recover my joy in life, and I learn to live the present moment.

ANGER *See also: APPENDIX III, INFECTIONS (IN GENERAL), LIVER DISORDERS, PAIN*

Anger is an intense affective excitement and a brutal way of expressing it through progressively increasing physical and verbal excitation, with screaming, the breaking of objects, aggressiveness, trembling, etc.

Anger is a spontaneous cry of alarm, a manifestation of an **inner revolt**, a violent dissatisfaction accompanied by aggressiveness. Before age two, it is a simple way of reacting or expressing an inner discomfort (cold, hunger, etc.), but later on it becomes, instead, a means of opposition and reaction to prohibitions, and can further become a means of affective blackmail and domination. These emotions invading me generally manifest themselves in my liver, by the appearance of toxins that can generate an **upset stomach**. My thoughts go wild, become jumbled, and become amplified to the point where **I can no longer see clearly**. My pressure goes up, and I start **seeing red**. What is bothering me so much and making me explode? I am experiencing great frustrations while being incapable of asserting who I am. I feel invaded by someone or something and I want to chase them away, to expel them; and I use my **anger** as a means of expression. I have difficulty in doing introspection and admitting that I have some things I have to change. I want to stick to my positions. If I am **angry**, it is important to find out the reason that is provoking this state. I may experience a feeling of weakness, injustice, frustration, powerlessness, misunderstanding, etc., that could be exaggerated by my great emotionality and my impulsiveness. Once I have identified it, I realize that the conflict repeats itself unconsciously and it can even originate from unresolved childhood situations; and once this has become clear, integration can proceed more quickly.

I accept↓♥ to open myself up to the **Love** that I can show **here and now**. I remain **vigilant** and pay attention to all the signals indicating any oncoming **anger**, and I no longer get carried away uselessly.

ANGINA (in general) *See also: THROAT DISORDERS*

Angina is characterized by a constriction in the throat, due to an acute inflammation of the pharynx.

There is something that 'just won't pass', a blocked emotion that is preventing me from expressing my true needs to the people around me. I feel that by constricting my throat (the *chakra* or energy center of creativity and **expression**), I can't express what I experience and feel for others, and I continue to uselessly focus my attention on this belief. I must find out what led me to think about that. I am usually able to find an answer in the last **48 hours** preceding the ailment. Is it a mild irritation (an inflamed duct) or a minor frustration **that I can't swallow** and that will subsist until I change my attitude and my thoughts? "There's no question that I will swallow *that* story", even if it "sets my throat on fire". It can also be dark and negative thoughts about someone or a situation. Is there something that I absolutely want to 'catch', a new job for instance, or an outstanding school result, that would enable me to avoid a situation where I have to justify myself, explain myself, give an account of myself, or would prevent me from feeling death prowling around me? My unexpressed emotions are boiling up. And when I do finally allow myself to say things, I can still feel uncomfortable or guilty. I don't give myself the permission to ask others for help.

Whatever the reason for this ailment, I accept↓♥ that it is time for me to remain open and to re-open this channel, **even if my raw sensitivity is hurt**. My basic needs must be satisfied and it is my right, along with everyone else's. I remain open to my needs and focused on my inner being if I want to avoid this sort of **angina** in my throat. I accept↓♥ to make requests in order to thereby open my **heart♥** to receiving life's gifts.

ANGINA PECTORIS / ANGOR PECTORIS *See also: HEART♥ / (IN GENERAL) / INFARCTION [MYOCARDIAL]*

Angina is derived from a Latin word, the verb **Ango** that means **to tighten, to squeeze**, to choke, which gave **Angor**, which means oppression and anguish. It is a very sharp pain associated with the main region of the **heart♥** (the energy center of **Love**). This temporary lack of oxygen in the muscles of the **heart♥** has all the consequences familiar to me: insufficient blood flow in this region, surgery, bypasses procedure, etc.

The **heart♥** often represents the motor or the **engine** of my system. **Angor** is the anguish of the **heart♥**. When I give too much **Love** with an attitude of attachment, my **heart♥** may tire of all these concerns and may no longer feel enough joy[18] in these situations (hence the diminished blood flow). If I am in a situation of **angina**, it may be that I take far **too much to heart♥** my life and the things I do and like. My worries are as exaggeratedly amplified as my joys: I become irritated and easily hurt myself, I feel dissatisfaction, sadness or irritation over a situation that, in sum, **is not all that serious**. I have the impression of being ***ridiculed***. It is as if **a war** is raging in my **heart♥**. Who is the person I want to 'hug' close to me permanently, and whom I can refuse to let go if that moment comes? My attention is constantly focused on this thing or this person. I want us 'to be together forever', but that may not actually be possible. Instead of detaching myself and going with the flow of life, I want to control, I want to keep everything. This is a heavy load to carry, and it brings uncertainty about the direction to take. The feeling of loss and emptiness when I let go can scare me, and it is very painful if I keep everything to myself and hide my emotions inside. I may receive a first alarm signal from my body following these states of being: spasms or pain piercing the **heart♥**. My heart♥ sends out an S.O.S. for me to become **conscious** of my inner feelings and of the fact that in a sense I am destroying myself with my discordant thoughts,

---

18. **Joy**: As blood is related to joy, then reduced blood flow expresses the reduced joy related to **Love.**

imperiling my inner harmony, and giving myself a 'bad **conscience**'. Great joys can also set off attacks of **angina** for, in such moments, the energy center of **Love** (the **heart♥**) opens wider and can activate a memory of great sorrows still present, and thereby set off an attack of **angina**. Maybe I do many things out of a sense of obligation, and not with joy and pleasure. So the joy stops circulating. It is as if I focused all my attention on others (their happiness and their ailments) instead of on my own well-being first of all. My ego is so present and **active** that it is separated from the totality of my being, which leads to an **emotional blockage**. It is an unconscious increase in self-esteem by focusing my attention almost exclusively on others. It is the Judeo-Christian principle of gift through sacrifice: "**Give unto others!" I become vulnerable, and the fear of opening myself up to those I Love manifests itself**. Nothing reaches me any longer, but the pains begin. Spasms, stitches of **heart♥** pain, cold extremities (hands and feet). My body is seriously warning me that something is amiss (this warning is generally more recognizable on the psychic metaphysical level than on the physical level). I may unconsciously want to leave my 'earthly life' because I have the impression I am being smothered by worries and I don't know how to get out of it, but that time has not necessarily come! I feel crushed and oppressed and I no longer feel like making any efforts. What do I fear, basically? It is interesting to **realize** that since **angina** manifests itself by a constriction of the blood vessels, I must ask myself if I am restricting or limiting the **Love** that others are giving me. Is it easy for me to accept↓♥ the help that is offered to me? Do I ***deserve*** everything that is offered to me? Or do I tend to want to control what is given to me, not knowing how I would react to an 'overdose' of **Love** and affection? I will tend to play the 'hot potato' game with my **heart♥**, because I immediately give back what I have received, not knowing how to accept↓♥ in my **heart♥** the gifts received. I may have the impression that far too much is being asked of me, that I'd have to fix all the difficulties of each and every person. This leads me to have an attitude of ***contempt***. All these situations however could well originate from my attitude toward myself: I may be a competitive type of person and I focus all my energy on myself, which is very demanding and pushes aside all my affective difficulties. My **heart♥** then suffers from not being on speaking terms with my emotions. I become **conscious** of the fact that life is an ongoing exchange. I give as much as I receive, like the contraction and dilation of the blood vessels, otherwise I will experience an imbalance, and my attention must return to this equilibrium that is necessary to a healthy life. This is a fundamental process in human existence, for I am a divine being and must express myself in this equilibrium.

The result of my becoming **conscious** is this: I accept↓♥ to stop taking life seriously and I remain open! This is easy, because I don't feel like dying but I **feel like living**, opening myself to **Love** and ceasing all power struggles. I focus my attention on the beautiful sides of life. I learn to **Love** myself as I am: my vital energy can thereby come back to life. Such are the first steps on the way to a serious recovery from this disease. I express what I am experiencing and I learn to accept↓♥ myself as I am. I take care of myself because my happiness can depend only on myself. I move from shame and ***hate*** to **Love**. A last point to note: watch all the expressions related to the **heart♥**: a '**heart♥ of stone**', a 'hard **heart♥**, he 'has no **heart♥**', he is '**heart♥less**', etc. Every such expression is an indication that something is afoot that requires my attention.

ANGIOMA (in general) *See also: BLOOD — BLOOD CIRCULATION, SKIN — PORT-WINE MARK, SYSTEM [LYMPHATIC]*

An **angioma** is not a tumor, but a malformation affecting the vascular system (lymphatic and blood vessels).

Because these vessels are ducts that serve to carry blood and lymph fluids throughout the organism, I have the impression that my life is not going in the direction I would like it to. I don't know what direction to take, I feel lost, I feel that I have lost control. Insecurity overcomes me and makes me imagine the worst; I don't know who I am and I scatter my energy. I am afraid of coming into contact with my emotions, which blocks the circulation of energy. I accept↓♥ to allow the movement of life circulate in me.

I accept↓♥ to welcome, and make peace with, all these long-rejected emotions. I learn to let the movement of life circulate in me and to respect it, as I choose to respect myself. I totally accept↓♥ what I am, **consciously** choosing to experience happiness in everyday life and knowing that I am protected. I fulfill myself in my best state through my vehicle of **Light** and **Love**.

ANGIOMA (simple skin) *See: SKIN — PORT-WINE MARK / STRAWBERRY MARK*

ANGOR *See: ANGINA PECTORIS*

ANGUISH *See also: ANXIETY, CLAUSTROPHOBIA*

Anguish is characterized by a state of psychic distress where I feel that I am **limited** and **restricted in my space** and especially **stifled** in my desires. I feel my space limited by borders that, in fact, **do not exist**.

"I am stuck". Or "I feel trapped". I can't express my anger. I consent to the fact that people invade my psychic space, and I manifest this by a sort of inner constriction. So I leave aside my own personal needs in order to please others first, to attract the **Love** I need (even if there are other ways of doing things). I experience a deep dissatisfaction. The **constriction** generally leads me to amplify my emotions and my general emotionality to the detriment of an adequate balance. Because I am living in a fog, my self-confidence is shaken, and despair and even the desire to stop struggling will then take hold. I feel an imminent danger, but I can't identify it. I am afraid of the future and of the efforts required to reach my goals. I am faced with a choice that seems impossible to make. The insecurity I feel is related to the fact that instead of believing in my own personal power, I place it in someone outside of me, whom I consider higher and more fulfilled than me. I want that person to protect me, as if I was too weak to take care of myself. I am searching for some meaning in my life. I feel at the mercy of a mortal danger, because I am searching outside of myself for someone or something I can lean on. I am filled with sadness and I feel stuck, tied up, ***compressed***, chained even. I no longer trust my capacities. What must have been the childhood situation where I felt constricted in this way, so that I am still faithfully reproducing this *pattern*[19] to this day? (Notice that **anguish** and claustrophobia are made synonymous by the word **constriction.**) It is natural for my body to fill my basic **psychic** needs: the need for air to live and breathe some space between me and other people, the freedom to decide and discern what is good for me. If, from now on, I respond **first of all** to what I expect from life, chances are good that I will let the expectations of others as they are: that way, I am more certain of being in agreement with them! And all that without violating their space[20], for I must remember that if I feel choked up, it may well be because I am smothering the people around me, consciously or not. **Anguish** also appears as a worried and oppressive expectation, an apprehension of 'something' that might happen, in a terrifying, diffuse tension, often nameless. It can be related to a **distressful** concrete threat (such as death, a personal catastrophe, a sanction). It is more often a fear unrelated to anything immediately perceptible or expressible. This is why the deeper sources of **anguish** are to be found in the child I once was, and are often related to a fear of abandonment, of losing the **Love** of a Loved one, and to suffering. When I find myself in such a situation, **anguish** resurfaces. Every time one of these fears arises, or whenever an imaginary or an actual situation is experienced, my unconscious perceives it as an alarm signal: wherever any danger is present, **anguish** reappears even more strongly. When I am a child, **anguish** often manifests itself by a fear of the dark and a tendency to live a solitary life.

From now on, I accept↓♥ to use discernment, to show courage and trust in life in order to respect myself and to let others be in their space, with no regrets. I banish any remorse from my life. I will thus see more clearly and get on with my life much more lucidly. I give myself the right to be in command of my life and my choices. I trust myself and I know that life gives me everything I need, insofar as I expect the best and accept↓♥ that I deserve it.

ANKLES *See also: JOINTS*

The **ankles** are a very flexible and mobile part of the body. They serve to support the body and, by their physical location, they sustain great pressures.

They are a sort of bridge, a link between me and the ground. It is through them that I am 'grounded'[21] in a solid base, that spiritual energy travels downward and upward, and vice versa, if I remain in contact with Mother Earth. They are also the place where I enact my capacity to advance, to stand

---

19. **Pattern**: A scheme of thought that causes events to repeat themselves in my life.

20. **Space**: This means to let others pursue their freedom of thought and action and respect them.

21. **Grounded**: In the sense of feeling familiarly connected to the earth and to the material, concrete, actual, practical world.

up and remain standing, stable and anchored. My **ankles** execute changes of direction and thereby represent my decisions and my undertakings that are made on the basis of my beliefs and my values. My **ankles** show me how I am able to rely on myself and my inner resources or, on the contrary, if I tend to rely, or even depend, on others. Any **injury** or **pain** in the **ankles** is related to my capacity for remaining flexible while changing directions. I don't know 'on what foot to hop'[22]! Should I stay, or leave? I am destabilized, having the impression that I can't measure up to certain persons I admire, like my parents for example. I have difficulty in detaching myself from them, especially my mother. If I fear what is coming, if I am inflexible about a decision to make, if I go too fast without thinking, if I am afraid of my current or future responsibilities, if I have the impression that I am unstable, then I risk slowing down the energy in my **ankles**. I may feel guilty of having taken a certain direction or feel I was forced into it. Like the caterpillar, I am afraid of coming out of my cocoon. Depending on the intensity of the energy blockage and my closing of the current of life, there may result a **sprain**, a **twist** or a **fracture**. I can't remain standing without my **ankles**. I may have to 'lean on' new ways of seeing things, and rely on new criteria that are more open and flexible. They take care of me and my inner being, they support me in life. If an **ankle** gives out or breaks, I no longer have a solid base, I need to change directions, I am experiencing a mental conflict. My **ankle** can no longer support me, and it is my whole body that is physically giving out. In a sense, my life is collapsing too, but this is more the image that something is amiss than my actual collapse as a person. Regarding the **sprain**, the twisted **ankle**, it is the energy that 'twists' in the **ankle** , and my support structure is deformed. Nothing is clear and defined any longer. The pressure is too strong and I don't know 'which saint I should trust'[23]. I am restricted in my movements, because someone is either preventing me or not giving me permission, or some other impossibility. I tend to rely on the judgment of others rather than on my own. I lack firmness. I need to solidify myself, to truly involve myself physically and emotionally in my relations with others. When I am faced with something very deep, a change that is **imperative** for my well-being, it is a **break** or a **fracture** that appears. I think that others are preventing me from advancing, but in fact it is I who needs to change directions. What is involved is my honor, my security, my goal and my direction in life. Any condition affecting the **ankles** is usually accompanied by **swelling**, which manifests the overflow of emotions that makes me stagnate instead of advancing with confidence and determination. **Edema** indicates that the fact of worrying and always dwelling on the same negative ideas makes me stay in place. If I have **weak ankles** that are easily injured, I must ask myself: "Do I have a poor capacity for supporting myself, and do I always need someone or an institution to take me in charge?" I 'restrain' my emotions so much that I risk '**straining**' an **ankle**. Whatever the ailment, the

---

22. **I don't know on what foot to hop**: I don't know what is expected of me regarding a person or a situation.

23. **I don't know which Saint I can trust**: I don't know whom I can trust or in which direction I should move.

period of immobility that ensues allows my body and my inner being to adequately integrate the aspect of my life that I must change, and also allows the coming marvelous transformation to take place in me!

I become **conscious** of the situation or the relation in which I feel ***chained***. I must also ask myself, considering that this ailment in my **ankle** is preventing me from performing certain tasks or a job, what benefits I am thereby deriving from this immobility. I accept↓♥ life and everything it places along my way. This will help me embrace life from its proper side! I am on the road that suits me best.

ANKYLOSIS (state of) *See also: JOINTS (IN GENERAL), PARALYSIS (IN GENERAL)*

Ankylosis is a state of numbness identified by the disappearance of movement, usually **temporary**, in one or several joints.

Ankylosis is partial, but can be total if I decide to become completely inactive; it is the first step toward a motor incapacity, a degree of paralysis of my thoughts. I must become **conscious** of the responsibility I am taking if I decide to stay there doing nothing, not wanting to feel or to move. What am I afraid of? Is it the unknown, what is in store for me, something new for me, that disturbs me? Is it something I don't want to do at all? Whom or what do I not dare trust? I can look at the body part involved in order to find additional information on the source of my **ankylosis**. For example, if it is in the arm, am I in a state where I refuse new life experiences? Do I feel mutilated? Do I feel like killing someone? If it is a shoulder, am I finding life heavy, or do I find that some person or some situation is 'quite a burden'? Is solitude or the necessity of facing the unknown congesting my thoughts? If it is a foot, what is the direction I don't want to take and to which I am becoming 'numb'? If it is my whole body, I am becoming numb in reaction to something or someone: it is a form of fLight. I am **Aware** of the fact that I am **accumulating** energy in this part of my body and that unconsciously, I am **anguished**. I want to stay put on my positions, and it is difficult to make me change opinions. I accept↓♥ that it is time for me to go ahead! From now on, I am **Aware** of my faults (or rather, of my responsibilities) and my life experiences, and I acknowledge them.

I lay down my weapons and I accept↓♥ to resume the movement temporarily interrupted, and I mobilize my thoughts once again by remaining open. I manifest a more creative spirit.

ANOREXIA (mental) *See also: APPETITE [LOSS OF], BULIMIA, WEIGHT [EXCESS]*

Anorexia, which is a more or less systematic refusal to feed myself because of my rejection of my own body image, is called **mental anorexia** (in popular language, only the term '**anorexia**' is used).

Anorexia is characterized by a complete **rejection** of life. It is a total disgust for everything alive that is in me and that can enter my **ugly** body to feed it. This feeling can even transform itself into hate. There exist several symbols of life: water, food, the maternal aspect (the mother), **Love**, the female side. It is the ardent and unconscious desire to escape from life, to detest and **reject** myself because I am experiencing an extreme fear of opening myself to the marvelous life around me. I am experiencing **discouragement** to such a degree that I wonder what could ever help me. I have an unconscious desire to 'disappear' in order to bother the people around me as little as possible. I therefore permanently reject myself. This can go as far as self-hate that leads me to punish and destroy myself. I live in shame and I would want so much to be Loved unconditionally as I am, and not for what I can accomplish. I deny my own needs and would want to go unnoticed. This leads me to live in secrets and lies. By living a 'hard life', I have the impression of redeeming myself. It is even easier if such was the treatment I received when I was young: a past of domination, punishment and reproaches leads me to act out the same behavior against myself. **Anorexia** and obesity originate from a deep feeling of unfulfilled **Love** and affection, even if the two disorders follow entirely opposite physical paths. Several food disorders are based upon the **mother-child relation** in which there existed, or still exists, a conflict. As a child, I want to flee far away from my mother, who is often anxious and wants to feed her children at all costs. I experience a duality between my attachment to my family and my desire for self-fulfillment, which forces me to separate from it. Furthermore, it is quite often an **annoyance over my territory**, which I have the impression of not having, of losing, of it not being respected by others. This territory may consist of my physical possessions (clothes, toys, car, house, etc.) as well as my non-physical possessions (my rights, my learning, my needs, etc.) or the persons around me (my father, my mother, my friends, my husband, etc.). I am experiencing a current annoyance with respect to someone or something **I can't avoid** and can't stand. I may wonder if I have the impression that someone is trying to kill me. Feeling this fear, I stop eating and I unconsciously want to provoke this death. I have the impression that my survival depends upon my capacity to cut myself off from others. By being as thin as possible, I will no longer be visible; I will disappear from sight and hide to be safe. I may simply reject the maternal image of my mother, especially if she is overweight. I want to avoid **at all costs** seeing my body develop and seeing myself start to resemble her more: I thereby want to kill my own image! Although **anorexia** is most often found during adolescence, it can also be found **in babies and in young children**. If I put myself in the baby's place, I realize that the refusal to eat can result from a troubled contact between my mother and me: I may have been deprived of the maternal breast and the warm physical ambience that should accompany suckling, or I experienced an artificial mode of feeding, dosed and applied too rigidly, the over- or under-feeding being imposed to follow an ideal weight curve, overlooking the changing individual feeding rhythms of this real baby. I may react to that by a progressive refusal to feed myself, by vomiting, weight loss, sleep disorders, food tantrums, etc. My mother is also full of remorse, which is related to death to some degree. It is important for me, as the mother, to respect the child's tastes and its own pace, and that I stop trying to be the perfect and over-protective mother. If I am a somewhat older child and I present **anorexia**, it is usually more mitigated and is characterized by a 'small appetite', being a spare eater who detests the chore of eating meals, having food whims with an obstinate refusal of certain foods, rarely finishing my portions, vomiting frequently and endlessly masticating the same mouthful. At this age, the table and its social imperatives play an important role, because meals are a family reunion under parental authority, where reactions or conflicts can occur. **Anorexia** is basically my need to fill an inner void of **affective nourishment**. **I need the unconditional Love and acceptance↓♥ of my inner mother**. **Anorexia**, contrary to obesity, is an attempt to make my inner void die of hunger and make it so small that it will disappear and will no longer demand anything at all. This is one of the reasons why I continue to see myself as fat (a mental fixation on size) although I am in fact thin and lean. In other words, I continue to see my affective and emotional needs as very great, and I feel overwhelmed by them. There is a life-and-death power struggle inside me. I need the attention of others to feel alive, so I adopt the behaviors and attitudes of a victim, where I force myself to change my physical appearance. I want others to 'fill me up', to satisfy my needs. However, as I myself do not give any of this **Love** that I need so much, and I refuse my emotions, my sensitivity and my child-like side, other people are just as hard on me. **Anorexia** can also be related to a feeling of being scolded by life and by **my mother**, the maternal symbol that nevertheless pushes me toward my desire for independence and individuality. That is why I reject the food **and my mother at the same time**, because I always had the impression throughout my childhood of feeling only her powerful maternal control. I therefore experience the feeling of being out of my own control over events, and I try, through exaggerated means, to regain this control. I may also have experienced this lack of control in a certain situation or in relation to some person, and I have the impression that the only thing over which I can have perfect control and that will give me a perfect state of well-being (in appearance) is the food that I choose, or refuse, to give my body. "I don't like the way my mother **Loves** me, and I detest her for that." "I want to remain a young girl or a young boy because I want to get as close as possible to a form of physical and inner 'purity'." (It is during puberty that **anorexia** generally manifests itself.) It is an absolute quest for youth. The fact of becoming very thin generally leads me to no longer feel any pleasures. I thereby cut myself off from all physical sensations related to sensuality or sexuality. It is like dying, I want to kill myself. As a young girl or a young boy, I refuse the sexual stages related to my age, being unable to control them, so much so that any attempt at sexual intimacy, discovery and abandon with an eventual partner (absence of maturity) are almost futile. If I experience all that very deeply, it is frequently because it is related to a deep sexual trauma, abuse or affective insecurity in my past. I may even feel myself attacked by the changes taking place in my physical body. This experience made despair occupy my physical body, and I 'closed the door' to my physical, spiritual and emotional desires.

Gradually accepting↓♥ my femininity, or my intuitive and emotional side if I am a boy, is essentially the first thing to do to resolve my **anorexic** condition.

I choose how I prefer to do it, but do it I must! I accept↓♥ a certain sexual intimacy, feminine and even motherly (for I have to learn to **Love** my mother!). I learn to **Love** my body and to **Love** others! I go slowly, for it is a delicate situation where I must open myself to **Love** and to the beauty of the world. I ask for help, if necessary. And especially, I remain open to what life has in reserve for me! Acceptance↓♥ and unconditional **Love** will be greatly appreciated. I do activities (sports or other) if possible. Here is an interesting aside. As an **anorexic** person, I may have the impression, inside, of being 'ringed in', as if I were caught inside a series of *hula hoops* isolating me from the rest of the world while intensifying my feeling of limitation in life. I remain open to notice any other such signs. I can envision myself getting free of these hoops and saying "Thank you!" for having helped me to become **conscious**, while knowing that now, they won't be necessary any more. I also visualize this image: on each inspiration, more **Light** enters in me to fill up my feeling of inner emptiness. I choose life, while ignoring what others may think of me. I give myself **Love**, the gentleness I need, instead of expecting it from others: hence the true satisfaction and the inner joy!

ANTHRAX *See: SKIN — ANTHRAX*

ANURIA *See: KIDNEYS — ANURIA*

ANUS

The **anus** is the orifice of the rectum, the place through which I release what I no longer need.

This is the place where I resolve my conflicts, my inner resentments. The problems here involve the fact of 'holding back' or 'letting go'; that is why, if I am a young child and I am constipated or soil my diaper, it is often to get revenge against my parents whom I consider authoritarian, manipulative or abusive. I really have the impression that someone is giving me s__! It is the place through which the main toxins of the human body are discharged. It is a hidden part of my body that usually corresponds to my unconscious part and sometimes serves to camouflage very hard feelings of violence, anger and bitterness. This can be the case if I experienced a situation where I was sexually abused, especially if there was forced penetration. I had to bare myself, whether in the physical sense (being undressed) or in the figurative sense (having to divulge a secret or express my true emotions, which carries a certain risk). There is something that makes me indignant and that I want to expel from myself at all costs, because I just can't digest what happened. Forgiveness seems impossible to give, and an alliance that can be different from my ***marriage*** is destroyed forever. I find myself with an identity conflict that burns me. The **anus** is located at the level of the pelvis, near the coccyx and the first *chakra* or energy center, the seat between the self and the world around me. It is linked to the energy base of the body. Some inner fears, stress and emotions are evacuated through this orifice. I can verify the following situations: "What am I trying to ignore to the point of holding it in? How far can I let myself go? Am I capable of relaxing and letting life guide me? Am I ready to experience new sensations toward life? From what, or from whom, do I close myself off? I may tend to hold back negative emotions to the point of imprisoning myself. I may cling to something or someone, which brings me much inner pain. I show ***obligingness*** when I would rather please myself. My difficulties involving the **anus** are often connected to my distorted relation to money.

I accept↓♥ to trust myself, while letting go of what I don't need any more and replacing it new ideas, positive attitudes and new projects!

ANUS — ANAL ABSCESS *See also: ABSCESS or EMPYEMA*

An **abscess** is an accumulation of pus, **frustrations** and **irritability** related to a **situation that I do not want to let go** (**anus**). Often, even if I try to hold it back, it escapes me in spite of myself.

This **abscess** will come out or manifest itself in any case. It is possible that I may be angry with myself because I don't want to 'evacuate', or give in to, certain mental fixations that are harming my current life. I may even be filled with vengeful thoughts concerning a situation in the past or someone whom I refuse to forgive. I felt myself belittled, ridiculed, shattered even. In my everyday life, I show this lack of 'letting-go' by the fact that there are some objects that I don't want to discard although they have no great value or usefulness.

This ailment tells me that I must accept↓♥ to trust in life and in what is beautiful around me. I rely on someone or something and, especially, I forgive the people around me. I let go, and I put my trust in life.

ANUS — ANAL FISSURA

Anal fissura are small **fissures** causing bleeding in the **anus**, which signifies some **loss of joy** in living that is related to a situation I must change.

If I am experiencing sadness that can '**splinter my rear**', I find out what is causing this sadness, and I accept↓♥ the changes in my life. I may feel weak, so I want to protect myself from the world outside. My vulnerability leads me to stagnate, to confine myself within well-established positions. I prefer to remain in certain unpleasant situations rather than take the risk of advancing toward the unknown. I feel torn in a situation: should I hold on, or let go? I hold on to what I have acquired. I want to be self-sufficient, to not need the help of others.

I now accept↓♥ to say to people who ask too much of me: "That's enough!" **I stop waiting for the others to move before changing myself.** I eliminate my frustration, my anger over a person or an event that annoys me or that I feel is making me fall between two chairs. I reclaim the place that was properly mine to take. I assert myself with my needs and I stop trying to please others instead.

ANUS — ANAL FISTULAE *See also: FISTULA*

An **anal fistula** originates from a situation where I am experiencing **anger** about what I want to keep but am unable to hold onto inside. It is as though I were trying to keep old scraps of waste from the past (old thought-forms, emotions, desires) but can't do it. I may even have feelings of vengeance against someone or something. I also hold back resentful emotions from the past. The manifestation is the **fistula**, a sort of channel communicating abnormally between an internal organ and the outer skin. I am unable to make up my mind to choose between the physical and the spiritual, between my desires and detachment (in the broader sense). I have the impression of not moving. I retreat into my inner world, in my dark thoughts, feeling incapable of communicating what I feel. I may experience a situation where I feel not quite ***married*** and not quite divorced, and this situation tears me apart. I would need to ***consult*** someone, but I prefer to ruminate in my corner. I have the impression of ***patching up*** this relationship, but everything isn't completely fixed. Should I cut this ***ring*** that ties me to the other person? I have the impression that some things are slipping away between my fingers.

I remain open in my **heart♥** and I willingly accept↓♥ to completely empty out these 'trash cans' of dark thoughts and unhealthy and vengeful ideas **right here and now**. I learn to freely communicate what I am experiencing in the moment, and my life then becomes far more joyful and balanced.

ANUS — ANAL ITCHING *See also: SKIN — ITCHING*

Itching is related to remorse and guilt over my recent past. Something is irritating me or tickling me, and I feel guilty about what I must keep in or let go. I am wearing a mask, hiding my true identity. My regrets and my anger may result from unsatisfying sexual relations, devoid of **Love**. I ask myself questions about certain events in the past, which I want to evacuate as hard as I can.

It is in my interest to accept↓♥ to listen to my body and achieve satisfaction in everything, because guilt only holds up my development, with no true benefits.

ANUS — ANAL PAINS *See also: PAIN*

Anal pains, called **proctitis,** are related to **guilt**. I hurt myself because I believe I am not effective enough to achieve my desires. It is a form of self-punishment, an irritation, the wish to condemn myself in a way that shows an inner injury, my sensitivity torn up following an event in the past that I have still not accepted↓♥. It may be guilt experienced about sexuality (mine or someone else's). I am experiencing deep distress that can cause blood loss and even hemorrhage, in some cases. I have punished myself for a very long time, and I retreat into myself.

I can accept↓♥ to become more responsible for my desires, to stop demeaning myself for what I am, and to stop preventing myself from living and uselessly punishing myself. I could stop being bothered by having my 'rear end on fire', and make a new start by better accepting↓♥ my past, present and future experiences, and thus drive ahead more in life. I stop destroying myself, and I accept↓♥ to see all the beauty that I manifest. I live for myself instead of always acting according to the desires and expectations of others.

ANXIETY *See also: ANGUISH, BLOOD — HYPOGLYCEMIA, NERVOUSNESS, TANTRUM*

Anxiety is a **fear of the unknown** that can be compared to a state of anguish. It manifests itself by certain symptoms: headaches, flushing, cramps, nervous palpitations, intense sweating, tensions, an increased rate of speech, crying and even insomnia.

If I am **anxious**, I may experience the 'shiver of anguish': this shiver comes from the cold, and reminds me that I am afraid. It is a sickness that grips my throat, makes me lose my self-control and my control over the events in my life, preventing me from using my **good sense** and my discernment. I may also feel either unbalanced or disconnected from the physical world over which I may have some control, and from my perceptions of the immaterial world, for which I don't always have any rational explanations or understanding. I no longer have control: the 'sky may fall on my head' at any moment! I constantly have a feeling of imminent danger, but which is undefined. I may be **anxious** in any situation: **I BECOME WHATEVER I FOCUS MY ATTENTION ON.** If my attention is constantly focused on my fear of this or that, I will surely experience **anxiety**, which can be more or less directly related to whatever resembles the fear of **death** or could remind me of it. Death, the things I don't know or cannot see, but which can exist, make this fear rise up in me. I have no trust in life.

Then, even if I fear the unknown and **unconsciously deny life and its process**, I now accept↓♥ to focus my attention on this: I am confident and certain that what is happening to me is all for the best, now and in the future. The symptoms will disappear, along with the fear of dying.

APATHY *See also: BLOOD / ANEMIA / HYPOGLYCEMIA / MONONUCLEOSIS*

Apathy is a form of insensitivity or nonchalance. I give up before life, I become indifferent and I have no motivation to change anything at all.

I live in constant ***dejection***; I have no interest in living. **Apathy** can appear following events that call into question my reason for being in this world. I am in revolt against so much injustice. I want to distance myself in order to avoid any further suffering. I live in the anguish that 'it might well happen again'. I may want to **leave** a situation by escaping it for lack of motivation or joy, or for fear of being disappointed. I resist, and I refuse to see and feel what is going on inside and around me, which drives me to a certain degree of insensitivity in order to protect myself. **Apathy** can also be related to deep shame and guilt. I thereby try to become insensitive to my inner being. I am like a robot, finding no meaning in my life. I live according to the norms of others. This way, I can remain disconnected from my deeper self.

I accept↓♥ to open myself up to life and to new pleasant experiences, which I maintain in order to find a new goal in my life. I take the necessary attitude. I allow my **heart♥** to guide me spontaneously. This is how I rediscover a taste for life, by letting all my senses enjoy every moment.

APHASIA *See also: ALEXIA [CONGENITAL], WORDS [SPOKEN]*

Aphasia is a language disorder of expression and/or comprehension, oral or written (**alexia**), due to a localized cerebral lesion. More generally, **aphasia** is a memory loss of the customary signs with which humans exchange ideas with each other. The language centers are located in the brain's left hemisphere, the rational side that is specialized in the functions of reading, speaking, counting, analyzing, reflecting, and defining relations. It corresponds to my Yang side (initiator, action).

I ask myself questions about my way of conveying my messages. Is my unconscious afraid of not being understood? Do I doubt my capacity for expressing myself? I am anguished at the prospect of expressing myself; I don't dare, for fear of 'making waves' around me. I therefore remain at a superficial level: I cannot communicate in depth, which allows me to avoid discovering things that might displease me. I feel in prison, and at the same time, it frees me from having to explain and justify everything. I fear being judged by my peers, and distrust makes me want to control everything.

I accept↓♥ the events of my life, in my **heart♥**, without having to rationalize everything. I take the time to consciously choose the right words to express what I need to say, banishing my fears, doubts and insecurities. I dare to be myself, I express my sorrows and disappointments, knowing that this is the most effective way to free myself of my secrets and my suffering; I thereby find inner peace again, and the desire to explore the world from which I had disassociated myself.

APHONIA

Our **voice** is the expression of ourselves, of our creativity. Too intense an emotion (distress, worry) can lead me to no longer know what to say or what direction to take, or how to interpret this direction in terms of the emotion experienced. It may be that this strong emotion was experienced on the sexual level and is resonating more directly in my throat or in my vocal cords because, in some way, my second center of energy (sexual) is related more directly to the throat, my fifth center of energy. In any case, my sensitivity (hyperemotivity) has sustained a shock, and I am no longer able to say anything! I am left gasping! If I dissipate my energy too much, for instance after an emotional shock, an inner 'vacuum' will be created by my dismay, and the sounds will be 'sucked' into this vacuum. It is as though I were swallowing my words into the back of my throat. It is therefore important for me to resume contact with the

breath of my inner communication. It is even possible that this experience may be protecting me because I am in a state where I must no longer speak, where I can no longer tell secrets. Am I using my voice and my vocal cords in a healthy manner? Should I remain silent for some time? It is sometimes said that words are silver but silence is golden. Or has someone reduced me to silence by force? I may generally feel powerless to express myself because I have the impression that I am "not worth much". I have the impression that it is better to shut up than to 'say something stupid'. I would like so much for people to listen to what I have to say, to recognize me for who I am, to respect me. Sometimes I feel so special, but this is of short duration and doubt settles in, my guilt reappears and I curl up in myself. Instead of living for myself, I live according to others, and as I don't always know what to say in order to receive the approval of others, I prefer to remain silent: either I decide to no longer speak, or my **vocal cords** decide of their own accord to no longer produce any sounds.

I accept↓♥ to express my emotions, my creativity and my ideas in the way I feel best, in keeping with my capacities.

APHTA *See: MOUTH — APHTA*

APNEA (sleep) *See: RESPIRATION DISORDERS*

APOPLEXY *See: BRAIN — APOPLEXY*

APPENDICITIS *See also: APPENDIX III, PERITONITIS*

Appendicitis is defined as an inflammation of the **appendix of the cæcum** (from the Latin for 'Blind') located at the base of the large intestine.

This illness originates from **anger related to tension or an acute situation** that I cannot resolve, that makes me 'boil' inside and feel indignant. It is most often an affective situation that unbalances my sensitivity and my emotions. My fear may have brought about this event because I was ruminating dark thoughts and worrying, which made it manifest itself. I feel an inner struggle between life and death. I am experiencing deep anguish and am facing a choice that is difficult for me to make because of the responsibilities that will follow from it. I prefer to retreat into my work or in things that must be done. I feel that I am in a *cul-de-sac* (which is the form of the **appendix**), because I have the feeling I am being oppressed, which triggers **fear**, **insecurity**, **lassitude and abandonment** in me. Most often, this annoyance is related to one or several members of the family or related to principles and ideas linked to the family. This may be a situation that concerns money, and especially pocket money. Maybe I should ***pocket*** an amount of money that I lost at the last minute. It may also involve something or someone I would like to 'add' or 'incorporate' into my life, but some circumstance is preventing this. For example, I may want my spouse to come and live with me, but he, or she, does not want to, or I don't have enough space to lodge him or her. There is an 'obstruction' to the flow of life, and I am repressing a multitude of emotions. I am crossing a new turning point in my life and I am afraid of the changes this will bring because I am experiencing a ***dependence*** on certain persons. This can even go as far as a fear of living. I no longer can effectively filter the new realities to protect myself from them. I see no other way out for my life. I have the impression that I can't get rid of, can't empty myself of something. I stock up on things until my **appendix** can't stand it any longer. I need to talk about what I am experiencing, I need to 'empty my bag', because I am having difficulty in digesting what is going on, I find it very disappointing. I feel I am in a dead end, and there is a situation that I find very rotten and hard to digest. I am afraid of life, and I hold back my spontaneity. I have the impression that I could be attacked at any moment and 'have my pockets emptied', materially as well as in **Love**. I can hardly eliminate the negative aspects of my life. The usual symptoms are heat and redness, related to inflammation, and pain, related to tension. I feel very **intense pain** when the **appendicitis** transforms itself into **peritonitis** (the bursting of the **appendix**).

I accept↓♥ to stop, to stand back and start living according to my needs instead of in accordance with the expectations of others. I let life take its course and I accept↓♥ the situations of my existence as what is best for me. I remain open in my **heart♥** and I lower my protective barriers gently and harmoniously. I take the time to relax and I fully taste life.

APPETITE (excess) *See also: BLOOD — HYPOGLYCEMIA, BULIMIA*

Food represents life, and is also related to **pleasure**, to a certain **joy in living**. Food thus fills my physical and emotional needs, and an excess can mean that I want to compensate to have more life in me, because I need **to fill an inner void**. It is a deep inner dissatisfaction with **Love** and a **hunger for Love** (like the 'thirst for **Love**'), a need to diminish a tension or simply to stay busy in order to not feel the need to think about myself. I judge my own emotions severely. I avoid looking within myself, and I find in food this feeling of freedom and satisfaction in fulfilling all my desires, whatever the quantity absorbed. It may be the case when I am in a state of hypoglycemia that is related to a lack of joy in my life or to an excessive desire for sugar (related to **Love**), which shows an obvious need for tenderness and affection. In children, it is easy to recognize their deficient[24] affective needs: they easily manifest a taste for anything sweet. Whether I am an adult or a child, it is always my inner child's **heart♥** that is wounded, and I must give more **Love** to my children, or receive some in order to fill my needs.

I accept↓♥ to become **conscious** of the fact that eating is directly related to the act of rewarding or consoling myself. Now, I remain open to this beautiful energy of **Love** to find a balance, a true communication, a recognition of myself, an exchange between what I am and what I need. Appetite finds its balance at the same time as when I am better fulfilled emotionally.

---

24. **Deficient**: Lacking in something that is needed.

APPETITE (loss of) *See also: ANOREXIA [MENTAL]*

As food is related to life, a **loss of appetite** can be attributed to **guilt** (I don't deserve to live, I am afraid and protecting myself) or to a loss of joy or motivation over a person or a situation. It often occurs following the departure of a Loved one (a death, a break-up, a move, etc.). I feel lost. As the wound is very severe, I keep it alive by destroying myself. I may also invest too much attention in a particular situation of my life, to the point of forgetting to eat. I refuse to go ahead, to have new impressions and exciting experiences that make me even more joyful. My emotions 'cut my **appetite**'. I thus push back my desires, my aspirations, my passions, my curiosity, my tastes. Often, my **sexual appetite** is also 'slowing down'. I refuse to absorb, to digest, to **partake of anything new** that comes up in my life because it doesn't suit me. I believe that others are crushing me or preventing me from living. In fact, I am the one who prefers to meld into the mass or to be absorbed (often by my partner or one of my parents). People 'have the shirt off my back"[25]. I punish or sacrifice myself, believing I don't deserve any better and wishing to be approved by others.

I accept↓♥ to remain open in my **heart♥** to adventure and life; I increase my own self-esteem and I am able to accept↓♥ 'new impressions' (new tastes) and go one step further. My appetite balance will return. ***As appetite is whetted by eating, LIFE comes on with LIFE!*** I accept↓♥ to take my place and to acknowledge this passion and these desires that ask only to express themselves outwardly, including through my creativity.

APPREHENSION

Apprehension is related to **doubt**, to fear about a situation or a person that makes me feel 'in danger'. Inwardly, I feel bewildered over what is happening to me. My mind is beginning to make up fearful scenarios from all sorts of ideas and I risk being off-centered.

From now on, I am focusing my attention on my inner being, and in my **heart♥**. I accept↓♥ the experiences that life brings me, while protecting myself.

ARMS (in general)

The **arm** is the part of the upper limb included between the shoulder and the elbow and is structured around the **humerus**.

The **arms** represent my ability to embrace life, to give and receive, my **capacity for greeting new life experiences** and for taking action. I use them to touch and to squeeze, to express my creativity, my potential for action and my **Love**. I can enter into contact with people, approach them and greet them in my world. I also show them that I **Love** them with joy and harmony. Because

25. **To have the shirt taken off one's back**: To let oneself be exploited by others without reacting.

of them, I move into action, I do my job or I fulfill my obligations. My **arms** therefore communicate and express my attitudes and my inner sentiments. The **arms** are very close to the **heart♥** and are linked to it. Thus, people feel that **Love** and energy emanate from my **heart♥** when I am open. Each hand contains a center of energy located in the palm, which represents one of the 21 minor energy centers (or chakras). The two energy centers of the hands are directly related to the **heart♥**. Thus, my **arms** enable me to extend my **heart♥** and to physically and energetically give out **Love**. The **arms** enable me to defend myself and protect myself against external attacks. That is why, if I instinctively cross my **arms**, I protect myself, I close myself off from certain emotions that don't suit me.

By opening my **heart♥** and my **arms**, I accept↓♥ to open myself to life, and I am able to give and to receive positively.

ARM AILMENTS

Arm ailments are related to a difficulty in acting and in manifesting **Love** in what I do, in my work or my everyday actions. It is an energy freeze, a **self-restraint** that prevents me from doing something for myself or for someone else. An **ailment** may originate from a situation I am experiencing that is reawakening a suffering related to prohibitions or to the fact of having been judged in the past, mainly by my parents. I may wish to imprison someone or something with my **arms,** or 'squeeze her, him or it with all my strength' in order to gain some control. Or on the contrary, I may have had to let go some persons I **Love**, and now I can no longer bring them back together or protect them (as the mother bird who protects her brood under her wings). I may be experiencing a conflict with a person whom I consider to be 'my right **arm**'. I am experiencing a situation where I received a 'slap in the face'. I may then feel **muscular rigidity**, **pain** or heat (**inflammation**). My **arms** become less mobile and more tense, my joints (shoulders, elbows), more painful. I know that the role of my **arms** is their capacity to take on the new situations and new experiences in my life. I may be in reaction against a new situation; I no longer find my work motivating; I am discouraged, frustrated or irritated because I can't express myself properly or because I have difficulty in implementing a project. A situation that I call a 'failure' may express itself outwardly through a **pain** or a **fracture** in the **arms**. I feel like 'dropping everything' because I feel powerless. It is generally the **bones in my arms** that are affected when I am no longer capable of doing as well as I used to, in a professional or sports activity in which I previously excelled. I no longer can take the people I **Love** in my **arms**; I refuse to admit that I have had more than enough of a situation that is harmful to me (**my arms are full**). Things are 'moving and shaking' in my life[26]! I must '**break the routine**' and if I refuse to see what I must change in my life, I may have to go as far as to **fracture** or **break an arm** in order to understand. Having **sore arms** generally means that I am taking on too much. It may also be something that I can't **take** or that I

---

26. I am feeling hurried by certain events in my life.

refuse to take. I may even go as far as to push back a physically or emotionally disturbing person or situation. I thereby create a space that will help me feel more secure and under control. I may no longer feel like communicating with others from the **heart♥**, I doubt all my capacities for getting things done. Going ahead in life seems difficult to me. Therefore, instead of holding out my **arms** as a baby does to show its need to be caressed and touched, in relation to the people it **Loves**, especially its mother and father, I reject the world that surrounds me. I close myself off by crossing my **arms** to better protect myself. I am experiencing a dilemma between accepting↓♥ that others come to me or refusing to be approached: I therefore want to push away. It may be someone I perceive as negative, who doesn't fit with me or my values; it may also be something positive (like abundance) that I refuse because I have the impression I don't deserve it. **Pains** are therefore an unconscious way of showing that I am suffering. I may have to 'let go' of a situation or a person I want to 'hold on to' at all costs. A difficulty with authority can manifest itself in the **right arm**, whereas my **left arm** will be affected if I experience a conflict in expressing my **Love** and my kindness. Men have a natural tendency to want to over-develop their **arm muscles**, which are a symbol of strength and power, and thereby denote their difficulty in, and resistance to, expressing the energy of the **heart♥** and their gentle sides. On the contrary, thinner and weaker **arms** indicate to me timidity in the expression of my emotions and a resistance to letting energy flow. I hold back from plunging into life and getting the most out of it. My **arms** correspond more to my inner expression. My **forearms** are more related to outward expression, to 'doing'. It is the beginning of the achievement of a desire. I 'roll up my sleeves' and I move into action! The softness present on the inner sides of my **forearms** manifests my sensitivity, and I may hesitate before expressing things physically in the Universe or before choosing how I will implement my projects. I may have to change my habits or my way of doing things, and that is so difficult for me, because of my rigidity, that my **forearms** will stiffen too. Do I get involved; do I set things in motion in my life? How far do I open up to myself and to others? Do I have the impression that I have difficulty in 'hugging' or 'embracing' certain situations or persons around me? How afraid am I of getting close to people? A situation bothers me so much that I am on the point of exploding! If I hold back from asserting myself for fear of the consequences, I risk **fracturing my forearm**. The **thickest part of the arm** is located across from the region of the **heart♥**. When it is in excess, there is an overflow of the **heart♥** that is kept secretly inside, for fear of expressing my **Love**. When it is bony and thin, am I able to accept↓♥ **Love** from others, or do I tend to isolate myself? In both cases, there is something that needs improving in my way of giving or receiving **Love**. Do I grasp too much so that nothing or nobody can escape me? I do more than is necessary to get people to like me. Do I want too much to protect others, or do I feel myself in danger? A **skin irritation** on the **arm** is related to a frustration or an irritation in what I am doing or not doing, in the way I express myself or in what can happen to me following the intervention of others. A **bruised**

arm indicates to me how hard I treat myself, or confirms my impression that people treat me hard and are pitiless.

I accept↓♥ to show more **Love** in what I do, to invest myself, to open myself trustfully to others, to hug the people I **Love** in my **arms** with **Love** and affection (the image of the father hugging his son as a sign of **Love**). I remember that the act of hugging someone is often therapeutic. I appreciate my best qualities of communication, tenderness and openness. I focus my attention on activities that are interesting. I get used to seeing the good sides of any situation. I do it while realizing that it is marvelous, that I am better than I thought. I change my ideas because I need to do so. I 'roll up my sleeves' and forge ahead, letting go of anything that is no longer beneficial for me and letting come to me everything that is most beautiful. I accept↓♥ life 'with open **arms**'!

ARMPITS *See also: ODOR [BODY]*

The **armpit is** a hollow space located under the shoulder, between the lateral face of the thorax and the internal face of the **arm**, containing many blood vessels and nerves. The **armpit** permits sweating.

It is related to my oldest and deepest forces and expresses how I enter into contact with them. Either I refuse my basic, so-called 'primitive' emotions (sexual, for example) or, on the contrary, they take up all the space. I have difficulty in advancing because I put aside what my inner voice tells me. Because my parents want me ***to seek shelter*** under their wings, I feel limited in my capacity to differentiate myself from them, to be 'me'! When the **sweat** is **abundant in my armpits**, my emotions are overflowing and I experience nervousness and anguish. There is a situation in my life that I can't stand and that I keep as a secret, 'under my wing'. If there are **swollen ganglions in my armpits** (**axillary adenopathy**), I am hiding my emotions and my impulses in the deepest recesses of my being. As I am not always able to contain them, this results in compulsive behavior and **ganglions** that swell. I am so afraid of asserting my true personality that I prefer to conform to others. However, I become dependent on them, and I am cut off from my deeper nature.

I accept↓♥ to 'come out of my shell' instead of staying hidden. I let go of whatever is no longer good for me. I allow my natural inner forces to express themselves, thereby giving myself all the self-confidence and the dynamism that I need to achieve my deepest desires.

ARRHYTHMIA (heart♥) *See: HEART♥ — CARDIAC ARRHYTHMIA*

ARTERIES *See: BLOOD — ARTERIES*

ARTERIOSCLEROSIS OR ATHEROSCLEROSIS *See also: BLOOD / ARTERIES / BLOOD CIRCULATION*

Arteriosclerosis, also called **atherosclerosis**, is a degenerative disease that originates from the formation of lipidic deposits (a sort of fat related to cholesterol) on the walls of the cerebral, coronary, renal or lower limb arteries. **Arteriosclerosis** is also a degenerative disease that originates from the destruction of the muscular and elastic fibers that form the arteries. Both diseases manifest themselves by a hardening of the arteries and the arterioles, which involve mainly an exhaustion and a loss of elasticity in their walls, a weaker capacity for dilation and blood circulation, an increase in fatty deposits, and therefore less **Love** expressed from the **heart♥**.

This progressive state manifests itself if I am **hardened**, if I am or become **inflexible** or **tense** in my communications and thoughts. It is the manifestation of a **very strong resistance** and a physical and inner **narrowness of mind**. The expression and reception of **Love** and joy become limited and restricted. There is therefore an imbalance between giving or sharing with others and receiving. I have fixed and pitiless ideas, I am often intransigent, rigid and without compassion; I also tend to see only the dark or negative side of life. I may unconsciously repress my emotions and say no to **Love** because I fear expressing myself. Maybe I am living too much according to the principles and morality that I was taught when I was young instead of living according to my own values. I remain imprisoned in this yoke because I feel safe. However, I stagnate instead of developing and growing. As my outlook on things is limited and even diminished by my fears,the same goes for my **arteries**. I am simply sclerotic[27], crystallized like my **arteries**. I feel confined at home. Instead of relying on my intuition to know what is good for me, I rely on outside points of reference. Maybe I have the impression of having made a mistake and I have judged myself severely. Where and when have I had a traumatic experience that makes me detest a part of myself to the point of repudiating it, and where I felt myself rejected? This disease is therefore probably related to an injury of **Love** or to a lack of acknowledgement of this **Love** in my life. What is the use of seeing what is good for me? Why express my feelings? Why involve myself or engage in a relationship if I risk being hurt? My body is indicating to me that I must change my behavior toward life. I am becoming **conscious** of the fact that what is accumulating in my **arteries** is the guilt, the bitterness, the shame and the regrets that I experience every day.

By accepting↓♥ to have a more open, tolerant and gentle attitude toward myself and what I am experiencing, the whole process of unifying my inner self and the outer world appears more clearly. I show joy, serenity and flexibility to those around me, and I abandon myself to the true expression of **Love**. The people around me will sense this change. I accept↓♥ to receive help. I must also develop more creativity on the physical level of matter. Life takes care of me. I express myself freely in order to avoid any further accumulations in my **arteries** and I push back my limits so that I can fully engage in my interpersonal relations.

ARTHRITIS (in general) *See also: INFLAMMATION, JOINTS (IN GENERAL)*

27. **Sclerotic**: Congealed, that does not evolve.

Arthritis is defined as the inflammation of a joint. It can affect each of the parts of the human locomotor system. Its most extensive form is **rheumatoid arthritis**, currently named **classic rheumatoid arthritis.**

It is characterized by inflammation, muscular stiffness and pain, which **correspond**, on the metaphysical level, to **closing**, **criticism**, **sorrow**, **sadness** or **anger**. Symbolically speaking, grace and freedom of movement are the main qualities related to a joint. When it becomes inflexible or hardens, **arthritis** is associated with a certain form of **rigidity** in my thoughts (crystallized thoughts), my attitudes or my behavior, so that all the deep emotions that I should normally be able to express are conveyed instead by the physical manifestation of this disease. Thus, **arthritis** occurs if I am too **inflexible**, **too demanding**, **obstinate**, **intolerant**, **very moralistic**, **critical**, **restricted or too proud** toward myself, others or the situations of my existence. A feeling of powerlessness usually accompanies the suffering that holds me back. I feel restricted by the system in which I live, and I criticize the authority that violates my freedom. Life is an eternal fight, a struggle of every instant. I experience the feeling of being **badly Loved**, of not being **Loved** and appreciated **at my real value**, which gives me much **disappointment** and **bitterness** toward life, and bad moods. I then show an exaggerated rational attitude. I often criticize anything at all because I am afraid of life and often feel a form of **chronic insecurity**. I feel **exploited**; I carry out actions more in order to please others than out of my true will and interest, so I end up saying 'yes' out of duty, whereas my true answer would be 'no'. I call myself a victim, but this suits me, because I can thereby attract attention. I feel powerless and I hold others responsible for my 'calvary'[28]. I may resent the whole world, and especially those I **Love**, but it is actually myself that I resent. I am afraid of the gentleness, the tenderness and the **Love** that inhabit me. I may have experienced a childhood trauma, and I now repress my emotions, without admitting what happened (obliteration) because "I suffered a lot in that experience and I permit myself (unconsciously) to blame and complain, so that others may understand how much I suffered." This manifestation is related to the **self-sacrifice** complex. **Arthritis** can also come from the way I treat myself or how **I treat** others with respect to criticism. **Arthritis** also causes a sort of **retrograde** action; I have the impression of being recalled to the rear, as if I was being told to do something else in a different direction, instead of going forward. Because my fear, my low self-esteem and my rigidity all conspire to raise deep emotions about the why, the how or the direction of my movements in life, I may have the feeling that I am constrained, restricted, immobilized or boxed in. I will then find it difficult to bend (my attitude), to be mentally flexible or capable of giving in. My **arthritic joints** indicate what I am experiencing, and they convey more information still. In the **hands** (fingers), the question is: "Am I actually doing what I desire and what I want to do? Do I have a good 'handle' on my own affairs? Are there any people with whom I don't want to shake hands?" I feel guilty, perceiving my life as a failure because

28. **Calvary**: A long and painful ordeal.

I have the impression of not being able to manage it. My freedom and my spontaneity in 'handling' what goes on in my world are limited by my rigidity and my hardness. I insist on things being done in a certain way, and I **refuse** any help from others. I find myself in an extremely rigid structure because I fear the unknown. In the **elbows**: "Am I inflexible to any changes of direction to be made in my life? Do I allow others to be free and to express their full potential?" In the **knees**: "Before whom or what do I have the impression that I have to kneel, and before whom or which I don't want to bow down?" In the **hips**, I am angry because the others don't see my needs. I would like them to respond to my expectations without having to ask them. As I use my pelvis in my movements, when there is a frustration or a feeling of powerlessness, I don't dare move, I cut myself off from the flow of life.

From now on, I accept↓♥ to test my true intentions about **Love**. I must change my way of thinking and adopt a new attitude toward the situations in my life. By remaining open to **Love** that is omnipresent (everywhere) and by expressing it more honestly, freely and spontaneously, my heart♥ will be radiant, and I will respect others as much as myself. Friendship, understanding and forgiveness are now available for me. I accept↓♥ that the only person over whom I have any power is me. I see myself as the creator of my life. The others are only a reflection of how I treat myself. By taking good care of me, the others will do as much.

ARTHRITIS — ARTHROSIS *See also: BONES (IN GENERAL), JOINTS (IN GENERAL)*

Arthrosis is a non-inflammatory and degenerative impairment of the cartilages with a secondary bone reaction. It is localized or usually generalized to the whole body. However, the joints most often concerned are those that are subjected to intense mechanical constraints, such as those of the spine (cervical vertebrae [of the neck], the lumbar vertebrae [lower back]), the hips, the hands, the knees, the ankles. The pain it causes is of mechanical origin and not inflammatory, and it usually appears after a sustained effort and disappears at rest (this disease is also called '**Wear-and-tear arthritis**').

When I suffer from **arthrosis**, it is as if I intensified my attitudes, my patterns[29] and my rigid thoughts. This disease is related to a **mental hardening**, to an absence of 'warmth' in my thoughts (cold and dampness accelerate the onset of **arthrosis**), often toward authority. I easily experience injustice and ***I accuse*** others for any and all reasons. My stiffness prevents me from bending, from giving in, just as in my life, where I no longer feel like bending before others. It is the exaggerated motivation to perform an action without seeking rest or balance (I go to the end of my limits without stopping to ask whether I am asking too much of myself), an **impression of being subjected to** a person or a situation that has now become intolerable, or a strong repressed reaction against some form of **authority**. I feel ***chained***, with the impression of being subjected to ***forced labor***, of being forced to do certain things of which I am

29. **Patterns:** Outlines, structures.

ashamed because 'I am worth more than that'. I am a perfectionist and I criticize myself all the time. I am bitter toward others who, I think, do not like me. I want to drop my weapons and resign, because I can't go any further. My sorrow is great because I am holding on to an event or a person from my past. I have difficulty in looking at reality straight on, and I flee my deeper emotions. I forget myself and I deny myself pleasure because I have convinced myself that I must take care of others before doing anything for myself. I am very intransigent and rigid toward myself. I have difficulty in accepting↓♥ the changes and the new opportunities that are offered to me, and which may raise questions about my old beliefs. My permanent stubbornness provokes constant tension.

My body is talking to me, and I really should listen to it now! I can integrate this disease by beginning to **consciously** accept↓♥ that I am experiencing anger and that my thoughts are rigid. The energy that flows through me is fluid, harmonious, **in movement**. By remaining open in my **heart♥** to this energy and admitting that I have something that I must change, I can reverse the process and improve my health! I am becoming more flexible and I accept↓♥ others as they are, without wishing to change them. Flexibility will then reappear in my physical body. I am deciding right now that I have the right to be happy. I am taking care of myself, and others are benefiting from it. I am living fully in the '**here and now**' and I am expecting the best for myself.

ARTHRITIS (gouty) *See: GOUT*

ARTHRITIS (in fingers) *See: FINGERS [ARTHRITIC]*

ARTHRITIS — RHEUMATOID ARTHRITIS

Rheumatoid arthritis or **classic rheumatoid arthritis** is an inflammation that simultaneously affects several joints at once. The immune system is so sick that it begins to self-destruct, attacking the conjunctive tissues of the joints (collagen), so that the risk of a generalized infirmity, with pain and swollen joints, becomes possible.

This is a straight-out attack on my own self; such is the inability of the powerful emotions of **rancor** and **pain to express themselves**. **Rheumatoid arthritis** is related to a **deep self-contempt**, a **long-repressed hate** or **rage**, a **self-criticism** so intense that it affects the most fundamental energy of my existence. I have gone through experiences where I felt very **ashamed** or **guilty**. It is the manifestation of a far more important **criticism of authority** or of whatever represents authority for me: an individual, a government, etc. **I refuse to bow down before this authority**, whatever the consequences! I have taken a dislike to anyone who has bothered me or hurt me. My mobility becomes limited, and I can no longer express myself freely (especially in the case of certain directions to be taken) because my joints are too painful. My body becomes rigid, like my attitudes. I can't express my strong emotions, and I have the impression of being constantly oppressed and subjugated. I then adopt behaviors of self-effacement, of self-sacrifice, and I ruminate over my emotions. I serve as a scapegoat by sacrificing myself to some cause. I have the impression that 'they're always on my back'. This disease may reveal to me a difficulty I have in performing certain gestures that I used to be able to carry out with much dexterity. Now, I have the impression of being more awkward or clumsy. I therefore depreciate myself with respect to this activity in which I used to excel, and I have the impression of losing dexterity, strength or precision. This disease is found for example in the seamstress who, after a number of years, has the impression of being slower and less skillful. Sports figures are often beset by **polyarthritis**, mainly because of the feeling of depreciation they experience because they are not at 100% of their capacities, or because their performances have diminished. These symptoms highLight how I can over-discipline myself because I am extremely demanding of myself. I allow myself no place for any mistakes. I refuse the sweets of life. My rigidity, my frustration and my inner anger make me ball my fists. They are very often channeled by the sports I practice. Once I have become less active or have retired from this sports career, the same frustrations will have to manifest themselves in some other way, and that is when **rheumatoid arthritis** may appear. It may also appear if I am compulsive, very **obstinate**, moralizing, or if I am experiencing some discomfort with respect to power. The latter manifests itself by my tendency to want to control everything, but I am not **Aware** of it. I tend to sacrifice myself for others, which often results from repressed aggressiveness; but just how far do I act with **Love**, while respecting myself? My inner and physical rigidity become aggravated because of this deep obstinacy in not wanting to change, and because of this guilt that is eating me up inside.

I am learning to accept↓♥ myself with all my strengths and weaknesses. Even if I have the impression of being less proficient or less effective, I look at all the experience I have acquired over the years. I acknowledge that it is a precious asset that makes me an exceptional person. The openness of my **heart♥** is essential, if I want to free up all the emotions that are poisoning my existence. From now on, I am reasserting my full power over my life, starting with **loving** and accepting↓♥ myself as I am. I am taking the place that is properly mine! I accept↓♥ to adopt new ways of being. I am reassessing my priorities in life and setting new goals that are more realistic, more in harmony with what I like and that give me pleasure and joy in life.

ARTHROSIS *See: ARTHRITIS — ARTHROSIS*

ASPHYXIA *See: RESPIRATION — ASPHYXIA*

ASTHENIA / FATIGUE (effort syndrome) *See also: BURNOUT*

Asthenia is similar to 'burnout', a form of energy and nervous exhaustion. However, it is different from fatigue, which is a natural phenomenon, for it does not originate from work or exertion and does not necessarily disappear with rest.

I feel at the end of my rope and my 'vital' energy is affected by it. It is an **illness of the Soul** interiorized over a long period of my life. The manifestation sets in at different levels (physical and inner), and several fundamental states or feelings re-surface: fear, deep sadness, amplified emotionality, remorse from past experiences, and even bitterness. I refuse the life that I am leading. I am experiencing discouragement and I don't feel like starting anything. Even if **asthenia**, whether it is somatic, psychological or reactive, can originate from several causes, I verify what is causing me to manifest this condition.

I accept↓♥ to be able to change this, provided that I find the deep cause that led me to 'lose' my previous determination to be and to do things, and instead made me develop a passive attitude of escape in the face of effort.

ASTHMA (also known as the 'silent cry') *See also: ALLERGIES, LUNG DISEASES, RESPIRATION DISORDERS*

Asthma is a respiratory illness characterized by breathing difficulties that can even lead to suffocation. When an **asthma attack** occurs, the reaction of the immune system to the allergy-causing substances (allergens) is so strong that it can block the body's respiratory system, lead to wheezing and even to death by suffocation. I need to take life into me (inhalation), but I can't give it back (exhalation), to the point that I start to panic (I easily **inhale,** but **exhale** with difficulty) so that my **respiration** – my ability to breathe – becomes very limited and insufficient because I let out a minimum amount of air.

I am experiencing enormous anguish, fearing for my own strength and wanting to run away. I hide myself behind a title, a diploma, an organization, any structure, in order to feel safe. This way, I feel choked by the power I give others, but still, it is better than to become autonomous and take my responsibilities. I can experience this situation as a **child** or as an **adult**. If I am a **baby** and I am **asthmatic**, I am experiencing an anguish that resembles that of my parents and it is ***horrible***. We resonate together in this, and I wonder if I have the strength to live. I wish someone would save me, would free me from this danger that is threatening me. I feel powerless and I live according to others. Is it because I am attached to certain people or things that I refuse to let go of? Am I choking myself with rage and aggressiveness, which I refuse to see to the point that it is 'seizing me by the throat'? Am I afraid of missing something, especially **Love**? Thus, **asthma** is basically related to the action of suffocating. I feel **held by the throat**, **walled in**, I **suffocate** and I **choke** over a relation with a Loved one or a situation. I refuse what is going on in my life and I always desire something else. With this attitude, I cut myself off from any feeling of freedom. I believe I must live in the obligation of things instead of free choice. I am constantly faced with an authority figure who prevents me from expressing myself and takes the wind out of my sails. I no longer feel free to speak and occupy my space. I can even experience disagreements that lead to quarrels and confrontations that poison my life and represent a threat for me. I am so scared that it makes me **gasp for air**. I have the impression that my whole life is in full ***effervescence***. I would so wish to magically find myself in my mother's womb, where I would be safe. However, this **Love** especially that of my parents, can be stifling: I may have the impression that my mother is too much of a brooding hen, which I fear, or a father who is too authoritarian and maybe also too motherly. I sometimes have the impression that for me to remain alive, I must absolutely not let it show that I am alive, but I must disappear. I would therefore like to take what is properly mine, but at the same time, that is dangerous. I use **asthma** to attract **Love**, attention or a form of **emotional dependency**. As **asthma** is similar to asphyxiation and allergies, I may feel I am being limited and **letting my vital space be invaded by others**, being easily intimidated by other people's power, used to the detriment of my own, wanting to please and doing things that don't suit me, and going as far as suffocating to signify my inner revolt against some situation. It is an excellent way to feel strong and to get what I want through manipulating others. As a person, if I don't want to see my limitations, my self-confidence will suddenly be replaced with worry and anxiety. I won't know how to deal with my emotions and I will feel great solitude. I feel crushed under the weight of my responsibilities, and I must shoulder them without anyone's help. It is interesting to mention that scientific studies have shown that the great majority of **asthma attacks in children** occur in September. This is quite normal because, as a child, I have just spent all the summer months playing outdoors in the fresh air, with my own friends. When school resumes, everything is ordered and timed. I may feel stifled by all this managed activity and the obligations of things to do (homework for example) or the things I can't do any more (such as going to bed later at night). To be at peace with life and be able to appreciate it, I must learn how to better recognize my strengths and weaknesses. Others will do anything to save me! I have the image of a person who is weak and who needs a lot of **Love**, without being ready to offer the gift of **Love** in return, like a child who cries to have his needs fulfilled, but does not have the maturity to share and be open enough to the divine gift. Life is a **mutual exchange, constantly balancing between giving and receiving**. All this of course is related to a **fear of the past**, a sort of stifling **Love** (generally maternal) that I have interpreted as such, a repressed sadness from early infancy. It is also a fear that goes back to the first breath I took at the time of my birth, where I felt suffocated or frightened (subconsciously) by **my mother,** or some other similar situation. Breathing thus symbolizes the independence of life, my individuality, the capacity to breathe on my own. I don't seem able to show a sense of independence, to live my own life, I feel rejected by the arrival of someone else; I have difficulty in getting hold of myself and freeing myself of my parental attachments (a repressive dependence, mainly toward my mother or my wife). **I can't imagine separating myself from this wonderfully gentle and reassuring image (my mother), getting married or seeing my parents' divorce without having a reaction!** When I manifest an **asthma attack**, I want to cry out my despair, my sorrow, my dismay. If I am in contact with a person, a situation or a thought that I absolutely cannot tolerate ("I am totally allergic to this"), and before whom, or which, I feel incapable of asserting myself, the **asthma attack** appears. When I see red or am ragingly mad, an **asthma attack** ensues.

I accept↓♥ to express what is stifling me and to occupy my space. I check to see if the ailment re-occurs periodically, and I change my mental programming accordingly. I now take my life in hand and give generously and quietly **without forcing** anything. I humbly recognize all I am capable of, no matter how small, and I especially accept↓♥ to open up with my heart♥ and work with the integration process that fits with what I really need. Everything will work out for the best, I *will* be satisfied, filled with **Love** and tenderness and enjoying normal, balanced breathing. I am learning to **Love** myself and to **Love** life. I am also learning to trust myself completely. On each inspiration, I feel more supported and reassured by life, and on each expiration, I learn to release control, to let go and go with the flow of life. I thus increasingly experience ***expansion*** and recover all the space that is rightfully mine. I learn to **Love** myself in my inner unity.

ASTHMA (infant)

Infant asthma is even more pronounced than **common asthma**. The **infant** is so afraid of life and living that already at this early stage, it refuses to be here. It is good that I speak to it in thought or in words with an open **heart♥** to tell it how much it is **Loved** and appreciated, and that I provide it with what it needs.

ASTIGMATISM *See: EYES — ASTIGMATISM*

ATAXIA[30] (Friedreich's)

Friedreich's[31] **ataxia** is a disease of the nervous system characterized by degeneration affecting the spinal cord and the cerebellum[32].

Its origin is generally a pattern of thought I have, as a mother. This mental pattern is so powerful that the engendered fetus (the child in gestation) picks it up and responds to it unconditionally (like a mother's **Love** for her child). I expect so much to have a child who will answer my dreams that it will end up feeling totally incapable of fulfilling me. If I am that child, I am afraid that I won't be able to perform all the ***tasks*** that my mother requires of me and that I won't be up to whatever I have programmed myself for. I am afraid I won't have the appropriate **physical vehicle** (a-'taxi'-a) at just the right time. I feel that my freedom is already affected, restricted. A blocking then manifests itself in my development. I want to isolate myself from the rest of the world. As a

---

30. **Ataxia**: Incoordination of movements.

31. **Friedreich** (Nikolaus) (1838–1927): A German neurologist who first described this disease in 1881. He was mainly interested in the hereditary forms of **ataxia**.

32. **Cerebellum**: Located at the base of the cranium; it is responsible for the coordination of the muscles necessary for balance and movement.

mother, I live in an imaginary kingdom where a certain social status must be maintained, and I don't like anyone disturbing the apparent calm that reigns there. However, regardless of the child's age, I must explain to her that I may have ideals for her, but that is because I **Love** the child and I want what is best for her.

Whatever my child's strengths or difficulties happen to be, I **Love** him as he is, so he doesn't have to become a 'superman'. I accept↓♥ to reconsider my priorities in life, what truly counts for me. If the child is still at the gestation stage, I can talk to it inside of me because, even at this early age, it understands the gist of what I am telling it. If the child is a little older, I take the time to speak to her: she will then feel all the **Love** I have for her and the healing process can then begin. Nothing can restore harmony between two persons like **Love** and forgiveness.

ATHEROSCLEROSIS *See: ARTERIOSCLEROSIS*

ATROPHY *See also: MUSCLES — MYOPATHY*

Atrophy is the diminishing in volume and weight of an organ, a limb or a tissue.

It shows me that there are a number of things that I am holding back from doing, expressing or manifesting, and which I don't dare carry out. Somewhere in one of the spheres of my life, there is a sensation of loss or diminishing that makes me vulnerable. I thus lose my reason for living, and I let myself waste away. As this is taking place at the emotional level, so too is my body accordingly doing the same. Why keep something I no longer need or no longer use? I sacrifice my dreams to the detriment of others. I may feel guilty of not having performed certain tasks well, and the limbs with which I carried them out can be affected. I also sometimes punish myself for not having attained my goals, which are often out of reach or unrealistic. It is important to go and see what part of my body is affected; this will give me more information. Take **muscular atrophy** (**amyotrophy**), for example: I become passive, not daring to move any longer because my gestures are 'always' judged to be bad, or they go unnoticed.

I accept↓♥ the fact that I long hid behind this defeatist attitude, but now, it only depends on me to pick myself up and move ahead. I stop belittling myself, I acknowledge my strengths and I put them to good use. I refuse all criticism and concentrate on my qualities and on what I have to do, knowing that I am constantly guided. From now on, I am rolling up my sleeves; I know I can get through this, whatever the situation. I have the capacity and the courage to face it with confidence and determination. I commit myself to respecting the **Soul** that I am, and I accept↓♥ to become the creator of my life.

AUTHORITARIANISM

A person who manifests **authoritarianism** is, consciously or not, strongly in reaction to some form of authority.

I firmly believe that it is the only way to make myself understood and make others understand 'how it works': *"That's how things work in this world!"* Unfortunately (especially for people wielding such power over many individuals), I show an excessively egocentric character. Anger is lurking in the background, mainly when I sense any resistance to what I ask for. I also 'turn a deaf ear' to what is said to me. As an **authoritarian** person, I may also **grind my teeth** or have **knee problems**. *"I am not about to bow down before anyone!"* Nothing stops me, no situations or circumstances, except possibly **those that directly and deeply affect my wounded heart♥**. As an individual, I greatly need **Love**, and the only thing that will allow **Light** in to brighten my sad life is to open my **heart♥**. The worst torture I can suffer as an **authoritarian** person is to kneel down before someone taller than me; it is usually here that physical ailments will manifest themselves. If the **heart♥** does not open up, life will see to it.

I accept↓♥ that my need for **Love** is great. The more I realize this, the more able I am to look for the means to fulfill this **Love** and heal my wounded **heart♥**.

AUTISM

Autism is the ultimate refusal to face the physical reality of the outside world, which brings about a form of retreat into my inner world, where imagination and fantasy prevail.

I am fleeing a situation or my entourage because I am too badly hurt or because I see my sensitivity being ridiculed. My sorrow, my sadness, my rancor, my fears or my despair are so great that I 'cut' myself off from the physical while still continuing to have this same physical body. I seek refuge in a mutism that represents for me my only escape, because the outer world seems hostile and threatening to me. I may wish to eliminate one or several persons from my life, so I ignore them and act as if they don't exist. The fact that I, as an **autistic** person, have 'shut myself away' voluntarily in my airtight 'bubble' means that every day, I receive thousands of items of information that are 'stored' and 'stocked' in my inner world, instead of being exchanged with other persons. I find myself in a black hole, on a road that seems to lead nowhere. I have the impression that the standards I must meet are so high that that it is easier for me to retreat into mute silence rather than constantly have to surpass myself and have to account for myself before others (parents, teachers, authorities, supervisor, etc.). I must be 'super-performing' when I speak. This makes me have to go and check things out dozens of times before I can say a word, because if I make a mistake, it would be catastrophic. I therefore force myself to shut up and keep my information to myself if what I am required to say is not perfect. It is as if my speech is trapped within myself, for I would like to say certain things, but the pressure on me is so great that I prefer to remain silent. As soon as I was born, I felt excluded, different, marginalized. My fear of being hurt or of not being up to the expectations of others leads me to retreat within myself. My ineffectiveness in achieving my dreams and ambitions forces me to live in an inner world to which nobody has access. I build a fortress around myself. In a sense, I am living in exile. This isolation that I experience highLights my own need for perfection in my own eyes, and reminds me all the more that I am 'less than nothing': I am a total failure because I don't even dare to try. Quite often, I may happen to be a hypersensitive child and, even in my mother's womb, I could already sense all my parents' anguish and uncertainty. They could see that the world in which I would soon be living was a hostile one. I decided to live in my head because the others are dangerous for me. My present inner states at that time were surely similar to those of my parents (as is always the case because we are in resonance). It is important for the parents to become **Aware** of their inner states that resemble mine (their incapacity to communicate in certain areas of their lives), so that each and every one becomes able to come out of their psychological prison. The members of my entourage must be able to communicate with me from inside themselves (from each person's inner world), to help me in connecting once more or better with the outer, physical world. Thus, by projecting me in my inner world, they will be more able to make contact with me and better recognize my needs and my fears, so that I am then able to show the confidence and the openness necessary for me to regain contact with the outer, physical world.

I accept↓♥ to build my inner security and self-confidence in order to be able to resume contact with the world around me. Even if there may be a certain risk, I decide to take the step, to go toward the others. Life is made up of challenges. I look at all the dreams, all the projects that are feasible for me, by accepting↓♥ to be reborn to myself and to life. I know I will always have the necessary support and the help I need. I stop criticizing myself. I know I am different, unique, that I have some precious talents and that I have all the freedom necessary to develop them, at my own pace and quite safely.

AUTOLYSIS *See: SUICIDE*

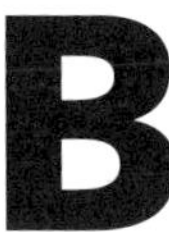

BACK (in general)

The **back** represents **the support of life**. It is the place that protects me from a person or a situation (I '**turn my back**'), if the need arises. If my burden is too heavy, if I lack support or don't feel enough support (affective, financial, etc.), my **back** will react accordingly and certain pains (stiffness) can appear. If I am fed up, my **back** can't take it any longer and the ailments appear. I sense that my survival is in danger and I have the impression that I am going to be 'dropped', either by the people around me or just by life giving me the slip. I can't **stand** what is happening to me any longer. I may even have the impression that I am being '**backed** against the wall'[1] in some situation, or of always 'having someone on my **back**'. I become **conscious** of the fact that I lean on something or someone outside of myself. As I don't trust them entirely, I find it difficult to move ahead. I experience frustration, feeling trapped and limited in the things I am able to get moving. I am no longer able to weigh things properly in order to make sensible decisions. My back may figuratively present a wide target, and so I am capable of taking blows, or else I humbly bow, out of respect or acceptance↓♥. For whatever reason, **a sore back** therefore indicates that I may want to escape from something by putting it behind me, because it is with my **back** that I bury the experiences that made me confused or hurt. I push back everything I don't want to see or let others see, thus acting like the proverbial ostrich. It therefore also hides away my past, anything unconscious or unknown. I can even bury my dreams and my desires that I no longer believe I can achieve. I am **deeply hurt**, still incapable of expressing my blocked emotions. I refuse to see what doesn't suit me! I may have received a '**stab in the back**' and I am experiencing this situation as a betrayal. If the pain is caused by a **slipped vertebra**[2], what is the situation that revolts me, or to what ideal do I aggressively aspire? I resist with all my strength because I am afraid of responsibilities. A supple but strong **back** indicates a certain mental flexibility and great openness of mind, contrary to **dorsal stiffness** that signifies pride, power and the refusal to give in. When I am comfortably seated, I may have the impression of being protected and quite safe. However, even if I use my **back** to bury undesirable things out of sight, and even if I want to 'play the ostrich', I accept↓♥ to see what is bothering me, and to express it. By acting in this way, I free myself from the burden I was carrying. If my **back pains** are **muscular** instead, they indicate a rigid attitude toward the situations I encounter in my life. I need to be supported, because otherwise I think I will have to let everything drop. The **postures** I adopt give some indications about

1. **Backed against the wall**: To have no way out, to be unable to escape.
2. Please refer to each specific vertebra under: **Back disorders.**

what I am experiencing and about how I deal with the situations in my life: if I am in reaction against authority and I want to stand my ground in front of someone or something, I will '**stiffen my back**' out of pride. If, on the contrary, I am feeling submissive, frightened or weak, I will **bend my back**; and the greater my concerns, the more my **back** will make me suffer.

I now accept↓♥ to release the energies held **back** in the places that hurt! I can better integrate the difficulties of living, through writing, dialogue or exchange. I choose the means that suit me best and I let life flow in me, so I can learn how to express myself more and assert myself when I need to do so. I accept↓♥ that life will sustain me in each instant, and I 'square my shoulders', knowing that I have the required strength to carry out all my projects. I accept↓♥ to rely on my inner resources. My intuition guides me in the actions to be done to reach my goals.

BACK DISORDERS — UPPER BACK (the 7 cervical vertebræ)

The **upper back** corresponds to the region of the **heart♥** and the cardiac energy center. It is here that I have the strength, or not, to bear my emotions[3].

Back ailments concern the first stages of conception, the basic needs and the most fundamental structure of being. The **seven cervical vertebræ** are mainly concerned in this region. The **cervical vertebræ** are related to communication (mainly through speech) and to my degree of openness to life. My naïveté can make me vulnerable in this regard. If I have the impression that people want to judge me, criticize me or hurt me, I may be affected on this level, and I will tend to 'clam up' like an oyster. The **cervical vertebræ** are linked to my capacity for communication, affirmation, voicing opinions, submission, and justice. The **cervical vertebræ C1, C2 and C3** will be more intensely affected if I depreciate myself about my intellectual capacities, whereas the **lower cervical vertebræ** will react to any injustice I may have the impression of experiencing in my own life or in the lives of others I see around me, and this revolts me. Each **vertebra** also gives me additional information about the source of my ailment:

C1 = The **first cervical vertebra**, called the **ATLAS** and bearing the number **C1**, serves as a support for the head. It is a pillar that keeps the head in balance.

If I worry too much (I "rack my brains") over a situation or a person, if I constantly fret and doubt, my head will get heavy enough to give me headaches, and **C1** will have difficulty in bearing the load. If I show narrowness of mind, if I refuse to look at all the facets of a situation, if I am rigid in my way of thinking, **C1** will react by stopping its activities, being no longer capable of pivoting. It will be paralyzed by my fear, my despair with life, my negativism, my difficulty in expressing my emotions. A **C1** in bad condition is generally accompanied by ailments affecting the

3. "I carry the world on my shoulders", mine and those of others.

head, the brain and the nervous system, such as migraines, amnesia, vertigo, nervous depressions, etc. Because it is the head that is affected by different ailments, it is my individuality that is being challenged. "What do the others think of me?", "How do I measure up?", "What point have I reached in my life?" I try to distance myself from my emotions. I play a game with myself so as not to have to look at myself straight on. I prefer to adopt rigid behavior to stay in my comfort zone, but sooner or later, I will have to turn my head to see what is going on around me and inside of me. I have a great need to communicate, but I often have the impression that I am not being listened to. I tend to have obsessional behavior and thoughts.

I accept↓♥ to listen to my inner voice, to keep an open mind and bring more calm in my life in order to diminish my cerebral activity, thus allowing me to see reality in a new **Light** and more confidently. I take charge of my life and I accept↓♥ to see myself in each of the facets of my personality. I reclaim my power and I achieve great things… for myself!

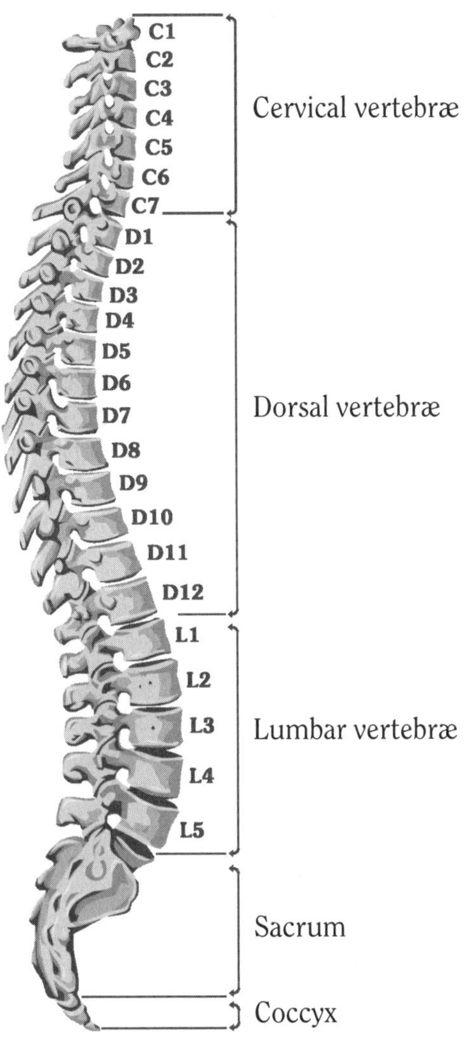

C2 = The **second cervical vertebra** works in close collaboration with **C1**. It is called **AXIS**. It is the pivot that enables **C1** to move. **C2** is related to the main sense organs, namely the eyes, the nose, the ears and the mouth (tongue). That is why they are affected when **C2** has an ailment.

This usually happens when I am going through a stage in my life and questioning myself about my personal development and the role that spirituality plays in my life. Opportunities present themselves to me to help me gain a new vision and understanding of life and of certain events I am experiencing. Am I truly ready to have the answers to my questions? If I am rigid in my way of perceiving life, if I refuse to let go of my old ideas to make place for something new, if I am always worrying about the next day, there is a high risk that **C2** will become just as rigid. I must be ready to go and plunge deep down into myself and contact the essence of my being. I still have some cycles to work through; I still have one or several bereavements to complete. My tears will often be dry when I repress my emotions and my sorrows, and disappointments and regrets remain buried inside of me. As the 'lubricant' (my tears of sorrow or joy) is no longer present, **C1** will no longer be able to join itself so easily to **C2**. There will be irritation and heating, just as in my everyday life. This happens especially in cases of depression or excessive emotionality (if there is a family conflict for example), of anger, bitterness, resentment or revolt, all of which is caused by the fear of moving forward, changing and taking my responsibilities; the fear of the judgments of others and myself, by a lack of self-esteem, which can even bring on a desire for self-destruction (suicide). What would happen if I allowed my deepest feelings to come out? I prefer to turn a deaf ear rather than truly know the actual cause of my different ailments.

I accept↓♥ to make contact with my emotions and stand by them, to take my place by expressing what I am going through, so that the flow of energy starts to circulate in my body again and so that **C2** can start working in harmony again with **C1** and everything runs smoothly! I accept↓♥ to reconnect with my creative force and let myself be guided by my inner voice.

C3 = The **third cervical vertebra C3** is an eternal loner. Because of its position, it can't count on anyone else nor work in co-operation with other **vertebræ**.

If my **C3** is not in good condition, I too may have the impression that I must muddle through all by myself. I may also withdraw into myself, live in my 'bubble' and avoid any form of contact or communication (oral as well as sexual) with my entourage. "Why waste my time? In any case, people never listen to me and never understand my ideas or my feelings!" I am separated from what I **Love**. Then come revolt, discouragement and distress, as my sensitivity is deeply affected. Anguish may take hold of me. The wear and tear of time does its work, and my dreams and dearest desires vanish little by little. I become irritable and bitter when I face a person or a situation I can't 'digest'. I am tired of having to prove my worth and sacrifice myself for others. If I fail, they will only confirm what I thought of myself – I am good for nothing. My life, in a sense, is a great masquerade. I tend to try to rely on someone else. I become anxious if I am afraid of not succeeding in a project, and therefore of not being recognized. I note that an ailment at **C3** can lead to ailments in my face (in the skin and bones as well as the nerves) and my ears and what is related to my mouth (teeth, gums, tonsils).

I accept↓♥ that solitude can be just as beneficial to renew myself, take stock and see more clearly in my life, as it can become a means to flee my emotions and the realities I find very difficult to understand. The choice is mine!

C4, C5, C6 = The **fourth, fifth** and **sixth cervical vertebræ C4, C5, C6**, are located at the level of the **thyroid** and are in close relation to it. The thyroid plays a major role in language, the voice (vocal cords), and any disharmony involving communication – when I am the one expressing myself as well as when other persons communicate with me – will lead **C4, C5** and **C6** to react. It may be because I took offense to what I heard, leading to indignation and anger. **C4, C5** and **C6** will react even more strongly if I furthermore do not express my opinions, my frustrations and my sorrows. My level of aggressiveness risks rising ever higher, which will close down the channels of communication with these three **cervical vertebræ. I swallow the wrong way** whatever comes up to me. I tend to ruminate over certain events for a long period of time. There can also appear ailments and pains affecting my verbal communication system as a whole: mouth, tongue, vocal cords, pharynx, ***tonsils,*** etc., and all the parts of my body located between the level of my mouth and my shoulders may be affected. If **C4** is especially affected, I look at what feelings I am always ruminating over, especially anger and guilt. I seek balance and justice. I have difficulty in finding solutions, often because I hesitate to express my differences of opinion. I cling to my memories, to my past. I flee my deep emotions instead of externalizing them. I avoid seeing what is going on inside of me, thereby avoiding discovering myself and flourishing. I destroy and punish myself; I sabotage my happiness that I do not believe I deserve. It is **C5** that reacts if I resist my entourage and reject their advice. I am afraid of being hurt with words or actions. I feel inferior to others, and so I will erect a wall around me. As I feel that nobody listens to me or understands me, I withdraw into myself. Compromises are not possible, for I avoid taking a position. I feel shame and in many situations, I prefer to remain silent rather than take responsibility for what I want to express. It is **C6** that will experience difficulties if I want to shape others according to my needs and desires. I expect too much of others instead of taking charge of myself. I am desperate, for I feel that only others can 'save' me, whereas I am the only one who has some power over my life. My old dreams are inaccessible, and I find this unfair. It reminds me of all the times I experienced this injustice when I was young. I feel like dropping everything, I am depressed because I am afraid that "the sky will fall on my head[4]". I carry the burdens of others so much that the fact of sacrificing myself this way is killing me little by little.

I accept↓♥ that each experience is an opportunity to grow and that there is a lesson to be drawn from everything. I must let things flow instead of persisting and resenting life. Otherwise, my head starts to 'boil' and I feel overloaded with all the tasks to be done and that I have the impression I will never manage to get done. I need to express myself, whether through speech, writing, music, painting, or any other form of expression that will enable me to 'reconnect' with my creativity and my inner beauty. All my senses will then be stimulated and activated, which will activate my thyroid and enable **C4, C5** and **C6** to function normally. The ailments felt in this region can then be resorbed.

C7 = The **last cervical vertebra C7** is greatly influenced by my whole moral side, my beliefs, my spiritual side and justice. If I live in harmony with the laws of nature, if I listen to the messages that my body and life in general send me, **C7** will function at its best. On the contrary, if I experience anger and am closed to the opinions and the ways of seeing things of the persons around me, if I rise up and oppose other ideologies than mine without keeping an open mind, **C7** will strongly react and may affect my hands, my elbows and my arms, which may become inflamed or have difficulty in moving. The functioning of my thyroid gland will be affected. Similarly, pangs of **conscience** over a word said, an act committed or a thought sent toward a person will also affect **C7**. If I experience intense emotions in my life, if I am disappointed or afraid of being rejected, or I find certain situations unfair, or if I hide under my shell to avoid being hurt 'again', **C7** may be affected. It is then easy for me to ***blame*** others for my misfortunes. How can I get out of this situation? My life is lacking in playfulness and spontaneity. My self-confidence is very weak, and I play the 'perfect quiet pupil' in order to avoid the wrath of the people around me. I allow others to decide for me. I feel too vulnerable and ashamed to communicate my needs. I prefer to isolate myself to hide from the looks of others. I carry a heavy baggage of unexpressed emotions. I cut myself off from my inner self. My intuitive and emotional sides are dissociated from my reason and are controlled by doubt. As I cannot trust my own power and my capacity for making decisions, I must rely on outside persons. Depression may appear, and I always feel stuck for time.

I accept↓♥ to learn to discern what is good for me and what is not. I must respect each person's point of view, even if it is different from mine. It is by opening my arms to others that I can learn the most, and become most able to make choices that will lead me to feel freer.

The **pains** in this region of the **back** come from **repressed** negative emotions that I drag like an unwanted ball and chain, which I refuse to see in me. I have high **expectations** of others, but have difficulty in expressing my

---

4. **That the sky will fall on my head**: That a catastrophe may happen to me.

true emotions, and so **anger**, a **fear of not being Loved** or a lack of affective **support** appear, and I feel I must think of everything and do everything. My level of frustration is high, and I sometimes feel more like turning my **back** to the world than facing it. I resist a lot by believing I can't support myself affectively, and I am convinced that if my entourage showed me more **Love** and support, everything would go far better. I may have such high expectations if I am a devoted mother or father, frustrated by the heavy burden resting on my shoulders. I then feel **responsible for the happiness of others**, which is becoming **heavy to bear**. I may even fear for my survival or for that of someone close to me. My body then sends important messages I must now heed in order to keep a good emotional balance.

From now on, I accept↓♥ to **Love** myself more, and I stop constantly judging and criticizing myself! I rediscover everything I had hidden and repressed: my ambitions, my desires and my goals in life, and I must accept↓♥ my **capacity** for achieving them. My confusion will dissipate, and I will no longer have to 'turn my **back**' or '**back up** against' a situation or a person, for I will have acquired the **certainty** that I can achieve everything I desire. I accept↓♥ to release all the energies that prevent me from fully flourishing. It is not surprising that I had difficulty in loving myself, for I was no longer myself. Becoming myself opens up wide the doors of life and those of my **heart♥**. I stop criticizing and I learn to express myself freely instead of repressing. I accept↓♥ that I need help from others, and I increasingly learn to ask. I thus respect more the person that I am.

BACK DISORDERS — MIDDLE BACK (the 12 dorsal vertebræ)

The **middle of the back** represents the large thoracic region of the body included between the **heart♥** and the **lumbar vertebræ**.

It is a region of **emotional and affective guilt**. The **12 dorsal vertebræ**[5] are mainly included in this region:

D1 = The **first dorsal vertebra D1** can react strongly when I push myself to the limit, either at work or in sports or in any other situations where I go to the limits of my mental, physical or emotional forces. It also does not appreciate a 'boost', whether in the form of alcohol or any sort of drug. Its sensitivity will be raw at that point. I am anguished and I build myself means of self-protection in order to protect myself from the people around me and avoid being hurt. This can manifest itself in my gestures or in my words: for example, I tend to push others away by my coldness or my hurtful words. By withdrawing, I prevent others from 'penetrating my space' or wielding too much power or authority over me. This can even manifest itself by a substantial weight gain, acting as my natural physical protection, because I unconsciously want to 'take up more space' and leave less for the others. It can also serve to camouflage my timidity, with which

---

5. **Dorsal vertebræ**: The way to identify each of them is by the letter **D** that designates ***dorsal***, followed by the sequential number of the **vertebra**. Another common way is to use the letter **T** to designate the ***thoracic*** **vertebræ**, which provides the same information.

I have difficulty in dealing. It will become even more prominent if I fear losing the **Love** of the people around me. I tend to be uncompromising, and disorder exasperates me. My closed mind and my fears affect the state of **D1**. I cut myself off from my emotions. My fear of losing someone's **Love** or the death of a Loved one paralyzes me. I don't dare do things or take my proper place. I must be vigilant and avoid shriveling up in myself, constantly mulling over dark thoughts, always fixed on the same ideas and frustrations. I tend to condemn myself for my past experiences. A **D1** in bad condition can bring about ailments in any part of my body located between my elbows and the ends of my fingers, along with respiratory difficulties (coughing, asthma, etc.).

I accept↓♥ to open myself to **Love**, respectfully embracing who I am.

D2 = The **second dorsal vertebra D2** will react easily and quickly like an alarm bell when my emotionality is affected. If I accumulate and stifle my emotions, **D2** will then send me a message and the '**back**ache' will appear. If I have the impression that I don't have my place in life and in society, that life is 'unfair' and I feel myself a victim of events, **D2** will be affected. I can be especially concerned by everything that touches my family, and I experience very intensely any situation of conflict or disharmony. I feel oppressed and psychologically (emotionally) as well as physically smothered. What is my place within my clan, especially in relation to my father? Have I experienced great wants with respect to him? Do I have too many responsibilities involving the family's safety and good functioning? I may have accumulated some old grudges. I may also be constantly stirring up past experiences and memories by trying to freeze my reality in past events, instead of looking to the future with confidence and living the present moment intensely. I may dread a new situation that brings on a fear of the unknown. Am I going to have too many responsibilities? Will I be supported, or will I have to muddle through on my own? How will the people around me react? If I doubt myself or my capacities, I may play the 'hardass' by becoming very authoritarian; I will thus have the **impression** of controlling the situation, but **Aware** all the while that I am trembling in fear, even to the point of anguish. I may also become irritable over a person or an event, and I react with mood swings. I doubt the others, and I prefer that they stay far away from me. That way, they won't hurt me! A **D2** in bad condition will often be accompanied by ailments and pains in the **heart♥** and in the organs linked to it, as well as in the lungs. This denotes a closing of the **heart♥** to a person or a situation, for I no longer feel like suffering.

I accept↓♥ to learn how to ask and how to trust my capacity for picking up new challenges. I let go of my past and turn to the future, knowing that I am now able to take my place in harmony with my entourage. I can also read the section concerning the **heart♥** to find other pathways for thought.

D3 = The **third dorsal vertebra D3** is mainly related to the lungs and the chest. I can go and see, under these two topics, the causes that can affect them, and this will give me a key to knowing why **D3** is also sending me messages. Also, everything that I can perceive through my senses and does not quite suit me will make **D3** react. As I am very sensitive to my entourage, I have developed a system where I know what is right, what is wrong, what is acceptable↓♥ or not. I may be frozen and rigid in my way of thinking and seeing things. I tend to judge any person, especially my mother whom I missed, or a situation that doesn't fit my definition of 'appropriate'. I may react strongly to what I consider to be an 'injustice'. I may become angry, or even violent, whenever I don't agree with what I see, perceive or hear. I may also build up a 'scenario' in my head, which produces a distortion of reality, often because of my fear of seeing reality straight on, and also because my ambient reality depresses me. I may develop excessive and unreasoned fears. Then my taste for life lessens, and I no longer feel safe. Sadness may engulf me, I no longer feel like struggling. Depression may gradually overtake me and I will want to cut myself off from this world that only brings me sorrow, frustration and anxiety. Sorrow takes over, and I curl into myself. I repress my emotions and refuse to face them.

I must learn to see life in a new **Light**. And accept↓♥ that I may not be living in a perfect world, but that any situation is 'perfect', in the sense that it enables me to draw a meaningful lesson from it.

D4 = The **fourth dorsal vertebra D4** is related to pleasures, desires and often unsatiated temptations. Sometimes my expectations are excessive, unrealistic even, and I become irritable and angry because my wishes are not granted and life is unfair. I resent life and the people around me. At bottom, I feel such a great emptiness, often affective, that I have depressive tendencies, and the only way I know to counteract this state of being and bring a little 'spice' into my life will be to create in it a state of excitement, either naturally or artificially. I may practice high-emotion sports (parachuting, rock climbing, etc.), or I may take drugs to bring me into a temporary state of ecstasy and well-being. I thus seek refuge in an imaginary world, sheltered from everyone. However, I am not safely sheltered from the emotions I have repressed and from which I have tried to escape. I may appear to be very free, but in fact I am imprisoned in my anger, my sorrows, my frustrations, my excessive resentment and my fear of being asphyxiated by the **Love** of others, which I have never been able to acknowledge and accept↓♥. I oppose myself, I remain distant and I maintain this gulf by my bad mood and my depressive attitude. I need so much to be Loved, yet I tend to reject others and condemn them, or even betray them. However, my true betrayal is directed against myself, which makes me stray from my mission in this world.

It is important that I acknowledge and accept↓♥ my emotions to be able to integrate them and enable me to fully live my life. When **D4** is affected, a difficulty in the gallbladder and the liver can also ensue.

D5 = The **fifth dorsal vertebra D5** is affected when I find myself in a situation where I have the impression of losing control and that my power is outside of me. I then feel destabilized, and rage rumbles in me. I may even find myself in a state of panic. This happens on the affective level with my spouse, a member of the family, a close friend, etc. This control sometimes hides under the guise of wanting to 'help' someone, 'guide' them or 'help them in their difficulties', but deep down, I am exerting control over this person by acting from a position of 'strength', however unconsciously. If things do not go as I wish, I may become frustrated, critical, impatient and even angry, and **D5** will react violently. I want to project the image of a 'tough, hard-boiled' character who is able to 'take on a lot'. But deep down, I know that I am taking too much on my shoulders, which leads me to experience insecurity and anxiety and to be revolted against my entourage whom I hold responsible for my misery. I don't feel that I am part of my family, and I feel guilty because I might help them more, but I am just incapable of it. I have great ambitions, which sometimes makes me move away from my deeper values and act in contradiction with them. I then rush into artificial relationships with people, finding disappointment after disappointment, for true, simple **Love** is not sufficiently present. I accumulate negative emotions, and I have difficulty in seeing the positive side of a situation, brooding over the negative. I live more in my rational mind, in my thoughts and my structures. I bury myself in my work and become dissatisfied with my life. I note that the bad condition of **D5** is often accompanied by various ailments affecting my liver and my blood circulation.

I accept↓♥ to listen to my inner voice, to renew contact with my essence and my true values, for calm to return in my life and so that I can see events clearly, flourishing and capable of experiencing true **Love**.

D6 = The **sixth dorsal vertebra D6** will react when I criticize myself and judge myself severely. I may have been raised in a very strict environment where the values and conduct guidelines had to be followed literally. Having grown up in this authoritarian and non-permissive climate, I may now have quandaries of **conscience** where I feel like having fun and taking some time for myself, but I judge it to be "not OK" and "I don't deserve it". I create useless worries for myself, for I never stop analyzing each of my gestures, words and thoughts in order to be certain that "I am OK". I am disconnected from my body and living in my head. Guilt is eating me up inside. Anxiety is very present, and I punish myself by cutting myself off from the world. I have difficulty in accepting↓♥ myself as I am. I feel I am a victim of life, powerless over events. I judge them severely, not wanting to accept↓♥ that they are there to make me grow, but seeing them instead as punishments and injustices. I refuse life and new experiences. I then feel frustrated and bewildered, resentful, envious and jealous of others. That is why a **D6** in bad condition is often accompanied by ailments in the stomach and the gallbladder, for the annoyances are many and I flee my responsibilities.

I accept↓♥ to be more flexible and permissive with myself, and I learn to see something positive in each event, knowing that every experience leads me to know myself better and to become a better person myself.

D7 = The **seventh dorsal vertebra D7** is a fierce worker. If I push myself to the extreme limit in the things I have to do in my life, not listening to my body when it needs to rest and relax, **D7** will raise a cry of alarm. I may thus be trying to forget or flee someone or a situation. I may want to forget my financial or affective worries. If I stop, discouragement and dissatisfaction over my life will risk surfacing again, which is something I don't want. I accumulate much anger and aggressiveness; everything is growling inside of me because "life has nothing good to offer me". I resist and persist to the point of stubbornness about certain ideas that obsess me. I refuse to allow my aspirations, my spontaneity and my creativity to see the **Light** of day, not knowing how to face them. As I allow others to tell me how to live my life, I am anguished and vulnerable, not in charge of my life. The disagreements that affect my family, and for which I feel responsible, eat me up inside.

I must learn to appreciate what I have and what I am, and to see all the abundance that is present in my life. I have the right to take some time for me; I have the right to feel emotions instead of letting them boil away inside of me. I give myself the right to experience my sorrow, my disappointment and my fears, for this is how I can accept↓♥ them and change them into something positive. I can do my inner tidying up as I go along, and enable **D7** to function normally. I resume contact with my body and with earthly life. This is how the illnesses that often accompany a **D7** in bad condition, and which often also affect the pancreas and the duodenum, may also disappear.

D8 and **D9 =** The **eighth** and **ninth dorsal vertebræ D8** and **D9,** which are located at the level of the diaphragm and are closely linked, are similar in all respects. This is why they are presented here together. They are affected mainly when I experience insecurity because I fear losing control over a situation or a person. I am domineering: I feel more self-assured when I perfectly manage all the aspects of my life, when I perfectly orchestrate any situation so that I know exactly what to expect. The uncertainty leads me to keep everything to myself. I hide in my glass bubble, not having to ask myself any questions nor make any efforts to change anything in my life. I experience all my emotions 'from inside'. But if this supposed balance is disturbed, **D8** and **D9** will strongly react out of fright, curling up in fear. By being withdrawn, I feel safer. I push away my emotions and repress my inner forces. **D8** indicates to me more especially that I am haunted by the fear of failure and that I have a situation to resolve involving my family. **D9** is related to the role of a **victim** that I assign myself. Despair may take over, and I am suffering from disquiet because I don't know what direction to take in my life and I am afraid of making a mistake. I hesitate to go forward, in part because I cling to the past, for I am afraid of abandonment and rejection. I have difficulty in seeing the

Light at the end of the tunnel, and I prefer to stay 'in place'. I may disdain life, and I am headed for an abyss of despair that I can overcome only by trusting in life and relinquishing the control that I wield. For it is by letting go that I gain mastery over my life. I note that a damaged **D8** may be accompanied by ailments in the diaphragm and the spleen (including blood disorders), whereas a **D9** in bad condition will be accompanied by an allergy or a malfunctioning of the surrenal glands or hives.

I accept↓♥ to allow my gentle and deep nature to emerge. I allow my child-like side to live together with my adult side, which now takes care of it.

D10 = When the **tenth dorsal vertebra D10** is affected, it often reflects a deep insecurity before which I feel unarmed and resourceless. My self-confidence is at its lowest, and I need a 'little nip' to help me find my courage and forget my worries. It may often be a greater than usual consumption of alcohol or drugs that will give me that 'little nudge'. Once I have resumed my normal state however, the 'bugs' are still there, and my life turns darker, because I only see the negative side of things. I am facing nothingness. Everything seems dark, and I refuse life, deploring my pitiful fate. I worry for trifles and become angry, but without being capable of manifesting it, which affects my sensitivity that becomes skin deep and makes me fly off the handle for trivial reasons, often with much aggressiveness. I am faced with nothing, and I don't know in which direction to go or what are the right choices to make. I feel I am a victim of circumstances, and that prevents me from taking charge of my life. I am bogged down in my emotions, which makes my communications with others difficult. I am seeking my place in life, and I can't position myself. A **D10** in bad condition is often accompanied by ailments in the kidneys, known as the seat of fear.

I accept↓♥ to trust myself, and I learn to see the beauty around me and within me. I have the courage to ask for help. I fully shoulder my responsibilities and I take charge of my life again.

D11 = The anomalies in the **eleventh dorsal vertebra D11** are generally found when my nervous system has difficulty in functioning. My very great overall sensitivity causes **D11** to deform itself, for I also deform reality in order to suffer less. I change it as I please so that it will be as I want it to be. I perceive myself as an ugly, unattractive person, full of defects. My negative self-image is such that I will find it difficult to establish durable relationships with my entourage because I have a great fear of being rejected. I willingly 'cut' myself off from my entourage because I have the impression that I am being invaded, and I no longer know what belongs to me or not. But this can only last so long, and sooner or later I must face reality. At that point, an inner tension will have set in, and I will have difficulty in dealing with it. It may become so intolerable that I may even have suicidal ideas, for I am living amidst misunderstanding and in fear of the future, because I feel **powerless** to change things in my life. I consider myself a 'victim' with hurt feelings. I am not up to the perfect and ideal image of myself that I want to project. I brood about the negative and I do little to extricate myself from this. I must learn to move and go forward rather than stagnate in a comatose state and mope around passively. Illnesses in **D11** often go together with ailments in the kidneys and skin diseases (eczema, acne, etc.).

I accept↓♥ to change things in my life, but I must be ready to put some effort into it and ask for help. I renew contact with my inner strength and I allow my creative energies to flow.

D12 = The **twelfth dorsal vertebra D12** is affected especially when I live in a bubble, withdrawn into myself. I tend to criticize, judge and easily jump to conclusions, not because I have checked them out, but only because my observations can leave me with false impressions that I interpret in my own way. This leads me to experience a lot of anger that 'eats me up inside'. My mind is very active. My sensitivity is 'skin deep'. I build myself castles in the air. I invent all sorts of scenarios and thus avoid my responsibilities. As I have difficulty in dealing with my entourage, I feel very insecure, and I am a perfectionist. I may brood over morbid ideas, being no longer able to absorb anything of what I see, feel or perceive, and envying what others have. I am suffocating because of all this aggressiveness, this sorrow and this feeling of abandonment inside of me. I wear a mask to protect myself against any other disappointments or disillusionments, especially in my affective relations. An ailment at **D12** is often accompanied by intestinal ailments, joint pains, deficient lymphatic circulation and also occasional ailments in the Fallopian tubes[6]. I learn to communicate, to go and check with the persons concerned in order to remove my doubt and my insecurity. I thus see more clearly in my life, and calm settles in me.

Ailments in the **middle of the back** are the clear sign of a difficult relation with life and the situations of my existence. I often have decisions to make, but I am constantly in doubt about them and about ***standing by*** them. This region of the **back** also corresponds to the movement of externalization of the energy of living that passes through me. This means that during a period of inner maturity (when I build up experience), several divine qualities such as confidence, **Love**, detachment (namely self-determination, mainly on the affective level) will be put to the test. My **back ailments**, including a **bent back**, can mean several things: guilt in situations where **I have no reason** to feel guilty, **bitterness** or **poor self-confidence** related to a life that I find very heavy to bear. I believe I must be the pillar and properly manage the structure that is already in place. I may feel that "they are always on my **back**" and that I am alone to do everything. If I have a **sore back**, this denotes a great feeling of **helplessness** in a current situation that is difficult to deal with and where I would need help. Not always knowing how to position myself in certain

6. **Fallope**, Gabriel: An Italian anatomist and surgeon (Modene 1523 – Padua 1562). Gabriel **Fallope** taught in Padua and made many anatomical discoveries, including that of the uterus tubes, to which his name was given.

situations where I have choices to make, I will often feel bitterness because I will very often make the needs of others pass before my own needs. I am touchy, which makes me close up. Despair may appear, for **I do not feel supported enough on the affective level** and I also suffer from insecurity. I tend to hold in my emotions and I live a lot in the past. I still cling to it, I go around in circles. I feel unstable and anxious. I have twinges of **conscience**. The goal to aim for is to more actively express the divine energy.

I accept↓♥ that I must be clear in everything, with myself and others, without conveying the feelings of a shaky past, and make place for a calm and serene **here and now**. I need help and encouragement. I need to connect with my inner being that always watches over me. My body gives me important signals. To ask for help is not shameful. On the contrary it is a sign of intelligence, for this help enables me to go forward. I see the importance of my own identity and I am prudent with my ego and my fears. I learn to communicate with my inner being through meditation or contemplation; I find many solutions and answers there. To be in contact with my inner being is to choose to experience the situations of life more adequately.

BACK DISORDERS — LOWER BACK (the 5 lumbar vertebræ)

Often confused with the kidneys and commonly associated with **backache**, this region is located from the waist to the coccyx. It is part of the **support** system. It symbolizes my security, my self-confidence and my trust in life. Pains in this region denote the presence of **insecurity**, **material** (work, money, goods) as well as **affective**. "I am afraid I am going to run out of…!", "I will never get there!", "I will never be able to achieve that!" express well the inner feelings experienced. I am so **concerned** by everything material that I feel sadness, because there is an emptiness, and this emptiness hurts me. There is a discrepancy between my desires and my actions. I may even base my personal worth on the number of material goods I possess. The **pains** at this level often appear following the loss of a job, a retirement, the leaving of a child, a separation, etc. I am experiencing a very great duality, because I want to have 'quality' as well as 'quantity', and with respect to my interpersonal relations as well as to my possessions. I tend to put too much on my shoulders and to dissipate my energy. I tend to do everything to be Loved, and I worry about what others think of me. I feel like a pillar and I can count only on myself. I may also wish to take on this role to enhance my own importance. It may also be a concern about another or several other persons. I may worry about them, and I may tend to 'take other people's problems on my **back**' and want to save them. **Lumbalgia** risks appearing at this point. My **powerlessness** regarding certain situations in my life makes me **bitter** and I refuse to submit, but I am afraid. This feeling of **powerlessness** (sometimes experienced in my sexuality), which can lead me as far as **revolt**, may lead me to develop **lumbago**. I don't feel supported in my basic needs and my affective needs and I feel incapable of taking on the material dimension of my life. The relations between things and persons are conflicted. I have difficulty in facing the changes and the novelty that present themselves to me, because I like to feel safe in my routine and my old habits. This often indicates that I am **inflexible** and **rigid** and that I would like to be supported in my own way. I can't be fully happy: there's always something dark in the picture, something hidden.

If I accept↓♥ that others may help me in their own ways, I will discover and become **conscious** of the fact that I have all the support I need. I thereby become more autonomous and responsible. I let go of the burdens that belong to others. I must acknowledge my worth in order to fulfill myself, instead of waiting for outside recognition. I must stop forcing myself to do things to project a good image of myself, because when I do so, I am trying to manipulate others and not acting from my **heart♥**. If it is a **pinching of the lumbar discs**, I am probably putting too much pressure on myself by doing things in order to be liked. As a period of rest is necessary, I take the opportunity to examine what is going on in my life and re-define my priorities. As I **don't feel supported**, I become **rigid** (stiff) with other people. Do I tend to blame others for my difficulties? Have I taken the time to express my needs?

I accept↓♥ that my sole support comes from myself. By remaking contact with my inner being, I am balancing out my needs, and I connect with all the forces of the Universe that are in me. These forces give me confidence in myself and in life, because I know that they bring me everything I need: physical, emotional or spiritual. I am supported at all times! The **5 lumbar vertebræ** are concerned in this region:

L1 = The **first lumbar vertebra L1** is affected when I experience a feeling of powerlessness in front of someone or something that doesn't suit me and I have the impression that I can't change, that I have to put up with it. I then become inert, lifeless. I spend lots of energy on things that are mostly minor, but which I amplify so much that they take on catastrophic proportions, which may even bring on a feeling of despair. I may experience insecurity regarding some aspects of my life, but for no good reason. I expect people to play dirty tricks on me. I want to control everything, but that is not humanly possible. I take others so much into consideration that I completely neglect my own needs and my freedom. I may also experience inner conflicts over what I want to do, but don't allow myself to actually do. I need to be close to people, but at the same time I also need some moments of solitude. This makes frustration, aggressiveness and anger surge up in me. These feelings harden my **heart♥** if I don't free myself of them, and make life bitter to me. An **L1** in bad condition can cause ailments involving the digestive (intestine and colon) or elimination (constipation, dysentery, etc.) functions.

I accept↓♥ the power I have to change the course of my life, and of mine only! I reorder my priorities so that I can better channel my energies.

L2 = The state of the **second lumbar vertebra L2** largely depends upon my flexibility toward myself and others. Solitude and bitterness, often caused by a pronounced timidity, are also important factors that can affect **L2**. I am a prisoner of my emotions: not knowing how to experience and express them, and as they are sometimes lively and explosive, I put on masks to protect myself and to prevent others from seeing what is going on inside of me. My ailment can become so great that I want to 'numb' my pain with drink, drugs, work, etc., and **L2** will then cry out for help. I don't want to be belittled and humiliated any longer. I tend to mope and live in a depressive state, which I actually appreciate in some small way because I am casting myself in the role of a victim, which doesn't force me to go into action and do something to change certain things in my life. I may blame my parents or certain events in my childhood for my current distress. I believe my survival depends on the **Love** of others. As for **L1**, a feeling of helplessness and also much sadness will affect **L2**. I am bitter about life because I am supposed to enjoy the pleasures of life, but often I don't allow myself to do so, because of my 'obligations' or my sense of duty, in order to show a good example. I must provide for my needs, but often also for those of other persons. I must learn that I don't have to be perfect. I may sometimes feel incapable or helpless when faced with a situation, having difficulty in letting go. An **L2 vertebra** in bad condition can bring about ailments in the abdomen, the appendix or the legs, where I may see varicose veins appear.

I accept↓♥ to let go of the anger or rancor that I feel about myself: I must only be true with myself and with others and simply express my sorrows, my joys, my doubts, my bewilderments and my frustrations, in order to be more open with others and so that **L2** will come back to life too.

L3 = The **third lumbar vertebra L3** is mainly affected when I experience tense or stormy family situations. There is often a conflict at the sexual level: either a rivalry existed or still exists, or extramarital relations produced or are producing children, or there are traumas related to a past or current incest. I refrain from saying or doing anything that might hurt or bother the others. But in so doing, it is to myself that I am doing harm. I play the 'good boy' or 'good girl' role by showing very great flexibility. But I become too easygoing, which brings me frustration, especially if I have to push aside my desires. And maybe I push myself aside also, especially because of my guilt and my timidity that lead me to reject myself. I judge myself severely, I have 'crises of **conscience**', grounded or not, which may amount to betrayals. **L3** also reacts if I avoid communicating my emotions because of my great sensitivity, not knowing exactly how these emotions will be received. I become 'paralyzed', powerless even, in my emotions, in my body and in my thoughts, which prevents my creativity from manifesting itself with everything it involves, especially communication and sexuality, which remain 'rigid' and 'frigid'. A bad condition in **L3** can bring about ailments in the genital organs (ovaries and testicles), in the uterus (in women), in the bladder or in the knees, such as arthritis, inflammation or pains.

To overcome discouragement, I accept↓♥ to reach out to others and to dare express my emotions, so my full creative potential can awaken and reveal itself.

L4 = When the **fourth lumbar vertebra L4** rebels, it is often because I am having difficulty in dealing with everyday reality. I may be indulging myself in an imaginary world, which can lead me to live passively, tired as I am of seeing what is going on around me and being very attached to the past. A little carelessness sets in. "Why care at all anyway?" I endure events more than I create them, which may leave me with a bitter taste. This is especially present in my work: I have ***enormous*** aspirations, but my fears prevent me from advancing and slow me down in the promotions I could earn. There follows an insecurity about money. I feel off-standard, different from the others. For example, it may be in my work or in my couple, which seems ill-assorted to me. I try to remain in a well-defined structure. It is the only way to win the approval of others, get their attention and maintain a positive image. Just as **L4**, I sometimes need to protect myself by becoming closed, for I can easily let myself be distracted or influenced by what surrounds me, especially by what people may say about me, and my sensitivity can be greatly affected. This also involves my sexuality, which I tend to deny. I also worry too much, and my discernment is sometimes biased or unsteady because my mind is very rigid; it prevents me from gaining an overall view of a situation and, by the same token, of the possible solutions or avenues for it. I then want to control, instead of listening to my inner voice. An **L4 vertebra** in bad condition can develop pains in the region of my sciatic nerve, of the uterine body in a woman and of the prostate in a man.

I accept↓♥ to listen to my inner voice, which gives me back my mastery over my own life. I retrieve my power to create my life as I wish, and I recover the taste to accomplish great things!

L5 = I may wonder what is happening in my life when the **fifth lumbar vertebra L5** is affected. Do I have an attitude of contempt or casualness toward a person or a situation? I may be experiencing a little jealousy, discontent or frustration, yet I already have a lot, life has pampered me, but still I have difficulty in admitting it. I belittle myself as compared to members of my family, my friends, my work colleagues, etc. I feel different also in my sexual fantasies, and so I live in silence. I am cut off from my inner beauty. My life is tainted by lust (at all levels) and I must learn to appreciate what I have and cultivate my interpersonal relations: I have difficulty, mostly on the affective level, in being true and feeling well, because deep inside I am experiencing great insecurity and I have difficulty in expressing what I am going through. I will therefore tend to be a little depressed, because I will often switch from one partner to another without knowing why this is happening to me, feeling 'OK' in what I am experiencing. I will invent all sorts of scenarios, and my attention will always be focused on the small unimportant details, which prevents me from advancing and going on to other things. A shadow of bitterness may darken my life and prevent me from enjoying it. My uncertainty, my distrust and the weight I carry on my back prevent me from advancing.

I learn to savor each instant that passes and to appreciate all the abundance that is part of my life. I live in gratitude and joy. An **L5** in bad condition can cause me pain in my legs, from the knees to the toes.

The **lower back** is also part of the system at the center of **movement**. If I am having difficulty in dealing with society, from the point of view of the directions to be taken as well as the support I expect from it, I may experience **frustration** or **resentment**. I don't want to take up the challenge with certain persons or situations. My **personal relations** with my entourage **suffer from it**. I may also have difficulty in accepting↓♥ that I am advancing in age. "I am getting old", and I must slowly come to terms with the notion of my **mortality**. Finally, the **lower back** is very closely related to the two inner energy centers, the coccyx and the second energy center that is more specifically related to sexuality. If I am experiencing inner or outer conflicts regarding the latter, if I have **repressed** my sexual energy, if I feel betrayed, a pain may appear in the **lower back**. The **5 sacral vertebræ** and the **4 coccygeal vertebræ** are related to this region. When the **sacral vertebræ** are affected, I may have the impression that I have no 'spine' and that I need someone else to support me. I am constantly being 'tested' by life in order to see where my level of integrity and honesty is. I have an enormous potential, but am I ready to make all the necessary efforts in order to reach my goals? The **lower vertebræ** are the following:

S1, **S2**, **S3** = As the **first 3 sacral vertebræ** are joined together, they will be presented here together. They form a whole. They react to the rigidity that I display, to my narrowness of mind about certain situations or certain persons, to my closed mind that refuses to hear what others have to say. I want to have control to feel strong and safe and, if I lose it, I will go into a stormy rage, and I may feel like 'kicking someone in the pants' because I am so frustrated and full of bitterness. All these feelings often have their source in my affective relations, which don't always go as I wish, or in a conflict with authority. My communications, verbal as well as sexual, are deficient, if not inexistent, and I am constantly being put in question. I have the impression of swimming against the current, and I feel in a dead end.

It is in my interest to take a moment off and take a clear look at my life, to think about what I want and build a solid base.

S4, **S5** = All desires have their source in the **fourth and fifth sacral vertebræ**. If I am able to manage them well, if I take the time to rest and do the things I like, **S4** and **S5** will work properly. However, if I am experiencing guilt, calling myself 'lazy' and confronting myself to my duties and my morality, judging my conduct 'not OK', then **S4** and **S5** risk reacting strongly. I have the right to do things for myself and sometimes enjoy a little escape, but I must prevent it from becoming a means of escape to avoid facing my responsibilities. It is at this point that laziness can become non-beneficial: for it then keeps me in a passive state of lassitude that prevents me from moving ahead. That is why, in extreme cases, my feet will also be affected. The only way to heal a **split** or **broken sacrum** is physical immobility and time. The **sacrum** is related to the second energy center that is located at the level of the first lumbar **vertebra**. An imbalance in this energy center can show up in the following physical ailments: in the genital organs, there may be infertility, frigidity or herpes; in the kidneys: cystitis or calculi; with respect to digestion and elimination: incontinence, diarrhea, constipation, colitis, etc. **Spinal deviations (scoliosis)** usually begin at this level and lead to **back pains**. The second chakra or energy center influences my relations with the people around me, and any dysfunction in it affecting my **sacrum** will be a sign of my stress, of my anxieties, my fears and my depressive tendency, which I must learn to manage. A difficulty at the level of my **sacrum** may manifest an inner conflict over what is ***holy***, **sacred**, my religious values. Am I in contradiction with these values, or am I feeling guilt for having set spirituality aside? Do I feel that I have to make many ***sacrifices***? I have a ***crucial*** decision to make, and I am feeling lost over what I must do. Who is supporting me in my decisions? The **sacrum** is linked to my child-parent relation, and may be affected because of a feeling of hate. I want to move ahead in life, but I hold on to my past or to familiar things or persons that provide me with an illusory feeling of stability, control and protection. My inner duality can dissipate only if I honestly identify and embrace my emotions; only then can they become a means of transformation.

The **coccyx** is related to the first chakra or energy center, the seat of survival. It represents the foundation of my sexuality, the adequate fulfillment of my **basic needs** (sexuality, food, protection, shelter, **Love**[7], etc.), which enables me to be stable. The **coccyx** is made up of **four coccygeal vertebræ** that are fused together. It represents my dependence upon life or upon someone else. When my **coccyx** is painful, the odds are high that my body is telling me to stop. It is my insecurity speaking up about my basic survival needs, such as having a roof, food, clothing, etc. Here, food includes physical needs, but also emotional and sexual ones. I need to feel safe, like a fledgling in its ***nest***. An ailment in my **coccyx** can result from my feeling of being dominated, of feeling that I am 'less than nothing'. I tend to ***crouch down*** in a corner as if I am being punished: I feel that part of me is dead, and I am watching life go by without truly taking part in it. I stay on in situations that should have stopped long ago, but my doubts and uncertainty keep the upper hand. Everyone needs **Love** in their lives. They also need to communicate with their partners through sexual relations. These needs are often denied and repressed, notably because of my moral and religious principles, which leads me to be dissatisfied. I may then feel impotent, in all the meanings of the term, and anger will brew within me. I want to escape any situation that hurts my sensitivity and makes me experience guilt. For example, if I must have my child raised by someone else, my **coccyx** will react very strongly. I may feel

---

7. **Love**: The **Love** referred to here is akin to **the Love of a mother for her child**. When my **coccyx** is affected, I may experience the fear of losing, or of not having, at least a **Love** similar to the one a child is entitled to expect from its mother. This is the sort of **Love** referred to here, not a **Love** relationship between two adults.

like a ***cuckoo*** who pops out of its hiding place for a few seconds and must then quickly retreat into its little house for long hours. I must put aside my pride, or rather my fears, in other words. I must place my trust in life and especially trust my own capacity for expressing myself and taking my affairs in hand. When I experience difficulties related to this facet of myself, I can confirm within myself just how far I am (I wish to be) dependent upon another person who, consciously or not, satisfies certain needs in my life. I am capable of carrying out my own actions, of being autonomous. It is possible that the persons to whom I am **attached** may be even more affectively dependent than myself and may thus need this sort of relation. Because the **coccyx** is related to the first chakra, an imbalance in this energy center can bring about physical disorders, most commonly involving the rectum or the anus (hemorrhoids, itching), the bladder (urinary disorders, incontinence), the prostate. There may also appear pains at the base of the spine, considerable weight gain or loss (obesity, anorexia) and bad blood circulation in the legs (phlebitis), the hands and the feet. These ailments indicate to me that I need to re-balance this energy center. If I sustain a **fall on my coccyx** causing pain, I wonder in what situation I have the impression of going in circles. I am in a *cul de sac*. I deny my impulses. As I fear my own emotions, I stiffen my back to project a good image, but life calls me back to order and brings me 'back down to earth', with 'both feet on the ground'.

I accept↓♥ to see just how much independence and vigor I am showing in my life. I must let go of any feeling of **worry** about my basic needs, and become **conscious now** of the forces that inhabit me and assert that I am the person best placed to ensure my own survival.

BACK — FRACTURE OF VERTEBRÆ *See also: BONES — FRACTURE*

The **fracture of a vertebra** generally results from an inner revolt, a reaction of mental **inflexibility** related to authority. I see life with such a narrow mind that I **attract** this **fracture** on myself. My thoughts are too **rigid**, I refuse to bend to certain new ideas that move me away from **Love** and bring me pain. I am intransigent, often very proud, and I need to develop more **humility**. My **back** is my support; to see it injured is uncomfortable. I have had enough of carrying all this weight on my shoulders. I WANT TO BE RECOGNIZED AND RESPECTED. There is a duality in me that is destroying me. I want to be focused, in contact with my essence, so I can know perfectly what is good for me. I want to be the creator of my own life. I feel stuck in a situation, and I must move forward to get free of it.

I accept↓♥ my present attitudes, knowing I can modify them now. Life is beautiful to live, with its flux of changes, and it is important I respect that. I remain open to life, knowing it is good for me. I let myself go with the flow of life.

BACKACHE *See: BACK (IN GENERAL)*

BACTERIUM (flesh-eating) INFECTION

Necrotizing fasciitis is commonly called the **flesh-eating bacterium infection**. This infection infiltrates itself into the different layers of tissues that cover the muscles (the *fascia*). It destroys the tissues and can cause death within 12 to 24 hours. It is recognizable especially by a high fever and a red and painful swelling that can start out from the location of a minor lesion (such as a cut).

I wish to change something important in my life, but I sense that my fortress is under attack from all sides. I find myself in a situation of inner conflict, a duality, where I can no longer pull back or change directions as I might want to. Will I have all the necessary protection and support for achieving my desire? My deepest convictions are being treated Lightly. Outwardly, people say that I have an 'iron hand'. Am I being faithful to my ideas, or am I just stubborn, even at the cost of risking self-destruction? I have difficulty in tolerating contradictions. My negative attitudes are 'burning me up inside'. I feel so many limitations and barriers that are being raised to stop me in one of my endeavors that I am beside myself, I am exasperated and I have 'goose flesh'. I may fear a separation, either in my personal life or at work. From my standpoint, this would have dramatic consequences for my future or for my reputation.

I accept↓♥ to be more flexible in how I deal with events and life in general. I stop trying to control everything. I develop moderation and detach myself from the opinions of others about me. By always seeing the good side of things, I keep my **heart♥** open, so **Love** can roam freely in me and around me. I learn to thank the Source for everything I receive, I clarify my goals and look at the situation with courage while accepting↓♥ to let go. I accept↓♥ to receive help from others and understand that when I let energy flow, I find the strength to reach my goals in peace and serenity.

BAD BREATH *See: MOUTH — BREATH [BAD]*

BALANCE (loss of) OR DIZZINESS *See: BRAIN — BALANCE [LOSS OF]*

BALDNESS *See: HAIR — BALDNESS*

BASEDOW'S DISEASE *See: GLAND [THYROID] — BASEDOW'S DISEASE*

BED-WETTING / ENURESIS *See also: INCONTINENCE [FECAL, URINARY]*

The fact that my child lets go during his sleep gives me information about certain emotions that he is experiencing in relation to parental or school **authority**. If I am this child suffering from **incontinence**, it may be a way for me to liberate emotions (that urine represents) that I hold in during the day, often for fear of being punished or for fear of displeasing others and no longer being Loved. I thus express a deep ***disquiet***. I am experiencing so much pressure during the day that I must let it go when night comes. This pressure quite often comes from my family or my school environment. It is as if I was rebelling against my parents who possess the 'supreme authority'. It is a small revenge, because it usually provokes anger in them. I am experiencing a conflict with the ***supervision*** I am given. Because I can't express myself during the day, I do it at night. There is a notion of secrecy attached to what I am experiencing: I want nobody to discover my secret and I want to keep it well, but it happens in spite of me, and it is usually at night, in the darkness of my room, while everyone is sleeping, that I will let go. I am afraid of crying in front of my parents, so I do it in silence. I thereby want to avoid their reaction to my crying, but I will have to face their reaction the next morning. Just as some animals mark out their territories with their urine, so I too, as a child, may unconsciously feel the need to do the same thing, as if to define my 'small child's territory' that I fear may be taken from me or may be transgressed, thus experiencing much insecurity. My insecurity will also be intensified if I am forced to sleep in the dark. As a child, I may experience an intense feeling of separation from someone or something I **Love**, and it is as though during the night, I were calling out for help because I need warmth. It is my feeling of shame and powerlessness that is crying out for help.

As a parent or an educator, I accept↓♥ to become **conscious** of the child's sensitivity to authority, to help her free herself from my overbearing authority with words of **Love** that she transforms within herself into increased trust.

BELCHING / ERUCTATION *See: ERUCTATION*

BILIARY CALCULI OR CHOLETITHIASIS *See also: LIVER DISORDERS, SPLEEN*

A **gallstone** is generally one or several deposits of cholesterol or limestone. In colloquial terms, we sometimes say someone 'has **stones in the liver**'. It comes from bile. This liquid secreted by the liver is used to digest food. Bile is stocked in the gallbladder and the **calculus,** or **stone** is formed in this same gallbladder (a single large stone or several small ones).

Bile is bitter and viscous and manifests the inner **bitterness**, the sorrow, the aggressiveness, the insensitivity, resentment, frustration or dissatisfaction I feel toward myself or toward one or several other persons. The **calculi** represent a pain deeper than the simple symptoms in the spleen, the liver or the gallbladder. It is crystallized energy, feelings and **very hard thoughts full of anger**, **bitterness**, **envy** and even **jealousy** that have solidified in the form of stones, and have been maintained and accumulated over the years. They may also represent a talent, a strength that I have never wanted to use because I didn't feel I was good enough, or I felt vulnerable or inferior. I accumulate my inner strengths instead of using them. I feel rage, but it is turned against me because I know my capacities deep inside myself. I decided one day to hide in order to protect myself from the outer world. I flee their judgment. The **calculi** may have remained 'hidden' since a long time, but a sudden and violent emotion can make intense pains suddenly appear 'consciously'. Often, I am ready to go ahead, to charge on and to open doors, but **something stops me**, limits me or smothers me, and my actions then are often carried out by fear. I then become frustrated by life, I manifest 'bitter' and irritating attitudes toward people, I can't make up my mind because I lack courage and my inner strengths are poorly channeled. I don't have control over myself. That is why I have **gallstones**. What is influencing my life? Am I too proud? What are my past debts (financial as well as emotional or spiritual) that I still owe, but had forgotten about or that I had deliberately omitted to reimburse?

Even if **calculi** are the expression of a **hardened life**, I must accept↓♥ to free myself of the past and to have **more gentle attitudes and thoughts**, a different openness to life by letting go of the past, of distant feelings and old bitter memories, thereby allowing myself to manifest true **Love**. I give myself the right to fulfill my own needs, even if this involves sometimes having to say no to others. The process of acceptance↓♥ in the **heart♥** will help me to see more clearly in my life and to better discover the road to improving my situation. I let all my talents express themselves gently; and this way, I can fully flourish.

BIRTH (how my birth took place) *See also: CHILDBIRTH / DELIVERY (IN GENERAL)*

Throughout the nine months of my gestation, when I was only a fetus, all my senses were already awakened, and I was **Aware** of everything my mother, my father and the ***people*** around me verbalized. I could also feel their emotions and feelings, especially those of my mother, with whom I was in very close and intense contact. The way in which I may have interpreted what I heard or felt during this period will have repercussions on my behavior in the future.

For example, I may have had the impression that "I made Mom suffer" during delivery, whereas quite likely, she may herself have contributed to increase the level of pain by her own anxiety, her fears and also by the fact that unconsciously she was again seeing her own **birth** that she may have found very painful. I may also have understood that it was because of me that my mother almost died. I will then bear throughout my whole life this feeling of guilt "for having hurt Mom", which I will then re-experience toward other persons. If I have the impression that I **was unwanted** or that they **wanted to keep me hidden**, I may live my life like a ghost. I may experience a great feeling of rejection, and I then tend to distance myself from my entourage. If I have had little contact with my parents, I may want to compensate by becoming overly close to people, 'like a leech[8]'.

Furthermore, the way in which my **birth** occurred, or the means used to facilitate it, will also influence the behavior that I reproduce in my everyday life and that refer, precisely, to **the way in which my birth took place**. This is especially true when I am experiencing great upheavals or great changes in

---

8. **Leech**: A person who imposes theirself discreetly upon others.

my life, where I don't control what is happening. Here are some examples of the situations encountered most often:

If I was **badly positioned** in my mother's womb, my **birth** was extremely difficult and painful. This may later lead me to go through a life of sacrifice, thereby continuing to punish myself and thinking that this is the only possible way. I tend to endure a lot of pain and frustration before extricating myself from certain situations.

If I was **born prematurely**, I will often show impatience: I want to finish a task even before starting it. I have the impression of not being complete, that something is missing in me. I constantly search for this 'something'. Furthermore, if I was **placed in an incubator** for a certain period of time, I will often re-live the same deep solitude and an impression of experiencing powerlessness over certain situations or certain persons, which leads me to isolate myself and to have a very low level of energy. I will be afraid of the dark, having been accustomed very early in my life to being in bright **Light** and noise. I may experience a feeling of intense rejection because I had the impression that my mother left me after my **birth** and that she 'expelled' me from my home. In this case, I will tend to place myself in situations from which I will be expelled, whether it is from my home, my work or my affective relationships. Contacts are rare or absent. I missed food from my mother for some time, and so I will tend to eat compulsively to avoid re-living this deprivation. I may have heard some people who came to see me at the hospital say to me: "How you must be fighting to survive!" While growing up, I will keep this impression of having to fight for my life and for good causes. Letting go or giving up then become for me synonymous with mortal danger. The fact of being **placed in an incubator** was for my survival, and survival is achieved mainly by putting on enough weight. Later on, I may have difficulty in losing weight because I registered **at birth** that I must preserve a certain weight in order to survive.

On the contrary, if I had a **delayed birth**, I will have difficulty in being punctual and in turning work in on time. I take my time and I often feel rushed in the things I have to do. I also like things to be done my way. I may show aggressiveness toward persons who want to make me feel guilty for my delays, for I will have the impression that it is because of outside events that I am delayed. I will tend to ruminate before acting, finding it difficult to make decisions. In my life, I may also tend to want to hang on to persons with whom I feel comfortable. Maybe my mother wanted to keep me longer with her, worrying about me and being so happy to feel me inside of her. Or was it I, rather, who wanted to remain fused with her?

The fact of being **born either too early or too late** therefore generates conflicted situations with time. I accept↓♥ to learn to take my time to do things well and also to take some time for myself, instead of always living in the future or in the past. I am learning to live in the present moment.

A **birth** that must be **induced** probably denotes that I was not ready to be born into this world; I will then experience many frustrations that will accompany me throughout my life. I may also develop distrust toward the people around me. **An induced delivery** or one done by **cesarean section** often leads the child to be frustrated or in an angry reaction, because it is not ready to be born: either he senses the mother's fears, or he is himself afraid. The **cesarean** break is drastic: the child is brutally removed from the mother's womb. It is therefore obvious that this exit that was too quick for him will result in frustrations. That is why we often see these newborn babies crying a lot in the first months following their birth. The fact that the delivery had to be induced sometimes means that it was the physician who decided the time of delivery. This may be translated in everyday life by a need for someone else to make decisions for me. I may also have a totally opposite reaction, not tolerating that anyone else make any decisions for me, not wanting "to leave my destiny in their hands". Only my opinion will count because, unconsciously, I remember that when I was **born**, I was not consulted about when I would be ready to be born.

If my mother needed an **anesthesia** to deliver me, I may tend to fall asleep at odd moments and I '**anesthesize'** reality, I don't perceive clearly, and I interpret events in my own special way, depending on the fears I have. It is a form of escape, just like a drug: by numbing myself, 'frosting' myself up, I avoid coming into contact with my emotions and my fears. I have difficulty in receiving caresses and I may have skin diseases. I may have a marked fear of pain and I may tend to be distracted at work, having difficulty in accepting↓♥ to perform tasks that require more time and energy.

If I found myself with the **umbilical cord wound around my neck**, I will feel 'smothered' by people or situations. My throat may be more fragile, I have difficulty in expressing myself, in communicating simply and affirmatively. I tend to feel myself 'held in a stranglehold'. This may denote the mother's despair over this child's birth, wondering if this baby will be born in the best possible conditions and if she should really come into this world. She does not want to let her go.[9] I may experience discomfort when I must wear a tie, a scarf or jewels because it reminds me, even unconsciously, that I once almost died with a **cord wound around my neck**. I will have difficulty in staying close to people, physically as well as affectively, because I have the impression that they are 'taking my air' and I especially don't feel like 'tying the knot' by getting married.

If the child was **delivered by cesarean section**, there are two possible scenarios: it may have decided to come out but it got stuck. The other possibility is that they went in to get it before it was ready to come out. In these cases, I will generally have difficulty in implementing projects to completion; any prolonged and constant effort is difficult for me. I am easily discouraged. I prefer people doing things in my place because I feel incapable of doing them myself. I may also feel that life or people are treating me unfairly, or that I don't get a fair return on the efforts I expend to get a task done. "Give

9. Patrick Drouot mentioned in one of his books that a high percentage (60% +) of persons born with the **umbilical cord** around their necks became **conscious**, during regressions into one of their past lives, that they had once been hanged.

to Caesar what is Caesar's, and to God what is God's"! The fact of having a **cesarean section** prevents me, as a mother, from delivering my baby through the vagina. I may have experienced a situation in my life where I felt abused, whether it actually occurred or whether I felt a horrible fear of it happening, it makes no difference. What counts is how I experienced it emotionally. In order to avoid remembering this painful event, the **cesarean section** therefore becomes an easier means for me to deliver my child. If I am this child, I may develop a hesitant, fearful behavior and have difficulty in engaging in life. I don't trust my decisions because I am afraid of making mistakes. Because I did not have this skin contact with my mother at the time of my birth, I may experience difficulty later on in appreciating sexuality through skin contact.

If I was born in **breech (or pelvic) presentation**, I often experience guilt, especially because I have the impression that I am causing people around me to suffer. I hold back a lot, and I have difficulty in letting go and trusting people. I then experience great inner tension. Everything I experience is difficult and seems to last for an eternity. I don't feel well-seated in life. It is as if I was placed backwards in this world, being unwanted or not feeling capable of meeting my parents' desires and expectations. I may also feel limited in my actions and my projects. It is as if people and the circumstances of life were conspiring to make me give up, or give way, in the new actions I want to undertake.

If the use of **forceps** was necessary, grasping and protecting my head in order to facilitate my expulsion at the time of my **birth**, I may suffer from headaches and cranial pains and I have the impression I am running into many difficulties in my life, especially at the outset of a project or a new relation. I will feel that I must stand up to the circumstances that come up in order to carry out my new project or my new relationship. I put great pressure on my shoulders and derive a perverse pleasure from taking on useless increased responsibilities. I feel 'forced' to do things, often with the impression that 'I don't have a choice'. I tend to wait until the last moment before doing things. I may often experience emergency situations where I need outside help, just as when I was **born**. Without this help, I will die. However, if as a baby I wanted to stay fused with my mother, I perceive outside help as negative, for it deprives me of contact with my mother.

I can ask my parents for the details of my **birth**. The very fact of becoming **Aware** of the difficulties experienced at that time will help me to understand and change the behavior that later derived from it, and which may displease me.

If I am a **twin**, I may wonder why my parents were in such a hurry to have children that they had two, or three, at once. Were they afraid of losing their child and they unconsciously had a second one to feel more secure? Whatever the reason, I thank them for having brought me into the world.

BIRTH MARK / HANGNAIL *See: SKIN — PORT-WINE MARK*

BLACKHEADS *See: SKIN — BLACKHEADS*

BLACKOUT / LOSS OF CONSCIOUSNESS *See: FAINTING*

BLADDER DISORDERS *See also: CALCULI (IN GENERAL), INFECTIONS (IN GENERAL), URINE [URINARY INFECTIONS]*

The **bladder** is the reservoir where urine is 'waiting' to be released.

It represents my 'expectations' toward life. It also symbolizes the fact of directly facing the truth contained in my emotions, in my whole affective world. The **bladder** functions well if I let my emotions flow freely in the process of my acceptance↓♥ of them. **Bladder problems** indicate to me that I tend to hang on to my old ideas, that I refuse to let go. I resist change because of my insecurity. I have difficulty in adjusting to a new situation. My **bladder** reacts if I want to escape the truth. I want to manipulate and control, especially in the sexual domain. My ailments show that I have been feeling anxiety for a very long time and that it is time for me to freely let go of my undesirable negative emotions. Thus, my **bladder** will prevent me from **drowning** in my own negativity. **Urinary infections** are an indication that I am experiencing many unexpressed frustrations, sorrow and insecurity. ***Hate*** may even inhabit me. I can question myself to find out what I am holding back in my life, and which it would be in my interest to let free. These feelings prevent me from undertaking things, from taking action. I am rather in a period of passivity and introspection. These feelings may be experienced in a situation where what belongs to me and what I consider to be part of my territory are being challenged. Take, for example, a situation where I feel nauseous every time I come back home and the house is all dirty and in disarray. I can't find my way in it (in my physical space as well as in my personal life). I am living in an ***immense*** chaos and I need to see more clearly in my life. I have the impression that people are trying to ***monopolize for themselves*** something or someone that 'belongs to me', they are ***encroaching*** on me. I don't know how to make people respect my limits. My life is disorganized, and I can't position myself because I have lost my reference points. To what family territory do I belong? The **bladder** also represents the domain of personal relations. It therefore often happens that these **infections** appear during the period surrounding a honeymoon, during a bothersome or conflicted relationship, or at the time of a break-up. A honeymoon or a first sexual experience may lead me to have various problems or even disappointments triggering anger or resentment toward my partner, as if he was responsible for my dissatisfaction. My fear of intimacy may be awakened. The break-up of a relationship is generally the outcome of things left unsaid, of emotions repressed inside of me. It is as if I was burying my psychological problems deep inside myself, provoking constant pressure. It risks **overflowing**. A poorly expressed creativity (including sexuality) brings on difficulties in my **bladder**. I must understand that by freeing myself from this pressure, whatever it is, I will inevitably experience a relief. **Calculi in my bladder** show me how hard I am on myself and that I am disconnected from my emotions. This causes me to feel confusion and doubt. If I have a **permanent need to urinate**, there is therefore a permanent pressure in my **bladder**. There is a constant overload of emotions. I feel overwhelmed by what is happening in my life. My urge to urinate is often a pressing one; therefore I am experiencing several situations where I feel hurried, in a state of emergency even. I can hurry to free all my emotions in order to avoid having to fully experience and accept them. Instead of having permanent enduring relationships with people, I tend to involve myself very little. I experience all sorts of new things, seeking full control over my actions, but having difficulty in involving myself and adjusting emotionally. Once a danger is passed, I feel the urge to urinate to release the accumulated stress. On the contrary, if the **quantity of urine is less** than usual (**oliguria**), my personal relations are 'dry', as if I was in a desert. This state is often caused by an inner rage that eats away inside. A **cancer** may develop if I decide to 'disconnect' myself from these so-called negative emotions and ***banish*** them from my life. By living only in my head, it is as though I were refusing to see the fire burning up my house. Instead of finding answers inside, I feel the need to always look outside.

I accept↓♥ to free myself from my old beliefs and make room for new things in my life.I accept↓♥ to invest some of my time and myself in my interpersonal relations, and I accept↓♥ to express all these emotions that overload my **bladder**. I let go of the past emotions I was clinging to. I am living in truth and simplicity.

BLADDER — CYSTITIS *See also: APPENDIX III*

Cystitis is an inflammation of the **bladder, generally infectious**.

Certain events or situations lead me to hold in my **irritation**, my **frustrations** and my **dissatisfaction**. I am so thwarted in my expectations that my **bladder becomes inflamed**. I am living under great pressure. **Cystitis** occurs very often when I am experiencing a breakup situation with my partner, a business associate or a member of my family. The distress experienced is great and I have difficulty in expressing my emotions. There is an affective struggle that is making me experience emotions of coldness and hardness. My silence holds a deep feeling of powerlessness because I feel tied up, chained and invaded. I prevent my emotions from expressing themselves. I direct my frustrations toward others. I may often want to play a mediator's role between two persons, often my father and my mother. Is this something I truly must do, or is it in fact interfering in their lives? A situation is burning me up, and the emotion linked to it wants to escape. Having a cystitis may be beneficial in a sense, because it usually disrupts sexual relations, which become more distant. I am experiencing a conflict, usually with my **Love** partner, and the underlying rage erupts suddenly and with excess. I have difficulty in finding my place, my space in the couple. I am burning impatiently over someone or a situation.

I accept↓♥ that it is essential to let go in order to free myself, because by holding back, I block my energy, essentially because I am afraid. Dissatisfaction over events, which produces nervous tension, will inflame my **bladder**. I accept↓♥ to fully live the present instant and I realize that by being open, I allow myself to taste some marvelous experiences. I am in action and moving forward.

BLEEDING *See: BLOOD — BLEEDING*

BLEEDING GUMS *See: GUM BLEEDING*

BLEEDING NOSE *See: NOSE BLEEDING*

BLIND *See: EYES — BLIND*

BLINDNESS *See: EYES — BLINDNESS*

BLISTERS *See: SKIN — BLISTERS*

BLISTERS (fever) / COLD SORES *See: FEVER BLISTERS, HERPES (IN GENERAL)*

BLOOD (in general)

In order for one's car to function properly, one has to get it the right grade of gasoline. The **gasoline** of the body is **blood**, which, in order for it to be effective, must circulate freely throughout the body.

If the gasoline contains waste or dirt, it might damage **the engine, which is the heart♥**. **The blood represents the joy of living, the craving for life**, and the impurities that can be found provoke sickness throughout the body. Depending on what I eat, the stomach produces energy that fortifies my **blood**, or makes me anemic; I have to choose the right grade of gasoline for my body, as I do for my car. **Blood** represents the energy that circulates inside me. It is the very center of the **heart♥**. **The red blood cells** transport oxygen from the lungs to the cells. They carry life and action. **The white blood cells (leukocytes)** defend the organism and represent who I am, my character. The **blood** circulation symbolizes the human being's desire to develop. Poor circulation indicates that **Love** is blocked; I can't express my feelings, I am in conflict with **Love**. A baby in its mother's womb is linked to her through the blood circulation system; the **blood** contains my whole genetic and hereditary baggage. Therefore if I have **blood** ailments, I can ask myself whether I have a conflict with a member of my **family**, my **blood line**, my **clan**: I might feel like a ***stranger***. Am I questioning my belonging on an emotional level?

The message from my body is: I let the **blood flow** in my veins, I let **Love** reach into my **heart♥**, I accept↓♥ to give and to receive, and I want to find my joy of living again. I leave room for new ideas because I am an ***exceptional*** person.

BLOOD DISORDERS *See also: BLOOD / ANEMIA / LEUKEMIA*

Poor **blood circulation** indicates a lack of joy in my life. I feel numb and my ideas are blurring. I feel like I have to fight to live. My **blood** is affected when I live more in my thoughts than in my emotions. I no longer have any joy in living. A disease affecting my **blood** is a sign of a deep, unaccepted↓♥ or unforgiven wound. I have the impression of living a ***clandestine*** life; I feel I am not truly part of a group or a family. I suffer from not having my place in my clan, in my family. Everything gets ***tangled up*** in my head, and I don't know any longer where I should go. As I don't respect myself, I am constantly short of breath and energy. I experience my relationships in a superficial way, where money, power, sex and appearances are paramount. I feel that I have always needed the ***consent*** of others to be 'OK'. I fret and worry all the time in my head, even for trifles. What I really want is to live from my **heart♥** and my sensitivity. I **spit blood** when my sensitivity can't take it any longer, when there is an overflow of painful memories from my past that are following me and that I absolutely need to clear away. It is as if my body needed a change of oil. I need movement, change, something new.

To rediscover joy, I accept↓♥ new ideas, I recognize the beauty surrounding me, I smile at life. I become **Aware** that I will live as long as I wish to live. It only depends on me! I renew contact with the gentleness and **Love** that inhabit me.

BLOOD — ANEMIA *See also: BLOOD / BLOOD CIRCULATION / LEUKEMIA*

Anemia is a diminishing of the level of hemoglobin[10] in the **blood**. At the center of hemoglobin is iron, to which are linked oxygen and carbon dioxide. **Iron-deficiency anemia** (due to a lack of iron in the **blood**) is the most frequent.

Blood represents **joy in living**, **Love** and **emotions**. This condition is related to a lack of joy, strength and depth in the **Love** I feel for myself and for others; to my doubts about my capacity for truly loving with strength and determination; **to a discouragement and a refusal to live**; or to the impression of being worthless and resistant to **Love**, hence this depreciation of myself as a person. I depreciate myself in what makes me live, what carries me in my life, especially my hopes and aspirations. I live my life in a "Yes, but…" mode, therefore with little or no interest, feeling myself restricted by everything. Thus, I think I can't achieve my deepest aspirations. I have the impression that I am going to ***collapse***, that my life or my family is ***falling apart***. What makes me live and upholds me isn't worth much in my eyes. I need to be supported by others because I feel that I am not strong enough to achieve my deepest desires. I may even feel despair and resignation. I feel undermined and weak, and I have such an impression of being drained of energy that I ***turn pale***. It is as if someone was 'sucking' my **blood**; I find myself in ***pieces***. I am smothering in my environment or often in my family, from which I feel apart. Why do I have to push myself to exhaustion to be recognized by the people I **Love**? I may also manifest much rigidity in facing life's events. I may even resent someone to the point of wanting to get rid of him, thinking that this will Lighten my burden. All these symptoms result from a great weakness in my **blood**. We can make a play on words by changing '**Iron**' for '**I run**'. Thus, the **anemic** person

---

10. The pigment of the red globules that transport oxygen from the lungs into the tissues of the body.

no longer feels enough joy and motivation to manage everything she has to **run,** and no longer feels capable of **running** to get whatever she wants. I feel that I can't do what needs to be done to fix a situation, or that what I have to do is not fair. But for what reason(s) do I refuse to use the energy of the Universe that is available to me? What am I afraid of? What 'makes my **blood** boil? Deep down, I feel that I wasn't Loved by my family and I may even, consciously or not, feel like eliminating or removing one of them. I am experiencing a conflict involving the **Love** of my 'clan'. I have no motivation because I don't know, deep down, what truly pleases me. I am not in contact with my inner self. The future becomes blurred, uncertain and dangerous. My negative thoughts about myself drain me of my energy. It is as if I was unable to integrate physical reality.

I accept↓♥ to say **yes** to this great energy that is ready to **lovingly** serve my life.I carefully choose the foods that will help me to nourish my body and my **blood** network and to regain my strength. From now on, I watch, I observe and I discover the joy all around me. It is everywhere: in my family, at work and among my friends. These beings of **Light** also are there to help me grow. I accept↓♥ to live my life instead of the lives of others. I acknowledge my deep desires.

BLOOD — ARTERIES

The **arteries** are the "vessels that conduct oxygenated **blood** from the **heart♥** to the organs".

These same **blood** vessels (as well as all the other **blood** channels, veins, capillaries, etc.) are the means for **Love** to manifest the divine qualities. They reside everywhere in the body and communicate with each part of it. The **arteries** are also related to what is called 'life'. They make the **joy in living** flow, and enable me to **communicate**, **express my emotions** and stay in contact with the Universe. They indicate now intensely I am investing myself in my life. If my nervous tension goes any higher, it will cause an emotional imbalance that may result from an inner conflict between my 'physical world' and my 'spiritual world'. I find myself in a situation where I can't be in action: for instance, I may want to leave home, but something is preventing me from carrying out this action. **Congestion** shows me that I am too involved in one aspect of my life or in an emotion that can be harmful to me, such as anger, jealousy, etc. When I am having a difficulty or when I stop expressing my emotions, I **close** (block) myself, which can result in various diseases related to the **heart♥**, such as angina pectoris, arteriosclerosis, thrombosis, etc. The joy of living stops circulating in me. I may depreciate myself in the actions I accomplish. Everything I want to achieve in my life demands too much effort and energy. It is hard for me to structure my work properly or give it solid foundations. All this can be the origin of an **arterial embolism in a limb**. My **carotids**[11] are affected if I feel I have to constantly defend my ideas or if I fear that the others

11. **Carotids**: Arteries of the neck and head.

are going to steal my good ideas. My frustration and my anger toward life can create an **arteritis**.

In order to allow energy to flow more regularly and thereby prevent the development of certain **scleroses**, which represent energy blocks, I accept↓♥ to be more constantly open to joy and to the circulation of this joy by remaining open in my **heart♥**, by accepting↓♥ to change my attitude and open myself to **Love**, so that this **Love** will be conveyed throughout my body.

BLOOD — BLEEDING

Bleeding can be compared to tears, to a loss of joy. When I suffer, the tears flow, my sorrow is so intense that it is as if I was crying **blood**. Where is my joy in life going? Why this sorrow, this aggressiveness that is making me see red? It may come from my questioning about my origins, my affiliation to my clan, to my bonds of **blood**. **Anorectal bleeding** (**blood in the stools**) shows me how much I hang on to the past. This has the effect of stagnating, or remaining in place. I feel backed against the wall (in general and also in my sexual life) and I blame others and the past for my current misfortunes. I curl in on myself, living in seclusion to avoid being hurt again.

I accept↓♥ my good fortune in being alive and I rediscover joy again. I free myself from all my sadness and I accept↓♥ to receive what life gives me.

BLOOD — BLOOD CIRCULATION *See also: RAYNAUD'S DISEASE*

Blood circulation is linked to the **heart♥** and to **blood**, a symbol of life. **Blood** passes through all the channels of the body: arteries, arterioles, veins, venules and capillaries.

These channels are essential for distributing **Love**, joy and life throughout the whole body. My **heart♥** (center of **Love**) accepts↓♥ to give **blood** (energy) to each part of my being, whatever its importance, without any discrimination. My **blood** represents my vigor, my pleasure in living and what I currently am in this Universe. All my circulatory difficulties are related to **blood** and to the totality of my being. If I experience an emotionally or mentally difficult situation, the energy that animates my being weakens. This weakness in my **blood** and my **blood circulation** means that I am emotionally retreating from a situation that currently affects me because I don't have enough 'energy' to go ahead. I am protecting myself from my overly energetic emotions because it is painful to feel them so present. I am not letting enough **Love** circulate in my life. I criticize myself severely, I am distressed, I am feeling great inner sadness. My joy in living and my good mood are declining, my ideas are becoming confused, my social life is unexciting, dismal and dull. I am closing myself off from life. I need to make lots of projects, ideas and sensations 'circulate'. Otherwise, everything will 'freeze' because of my worries, my sorrows, my fatigue or my anger; an over-excitement or an obsession that unbalances my **blood circulation** will have the same effect. The lack of joy therefore leads me to escape my responsibilities. I have mental blocks that make me avoid certain situations. It is a way of saying **no** to life, unconsciously wishing for death. Thus, several patterns risk re-surfacing (control, going slack, indifference toward life, an exaggerated need for attention, a desire to die). **Blood circulation** disorders appear first in the hands and the legs, in the most external and active parts of my body, those that move me about in the Universe. Poor **circulation** affecting my **legs** is related to my emotional control, to the emotions I can count on and that I want to hold on to. When my **hands** are affected, it is an expression of my emotions and a desire to stop what I am doing. In both cases, my **cold extremities** tell me that I am retreating within myself, relinquishing full emotional participation in my world. I no longer want to go along with the ***party*** and I am keeping my distance! A **blood clot** represents a well-guarded secret, an event where I felt I was being betrayed or cheated, and rather than let the associated emotions flow freely, they have hardened and are showing up in the form of a **blood clot**. The different **blood disorders** are **atherosclerosis**, **arteriosclerosis**, **increased cholesterol levels, thrombosis**, **embolism**, etc.

I accept↓♥ to fully face myself and especially to observe my attitude toward life! Isn't life extraordinary enough to want to fully benefit from it? I open my **heart♥** to **Love**, I take charge of myself and I let life guide me. Whatever happens to me will always be for the best.

BLOOD CELLS / GLOBULES / HEMATOCYTES *See: BLOOD (IN GENERAL)*

BLOOD — CHOLESTEROL[12] *See also: BLOOD / (IN GENERAL) / CIRCULATION*

Cholesterol is linked to the **blood**; it symbolizes the **joy in living.** It comes from certain non-vegetal foods. Our organism transforms it in the liver. It is an essential constituent of the cell walls. When it is in excess, it progressively reduces the diameter of the blood vessels.

Why? Because I no longer have the joy of living! In my deepest inner self, I believe that I have no right to be happy and joyful, and **this joy circulates badly!** I take a look at my 'reasons for living' – *Is my life running along the lines that I wish*? I can ask myself whether I do too much or if I worry too much, especially as far as my mother or family are concerned. I might have an increase in my **cholesterol** level after certain events, for example: after retiring, because I have no joy for living as I did when I was with my work colleagues or with people I met through my work. This can also happen when someone I **Love** and who brings a **Love** of living disappears from my life. Here, instead of developing diabetes, which is a deep sadness; my body interprets the event as a lack of joy in living and increases the **cholesterol** level. It might also be when I lose a pet, or any other kind of situation, **conscious** or unconscious, where my joy in living decreases. I often also feel unsafe. I experience a situation as **dramatic**. It could be a case where **I want to undertake a project**

---

12. **Cholesterol**: There are several types of **cholesterol** including **LDL** (**L**ow **D**ensity **L**ipoproteins, also called 'bad' **cholesterol**) and **HDL** (**H**igh **D**ensity **L**ipoproteins, also called 'good' **cholesterol**).

or build something that is dear to my **heart♥** but that nobody can help me to achieve. **I can therefore only rely on myself and this greatly affects me**. If I let this situation get any worse I could have a **heart♥ attack**. In fact, if I don't resolve the situation that makes me experience this lack of joy, it will affect the area in my life that is **Love**. When my joy diminishes, I feel as though there is less **Love** inside me, and that's why my **heart♥** is affected. A **high cholesterol level** also points out that I find it difficult to be truly involved in life. I am like an actor playing out a role at the theatre: I belong to the play, but I don't fully enact the emotions. I play a role to please others, when I should be pleasing myself. I have become hyper-altruistic to avoid being judged as an egocentric. I have the impression that my dreams are unacceptable and impossible to realize. I am searching for my own identity. I no longer identify myself with my family, which I see as broken up and destroyed. This can be my biological family or a group that I or my work colleagues belong to. I want the group to cohere closely together and live in harmony, but I feel unable to intervene. Most of the animal **cholesterol** (from meat and milk products) appears because of the overly rich food we eat in Western society. My food contains a lot of **cholesterol** and represents a certain selfish satisfaction of my appetite. I feel good, without thinking that this excess could very well change and even destroy my health! It is an illusion to imagine that I am pleasing my body. I can check to find out if I like myself in an 'egotistic or egocentric way'. By swallowing these foods containing too much **cholesterol**, I renounce the joys of living. I will pay for this one day. Do I actually want to be sick?

I accept↓♥ to change immediately by letting joy flow inside me, like a child who is enchanted by the beauties of life! I can neutralize my fear of living the joys of life and I accept↓♥ that this can be part of my life. I accept↓♥ to be myself, to fulfill my dreams. I will savor every moment, and I have the right to be happy.

BLOOD CIRCULATION *See: BLOOD — BLOOD CIRCULATION*

BLOOD COAGULATED (in veins or arteries), CLOTS *See also: BLOOD — THROMBOSIS*

Blood represents joy circulating in my body.

When it **coagulates**, it forms a **clot**, a semi-solid mass. This clot is necessary to stop a hemorrhage when **blood** vessels are ruptured. When **coagulation** is **deficient**, the emotional injury that manifests itself through the hemorrhage seems impossible for me to overcome and to heal. In a sense, it is as if I was letting myself die: my powerlessness, my 'lack of power over my life' generates despair. I am always in the past. My deep energies are unbalanced. When a **clot** forms spontaneously (**thrombosis**), for example because of poor circulation, it can produce an **occlusion**[13] or an **embolism**. It is as if I decided to put a cork that has the effect of cutting off all circulation. This **clot** may symbolize a well-kept secret, a lie, or some cheating that was never expressed.

---

13. **Occlusion**: A total or partial obstruction.

I accept↓♥ to allow joy to pulse in me, I am awakening to a new life. I acknowledge my power and my rightful place. Each situation, each difficulty in my life brings me more wisdom and **Love**. I have everything I need to change my life: I only need to make the decision!

BLOOD — DIABETES MELLITUS *See also: BLOOD — HYPOGLYCEMIA, DISEASES [HEREDITARY]*

Diabetes is defined as a disease that has an over-abundance of a urine substance. When one uses the sole term **diabetes**, it means **diabetes mellitus** ('**sugar diabetes**'); the terms **juvenile**, **lean** and **infantile diabetes** are also used). It is caused by an insufficient secretion of insulin by the pancreas, which cannot maintain sugar at a sufficient level in the **blood**. So there is an excess of sugar in the **blood**, yet the **blood** cannot adequately use this sugar in the **blood** flow. These excess sugars are detected through an increase of **glycemia** and the appearance of sugar in the urine.

As sugar is linked to Love, tenderness and affection, diabetes reflects various feelings of inner sadness. This is **Love** sickness, a sure lack of **Love**. I therefore need to control my environment and those around me, because of my previous wounds. I am experiencing an emotional abstinence. Yes! **If I am diabetic, I usually experience repetitive sadness, repressed emotions stamped with unconscious sadness without any gentleness, which makes me *harder*.** Gentleness has disappeared and has been replaced with ongoing pain. I then start eating sugar of every possible variety, pasta, bread, sweets, etc., to compensate. This can sorely affect my emotional, social or financial life. I have the impression that I must 'take it', I am ***forced to struggle and take on life***, people or events. I try to compensate in every possible way. I restrict myself in many ways. I become bitter toward life, which is why I find myself bitter, and I compensate by a more 'sugary' state. I am full of regrets for what was and what could have been; I think that I am not worthy of happiness or pleasure.

As I have trouble receiving **Love**, I feel suffocated and overloaded, stuck in an excessive and uncontrollable situation. This situation that I can't seem to manage leads me toward compensatory food habits and overweight, which provoke **diabetes**. I have a great need for **Love** and affection, especially from my father, but I don't know how to act and how to react when I do receive this. I find this unfair, I doubt, or don't trust, any authority exerted over me, whether by my father, by my boss or by a person representing authority in my religion. I find it difficult to receive **Love** from others, and life has no pleasure for me. As I can't accept↓♥ the 'little **sweetnesses** of life', I become **diabetic,** which consequently forbids me to eat the 'little sugary things' I used to eat. I find it difficult to let myself go and express true **Love**. I may not be able to express joy, **Love** or passion openly, because of a particular situation that imprisons me. My expectations are often excessive, as I want people to fulfill my desires. These expectations make me frustrated, angry about life and make me close myself in. **I experience a lot of resistance when I am confronted with a**

situation that I want to avoid and feel compelled to suffer and I **refuse to give way**. I just **can't give up** like that!

For instance, it might be a separation, a change of house, an exam, etc. The emotions experienced in this kind of situation are often linked to the loss of a Loved one, a deep solitude which can even make me feel despair. My family, or what represents my family, is usually involved. **A feeling of disgust, loathing, or scorn toward this situation, is linked to this resistance**. Since this situation arose, and because of all the different constraints, it is difficult for me to find the gentle sweetness that I need. Even if time goes by, the lack and the pain still resist and persist. I have lost my best friend, or a close companion, or one of the few persons in whom I could confide and who knew me well. I resist because, without realizing it, I am frightened of something or someone, I have become paranoid[14] about it. Consciously or not, I think about this constantly. I have the impression that I have to face a serious ***adversary***, and I don't know who will turn out to be the 'strongest'. Will it be stronger than me? Is it inside or outside of me? This situation is very ***nerve-wracking*** for me. I am reluctantly 'ready to fight'! That is the reason why my high **blood** sugar level constitutes the reserves that are necessary for me to 'be ready at all times' (it is the sugar in the **blood** that furnishes the energy that my muscles need to fight). If I am in conflict with authority, is it possible that I derive some pleasure from resisting someone or something, or a principle?

Hyperglycemia appears at this point. I might feel helpless. This means that I am unable to undertake any kind of action, to **get to the end** of what I have to do. A lack of energy stops me from going forward. I feel pushed to do things that I want to **resist**. Biologically, the sugar contained in my body is what produces the increase in energy that makes my body move.

The sugar level increases in my **blood** because this is the one that can be transformed and used the quickest. I therefore become strong and 'powerful', which enables me to accomplish things quickly and efficiently. I need to take control of myself now. I need to change the situations that affect me, starting with **Love** and joy in all things. Sugar is related to sweetness and **Love**.

As **a child who has diabetes**, I fear that one or both of my parents will not trust me or will be disappointed in me. I am afraid of flourishing, of becoming myself. I need gentleness and affection, but I don't know how to go and find what will meet these needs. I am insecure, but I don't know how to express this, so I toughen myself. I feel strained before the sheer scope of a task, and I would rather not have to face it. I worry all the time, and I am going in circles. It is as if I had no hold on my life, as if everything was imposed on me. I am anxious because I don't know who I am. I don't know how to trust myself. I still haven't accepted↓♥ my 'I' as a human being. I feel insecure and unsettled before the life that awaits me. I resist aging and becoming a 'grownup'. **Diabetes** (or **hyperglycemia**, too much sugar in the **blood**) and **hypoglycemia**

14. **Paranoia**: A mental disorder characterized by illusions of greatness and of persecution.

(not enough sugar in the **blood**), both of which are related to a lack of joy, are directly linked to the **Love** that I am capable of expressing toward myself and others. In the case of **gestational diabetes**, which usually appears in the second half of pregnancy, I must ask myself the same questions as those asked by a person suffering from **diabetes. I may consciously discover a deep sadness, reluctance or resistance.** This pregnancy may activate and amplify in me the more or less conscious memory of these feelings experienced in my childhood, and make me develop **diabetes.** After the child is born, the return to my normal state indicates to me that these feelings have disappeared or that their importance has greatly diminished, which restores the **blood** sugar level (glucose). As a mother, I must ask myself if I don't feel that I, too, am tiny and dependent like my little baby right now. Sometimes I am incapable of taking my place, which greatly distresses me. Now, is this baby going to be still another person who will invade my space? I already find it hard to accept↓♥ myself as I am. The fact of being pregnant modifies my body, and I find it difficult to be in harmony with this new image that I project. I see myself as a lazy, passive person and I persecute myself instead of giving myself **Love** and compassion. If I am **diabetic** and I must receive injections of insulin, I must ask myself what this dependence is related to on the affective level: am I still dependent upon one or both of my parents? Do I give others as much **Love** and affection as I need to receive myself, or do I feel too 'empty' and alone to be able to give such **Love**? Who or what am I ***hanging on to***, or ***clinging to***? There is so much **Love** available; am I truly **Aware** of the **Love** that people have for me? People **Love** me, and from now on, I must see it. If I am a child, it is time for me to take initiatives and go ahead. Several opportunities present themselves for me to improve my living conditions, but I resist them because they will also have the effect of bringing substantial changes into my life. I am tired of always living hand-to-mouth. I may not feel supported by my father or whoever represents him, or he shows no interest in me or in my activities. I feel his indifference. If I am a woman, or if I am a man with a highly developed feminine side, I desire to become more active and independent. However, I know that this will bother the people around me, and I am afraid it will estrange me from the people I **Love**. Besides, I have trouble in accepting↓♥ their advice because I believe it curtails my freedom. My ego sometimes erupts, which takes the form of violent fits of anger or staking out rigid positions.

I accept↓♥ my past for what it is, in a detached way. I open myself to life, knowing that it holds only beautiful moments if I am ready to accept↓♥ them. I believe in myself and I don't need anyone to lean on: I have all the courage and determination necessary to create my own happiness. It is by opening my **heart♥** that miracles will happen! Letting go of my **resistance** liberates me from my frustrations, and I can live in harmony with life and its seasons. I learn to feel safe when looking for affection and tenderness, and I can feel **Love** coming from those near to me. I become **Aware** of my own worth. I become more spontaneous and let my inner child fill up with gaiety and self assurance. I thereby no longer destroy myself, and I give myself a safe, pleasant life filled with sweetness.

BLOOD — GANGRENE *See also: AMPUTATION, INFECTIONS*

Ischemic **gangrene** is the result of a stopped **blood** flow in one or several parts of the body, which causes the death of the tissues in the affected areas.

Blood flow is related to the expression of my **Love** to, or its withdrawal from, the Universe, and also to my joy in living. If, for instance, **gangrene** affects my legs, it is therefore because the withdrawal or the cutting off of **Love** within me is so deep that it completely stops any forward movement. Usually in such a case, fear for the future and insecurity about what is in store for me are quite present. I destroy and poison myself by my deep-rooted guilt, shame or sorrow, and part of me is dying. I feel deeply soiled. I stagnate instead of evolving; I move back instead of advancing. I have lost my creative power.

Life is leaving me, joy is no longer here. As I am destroying myself, so am I wishing it upon others, being under the impression that I hold some power over them and wanting them to feel just as powerless as I am. In the case of **dry gangrene**, the **blood** no longer irrigates the tissues. I must therefore regain contact with myself and with the joy that must inhabit me regarding the side of my life that involves my affected body part.

In the case of **moist gangrene**, which also results from an infection, I am facing poisonous thoughts and thoughts of death for myself or for life. **Gas gangrene** (rarer) is due to the bacterial infection of a wound, generally by bacteria developing in an environment devoid of air or oxygen. As a result, nauseating gases, emanating from the proliferating infectious germs, form under the skin. Not only are the ideas of death from one part of me present, but also a deep rejection of the same part of me that makes me experience this situation.

I accept↓♥ to better integrate **blood** and **Love** in the expression of who I am, in my life. I learn to accept↓♥ myself as I am and to rediscover the joys of life. I become the master of my life.

BLOOD — HEMATOMA *See also: ACCIDENT, BLOOD / (IN GENERAL) / BLOOD CIRCULATION*

A **hematoma** results from a hemorrhage causing an accumulation, a collection of **blood** in a tissue or an organ.

As a **hematoma** almost always occurs after a trauma, I must ask myself what fear or what guilt feeling is preventing me from allowing joy to flow freely in my life. It may be a punishment I am inflicting on myself. I feel myself in the middle of a disaster. I am trying to regain contact with my full potential.

The accumulation of **blood** indicates to me that I must put more joy in my life, and the affected body part informs me of the side of my life that will most benefit from showing this joy.

BLOOD — HEMATURIA *See also: ADENOMA, BLADDER / DISORDERS / CYSTITIS, URINE [URINARY INFECTIONS]*

Hematuria is the presence of **blood** in the urine in a microscopic[15] or macroscopic[16] form.

As urine represents my old emotions that I release, and as a loss of **blood** indicates a loss of joy, then **hematuria** symbolizes a more or less intense sadness about my past emotions that are tearing me up inside. It has been a long time since I had a good laugh. I would like to go far away, leaving my heavy responsibilities behind me. I feel immature in some areas of my life, but deep down, I know I can become a leader. I can no longer see clearly in a situation that often involves my partner and where I feel stuck. It is as if **Love** has been torn and destroyed. I then become rigid and on the defensive. I am confused and I doubt my decisions because I no longer have any self-confidence. I may experience a conflict with a member of my family I would like to get rid of. I must identify all these events that tore me up emotionally, in order to be able to find gentleness and understanding and to let healing take place.

I accept↓♥ to take some time to examine the changes I need to make in my life. I also accept↓♥ right now to convert my ideas and my dreams into physical actions. That is how joy will flow in me again.

BLOOD — HEMOPHILIA *See also: BLOOD / (IN GENERAL) / DISEASES / BLOOD CIRCULATION / DIABETES, DISEASES [HEREDITARY]*

Hemophilia is a hereditary disease linked to a **blood** coagulation disorder. It is transmitted by the mother, and only boys develop this disease. Daughters do not present it (except sometimes for some minor disorders).

Because my **blood** has difficulty in coagulating, a cut or an injury can cause **blood** losses that are difficult to stop, which can put my life in danger. Even if this disease is known as hereditary, the fact still remains that I must become **conscious** of something involving joy. The least accident or incident risks putting my life in danger if I don't intervene quickly. I need to become **Aware** in my life of whatever can make me experience despair to the point where I could die from **blood** loss. I don't feel safe in my affective and social life. I have never truly integrated the outside world. I am living in stark solitude and with the feeling that I am incapable of making a success of my life. Everything I undertake 'turns to vinegar'. I was hurt a lot in my past, and I feel forced to always be on the defensive. A 'menace' looms over me. I react disproportionately when I am thwarted. I always have a doubt following me and preventing me from being autonomous and moving ahead. There is a

15. **Microscopically**: That is not visible to the naked eye in the urine: that is detected only under the microscope.

16. **Macroscopically**: That can be detected in the urine by the naked eye, either by its reddish tint or the traces of blood that may appear in it.

duality: I want to be autonomous, but I am dependent and I want to be coddled. I live according to others instead of following the impetus of my **heart♥**. I can examine in what respects **diabetes**, when seen in a certain **Light**, can resemble what I am experiencing.

I accept↓♥ to trust myself. I charge ahead instead or remaining on the defensive: I know that if I follow my **heart♥**, I am always guided and protected. I welcome **Love** and gentleness into my life. I have more joy in my **heart♥**.

BLOOD — HEMORRHAGE

A **hemorrhage** is characterized by a loss of **blood** from a **blood** vessel.

This uncontrolled effusion of **blood** is often associated with emotional distress or trauma. My emotions, held back for too long, such as aggressiveness and anguish, become uncontrollable inside, and suddenly erupt. I may experience events that don't go according to my expectations or desires. Having reached the end of my rope and mentally exhausted, I let go, and a great part of my joy in life suddenly leaves my body. My great emotional wound, still open and raw, shows itself as a **hemorrhage**. I may have been ***humiliated***, attacked in my innermost self, and I was unable to defend myself. I feel crushed, ***massacred***, powerless, and I am feeling a lot of aggressiveness. I am living dangerously because life isn't worth much anyway. I am losing my strength and my joy in living. It is as if I was repudiating myself. I am searching for stability in my life. My family is broken up, and this saddens me a lot. It is important to see what part of the body is affected to have more information about what I am experiencing. For example, a **uterine hemorrhage** tells me that I am experiencing a loss of joy involving my family, my home. A **stomach hemorrhage** tells me that there is a **blood** overflow associated with an emotional shock that I just can't 'digest'. I am eating away at myself inside; I am losing my joy in life. Resolving this situation of bereavement is a matter of urgency, so that I can regain better **blood** circulation. **Post-natal blood losses** are normal. However, when labor is prolonged, the uterus is too distended and a **hemorrhage** may occur, often associated with anxiety, an emotional upheaval or trauma, or even with **post-partum** physical or moral lassitude. I hold in for some time, I become tense and I let go all at once; it is the resistance barrier that falls, along with my vital energy. I find myself alone, and I am confronted with myself. Previously, all my attention was focused on the baby in me. The **Love** I felt inside of me is replaced with an emptiness that others can't fill. In a sense, I am separated from myself.

I accept↓♥ to become **Aware** of the fears associated with childbirth, I learn to breathe better and focus my attention on the '**here and now'** to stay in control of my emotions, contracting and uncontracting my uterus, and I free my child calmly by trusting myself. Listening to my body, I can see a message that will help me to live better in harmony. I accept↓♥ to let go and express my emotions more freely. Feeling freer, I focus my attention on the joy within me and around me.

BLOOD — HYPOGLYCEMIA *See also: ALLERGIES (IN GENERAL), BLOOD — DIABETES, BRAIN — BALANCE [LOSS OF]*

Hypoglycemia is characterized by an abnormal diminishing of glucose[17] in the **blood,** most often by an insufficient supply of caloric energy or by an excess of very sugary food, sometimes by an excess of insulin[18] treatment. The part of the pancreas that secretes insulin is over-activated. As a result, the cells and the muscles are deprived of energy-rich glucose. This situation is the obverse of what we see in diabetics. It is caused by an excess of insulin or of exercise.

Sugar represents a form of **reward**, of **affection**, of **gentleness** and **tenderness**. It is the manifestation of **Love**, according to metaphysics. Currently, am I seeking this **Love**? Am I expecting it from outside? Do I eat sugar to fill this gap? Several manifestations are related to **hypoglycemia**: it may manifest itself because I am giving so much to others that I have nothing left to give myself. My life is unbalanced, and I feel like dropping everything and running away. This shows me the need to begin by loving myself and respecting my own needs. **Hypoglycemia** comes from my strong emotions, from a deep sadness causing me to feel anguish and even hostility and an ***aversion*** to others. Do I have expectations to which others are not responding and which remain unsatisfied? I refuse what comes from outside, especially from the person in authority, and I am feeling greatly annoyed. I may also feel intense fear of something or someone who ***disgusts*** me and whom I prefer to avoid. I may be disgusted by my physical body that I constantly see in the mirror. I must **resist** with all my strength to try and avoid this ***horrible*** and ***odious*** thing that ***disgusts*** me and that I find ***repulsive***. My strength is ***diminished*** by it. It may be an object as well as a gesture, or something that was said and that made me feel like throwing up. This thing or person I find ***repulsive*** is also ***abject***! I may react by stopping to resist, so that the 'thing' will stop as quickly as possible. If I am being threatened with physical violence, then if I stop arguing or retorting, the other party is more likely to quickly relent than if I persist, even if what I am enduring and imposing on myself is intolerable. I get to the point where the sLightest act in my life is ***tedious***. I feel like ***tossing*** everything overboard. **Hypoglycemia** can also appear when I am experiencing excessive inner tensions or pressures over which I believe I have no control. My life is unbalanced and I am wholly disoriented. A food allergy can also be the 'physical' cause of this lowering of my **blood** sugar. I must therefore carry out the necessary physical verifications and find out to whom, or to what, I am allergic. When I am in a situation of **hypoglycemia**, I become weak, which reminds me that in certain situations I like to feel weak and a victim, and thereby get people's attention. This is easier than to keep a straight back and fight for what I believe in. I have been playing hide-and-seek, but I must accept↓♥ to take the reins of my life in my own hands.

---

17. **Glucose**: A form of sugar in the **blood**.

18. **Excess of insulin treatment**: Because insulin helps to diminish the glucose (**blood** sugar).

I accept↓♥ what happens to me and I know that by giving more of myself, I will then be able to give more and **Love** others. I can't give to others what I don't give to myself. I decide to make my life more joyful. I meet my expectations. My body is a wise, loyal friend to whom I am receptive. I accept↓♥ my role as a leader, instead of following others.

BLOOD — INFECTIOUS MONONUCLEOSIS *See also: ANGINA (IN GENERAL), FATIGUE, HEADACHES, INFECTIONS (IN GENERAL), SPLEEN*

Infectious mononucleosis is an infection characterized by an increase in the lymphocytes that are part of the **blood**'s leukocytes, or white globules. This disease is found mainly in adolescents and young adults. It is also called the '**kissing disease**' because it can be transmitted by saliva.

If I am an adult and I have this disease, I try to find out what may have affected me, as if I was an adolescent, or what it reminds me of from the time of my adolescence. I want to live fully, I sense a change in me and **I feel that I have to constantly fight to obtain what I want**. My system of defense has evolved to compensate for the attacks and limitations that I had the impression of receiving from life. I feel I am ***alone*** to face the obstacles that come up before me, far from my clan. I want so much to feel ***accepted↓♥*** by my family, my friends, and society! Just like a wolf, I want to be part of the ***pack***. But I feel so alone, like a ***scrap*** of waste in society. I disparage myself and I get to the point of wanting to push other people away, but at the same time I need to hang onto them. This brings about an inner duality and great tension. I develop **mononucleosis** when I feel guilty over a situation or when I want more permission, when I criticize people or life in general. I have a deep **Love** sickness. **Mononucleosis** has a link with problems involving the **spleen**, for this organ then increases in volume.

I accept↓♥ to clean up my life and to put more **Love** in it for myself and for others. I get back my courage and my self-confidence, and I can then recover my energy and my joy in living, which will enable me to experience more **Love**.

BLOOD — LEUKEMIA *See also: BLOOD / ANEMIA / BLOOD CIRCULATION, CANCER (IN GENERAL)*

I have **blood cancer** or **leukemia** when my white globules proliferate out of control.

Blood cancer is joy that is no longer flowing freely in my life. I have hate deeply hidden in me, often directed at one of my parents. I am destroying myself and refusing to fight. If I am a child with **leukemia**, it is because I am refusing to be re-born, I am deeply disappointed with what I see on earth. Growing up represents a danger for me.I see all the pressure put on me to succeed, and it is too much for me. I want to go away and leave this body. **Leukemia** often appears after the death of a Loved one (it can even be an animal that I especially liked). It may be a distance that has opened up between me and one of my parents, often the father, and which I find very painful to live through. I have the impression that I have to join another family or another clan in order to be defended. Whether I am a child or a little older, I want so much to please the family and meet their high expectations that I will 'kill myself' to get there. This form of **cancer** is directly related to the expression of **Love** within oneself. It may also appear after a significant event for me, which made me depreciate myself. This depreciation affected my whole being, and I feel it very intensely and deeply. Take the example of a young boy who was rejected for a place on the village or neighborhood hockey team. It is a tragedy! It is as if life no longer had any meaning and was no longer worth living. I am only good for **bits and scraps**, I feel ***pathetic***. I seek my place in a group or in my family. I no longer have any motivation, so I no longer want to build a life for myself. I may have the impression that I have to constantly over-protect myself to obtain what I want. I may feel defenseless (**children** and **the elderly** are the ones most often affected, by the way). I may have experienced intense frustration and I violently choked off my emotions. If my **Love** or my desire to live has been hurt in any way, my attitude in loving may become distrustful, confused and alienated. I then want to insulate myself from all feelings. Instead of living with my emotions, I ***pretend***. Life no longer has any meaning. I may feel I am a slave to another person. I have lost my deep identity, I no longer feel like defending myself. **Love** is absent, especially my father's. I replace **Love** with money, to some extent. My ego is 'worn out'. If I am older, already retired for example, I may realize that it is now too late to achieve my ambitions. I am experiencing disappointments with my projects: either I have too many of them, which is too heavy a burden and I won't be able to complete all of them, or I have the impression that it is now too late to complete any of them. I have ***rage*** in my **heart♥**.

I accept↓♥ to go with life instead of against it. I take the best available means for me to change surviving for living. I am thus more at peace with myself and I no longer feel the need to defend myself beyond measure. I let go of the past and undertake to be true at all times. I renew contact with my deep desires. I have the courage to show my deepest emotions. Whether I am a child or an adult, I must live in truth and authenticity to regain contact with the life that inhabits me.

BLOOD — LEUKOPENIA

Leukopenia is a lowering of the white globules, an imbalance in the **blood**. The white globules then become little soldiers who drop arms.

I no longer feel like struggling: I am too sad. It may be a form of escape, for I force myself to go on in the same order, thus preventing myself from experiencing new things in order to always feel safe and in control over the situation. I am emotionally impoverished, and I need to be together with my family, in calm and harmony.

I accept↓♥ to take care of myself to rebuild my inner strength and find a greater taste for life and all that is exciting about it.

BLOOD — PHLEBITIS

Phlebitis is defined by a blocking of **blood** in the veins, mainly in the lower limbs, caused by a clot induced by an immobilization (plaster cast), a varicose[19] pathology or a **blood** hyper coagulation.

Blood represents the free circulation of life in the veins of my lower limbs. My means of locomotion is therefore limited, irritated and defective, because this blocking of **blood** indicates to me a loss of joy related to the legs, which transport me toward the different destinations in my life. **Phlebitis** appears when I experience a brutal event in my life that gives me a great feeling of confusion and limits my freedom. I feel like 'biting someone enough to make them **bleed'**. As the **blood** is no longer flowing back upwards in my legs, I feel compelled to 'pump up the spirits' of someone, often my husband, whose "morale is always low" and who sees everything darkly. Depending on whether it is the left leg (my inner self) or the right one (my outer self), or both legs, the loss of joy will identify for me at what level or in what direction I hesitate or refuse to advance, to accept↓♥ a new destination. I fret about certain situations that life presents me with. I therefore experience a stopping, a slowing down because of an emotion, a feeling that limits my joy, my pleasure in living. I may experience frustration with my sexuality. I tend to blame others and ***despise*** them; I hold them responsible for the deprivations I may be experiencing and for taking away my joy in living and in moving forward. I feel 'unsteady on my legs', unstable. My doubts weigh heavily. I feel powerless. Do I ***deserve*** to be happy? I feel that I am marking time, that nothing is moving. Or could it be that this is actually what I want?

I accept↓♥ to let go of the sadness, the discontent and the frustration that I am experiencing, and to act responsibly for what happens in my life. I accept↓♥ to have the power to create my life as I want it to be; however, I must accept↓♥ that I have a right to happiness and that I deserve having joy and peace illuminate my road. I turn back to myself, at the **heart♥** of life and truth.

BLOOD — PLATELETS *See also: BLOOD / COAGULATED / THROMBOSIS*

The **platelets** are blood cells that play an important role in coagulation.

When the number of **platelets** falls below normal (**thrombopenia**), I must ask myself what can be the source of my difficulty in integrating in my family or in a group with which I identify. There are conflicts where the relations that already exist in this group are precarious and risk breaking up if the persons involved do not decide to ***act***. I would want to intervene to be able to 'stick things back together again', but something is preventing me from doing this. I feel fragile in this situation, for I don't want to hurt anyone. I feel alone on my side, fallen between two stools and powerless.

I accept↓♥ that I have power only over my own life. I remain neutral about the decisions of others, especially those that affect the members of my family.

19. **Varicose**: Swollen or enlarged (veins).

I know that we are all guided in our choices, and I allow the Universe to take care of the people I **Love**. I take care of myself without letting myself be influenced by the statements or the conflicts of others.

BLOOD — SEPTICEMIA

Septicemia is a severe infection (a generalized poisoning) of the **blood**.

It is what we call fretting or **plaguing one's life**. I play the role of a victim, but I really should ask myself: "By whom, or by what, am I letting my existence be poisoned or contaminated?" I am stagnating in a situation, I feel myself 'rotting'.

I accept↓♥ to take full responsibility for my choices, and I become **Aware** of the joys of life.

BLOOD — THROMBOSIS *See also: BLOOD / BLOOD CIRCULATION / COAGULATED*

The **blood** circulating in my veins represents my joy in living. A **thrombosis**, which is defined by a formation of **blood** clots in a vein or an artery, provokes a block preventing the **blood** from circulating freely.

This condition shows that there is also a block in the freeing and circulation of **Love**. Feeling alone, I am saddened and I have the impression that the difficulties I am running into are too heavy to bear and that I am unable to overcome them. I lose my joy in living. My life seems to be stagnating, I feel neglected, abandoned and misunderstood. I feel that I no longer have any **Love** in me, I become inflexible; I am increasingly firm in the way that I act and think, which provokes the hardening of my arteries. I fight against any change, and I stay put on my positions. Is there a situation or a belief that I hang on to and don't dare let go of? This manifestation affects my whole body. It is interesting to note that a **thrombosis** often manifests itself in the **veins**. I may be in a situation where I find it difficult to receive, especially help (either psychological or material and financial) from others. I think I am able to do everything by myself. I hold back **Love**. When the **thrombosis** appears on my **legs**, it indicates to me a fear of moving forward, a tendency to stay 'frozen', or to slow down. I may feel myself 'rooted to the spot'. It can also indicate the insecurity I feel over seeing a **Love** leaving me or seeing myself leaving this **Love**. By trying to hold it back in this way, I increase the odds of seeing it die. I may be feeling 'stuck' in my emotions.

I accept↓♥ to increasingly open myself up to life and I accept↓♥ these changes as signs of my development. I allow my frustrations to express themselves, and I thereby become more active and creative.

BLOOD — VARICOSE VEINS

Varicose veins (**varices**) are usually located in the legs. They are the result of dilated **veins**: the **blood** can no longer flow freely back up to the **heart♥** because the valvulæ in the veins no longer function normally.

My legs enable me to advance in life, to move from one place to another. **Varices in the legs** indicate poor circulation. I can therefore conclude that the place where I no longer am suits me, or that I don't like what I am currently doing. I no longer find any joy in it. It may be an affective relationship, or work that has become tedious. It may be at home, where I am depreciating myself in the eyes of the family. I am seeking my place, my 'little nest'. I can no longer advance in a specific direction, but I don't know how to withdraw from it. My life is full of dissatisfactions; it is dull and without passion. I then become '**avaricious'** of my smiles and of my gaiety. I always want more! The structures in which I make my way no longer suit me. Blood represents my joy in living and the circulation of **Love** in my world, and my veins are its means of locomotion. The **blood** in my veins is on its way back to my **heart♥**, bringing back with it all the **Love** it has received from the Universe. **Varicosity** may indicate that a deep emotional conflict is directly related to my capacity to **Love** myself and to receive all that **Love**. I am no longer true to myself. The direction I have taken or the ground on which I stand are no longer giving me what I expect, emotionally speaking. This blocks and muddles my 'emotional movement'. I have the impression of dragging an enormous weight, like the prisoner who must constantly drag along his ball and chain. This weight will often be a financial one, with money causing me many headaches, and the temptation of avarice looming in my future. In general, I have the impression that I suffer situations more than I create them. I live under a feeling of obligation, with all sorts of things I 'have to do', which prevents me from being myself and doing things for myself. **Varicose veins in the legs** often appear during a pregnancy, which shows that certain fears are linked to this condition; as a pregnant woman, I am afraid of sharing this **Love** with another person, of losing my individuality in my new role as a mother, and of all the responsibility involved in taking care of a child. What place will I hold with this child and my spouse? Will I have all the help and support I will need? The burden of my responsibilities will get even heavier. I feel overwhelmed, and I am afraid of not doing everything, because I tend to amplify the small details. That is when discouragement may occur. I don't feel sustained and supported (it is interesting to note that the wearing of compression **stockings** for support is recommended for women who have **varicose veins** or to prevent them from appearing). I have the impression that I give far more than I receive in return. To re-balance this situation, it is important for me to learn to like what I do.

I accept↓♥ my freedom to choose and to move about as I want. I make myself respected, and I express my needs. I ask for help if necessary. I no longer need to justify myself. I live from my **heart♥** and I take care of myself. I fully enjoy life.

BLUE BABY *See: CHILD — BABY [BLUE]*

BODY (in general) *See: APPENDIX I*

BOILS (vaginal) *See: SKIN — FURONCLES [VAGINAL]*

BOILS / FURUNCLES / CARBUNCLES *See: SKIN — FURUNCLES*

BONE(S) (in general)

The **bones** are the solid framework of the body, the pillars, the tree of life. Within the **bone** itself there exists the marrow, the deepest core of my being, which gives birth to the immune cells that have the ability to protect me.

The energy of the kidneys (linked to fears and insecurities/self-confidence) nourishes the **bones** and the marrow. The **bones** concern my structure, the ***fundamental*** framework on which my entire being is constructed, the **support** for my whole emotional body. They are thus also related to the structure of laws and fundamental principles with which I must deal every day and that are applied by authorities (police, teachers, parents, etc.) to provide support and for peace and order to prevail. When I am a child growing up, I position myself toward authority and often, once I have reached the size where I am now as tall as my authoritarian mother, my attitude toward her will change significantly.

I accept↓♥ to stop being afraid, and I learn to **trust myself**.

BONE DISEASES

Ailments or **diseases** of the **bones**, including **bone cancer**, reflect a rebellion against the authority that I have been resisting, feeling powerless to act against a particular situation dictated by certain existing laws or principles. I have the impression that someone is bilking my efforts. I oppose authority. I can ask myself if I feel deeply upset in my basic beliefs, in my deepest convictions. I am very **disappointed** with several aspects of my life and with society in general.

I may even feel ***distressed***, being so affected by certain situations. If an ailment or a disease affects my **bones**, I must ask myself regarding what facet or aspect of my person I am **depreciating myself**, almost wanting to make it ***disappear***. My worth as a human being is at issue. I feel like a piece of ***trash***, of waste. Do I feel myself being ***annihilated***, ***broken***, ***shattered***, and destroyed by others? Either I depreciate myself and I find it difficult to make people respect me, or I am hiding behind an image that shows only my positive side. I prefer to appear hard and cold: it gives me the impression of being in control, while in fact I am trembling in fear at the idea of making contact with my emotions. I feel weak, defenseless, ***shiftless*** even. Feeling myself inferior, I have trouble standing straight. In a sense, I feel I am already dead. I am worthless, I am nothing. I am structured on nothing. My life revolves around emptiness and loss. I am not allowed to make mistakes. I am very ***austere*** in my everyday life. Have I ***violated*** or transgressed some law, and I am now feeling guilt and remorse? I may want to hang on to the image I give of myself in order to gain some superficial self-esteem. I would so much like to be a***ccompanied*** in what I am experiencing. If I notice and analyze what part of my skeleton is affected, I will have a good indication about which aspect of my existence is involved. In what area of my life, or to whom do I have the impression that I have to submit? I am rebelling against the organization of society and I want to circumvent the prevailing laws. If I **break a bone**, I must ask myself what is '**broken'** in my life and that I resist so much that I have to break a **bone** to help me to stop, in order to become **Aware** of it. A condition affecting my **bones** shows me how I sometimes feel like I am de-structured. My body is sending me an **SOS**.

I accept↓♥ to allow myself more flexibility and to stop pressuring myself for no reason. I take the time to look inside of me and, if need be, I ask for help in order to see more clearly in the decisions I must take. I trust in the fact that everything is in place and that I am guided. Like an ***architect***, I too can build my life with all the elements I want.

BONES — ACROMEGALIA

Acromegalia is characterized by an exaggerated growth of the **bones** in the extremities and in the face. The growth hormone is therefore being secreted in far greater quantity than the normal level.

If I am in this situation, I ask myself in what situation I felt I was too little to undertake or complete a project. Where did I feel too small, too slender and too weak to be able to take my place and make people respect me? My body's answer was to grow excessively in order to help me in taking my place more easily. I thank it! I wanted to impress, to show I was the strongest. I may have felt I was abandoned by one of my parents, and the anxiety of being hurt again makes me be distant from the people around me. Though I may feel that my body takes up a lot of place, I try by all means to stay remote from the life around me. I perceive the world as cold, and I need a life preserver. "What person or institution could take charge of me and allow me to never again need to worry about the future?" I doubt my power and I seek the truth. I compensate by becoming dependent on a substance, money, food, etc.

I accept↓♥ to re-examine the structures I have given myself and those that society has tried to impose on me. As my physical growth is great, it is now time for me to grow just as much emotionally and as a person. I trust life and I decide to engage in it. My new thought structure (**bones**) now includes respect for myself, my emotions and my differences.

BONES — DEFORMITY

Bones can become deformed because of the pressure I put on myself or that I feel I have to endure. I am mentally more rigid, and this manifests itself by anger. A **deformity** expresses what I couldn't shout loud and clear. I often experience a family situation that chafes at my sensitivity, and I would like to preserve harmony, but this is asking a lot of me. I feel compelled to submit, and so does my body. It is important to see where the **deformity** is located, and thus identify the specific emotional correspondence of this part of the body.

I accept↓♥ to be more flexible about my principles for living. My openness of mind will enable me to appreciate different facets of life and to discover that **Love** is present in different guises.

BONES — DISLOCATION

The word **dislocation (dis-location)** means a '**loss of location**', as though I were off-track or in a lane going in the opposite direction to everything going on. A **dislocation** is related to a deep feeling of **imbalance**. At the joint, the **bone** moves and completely 'comes out' of its socket. A **dislocation** shows me just how far I am not, or do not feel I am, in the right direction. As the **bone** is linked to the core of my being, to my fundamental energy, a **dislocation** indicates a deep change in the deepest energy of my being. Do I still have my place in the world? What is bothering me to the point of feeling so confused? I have reached a stage in my life where my structures are changing. My values are changing, and I want to reinforce my bases. I may feel that I am entirely 'outside the track'.

I verify and I accept↓♥ to become **Aware** of what I really need to understand, which will enable me to go beyond my current limits and discover something new in my life. The **dislocation** is painful enough for me to become **conscious** that I must change so that I won't have to experience it again.

BONES — FRACTURE (osseous) *See also: BACK — FRACTURE OF VERTEBRÆ*

The **bones** represent the structure of the laws and principles of the world in which I live. The existence of a **fracture** is an indication that I am currently experiencing a deep inner conflict. It may be related to revolt or reactions against an authority from which I want to cut myself away. I feel constricted and I want to come out of my prison. I feel that I constantly have to prove myself to show my worth. By resisting too much and being impatient with myself and others, my bones can't take it any longer, and fracture themselves. This **fracture** tells me that I can't go on like this, and that a change is imperative. The **location of the fracture** informs me of the nature of this conflict. If the **fracture** took place in an accident, I need to see how guilty I feel about this situation. Why go so hard on myself to the point of **fracturing a bone**? **Bones** also represent support and stability, and a **fracture** may be a warning for me to separate from my past, to let it go with flexibility, to avoid useless stress and proceed to the next stage in my development. A break is necessary and makes me question myself. It may involve a personal or a professional relation. It may also be to free myself from an ideology or a way of doing or thinking that no longer suits me. Do my standards for myself or society make me demand perfection to the point of being rigid? Have I focused more attention on physical activities to the detriment of the spiritual aspects of my life? A **skull fracture** tells me that I am experiencing a situation where I am "always breaking my head" and it seems unresolvable. I feel stuck and frustrated. It is enough to make me 'beat my head against the wall'!

To find this inner freedom, I become **Aware** of what bothers me. I accept↓♥ to **Love** myself enough to express what I feel. By finding my inner freedom, I find my freedom of movement. I decide for my life. I focus on myself and on my unlimited potential.

BONE MARROW *See also: BLOOD / (IN GENERAL), DISORDERS*

Bone marrow is a tissue present in the **bones**, and responsible for producing all the elements that make up the **blood** (white and red globules, platelets).

A condition affecting it shows me how I can't hang on to anything any longer and that nothing is running as I would like it to. I can't give any meaning to my life. My disappointment with who I am or whom I have become is so great that I don't feel worthy of living. I have the impression of descending into the pits and not being able to climb back out of them.

I accept↓♥ to need help and I dare to ask for it. I consider the missing elements for my happiness. I understand that I am the creator of my destiny. I decide to overhaul my basic structures and adjust to certain facets of myself. I am also saying yes to life; yes to examining my inner injuries and learning the life lessons that will enable me to connect with **Love**, peace and the joy of living.

BONES — OSTEOMYELITIS

Osteomyelitis is an infection of the **bone** and the **bone** marrow, which usually affects a part, located close to a joint and appears most often in children or adolescents. **Osteomyelitis** is found mainly in long **bones** such as the tibia, the femur or the humerus.

The energy contained in my **bones** is manifested by my joints. An infection involves an irritation that creates an inner weakness. I feel anger and frustration toward authority and the way in which life is structured and 'regimented'. I may also have the impression of not being **supported**, often by my father. I find him indifferent and I, in turn, tend to adopt the same behavior. I am constantly on alert. I distrust myself and everything around me, which fosters a degree of passivity. I compensate by being controlling and sometimes autocratic.

I accept↓♥ to have to learn to trust, to let go and to accept↓♥ that the Universe supports me. The infection only serves to **illuminate** certain conflicts that I am currently experiencing. If the **osteomyelitis** comes from a previous injury, then it is possible that the original causes of this injury may not yet have been treated.

BONES — OSTEOPOROSIS

Osteoporosis involves a loss of the proteic framework of the **bones**, which become porous.

It involves a loss in the intention of the desire to 'be', a loss of interest and motivation for being 'here' at the deepest level of oneself. "I am no longer what I was". I am experiencing discouragement. I am ***alone***, and tired of always having to fight authority or human laws. **Osteoporosis** usually appears in women after menopause. Because it is the **bones** that are affected, namely my basic structures and beliefs, I can ask myself what are the beliefs I hang on to and that maybe I should change, because now I can't have children any longer. I can still be just as 'useful' and 'productive', not for procreation but in other personal, social or professional areas, which can be just as status-enhancing and enriching. There are many things I don't ***dare*** to do any longer, thinking that they're 'no longer fit for my age'. I must therefore overcome this **tendency to depreciate myself**, believing I am useless or 'good for nothing'. I lose my feminine identity, I see myself as less desirable than before. As I can't remain young, I want to fade out progressively, without leaving any trace. By constantly criticizing myself and others, I prevent myself from fully living my life. The guilt I feel may come from my religious beliefs. I look at my life and I may feel that it is a failure. Sometimes a feeling of ***grief*** overcomes me. I have the impression that my life is in decomposition. I don't know how to organize my life that is rapidly changing, and courage is giving out. I have the impression that my death is approaching, and my negative thoughts are going to annihilate my creative energy.

I accept↓♥ to change my way of looking at it, and to develop more tolerance toward myself. I look at all my fine achievements. I accept↓♥ having reached a new stage in my life and being able to change these structures that controlled me all my life. I look to the future, I analyze what I really like to do, and I undertake new projects. I overcome my ***timidity***. I must trust in life and find new sources of motivation. I am now the master of my life!

BONES (cancer of the) *See also: CANCER (IN GENERAL)*

If I have a **bone cancer**, I am experiencing a very deep conflict where I feel that I am worth nothing and am less than nothing. I have the impression that I am worthless, and I am so filled with emotions that I keep inside of me those that **soak me to the bone**. Another way of expressing it is that I feel deeply depreciated. I am living in ***abnegation*** of myself. I give up who I truly am. I may be in a situation where my structures and my principles are fundamentally shaken and questioned. This situation may have taken me by surprise, and I feel **caught like a rat**. Because I feel constrained by what is around me, I revolt.

I accept↓♥ to acknowledge my qualities. It is by becoming more open and flexible that I will be able to deal more easily with the unexpected and the unconventional. It is by learning to express the emotions that I experience, which I often feel very intensely, that I will be able to heal and that my **bones** will be able to regenerate themselves.

BONES (cancer of the) — EWING'S SARCOMA[20] *See also: CANCER (IN GENERAL)*

It is a form of **bone cancer** that is more likely to affect me between the ages of 10 and 15, though it is rare. As this **cancer** affects the **bones** of my legs, this means a great fear of advancing in life. I am afraid of not having everything I need to face the future. My body cries out in pain from the insecurity that inhabits me. I think I am not able to enter the adult world.

I accept↓♥ to trust in life, knowing that it will provide me with the opportunities I need to live in society.

BOREDOM *See also: DEPRESSION, MELANCHOLY*

Boredom manifests a deep sadness, a great sorrow. As soon as I say that **I am bored**, it is because I am not using my strength and my potential. Why do I always need the company of others as a stimulant? What is this sorrow that is pursuing me and that I am trying to escape from? **Boredom** is melancholy that, in the long run, could lead me to a **nervous depression if I do not react**. It is as though I were living in an endless night, with no hope of ever seeing the sun one day. Melancholy is related to a lack, an emptiness that I feel in my life. I become **Aware** of this state.

I accept↓♥ to let myself be guided by my higher self, because all the resources are in me. I accept↓♥ to listen to my inner voice. Meditation and energy treatments can help me. It is my prerogative to direct my life, for I am whole and autonomous in my world.

BOUILLAUD'S DISEASE *See: RHEUMATISM*

BRADYCARDIA *See: HEART♥ — CARDIAC ARRHYTHMIA*

BRAIN (in general)

It is the energy generating station and the central unit processing all the information in the marvelous human machine: by itself, it has 30 billion neurons, each of which has a special power.

It is the command center with respect to my autonomy and my control over my life. The **brain** is related to the seventh chakra (the crown chakra), or energy center, and to the pineal gland, also called the epiphysis of the **brain**. It has two distinct hemispheres. **The right hemisphere**, the Yin[21] of the Chinese, represents the female side (introverted), creativity, the wholeness of situations (an overall view of things), intuition, perceptions and art; it is the **receptive** hemisphere. It manages experiences, the 'why' of things, the

20. **Ewing** (James) (Pittsburgh, Pennsylvania 1866 – New-York 1943): An American physician and histologist, he studied the histology of tumors and lent his name to a sarcoma of the long **bones**.

21. **YIN**: It is the name given in Chinese medicine to affective or female energy. Rational, or male, energy is called **YANG**.

sensations and what is sensed, and my perceptions of the inner world. It is nourished by experienced facts. It is oriented to affectively meaningful knowledge. The **left hemisphere**, the Yang, is the one that **gives**, that 'dominates', that is extraverted, aggressive, rational and logical and analyzes everything. It is related to the perception of the outer world, to concepts, words, numbers and reasoning. It manages the 'how' and works out detailed plans. It is nourished by acquired knowledge. It is oriented to time, facts and know-how. Each hemisphere controls the opposite half of the body (the right hemisphere controls the left side, and vice versa). The crossover point of the nerve fibers toward the opposite side is located in the spinal bulb (at the top of the neck) and descends along the spinal cord. This is why people who have a cerebrovascular accident in the left side of the **brain** will often suffer paralysis in their right side (see C.V.A.). Another crossover point is located at the level of the optic nerves of the eyes, the seat of the chakra, or energy center, of the 'third eye' located at the root of the nose between the eyebrows. A balanced development must accommodate the overall functioning of both hemispheres.

The **brain** is the organ that represents the seat of thought, knowledge, my HIGHER SELF, the center of the Universe, identification with all forms of divinity. Socrates said: *«Know yourself, and you will know the Universe and the Gods»*.

BRAIN DISORDERS

The problems of my **brain** indicate that I tend to try to **understand** with my head and my rational side (left hemisphere) all the situations I experience. I push aside my emotions (right hemisphere) with which I am afraid of coming into contact, trying to convince myself that they are useless or that they may be more harmful than useful. I have acquired a great rigidity in my way of thinking and I absolutely want to always be in the right! There are items of information or new elements that come to my attention but that I don't want to take into consideration. I feel ***clumsy*** and I may experience much ***confusion***. It is therefore difficult for me to change my opinion and to admit that I may have been mistaken. A **cerebral embolism** shows me that I feel caught in a situation that I have been ruminating over and that I want to escape at all costs, even if it means leaving this world.

I accept↓♥ to set aside my overly 'adult', serious and rational side and recover my 'child-like' side that likes to laugh and have fun and shines with its naïveté and its desire to learn.

BRAIN (abscess in)

When an **abscess** reaches my **brain,** it is because it comes from an infection in my sinuses, from my middle ear or from some other part of my body.

This indicates my anger about taking control of my life and my fear of losing control over my autonomy. I find it difficult to properly analyze all the elements of my life, for everything changes very fast and I become passionate very fast.

I accept↓♥ to trust the divine power within me to move toward the solutions that help me discover my full potential.

BRAIN — ADAMS-STOKES' SYNDROME *See also: BRAIN / EPILEPSY / SYNCOPE, VERTIGO*

The **Adams-Stokes'**[22] **syndrome** is a neurological accident that is due to a sudden diminishing of cerebral irrigation.

Because the **heart♥** beats are diminishing, I must ask myself what situation I want to escape because I don't know how to manage it. My sorrows are great and deep and I hang on to certain painful memories. It is hard for me to feel moments of joy, because there is an unfinished bereavement (affective or occupational). I easily accumulate bitterness, I am obstinate, I don't want to let go. I push back deadlines that could let me go on to something else, but I am afraid of the unknown.

I stop rationalizing this sorrow and accept↓♥ to resign myself to the situation. I accept↓♥ to let go of everything that I can't control and that is harmful to me. I focus my attention on the good things in life. I open my mind to accept↓♥ that the past is behind me, and I choose to move forward, knowing how to draw the lessons from my past experiences. I thus make peace with the history of my life. I allow life to flow in me and in each of my neurons. I accept to stay receptive to new experiences that will allow me to discover sharing, joy, happiness and giving and receiving **Love**.

BRAIN — APOPLEXY *See also: BLOOD — HEMORRHAGE, BRAIN / CEREBROVASCULAR ACCIDENT (C.V.A.) / SYNCOPE*

Apoplexy (or **cerebral attack**) is a common term referring to a **parenchymal hemorrhage**. **Apoplexy** is the sudden and more or less complete suspension of all the **brain** functions, characterized by a sudden loss of **consciousness** and voluntary mobility, with a persistence of circulation and respiration. It often results from a cerebral hemorrhage.

An **apoplexy attack** is the sign of an extreme need to **resist life** and **change**, a **rejection** and **negation** of several aspects of my life and my being. I am feeling very indecisive, hesitating to make changes in my life. Blood, the vehicle of joy in living, can no longer properly irrigate part of my **brain**. This part stops working, and paralysis ensues. During an **apoplexy attack**, I am incapable of expressing in words or gestures what is making me furious. I am worried and confused. I become **Aware** that I tend to want to fix and control everything for others. I interfere in other peoples' lives. I exceed my limits by wanting to do too much. Being like this, I focus all my attention on others, but I forget myself. I flee myself. That's why I refuse others interfering in my life (as I do in theirs). An **apoplexy attack** often occurs when I am older; it shows my fear of ageing, my insecurity about the emotional and financial support I will get

---

22. **Adams-Stokes:** Robert **Adams** scientifically described the syndrome for the first time in 1827, followed by the Irishman William **Stokes** in 1854.

from my family. If I resist life, I agree to give up and to stay closed. I prefer to die: it is easier, and destruction is my only salvation. It is defeat! This paralysis stops me from fully expressing my vital energy and creative potential. My activities are now limited.

If I want to regain the joy that nourishes my life, I accept↓♥ to open myself to intuition and **Love**, and to express more of what I feel. Mainly, I begin to trust more in life. I focus my attention on my own values and qualities. I allow this Life to grow in me. By spreading peace, **Love** and well-being, I help others to feel better, in the freedom and respect of all.

BRAIN — BALANCE (loss of) / DIZZINESS

On the physical level, **balance** is maintained by the distribution of my weight in my body, which allows me to move about without toppling over to one side or the other. **Balance** control takes place in the middle ear, in the labyrinth. The movement controls come from my **brain**: from my visual system or my proprioceptive[23] system, or my vestibular system in the middle ear, and mostly from the **cerebellum** that integrates them all together.

When my **brain** feels **rushed** and **overwhelmed** by situations or events, it is drawn in all directions at once and **loses its balance**. My ideas are scattered, and I can't think clearly. **Loss of balance** or **dizziness** is sometimes related to **hypoglycemia**[24]: I lack sweetness in my life. This escape may be related to a situation or an individual that I feel is changing too fast for me. These spells of vertigo occur when my reality becomes overwhelming, because I held on to false ideas that surfaced as a result of my expectations, which are not always met. I then lose my sense of **balance** and harmony. My discernment is affected, and I feel my life 'all upside down'. Though **dizziness** may result from various physical causes such as **hypoglycemia** (lack of sugar in the blood), **hypotension** (low blood pressure), **slowed heart rate**, an **ear problem** or a **deficit in kidney energy**, this ailment is related to **escape**. In fact, when I feel rushed I try, consciously or not, to 'make myself dizzy' so I can forget what I am experiencing. My energy is spread and scattered, which gives me the feeling of no longer having any power over my life. I want to take a roundabout route, but I know that at the end of the road, I will just have to face whatever scares me. A **labyrinthitis** indicates that I am losing myself in details, tasks or activities that are secondary for now. I no longer see clearly in my life, I feel that I am in a labyrinth. One part of me is resisting the coming changes. I feel engaged in an undertaking and I can no longer stop, or at least slow down. I no longer control the situation, and this raises anxiety. Uncertainty paralyzes me. Doubt makes me cling to persons or things. I repress my emotions and this makes me live superficially.

---

23. **Proprioceptive system:** Made up of sensitive microscopic receptors that inform me about my joints, my muscle tone and the positions of my joints.

24. **Hypoglycemia**: Lack of sugar (glucose) in the blood. (See: BLOOD – HYPOGLYCEMIA).

I accept↓♥ to become **Aware** of the fact that I am going in too many directions at once, and I give myself the time I need to regain my **balance**. I also listen to the messages my body sends me and I accept↓♥ to give myself my 'own sweet time'. I take the time to savor everything that is beautiful and good in my life. I clearly identify my priorities and assert my choices with conviction. I continue to advance, knowing that I am the Master of my life. I no longer have to wait for the approval of others, especially that of my parents. I accept↓♥ to be different and that I deserve to be happy. I open my **heart♥** to receive **Love** and joy in my life.

BRAIN — BRAIN CONGESTION *See: CONGESTION*

BRAIN — CEREBRAL PALSY

Cerebral palsy often appears at the time of birth and manifests itself by an anomaly in the **brain**. The **cerebral** tissue is partially or totally paralyzed, depending on the nature of the trauma.

I often wonder why, as a child, right from birth, I was already suffering from this **paralysis**. I may assume some previous karmic cycle[25], some 'pre-birth' pattern or experience so violent, or a mental trauma so intense, that it caused a complete closure, a stopping of all forward movement, preventing progress. In a sense, I am a prisoner of my past, of a structure that limits me instead of making me grow and develop. I may feel paralyzed, forced to follow a road that does not suit me. It may be the expectations of my parents for me, those of society or even those of my family lineage, hoping somehow to repair the mistakes of the past. As if I could 'save face' or shore up the family's reputation. Can I really carry out such a mandate? **Cerebral palsy** is a condition still defined as irreversible (I say 'still' because we can't predict the medicine of the future) and I can't be freed from this, despite the unconditional **Love** and attention of the people around me. When healing happens, it is more on the spiritual level.

BRAIN — CEREBROVASCULAR ACCIDENT (C.V.A.) *See Also: BLOOD / (IN GENERAL) / ARTERIES / BLOOD CIRCULATION, INFARCTION (IN GENERAL), TENSION [ARTERIAL] — HYPERTENSION*

This type of **accident** is related to blood circulation and the blood vessels. It results from a hemorrhage or an occlusion by a clot, whether its origin is arterial or comes from the **heart♥**.

It may manifest itself in several situations that are all related to **Love**. This sort of **accident** is a very strong reaction, a **categorical 'no'** to a balance, or some other sign that tells me from what angle this fear appears in my life. I may have the impression that I am losing the means for managing my life. In the case of **hemorrhagic cerebrovascular accidents**, it is an artery that bursts,

25. **'A previous karmic cycle'**: For those who believe in reincarnation, this means that it may originate from a cause related to a previous life.

which produces a blood effusion in a part of the **brain**. I may be feeling a tension so great in my family or at work that the accumulated tension is released by this bursting of my joy in living (the blood) that symbolizes all the sorrow I have been experiencing in this situation.

Depending on whether the **accident** occurs in the right part (the intuitive side) of the **brain** or in the left side (the rational side), I accept↓♥ to identify more specifically the message my body is giving me, to re-make peace with myself and recover more quickly. I visualize my **brain** bathing in a liquid made of white and golden **Light**, to allow all my nerve cells to regenerate themselves or distribute the work differently, so that I can recover my health more rapidly.

BRAIN — CHRONIC VEGETATIVE STATE *See also: CHRONIC [ILLNESS]*

When I am in this state, I have no detectable **conscious** activity. I live in a state generally described as **vegetative**. My **brain** is affected following a prolonged circulatory arrest or because of a cranial trauma.

As my **brain** corresponds to my individuality, I experience great fears or guilt, to the point of unconsciously wishing to escape life. I feel incapable of carrying out projects to completion, of producing great achievements. Seeing my power as limited, I reach the point where I want to 'disconnect myself' from this world that I find unfair.

Being in this state, I accept↓♥ that the fact I am still alive allows my Loved ones to gradually make peace with my departure from this world and to express their **Love** to me, while I can begin to calmly prepare myself to leave this world for higher realities and planes of **consciousness**.

BRAIN CONCUSSION

A **cerebral concussion** is a shock sustained by the whole **brain** during a cranial trauma, resulting in a temporary coma.

A **concussion** is a form of escape, a sudden and indirect way to stop and frankly observe what is going on in my life. A **cerebral concussion** makes me realize that unconsciously, I hold on so much to old ideas or attitudes that they collide with the new ones trying to find their place. I may also be clinging to someone or something: I leave to others the responsibility for my life. I define myself according to others instead of being myself. I feel safe if I feel close to someone, but this attachment ends up smothering me because deep down, I want to live my own life, not the life others want me to live. I may escape my emotions in alcohol, drugs or gambling, but sooner or later, I will have to face reality. There is a jolt in my life, I feel shaken up by a person or by something they said. There is an endless struggle that affects me to the highest degree. I am being indirectly made to stop and examine my life and consider in what directions I now want to move. I return to my priorities. Also, my head may be 'too full of ideas', I am over-extended, I need to come back to earth. There is a scramble, and a shock ensues. The **concussion** follows an injury to the head or an accident that 'shocks' the head, the **brain** and the mind. My body is temporarily 'gone' and unconscious. What point have I reached in my life? What direction will I take? Is my mind scattering in all directions at once, with no true orientation?

I accept↓♥ to come back on earth, to reality, in order to 'realistically' and more adequately resolve the situations I am currently experiencing. It is possible to avoid a **concussion** if I accept↓♥ to stay very open to what is going on in my life.

BRAIN — CREUTZFELD-JAKOB'S[26] DISEASE OR 'MAD COW'S DISEASE'

Creutzfeld-Jakob's disease is a very severe cerebral disease that is lethal in a few months, affects persons in their fifties and older, and produces a clinical picture of dementia with a major neurological impairment. In humans, it is a rare transmissible disease: **transmissible spongiform encephalopathy**. It is a dementia, an impairment of the person's 'intellectual' or cognitive (knowledge) functions. It is very similar to an infection by prions (infectious particles) transmitted by eating meat from diseased cows, informally called '**Mad Cow's disease**'.

This disease manifests itself when I ask myself questions about my life: I am anxiously confused. I am living my life on the surface, like an automaton or an animal. I like it when everything is set and there are no surprises. I avoid suffering and pain in all their forms. I prefer to keep a distance from people and face my own emotions. I thus lay aside my capacities and my full creative potential. I escape a bothersome reality. Over the years, an indifference toward life in general has set in. Am I still comfortable with this way of functioning? Is life trying to give me more, but I have closed the doors because I think I don't deserve more? The absence and the superficiality in which I live make my life uncomfortable. I hide behind a title, an office, a book, a sport that I push to excess, etc. I don't hesitate to use a certain cruelty in getting what I want. I am a little '***cannibalistic***', and I am indifferent to the harm I may be doing to some persons. I refuse to engage totally in life. As I fear being hurt, I avoid human contacts. There is an absence of communication with my own emotions and the persons around me. I prefer to 'sleep' out my life, and my **brain** does so as well.

Instead of rejecting myself and the rest of the world, I accept↓♥ to connect and communicate with the world around me. I accept↓♥ to let all my senses flourish in order to live the most experiences possible. Whatever emotions appear, I am constantly protected. I allow the joy of living to settle in all the cells of my body and especially in those of my **brain**. I discard my escape mechanisms, and embrace life and all the experiences it may want to offer me. By accepting↓♥ my full potential, I discover my true worth and can thus do things with joy and motivation on the way to self-fulfillment.

---

26. **Creutzfeld-Jakob:** These are the names of the two German physicians, **Creutzfeld** and **Jakob**, who first described the disease in 1920.

BRAIN — ENCEPHALITIS

The **brain** (or **cerebrum**) includes the **brain**, the cerebellum and the brainstem. The **brain** is the highest part of my nervous system that controls my whole organism.

The **cerebrum** therefore represents my individuality at its highest level. Though my head also generally represents my individuality, the **cerebrum** represents my inner individuality. When there is an inflammatory disease in the **cerebrum**, it is called **encephalitis** (the Spanish Flu epidemic in the years 1916–1920 is legendary). This corresponds to anger about who I am. I say 'no' to life for the changes it presents to me. I fear losing my individuality, my experience of who I am. I fear losing control of myself and of what happens to me or of what might happen to me. I feel limited in my self-expression. I feel incapable when I can't analyze my life, and everything is fuzzy.

I accept↓♥ to open myself to new facets of myself and to trust in life. I replace rigidity with flexibility, the strict control of certain parts of myself with openness, in order to discover new facets of myself. I give myself the **Love** and understanding I need, and I allow inner peace to settle in me.

BRAIN — EPILEPSY

Epilepsy is caused by poor communication and also by hyper excitability among the cells of the **brain**. The resulting accumulated nervous influx creates an overload and the formation of shock waves that attack the other parts of my **brain**. **Epilepsy** attacks can be of different intensities.

Thus, I may be among the persons who are simply 'in the moon' for a few moments, with a loss of **consciousness** of a few seconds: this is called '**petit mal'**. This indicates that I want to escape from a situation, finding my responsibilities too great. This makes me feel much anxiety and impatience. My **brain** overheats because I focus my attention too much on my rational side instead of living more spontaneously. I am cut off from my emotions and don't know what to do with them. An **epilepsy attack** brings to **Light** a great violence turned against myself, and shows me how I tend to punish myself because I judge myself severely. I may be among those who lose **consciousness** completely and have rather strong convulsions for 5 to 10 minutes, which is generally called '**grand mal**' To experience such a situation, it is surely because I believe that life only brings me rejection, violence, anger and despair. I feel that I always have to be fighting. I feel persecuted. I feel guilty of the aggressiveness that rises in me and I repress it. I also repress all the feelings that want to express themselves. My uncertainty makes my head full of ideas, but they are all a little muddled. This brings great instability in my life. I have the impression of living in a prison, feeling that I have had to submit to the people around me, my freedom being thus bullied. I feel myself under the ***hold*** of someone or something greater than me. I must fight against an enemy that I sometimes don't even know! I resist so much that my body must, at some point, release this overload of emotions and frustration. I feel intense anguish that makes me lose control over my orders. I fear losing someone or something that is 'mine' and being separated from them. A wind of panic blows through my life because I feel I no longer have any control over my life. I protect myself by losing **consciousness**. As my relations with others and with society are very difficult, I want to temporarily cut myself off from them completely, to allow me to 'catch my breath'. This shows the deep duality that I am experiencing and the impression of being caught in a trap. I like to punish myself and treat myself roughly. Instead of listening to my intuition and living the present moment, I live in my head and I give priority to my thoughts and the things I force myself to do. My 'nerve circuits' overheat. I want so much to control the people around me that my body gets out of control, precisely to make me **Aware** of the fact that the only mastery I can have is over myself. I have had enough; it demands too much effort from me. I reject this life that persists in making me suffer. I want to become insensitive by curling up in myself. It is often despair or anger that prompt me. At the same time, I will feel persecuted by life, letting it bring some violence to me. Self-rejection is extreme, and it results in a conflict of individuality. During the **epilepsy attack**, my body stiffens to protest against these injuries, and the convulsions surge and break, like powerful waves that allow me to release my long-repressed anger, bitterness and aggressiveness. I have no other choice but to let myself go with the intense feelings that inhabit me. I escape into unconsciousness from these situations that make me suffer so much, because I am afraid, upset or suffering. At this point, my mind has no control. I have the impression that I am fighting a ghost. During an **attack**, I observe the movements carried out, which express what I previously couldn't, or wouldn't, manifest in words or gestures. It is like a liberation. **Epilepsy** thereby tells the people around me of my great need for **Love** and attention. The deeper cause of **epilepsy** often goes back to early childhood and may even go back to the time of pregnancy: as a child, I felt highly guilty; it has followed me all my life, and I see my life as a daily struggle. It may also be abuse, sexual or other, or perceived as such, or a previous rejection experienced in early childhood as a **separation**. The fact of feeling separated from someone involves a loss of physical contact with that person. It may be my relationship with my father whom I wanted so much to be close to and do things together. Or it may be my own children, from whom I don't get as much news as I would like to, or with whom I have lost contact. An **epilepsy attack** can therefore become a means for obtaining or gaining more attention, and to reinforce my sense of superiority. As **epilepsy** indicates an overload of the **nerve circuit**, it shows that what I must deal with in my everyday life is taking up too much place; a situation comes up where I must choose. This feeling of being overloaded may result from events that I amplify (exaggerate) in my mind. This exaggeration may lead to arrogance by leading me to think that I know more than anyone else. I may also tend to be overly abstract or show too great an adherence to the psychic realms. I thus avoid dealing with objective reality. **Epilepsy** may also result from a holy fear I have (of death, sickness, losing someone, etc.). A feature of motricity, as if to prevent me from advancing, adds itself to my fear (for instance: if I must go to a funeral [death] but don't want to go). It is impossible for me to do anything right now!

I become **Aware** of what is going on in me, and I accept↓♥ to no longer concentrate my efforts only on the negative, and to see how much **Love** and beauty the world brings me. My body is telling me, through these **epilepsy attacks**, to wake up and stop living in my mental prison. I accept↓♥ to let go and live my life fully and more spontaneously. I leave control to others. I release all these emotions I want to share with others, knowing that it is the only way to get out of this prison that I had built. This is how I will find my truth and my rightful place.

BRAIN — HEMIPLEGIA *See also: BRAIN / [ABSCESS in] / CEREBROVASCULAR ACCIDENT [C.V.A.]*

Hemiplegia is a paralysis of one side of the body (left or right) caused by a **brain** lesion. It can occur after a great shock, physical or emotional, such as the death of a Loved one ('my better half'), which often brings on a very deep state of despair and a highly affected sensitivity.

I have the impression that I have been ***shot***. An explosion of rage may also be the cause. For example, I may have been raised by two ***mothers***, and that did not suit me at all. My body is telling me that one part of me can no longer act, that it no longer has the strength. Is it a feeling of powerlessness over an annoying situation? I feel torn in half: they want to tear away from me something or someone dear to me. I constantly need help because I can't shoulder the obligations of my everyday life. I do things part way, and it bothers me. I may also be living my life half-heartedly. The side that is affected tells me if it is mostly my affective side (left side) or my rational side (right side) that is involved.

I accept↓♥ to take the time to heal my injuries, knowing that any experience, however difficult, leads me to become a more **conscious** and a stronger person.

BRAIN — HUNTINGTON'S DISEASE OR CHOREA *See also: BRAIN — TICS*

Huntington's disease[27] or **Huntington's** (or **hereditary**) **chorea** is a rare disease, defined as hereditary, affecting the nervous system and muscle contraction. It usually appears between ages 35 and 50, causing jerky movements and progressive cognitive deterioration. This disease brings mental disorders such as impulsiveness, aggressiveness or depression.

I live in an emotional desert, feeling completely cut off from others, especially my partner. I feel a great emptiness. I am haunted by my desires that I believe to be impractical. I am seeking my identity. I go out 'hunting' for

---

27. **Huntington** (George) (1851–1916): An American physician established in New York. He practiced in Long Island and in 1872, he described the chronic family forms of **chorea**. **Hereditary chorea** bears his name.

relationships, especially if I am living alone. But these relationships are superficial, just on the surface. Other persons seem inaccessible. As they don't fulfill my desires, I become frustrated and spiteful. I go left and right, pouncing on anything that goes by, thinking every time that I have found what will make me happy. But I only go from one disappointment to another.

I accept↓♥ **here and now** to take myself in charge. I learn to know myself, to recognize the emotions that inhabit me and the power I have to change my life. Instead of waiting for others, I put things together in order to reach my goals. Instead of wanting to lean on others, I connect myself with my inner power. I go at my own pace. I am attuned to my senses and I take the time to savor each instant of my life, even in the smallest things. This enables me to better reconnect with earthly life, and it provides me with greater balance.

BRAIN — HYDROCEPHALIA

Hydrocephalia is an excess of cerebrospinal fluid in the cavities of the **brain**.

I constantly ask myself questions about the place I occupy here on earth. I feel abandoned, and sometimes I even feel I am not on the right planet. I have a deep sadness in me because I have the impression that I shouldn't have been born. It is difficult for me to face reality. I sometimes think that I would want to go back up there, because I don't feel in harmony with my environment. My unchannelled emotions continue to become congested and are on the verge of 'overflowing'.

I accept↓♥ to let my thoughts and emotions roam, helping me to get in better contact with my body and the ambient world. I am sure I have a role to play here, and I accept↓♥ to discover it and take it on. I live in the joy of the moment!

BRAIN — MENINGITIS

See also: HEAD (IN GENERAL), SYSTEM [IMMUNE], INFLAMMATION

Meningitis is an infection of the cerebrospinal fluid, resulting from inflammation in the membrane covering the **brain** and the spinal cord. It indicates a weakness in the immune system and its incapacity to protect itself.

Meningitis warns me of a weakness and an incapacity to fight against very strong external pressures, especially of an intellectual nature. It is often because I find it difficult to protect myself. Being hypersensitive, I experience everything more intensely and I am affected more deeply, especially by things that seem ordinary to others. I have so many ideas rushing around that they 'compress' my **brain**. I am always 'racking my **brains**'. This is in addition to all the feelings of aggressiveness and frustration that I am incapable of verbalizing I am ***annoyed***, but I don't know how to ***defend*** myself. Part of me is nonexistent, almost dead, for I disavow it or hide it from myself and others: it is my whole creative, extravagant, sensitive side. I prefer to merge into the crowd and remain unseen. I feel in prison, but at the same time, I prefer this to looking at my face in the mirror and discovering who I really am. Instead of trying to see what is going on in my **heart♥**, I prefer to remain in my head. It is a way of protecting myself. I am hypersensitive, and I tend to take everything on my shoulders and to want to fix the problems of the whole planet! I am afraid of 'losing my head', of 'having my head cut off', that my 'head will explode'; as for example when I think I am going to lose my job. When I was a child, I may have been very surrounded and overprotected by my ***mother*** and now, I must ***defend*** myself. I may also sense that **Love** is denied in the house where I live, or that something or someone there is 'seriously grating on my nerves'. This disease sends me the message that I must protect myself from blows coming from outside and to not feel guilty for the behavior of others, while acting responsibly for myself. Otherwise, **revolt** rumbles, I am angry and fright seizes me. As the **brain** governs the whole body, **meningitis** involves a deep inner weakness that attacks me at the deepest level.

As **meningitis** imperils the command center of my body, the **brain**, it is imperative for me to accept↓♥ to make the decision to live and to get my act together, to 'hold my head high' and release in myself this inner force that will enable me to pursue a rich life filled with marvelous experiences. I learn to trust, and I accept↓♥ to go and see in my **heart♥** the treasures to be found there. I also look at all the emotions I have held back for so long, and I accept↓♥ to let them go. I discover the talents I have inside. By reconnecting with my creative and artistic side, I allow my **brain** to 'catch its breath' a little. It will thus have an opportunity to rest, and my level of stress and inner pressure will therefore diminish. I learn to 'be', quite simply. I thus become the master of my life again.

BRAIN — PARKINSON'S[28] DISEASE *See also: NERVES (IN GENERAL), TREMORS*

Parkinson's disease is a deterioration of the nerve centers of the **brain**, especially in the regions that control movement. Tremors appear and usually affect the hands and the head.

When I tremble and ***vibrate***, it is because I sense or see a danger threatening me or someone I live, whether it involves a fear of losing control (that I am losing increasingly often!), insecurity or an incapacity to move ahead in life. I also feel powerless or incapable of being the best. I find my life very ***chaotic*** and I need more stability, but I seem to be finding it difficult to reach this state. I ***nod*** my head as a sign of despair. I am afraid of the future, of no longer living, so why then finish anything at all? I may also have experienced a trauma, abuse or other difficulties that left traces, and about which I feel sorrow, frustration, guilt, rage and depression, which lead me to exhaustion and discouragement, and that I want to escape rather than face and resolve them. I may have felt limited by my overly severe education, where performance was paramount. I was probably a very ***agitated*** child. When I am in perfect health and I tremble, it is often because I am nervous and afraid of performing a task because of my

---

28. **Parkinson** (James): This English physician (1755–1824) described the *trembling paralysis* disease that now bears his name.

lack of self-confidence. I always ***fear*** the worst. These same tremors may reach the point of appearing more frequently and automatically, and will later be diagnosed as a case of **Parkinson's disease**. Therefore if I am affected, it is quite probably because I experienced many situations where a certain way of doing things was imposed on me, which made me feel inner nervousness. I ***was prevented*** from being myself. It may also have been a situation where I had to hold back a gesture. When I am 'full of nerves' or I want the pain to ***stop***, my overloaded body can't take it any longer, and the overload causes permanent reactions in it[29]. It is as if my accumulated hate was making my whole body move. The gesture that I was forbidden to make wants to manifest itself, as if to show that I am alive. I have the impression that I am in a car that is parked and can't move forward. I must stay in place, which greatly irritates me. I am slowly destroying myself, producing deterioration in my current nervous function. A powerlessness in the motricity of my **upper limbs** (especially my arms and hands) often originates from a situation where I wanted to repel a person, a thing or an event or, on the contrary, where I wanted to ***grasp*** and hold someone or something and I felt incapable (physically or psychologically) of doing so. This may have caused serious consequences, possibly resulting in death. This happens when my spouse is on the point of leaving their physical body and I want to hold them back with all my strength. Being still under the impression that I had failed to do so, it is as if my body had registered stress and that, seeking release, it started to move 'without my permission'. If my **lower limbs** are affected (my legs and feet), it is with these that I would have wanted to either repel, or bring back to me, the person, the thing or the event concerned. I feel like escaping this situation where I feel overwhelmed and that I see as providing no way out. I tend to want to control everything, and the disease reminds me that I can't have any control over others. I can't even control my own limbs! I desperately want to control others, but I become **Aware** that I can exercise mastery only over myself.

I accept↓♥ to get my act together and learn how to control MY life and not the lives of others, by trusting in life and telling myself that I deserve to live. I let myself be guided by **Love**. It is much easier to let others be free. Instead of trying to prove anything to others, I accept↓♥ to show my inner world to the rest of the world, with all the emotions that have accumulated over these many years.I am myself, with my child's **heart♥**, and I am now living my life spontaneously.

BRAIN — SYNCOPE

Syncope is diagnosed by a complete, reversible, but brief loss of **consciousness**. The loss of **consciousness** comes from a lack of oxygenation of the **brain**. It may result from a heart♥ arrest, but not necessarily so. It may come from a form of asphyxia, or be related to blood vessels that dilate brutally after an emotional shock, leaving little blood for the **brain**, and therefore little oxygen.

29. This disease, it is interesting to note, mostly affects men, who are more YANG by nature and therefore in action, which necessarily involves movement.

It is the spirit that leaves my body for a short moment. It is as if I chose to withdraw into myself and shut myself off from the physical world; I am in revolt, no longer knowing how to face a certain situation. I have lost hope of being freed from it. I want to withdraw from life because what is going on is too much for me. Instead of following what my inner voice dictates, I prefer to follow what others expect of me. The **syncope** is a sign that I must 'wake up' and really do what brings me pleasure. This state can't be compared to that of a yogi[30], for the latter fully masters a discipline that aims at freeing their spirit from all bodily constraints in a harmonization of movement, rhythm and breath.

I accept↓♥ to become **Aware** of what made me thus take leave of my physical body, of what anguish, what inner feeling of panic produced such a situation. I know that in all circumstances, I am guided and protected, and I accept↓♥ to remain fully **Aware** of the life that is in me. I thus regain my place in this world and I can now breathe great lungfuls of air!

BRAIN — TICS

Tics, defined as the sudden execution of repetitive and involuntary movements, display a disturbance of nervous tension and an imbalance in the **brain**.

If I have one or several **tics**, the odds are high that I am a very emotional person, that I repress much aggressiveness and that when I was young, I perceived the education I received as rigid and perfectionist. In this way, I display the concern and the bitterness that I feel inside. I may experience a situation where I feel in a ***dead end, backed*** against the wall. I don't have the time, a danger threatens me. Something is on the point of exploding (maybe my own emotions!), a family secret wants to come out. If I am a boy, I may have been affected by actions that someone representing authority to me asked me to do. This could explain why almost 4 times more boys than girls have **tics**. Girls are generally more receptive to authority and therefore less affected, again in general, by this factor. I may have been annoyed by certain movements I was prevented from doing when I was younger (for example being forbidden to move in church) and now my body moves in spite of me, as if in rebellious reaction against what I was previously forbidden to do. I may even have had the impression of 'losing face' before someone, which generates **tics**, especially in my **face**. My face wants to push back the danger, the aggressor. I was irritated, annoyed or ***bothered***, and now, it is my own **tics** that are bothering me. I have **jaw tics** if I was often told to "shut up" when I was a child. The accumulated and unexpressed rage is released: a **tic** is like speaking in silence. Unusual **eye blinking** may remind me of an experience where someone 'gave me the glad eye', or means that I am vainly seeking someone else's attention and look.

---

30. **Yogi**: A person who has reached a certain stage in their spiritual development. Through the practice of meditation, they can consciously leave their body for a variable duration. Certain persons can even slow down or practically stop their **heart♥** beats and then resume their normal **heart♥** rate.

I accept↓♥ to become **Aware** of this state, to clear up the blocks of the past and clearly express my needs.

BRAIN (tumor in)

A **tumor** is an excessive proliferation of abnormal cells in the **brain**.

A **tumor** is related to **repressed emotions**, **deep remorse** and **past sufferings** that I turn against myself. The **primitive**[31] **tumor** that develops from **brain** cells means that my information-processing center is still registering certain ideas, beliefs or mental schemata **that no longer have any reason to exist**! The **tumor** results from a violent emotional shock related to a situation or a person that I **liked a lot** or to something that made me suffer a lot or about which I still feel hate, resentment, fear, anger and frustrations. It may have been about my father who depreciated me. I always had to surpass myself and find solutions, and my head 'overheated'. If my **tumor** is located in the upper part of my **brain**, in the middle or in the hypophysis (pituitary gland), it is often because I experienced an emotional shock or because I have a great fear involving my spirituality, my intuition, etc. I am very **obstinate** and I refuse to change my way of seeing life and dealing with current reality. It is a deep mental conflict for me to be here now, to accept↓♥ my life and everything that goes with it. I am **rigid** and **frozen** in my thoughts, I am confused inside and I find it difficult to take stock. I am distracted, I am absent and I often live in denial. I think that my intellectual capacities are insufficient for finding a solution to my special situation: I must surpass myself at all costs! I generate a mental energy that doesn't fit my deepest needs and that is poles apart from my divine desires. My body reacts strongly, and then an out-of-control production of certain **brain** cells suddenly appears. This is a critical and dangerous state, and I must change my closed attitude and unlock my **heart♥** if I want to stop this **tumor**.

I must become **Aware** that I need to make a radical change in my life, and this is the ideal moment to do it. I must detach myself from the past and everything negative in it, and focus my attention only on the positive and what I truly want to do with my life. From now on, I accept↓♥ to see life in a more open and flexible way. It is in constant transformation, always straining toward the better. It is my self-confidence that will enable me to reach this goal. I accept↓♥ to listen better to my inner voice, to be more spontaneous, and I let go of the control of my mind.

BREAST(S) (in general)

The **breasts** represent my **Awareness** of who I am and my generosity toward myself and others. They are the symbol of maternal beauty. Depending on their condition, I can see the balance that prevails in my life between giving and receiving, between my female and male sides. A good balance or exchange leads me to be truly fertile in all the areas of my life. My affective life is thus in good

31. See the footnote about **generalized cancer** in the "**Cancer (in general)**" section.

harmony with my rational side. A person with **large breasts** (whether a man or a woman) has often begun, from the earliest age, to 'mother' others in order to feel Loved. Even if I have this ability to take care of others, I realize that I often act like this because I am afraid of rejection and because, feeling admired for this side of me, I thereby attract the gratitude of the people around me. Maybe I am the one who needs to be mothered. On the other hand, if I have **small breasts**, it is possible that I may doubt my capacity as a mother and that I always feel the need to prove that I can. The **left breast** represents the more emotional and affective aspect of my maternal side, whereas the **right breast** is associated with a woman's role and responsibilities in the family or in society[32]. If my **breasts** are **soft** and **pendulous**, I would be well-advised to become firmer in my way of speaking and acting. The **breasts** also represent femininity in women, as well as seduction. They are often overly admired. The emergence of **breasts** amounts to becoming a woman. They evoke many reactions in a woman. I may fear becoming a sex symbol, or being ridiculed. I may experience shame or embarrassment, or feel belittled. I may not want to have children because, consciously or not, it reminds me of a past 'shock'. It is possible that I may experience certain fears about being at once a woman and a mother. Or do I have the impression I may not have been up to my role, either as a woman or as a mother?

I choose to accept↓♥ receiving as much as giving and I accept↓♥ my femininity.

BREAST DISORDERS (pains, cysts) *See also: BREASTS — MASTITIS, CANCER OF THE BREASTS*

When I feel **pains in the breasts**, I must ask myself whether I am adopting an over-protective or dominating attitude toward my children[33] or toward my spouse. Am I afraid, or did I ever actually experience having a dearly Loved one taken away from me? I may have been physically separated from that person, or it may have been a break-up of a personal relationship because of insufficient communications or sharing. My unfulfilled need to be related to things and people leaves a vacuum in my life. I was repudiated by someone close to me and I am suffering a lot. Or maybe I repudiated someone close to me. I am anguished and I think too much. I feel that my freedom is being infringed upon. I am not very preoccupied with my emotions, and I end up wanting to dominate and to be possessive. I pass bloody judgment on others and I don't want to hear what they have to say. I want nothing to escape me. I doubt my worthiness, I tend to easily become passionate in **Love**, and I lose myself in my

---

32. According to the ***Total Biology of living beings***, being left-handed or right-handed has an impact on conflicts related to ailments affecting the **breasts**. This theory is not noted here. This interpretation is valid, as well as the one stating that the right side is related to rationality and the left one to the affective and the emotions. Both ways of construing this interpretation merit consideration.

33. **What represents my children**: It may be a project I have undertaken at work and that I look after as if it was my baby; a member of the family, a nephew, a niece or another child whom I consider **like** my own child; my parents, now that they are in my care and need attention **like** children.

relations to compensate for my lack of self-confidence and self-esteem. The joy that I might feel is diluted in my old sorrows or worries, which have followed me for several years now already. My anxieties and my insecurity are stronger than my desire to take myself in charge. I have the impression that I am living in sin. I put all my power in my rational side to get away from my emotions. Nevertheless, my emotions are still present, and my breasts may become **hypersensitive**, letting all this inner pain and sorrow show through. A **cyst** may appear if I feel guilty over a pregnancy or if I sustained an emotional shock. For wanting too much to protect the people I **Love**, I am preventing them from living their own lives, I am making decisions in their place, I am becoming a **mother hen**.

I accept↓♥ to let those I **Love** become autonomous so that they too will become responsible persons. I allow my true personality to emerge. I deserve what is best. By letting go of my anxieties, my worries and my resentments of the past, my **breasts** will return to perfect health.

BREASTS — BREASTFEEDING DIFFICULTIES *See also: BREASTS — MASTITIS*

Breastfeeding difficulties result, among other factors, from **fissures at the ends of the breasts' nipples** or from an **insufficiency of milk**. I have difficulty in accepting↓♥ my role as a mother. I feel that this child is infringing on my freedom. I perceive myself as a 'milk-producing machine'. I have difficulty in building up this mother-child tie that seems so extraordinary with most women. But it is not like that for me, and I wonder what 'my problem' is! I am becoming anguished because this child depends on me for living. I must ask myself: how can I give **Love** to my baby through the act of breastfeeding when I feel unworthy of the child? Then, I try to go at double speed. I have poor self-esteem and I don't give myself the **Love** and tenderness I need so much – how can I give my baby what I can't give myself? I want to do a lot to feed this child, I am giving it a lot, I am giving tremendously, and I am totally forgetting the woman in me who has left the whole place to the mother; and as a result, I am feeling overwhelmed because I am trying too much to do it well, for I don't feel up to the task and I am breaking down. How can I be a Lover for my spouse and a mother for my baby? I must learn to adjust to this new situation and dose things a little. The **little food** (milk) I have for my child may indicate that I have been receiving little affective nourishment myself (affection, tenderness, attention, etc.) from my spouse since the arrival of this baby who has been 'taking up the whole place' and getting all the attention. This may also remind me of my relationship with my own mother, where I felt a coldness, an emptiness, a lack. The fact for me of now having this mother's role reactivates my early emotional sufferings with my own mother. How can I be a good Lover and a good mother at the same time? How can I organize the intimacy with my child so that I can feel well in it?

I accept↓♥ my body and my person as they are. I take my place and the space I need and that are rightfully mine. I consider myself with **Love** and gentleness. I accept↓♥ to share this **Love** with my baby, knowing that it is in my life to help me become a better person. It brings me joy and unconditional **Love**. This helps me in gaining greater mastery over my life and in enlarging this feeling of freedom that inhabits me.

BREASTS (cancer of the) *See: CANCER OF THE BREASTS*

BREASTS — MASTITIS

Mastitis, which is an inflammation of the **breast**, makes it very painful and may appear during breastfeeding, which must then be interrupted if pus is running from the nipples.

Again in relation with pregnancy, I may be feeling very fatigued after childbirth (or for other reasons) and I experience a malaise that stops me from breastfeeding without feeling any guilt. It may also be because I have the impression that I am being too 'mothered', either by my spouse or by somebody else around me. These pains in the **breasts** may also show that I am going too hard on myself. I feel that I must **sacrifice** myself for my family, for my work, or for a cause that is close to my **heart♥**. I can't take it any longer, I am aggressive and the frustrations are accumulating more and more.

I accept↓♥ to acknowledge that my way of functioning is preventing me from flourishing. I carefully examine all the qualities that I have. I ask myself why I needed so much to feel useful to somebody. By accepting↓♥ my worthiness, I have nothing to prove to anyone. By giving myself more **Love**, I can also give it to others, but freely, without any expectations or any desire to control them. These are entirely free gestures, done quite simply, as a child will do. I am capable of saying yes or no, according to what is good for me. I accept↓♥ to let others freely make their own choices and I learn to **Love** myself. I recognize that all of us grow through our own unique experiences.

BREATH (bad) *See: MOUTH — BREATH [BAD]*

BRIGHT'S[34] DISEASE *See also: KIDNEYS [RENAL PROBLEMS]*

Bright's disease is also called **chronic nephritis**. It is a serious inflammation of the kidneys, accompanied by edema[35] (swelling and failure to eliminate urine). Usually, the kidneys degenerate or die rather quickly. It goes deeper than kidney diseases in general (sclerosis).

I am suffering, and I am experiencing a **frustration** or a **disappointment** so intense about a situation where I have a feeling of loss, that I have reached the point where I consider my life or myself personally **as a total failure** (the

---

34. **Bright (Richard)** (1789–1858): A British physician who was the first to study chronic nephritis or renal failure.

35. **Edema:** An abnormally high retention in the tissues of the organism. Also commonly called: 'water retention'.

kidneys are the seat of fear). I am afraid of not being suitable enough, good enough or **bright** (intelligent) enough.

I accept↓♥ the fact that I am unique and that I have always tried my best. I become more **conscious** of the fact that an openness of **heart♥** is necessary if I want to show a change of attitude to heal this condition.

BRONCHI (in general) *See also: LUNGS*

The **bronchi** are the ducts through which air enters into my lungs.

They represent life. A discomfort or a pain in my **bronchi** usually means that I am struggling in life and I am feeling less interest and joy in my life. The **bronchi** represent my vital space, my borders, the territory more especially related to my couple, my family and my workplace. If I sense that I am going to lose my territory or someone linked to it, my insecurity will set off an ailment in my **bronchi**. Fear may manifest itself when there are ***altercations*** or quarrels precursory of more serious conflicts. There is an imminent danger. Wanting to appear strong, I endure certain events without flinching. I may feel that I am lacking air and I will be ***asphyxiated*** and lose myself. I feel that ***others*** are smothering me. I tend to be ***jealous*** of them. I worry about what others think of me; I can't stand ***what people may say***, because I am afraid they will laugh at me and ***slander*** me. I am no longer ***cheerful***. I would like to be able to fill up my lungs and drum my chest like a gorilla to impress the others and make the threat go away. Often, it may be my couple that is in danger. Among men, it is often work that is involved, for instance in the fear of being fired; for women, it is the family that is more often involved, as in the case of a sick child.

I accept↓♥ to trust; I know that if I have clearly demarcated my territory and demand respect for it as I demand respect for my rights, nobody will be able to 'invade' me because everyone's space will be clearly delimited and everyone will be able to live in respect and harmony. I try to determine what person or what situation is associated with this pain, and what I must do to change that. It will be beneficial for me to create situations that promote laughing and relaxation.

BRONCHI — ACUTE BRONCHITIS *See: RESPIRATION — TRACHEITIS*

BRONCHI — BRONCHITIS *See also: LUNG DISEASES*

Bronchitis (-itis = anger) is characterized by an inflammation of the mucous membrane of the **bronchi**, the tubes conducting air from the trachea to the lungs.

It is a disease essentially related to respiration, the act of taking in life and air with desire and enjoyment (inspiration) and then ejecting them temporarily with detachment (expiration). Inflammation means I am feeling **anger**, **frustration** or **rage** over repressed emotions, words I need to express and release a stifling situation where I feel harassed, a conflict marked by aggressiveness and criticism, (upheaval in the family, quarrels, etc.). It is often a family atmosphere that is charged with tension, silences and lies. My freedom is being curtailed. I lack time for myself. I can't catch my breath and breathe. I no longer trust the others. I want to be close to the people I **Love**, but at the same time I am suffocating, which makes me experience great inner heartbreak. If this conflicted situation involves very intense quarrels and confrontations, I may even develop a **cancer of the bronchi**, which is the usual form of '**lung cancer**'. There is an inner turmoil, a disruption that prevents me from manifesting my true being and getting proper respect for my rights. I try to communicate with the people closest to me, but I can't achieve a certain inner peace. It is as though life were making me exist exclusively cut off from one person, who is usually my mother. The family situation is too difficult. I then feel a certain discouragement with life, and I stop struggling to pursue my way. I have little joy in living, and I feel a deep lassitude and inner dissatisfaction. I want to be independent, but I feel great insecurity. What are my own limits? My situation is untenable: my feeling of powerlessness and my inner pain lead me to resist the impulses of my **heart♥**. A **cough** indicates that I want to free myself by rejecting something or someone that bothers me and makes me angry. If I am a **child**, I may feel insecure or anxious about what is going on in the family. I may feel very sharply my parents' sorrow or their repressed anger, and I have the impression that I must bear all that, being too young to differentiate myself and detach myself from what is going on. I feel I am under the hold of my parents, living in an emotional prison.

If I don't want to suffer from **chronic bronchitis**, I must change my way of seeing life, **my attitude**. I was born in a family where each member is going through experiences similar to my own. My parents, my brothers and my sisters are all learning, too, as well as they can manage. I therefore accept↓♥ to start seeing joy and **Love** in myself and in each experience in my life. I accept↓♥ that my personal happiness is my own responsibility and I stop believing that others will make me happy. Making my own decisions and breathing on my own: such is the first step toward my independence!

BRONCHOPNEUMONIA *See also: LUNG DISEASES*

Bronchopneumonia is a respiratory inflammation that affects the bronchioles and the alveoli of the lungs.

It is directly related to life, to the fact that I feel diminished and limited by life itself. I feel it is unfair to me, which makes me angry. I feel that I am not breathing fully, and I have no doubt accumulated some sadness, which has made me angry against life. I am angered by a situation that I am going through and where I refuse to shoulder my responsibilities. It is a **more serious** infection than a simple bronchitis or **pneumonia**, because **the inner pain is deeper**.

I accept↓♥ to breathe life in a new way and with a different approach, full of **Love** and joy.

BRUISES *See: SKIN — BRUISES*

BRUXISM *See: TEETH [GRINDING]*

BUERGER'S DISEASE[36] *See also: ARMS, BLOOD — BLOOD CIRCULATION, CIGARETTES, INFLAMMATION, LEG, NUMBNESS*

Buerger's disease or **thromboangiitis obliterans** is a disease that involves a more or less marked obstruction of circulation in the arms and legs, caused by an inflammation of the walls of blood vessels. It mostly affects the arteries, but also the veins. It develops toward cutaneous lesions and amputations caused by thromboses. Very rare and serious, it can prove lethal over a few months. This disease mainly affects people originating from Central Europe (as genetically defined) and smokers. The cause of this inflammation is often the irritating agents introduced into the blood by cigarette smoke.

My body is indicating to me, by the numbness in my arms and legs, that I am trying to become insensitive to situations in life, which are related to the arms, and to what is in store for me in the future, which is related to the legs. I want to protect one of my parents, often my mother, from suffering because of certain actions or words expressed by her spouse.

I accept↓♥ to seriously consider the message my body is sending me, and I accept↓♥ to see my life more clearly. By ceasing to smoke, I will only feel better.

BULIMIA *See also: ANOREXIA, APPETITE [EXCESS], WEIGHT [EXCESS]*

Bulimia is a compulsive disease, an uncontrollable need to absorb food in great quantities, a nervous imbalance because I am in **total reaction** against life.

Bulimia presents the same inner causes as obesity and anorexia. I eat excessively to satisfy myself completely or to find a form of **Love** and affection (food symbolizes life, **Love** and emotions). I am trying to emotionally fill a deep emptiness in myself, a self-hate so great (disgust, contempt) that I want to fill this void at all costs, preferring to let myself be dominated by food (life) rather than open myself up to life. I disavow part of myself or a situation, and I experience sorrow or anger because I feel isolated, separated or rejected. I totally reject my body; I refuse to live on this earth. I no longer want to suffer all these frustrations and anxieties. I am afraid of losing what I have, and I feel insecure because I may be different from the others. I no longer feel able to embrace life. I don't have everything I want, or don't have **enough control** over my desires and emotions. I constantly seek the crying need to feel stronger than food and my feelings and emotions. I therefore prefer to make myself vomit rather than be in good health, because I deeply despise myself. I am suffering an intolerable inner conflict. I would like people to approach me and allow me to share their emotions and mine, but at the same time it disturbs

36. **Buerger's disease**: Also called 'Leo **Buerger's disease'**, after the name of the physician who first described it.

me so much that I want to reject them right off so as not to be affected in my intimacy and to keep control over my emotions. The gaze directed at me, either by myself or by others, causes a conflict about my own identity and the image that I project, which often disgusts me. I tell myself that I am nothing and that I merge into the mass, I am submerged, which sometimes suits me. However, I would also like to take my place, pull my weight and be different! I generally feel a deep depression, despair and anguish that I want to soothe, a frustration for which I am trying to compensate. I have an image of myself that I want to rehabilitate: I would want so much for it to be perfect! **Bulimia** is strongly related to the mother (source of life), to the maternal side and to creation. Am I in reaction against my mother? Do I feel that I was controlled and intimidated when I was little, so that by eating like this, I am trying to escape my mother, neutralize her (in the metaphysical sense), or leave this planet? Do I feel joyful by acting like this? Is it possible that I may have experienced the weaning stage, when I was a baby, as an abandonment? As if I was being 'torn' from my mother? If such is the case, I have the impression that I am going to 'die of hunger', hence the need to eat great amounts of food to fill the void and diminish my stress. I feel lost, at the mercy of predators.

As a **bulimic person**, I must remain open to **Love**. The necessity of accepting↓♥ that there is something for me to understand, in this depressive state, leads me to **Love**, and I learn to **Love** myself and accept↓♥ myself more as a channel for divine energy. I am on this earth to accomplish a mission for myself, with my mother and the people I **Love**. Why not appreciate the beauty of the Universe? I accept↓♥ my body as it is, my ego and its limits, and food as a gift of life. I accept↓♥ **Love** for myself and for the others, and I discover the joys of being in this world. That's all.

BUNIONS / CORNS *See: TOES*

BURNETT'S SYNDROME *See: MILK — ALKALI SYNDROME*

BURNOUT / EXHAUSTION *See also: ASTHENIA, DEPRESSION*

A **burnout** generally manifests itself after I have given up a struggle where I unsuccessfully tried to express a certain ideal. The time and energy devoted to trying to implement this ideal were so great that I 'burned the candle from both ends.' I exhausted myself and made myself sick. It is a **deep inner emptiness** because I refuse a situation in which I want to see some real, concrete and durable change, either at work, in my family or in my couple. I am a devoted perfectionist and I want to achieve my ideal. It may also be a part of me that I don't accept↓♥. I feel I am fighting the whole of humanity because it seems to be functioning at cross-purposes with my deep expectations and convictions. It is as if I was seeing a collective lie, a heedlessness or a carelessness that is clashing and affecting my deeper truth. "Why go on? I am giving up; it is just too much for me!" **Burnouts** are very frequent among teachers and nurses, in reaction to their respective work organizations. A feeling of powerlessness before an unachievable ideal is very present. It is a form of compulsion, because I want **at all costs** to change the system with approaches better adapted to modern times. At the same time, I may have difficulty in adjusting to the new technologies, which I perceive as aggressive. If I feel that I want to save the world, I must verify my attitude right now. A **burnout** is also an illness of **escape**. I can ask myself: "What am I trying to escape by working to excess? Am I afraid of having to face myself? Do I need a reason to no longer be with a spouse whom I can't stand? What am I trying to prove, while avoiding the fear of failure?" My great need for recognition and my fear of criticism impel me to work more and more, until the day when I just can't go on any longer. The symptoms of **burnout** are clear enough: mental and physical fatigue, lowered vital energy, incoherent thoughts! **Exhaustion** occurs, and then, calm and rest appear, so that I can recharge my energy.

I accept↓♥ that I don't have to please everyone! That is a dream, and true reality is knowing that I do my best by applying 100% of myself, and I recover serenity, inner peace and real **Love** in action.

BURNS *See also: ACCIDENT, SKIN (IN GENERAL)*

A **burn**, from various sources (heat, cold, etc.), causes a lesion in the skin.

Skin is the limit between the inside and the outside, the border between my inner world and the world around me. Something is **burning** me up inside: a deep pain, deeply repressed, gloomy and violent emotions (anger, sorrow, despair) that I turn against myself in the form of **guilt** and **self-punishment** (**burn**). A **burn** may involve several levels of the body (skin, soft tissues, body fluids, sometimes the bones). An 'emotional' or 'mental' **burn** manifests itself physically in a very strong and aggressive manner. I check the part of the body that has been burned. For the **hands**, it is probably because I feel very guilty of doing something related to **a current situation** and because I persist in stubbornly facing someone or a situation. The **feet** concern the future and the next direction of my actions. I may fear being introduced to a new person or a new situation because I am **burning** to know them. Maybe I fear that my projects will go up in smoke. I may also have a **burning desire** to find myself with a person I **Love**. I may '**play with fire'** in a special situation in my life, and I need to be more vigilant about whatever I say and do. I may also verify the type of **burn**: liquids (boiling water, gasoline) may be related to a **violent emotional reaction**, whereas a **burn** with a more solid substance (embers, metals, etc.) involves a **burning** (combustion) on the **mental or spiritual** level. **Mild burns** remind me to go more slowly and to focus my attention on the present moment instead of dissipating my energy by applying it to several things at once. A **more severe burn** manifests more violent and destructive emotions. I feel '**burned'** by someone or by a past or present situation that is crystallized in me. I examine what emotions I am experiencing as '**burning'** me inside. I feel stuck, as if my freedom was curtailed. I accuse the others, but I am the one who needs to take on my responsibilities and respect myself, in order to bring others to respect me too. There exist different types of **burns** that are classified according to their depth. Thus, everything stated above holds true with more or less intensity, depending on how deep the **burn** is. Thus, **first-degree burns** that affect the superficial part of the skin, such as a sunburn, may involve annoyances in some situations of my life. **Second-degree burns** more often concern sadness about some aspects of my life that I feel are important. **Third-degree burns**, which affect the skin to its full depth, may attack a muscle, a tendon or an organ. These **burns** correspond to intense anger and aggressiveness that pierce my natural protections, physical as well as psychological. In cases of severe **burns**, the physical effects cannot be reversed. However, all the divine qualities (**Love,** tenderness, respect, etc.) can manifest themselves to enable me to integrate the experience of a severe **burn.**

Instead of seeing only the difficulties and problems of my life, I now accept↓♥ to see **Love** in each situation of my life. **Love** is everywhere, and I remain open to draw the lessons from my experiences. This is the normal integration process at the level of the **heart♥**. I can therefore heal my inner and outer injuries alike.

BURPING, BELCHING *See: ERUCTATION*

BURSITIS / SYNOVIAL EFFUSION *See also: ACHILLES' HEEL TENDON, ARM AILMENTS, ARTHRITIS (IN GENERAL), ELBOWS, INFLAMMATION, KNEE AILMENTS, SHOULDERS*

Bursitis (also called **hygroma**) is an inflammation or swelling of the bursa in the joints of the shoulder, the elbow, the patella or the Achilles' heel tendon (near the foot). This bursa, which resembles a small sac, contains a fluid that reduces friction in the joints. The bursa thus provides fluid, easy and gracious movements.

Bursitis is often related to what I experience in my work. It indicates **frustration** or **intense irritation**, **contained anger** over a situation or a person whom I really feel like 'punching', in the case where the ***arms*** are affected (shoulder or elbow), or 'kicking', in the case where the ***legs*** are affected (patella or Achilles' heel tendon), so enraged am I! My thoughts are **rigid**, and something absolutely does not suit me! I have had enough and, rather than express what I am experiencing, I contain my emotions. It is possible to find the cause of my desire to hit by examining what I can, and cannot, do with this painful arm. If my left side is sore, it involves the affective level. On the right side, my responsibilities and my 'rational' side are involved (work, for example). I feel the pain even if I hold back from striking anyone. I must find a more adequate way to express what I feel. I can also examine my life and ask myself if it still has any meaning; are there still things to be done that excite me, or am I deeply bored? I am feeling irritation. I may even have the impression that people are profiting from me. Do I have the right to be happy? I expect a lot from others, but I should also contribute some things myself, in order to attract what I want in life.

Instead of leaning on others, I accept↓♥ to take charge of myself; otherwise, I will remain in this state of inertia. I find the cause of my pain, I remain open and I change my attitude by better accepting↓♥ my feelings and my emotions. I can then transform them into **Love** and harmony, to my advantage and for the well-being of others. My body is only telling me to adopt a more positive attitude, so I can adjust to the new situations that come up.

BUTTOCKS

The **buttocks** are the fleshy part of the body on which I sit and take place, **MY PLACE**. They symbolize my **power**, my foundations. They refer to my feeling of confidence based on the fact that I feel safe. It is my inner authority, my feeling of pride. When I tighten my **buttocks** or walk with my **buttocks tightened**, I am feeling threatened, I am afraid of losing control, I am holding in. It often happens that my **buttocks** are tense when I feel watched by a person in authority before me, or when I am afraid of 'not being OK' or 'up to the mark', with my parents, for instance. I'd like to '**spank'** this person, but I can't do it. I don't want to be noticed, because that could lead me to change, to accept↓♥ past or later things, events or situations that I am not ready to come to terms with. Am I able to 'establish my seat of authority'? Or am I in reaction against it because, as a youngster, I was given a **spanking** or someone dared to lay their hands on my **buttocks**? On the other hand, if I walk with my **buttocks** very relaxed and with a very pronounced swing of the hips, then I am taking my place, mine and that of others. I like power because by directing, I ensure my control. I don't have to change: I try to force others to change! I become **Aware** of the fact that I am clinging to my past, my ideas, my old wounds, and may even feel resentment or anger. How far do I want to evade my responsibilities? Why would I doubt my inner strength? I feel unstable, and the gaze of others bothers me a lot. I am distracted and 'soft' about the decisions I have to make. I often feel that I am 'falling between two stools' or constantly have someone 'sticking close behind'[37].

I accept↓♥ to let go and move forward, and open myself to new experiences in life. I accept↓♥ to develop my social power congenially with my entourage.

BUZZING / RINGING IN THE EARS *See: EARS / BUZZING / TINNITUS*

37. **To have someone sticking close behind:** To have someone behind me who is either watching me, pursuing me, or from whom I want to flee.

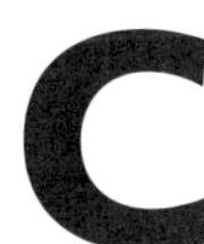

CÆCUM *See: APPENDICITIS*

CALCANEUM *See: HEEL*

CALCULI (nephritic / renal) *See: RENAL CALCULI*

CALCULI / STONES (in general) *See also: CALCULI / STONES (IN GENERAL), RENAL CALCULI*

A **calculus** is a stony concretion that is formed by the precipitation of certain components (calcium, cholesterol) of bile or urine.

A **calculus** is the accumulation (or 'additive effect') of false ideas, hardening one's position, withdrawal, frustration, or mistaken notions about reality, which can be illustrated by the expression 'making a **calcul**ation mistake'. It may also be repressed emotions and feelings; a concentration of thoughts like a mass of energy that solidifies and crystallizes to the point of forming very hard stones in the organ where the cause of the disease manifests itself. As I feel inferior to others, I cultivate sorrow and feel bitter about life. My stubbornness makes me move away from my real needs. I have the impression that someone is ***encroaching*** upon me, on my 'territory'.

I accept↓♥ to trust in life and I know that I can 'count' on my divine power that will enable me to see events with a greater openness of mind and quite safely.

CALF *See: LEG — LOWER PART*

CALLOSITIES / CALLUSES *See: FEET — CALLUSES AND CORNS, SKIN — CALLOSITIES*

CALLUSES / CORNS *See: FEET — CALLUSES AND CORNS*

CANCER (in general) *See also: TUMORS*

Cancer was one of the main diseases of the 20th century. These abnormal **cancerous** cells develop, and the immune system, which cannot distinguish the healthy cells from the unhealthy ones, does not react to their presence, and the cancerous cells thus proliferate rapidly in the body.

Humans often have **precancerous** cells present in their organism, but the immune system, which is the body's natural defense system, usually deals with them before these cells become **cancerous**. Because these abnormal cells develop incessantly and uncontrollably[1], they can hinder the healthy functioning of an organ or tissue and can thereby affect the organism's vital parts. When these cells invade different parts of the body, this is called **generalized cancer**[2]. **Cancer** is chiefly linked with **suppressed emotions**, **deep resentment**, and at times with something that dates back to an issue or a situation that still perturbs me today and about which I **never dared to express my deep feelings**. Even if **cancer** can show up soon after a difficult divorce, the loss of a job, the loss of a **loved** one, etc., it is usually the **result** of many years of **inner conflict**, **guilt**, **wounds**, **sadness**, **resentment**, **hate**, **confusion** and **tension**. I live with **desperation** and **self-rejection** that wear me down. I feel a little like a dunce[3]. I constantly ruminate the same feeling of failure. What is happening on the outside of me is a reflection of what is happening on the inside of me, the human individual being represented by the cell, and the environment or society by the tissue. More often than not, if I have **cancer**, I am a good loving person, devoted, very attentive and full of kindness toward my entourage, extremely sensitive, sowing **Love** and happiness all around me. During all this time, my own personal emotions are suppressed in the deepest part of me. I comfort myself and fool myself by seeking satisfaction outside of me rather than looking for it within, because I have **very low self-esteem**. So I take care of everyone else, **putting my own needs last**. I feel powerless to change my life. This helplessness derives from the impression that I have no power over my life. I leave this power to an authority greater than myself and located outside of me. I am not in contact with my own body and emotions. I am lost, for I define myself through others. I have no identity. I am a stranger to myself. I leave my place to others; I therefore let go of my healthy cells, which represent my identity, and they are replaced by foreign cells that do not have their proper place inside of my body. But as the well-being of those around me comes before my own well-being, I decide that I am worthless and that I can allow others to invade me. I hesitate to take charge of my life, believing I am incapable of doing so. Since life seems to have nothing more to give me, I surrender and lose the desire to live. Why struggle? If I go through a lot of **strong emotions** of **hate**, **guilt** or **rejection**, I will experience a very powerful reaction (like the cell): my healthy cells will turn against me and my unhealthy cells will prevail; I will even feel responsible for the suffering and problems of others and I will want to **destroy myself**. The **cancerous** cells live in isolation, exactly as I do when, faced with a situation that I find difficult to accept↓♥, I withdraw inside myself: I say little about it and I repress the emotions that are

---

1. According to the work of Doctor **Ryke Geerd Hamer**, **cancer** is the development of specialized and organized cells originating from a special program produced by the brain in response to psychological overstress.
2. In the case of **generalized cancer**, there is often a question of metastases, which are **cancerous** cells that originate from other **cancerous** cells located elsewhere in the body and that were transported by the blood or lymph networks. It seems that there exists little or no evidence to support this hypothesis of **cancerous** cells transporting themselves from one location to another. It could be the case, rather, that **the initial cancer originating from a conflict** has made manifest and **uncovered another conflict** which, in turn, is provoking another **cancer**, and so on.
3. **Dunce**: Someone who is miserable, with poor self-esteem.

poisoning me. "I am angry at life"; "Life is too unfair". I play life's 'Victim' and soon become the 'Victim' of **cancer**. It is usually hate toward a person or a situation that will 'eat me from the inside', that will induce cells to self-destruct. This hate is deeply hidden inside my being, and I am not even **Aware** that it exists. It is hidden behind my 'good person's' mask. My body slowly disintegrates, just as my **Soul** is: I need to fulfill my unsatisfied desires instead of trying to please everyone else. I must offer joy and 'little acts of tenderness' to myself. I have accumulated resentment, inner conflicts, guilt, and self-rejection toward myself because I have always functioned in accordance with others, and not in accordance with what I want. The exemplary patience that I present to others is very often associated with low self-esteem. I avoid giving myself **Love** and appreciation because I don't believe that I deserve it. My will to live becomes almost nil. I feel useless. "What's there to live for?" It is my way of putting an end to life. I am destroying myself, which is a **disguised suicide**. I have this feeling that I 'missed my chance with life', and I see this as a failure. Death may appear, even unconsciously, more beautiful than the life I am leading. I need to redefine who I really am instead of identifying with the image that others want me to project. I need to drop my masks. I may be anxious for a moment, but it is essential for me to regain mastery over my life. And I will discover that I have all the courage and all the strength required to accomplish all my dreams. The part of my body that is affected enlightens me as to where my problem or problems originate from: this tells me what kind of mental maps I am dealing with, or the attitudes I need to adopt in order to overcome this illness and make it disappear. I must **resume contact with my inner self and accept↓♥ myself as I am** with my qualities, my shortcomings, my strengths and my weaknesses. I accept↓♥ to let go of my old attitudes and moral habits. **Accepting↓♥** my illness is essential for me to be able, then, to 'fight' it. If I refuse to accept↓♥ the disease, how can I then heal from it?

I accept↓♥ to remake contact with this part of me from which I had cut myself off, in order to also resume contact with life. **I open my heart♥ and become consciously Aware** of all that life has to offer me, and of how much I am part of it. Even if **cancer** seems at first sight to be playing the role of the evil enemy, I realize that it is a catalyst to help me make important changes in my life. The fact of receiving a holistic treatment, massage or any natural technique that I am comfortable with, will have a harmonizing effect that will enable me to open my **consciousness** to all the wonders of life and the beauty that surrounds me and that will help to reinforce my immune system. I accept↓♥ to come to terms with the different emotions that inhabit me. I regain mastery over my life. Only I know what is good for me! Only I can decide to heal. I accept↓♥ to be able to heal, for I have many things to accomplish and many dreams to fulfill. I accept↓♥ to live in the present moment, accepting↓♥ my whole past as a period for learning to discover myself, to know who I truly am. By allowing life to flow in me, my cells will be well nourished and will replace those that I no longer need.

CANCER of the BLOOD *See: BLOOD — LEUKEMIA*

CANCER of the BONES *See: BONES — (CANCER OF THE...)*

CANCER of the BREASTS *See also: BREAST DISORDERS*

The **breasts** represent femininity and motherhood. This sort of **cancer** generally indicates certain attitudes and thoughts deeply rooted since early childhood. Since the 1960s, in certain parts of the world, women have been asserting themselves more, taking their place in society and wanting to move forward. I may therefore find it difficult to express my true feelings and find a balance between my role as a mother and an accomplished woman. These deep inner conflicts torment me as a woman who is seeking a proper balance. It has been discovered that this type of **cancer** generally comes from a **strong feeling of inner guilt** toward oneself or toward one or several of one's children: *"Why was he born? What did I do to have him? Am I a good enough **mother** or **woman** to take care of him?"* All these questions increase my level of guilt, leading me to reject myself and increasing my fear that others may reject me. I must remember that "**Love** for my child is always present, but that my thoughts are very powerful and I must be vigilant". If I judge myself too severely, all my anger and rejection will be amplified, and my emotions will be 'evacuated' through my breasts, which will become the symbol of my 'failure'. **Breast cancer** will thus help me to become **Aware** that I am experiencing a conflicted situation, involving myself or someone else and related to an element that is part of my vital space, of my 'little ***nest***'. It will often involve my children, my 'fledglings', or someone whom I consider as such (for example, my sick mother whom I sense to be helpless, like 'a little child'). At all costs, I want to give my child everything, and I also want her to take everything I give her. Otherwise, it is doubt and guilt that will take control. I may also fear that my '***nest***' (home) could come apart. I may also have a great fear or great stress about the survival of one or more of my children. I am afraid that if something happened to me, their father might not be able to take care of them and nourish them emotionally. In a broader sense, the '***nest***' can encompass my spouse, my home, and my brothers and sisters, especially if they live under the same roof. It is therefore about the family, what historically could be called the '**clan**', that I fear there might be a collapse or a breaking apart. There is a fear, a thought that constantly comes to mind and is ***unthinkable***, of discovering, for instance, a betrayal by my spouse. I would like to be able to take care of everyone and 'feed' them, but that is impossible and it tears me apart. Men as well as women may develop this sort of **cancer**, which is often the male's inner conflict in accepting↓♥ his own divine feminine nature. Certain men sometimes manifest their female and maternal side almost as much as women. As a **man**, I will never be a woman, but energy-wise, I may be as female as she is, or even more so. That is why **breast cancer** in me, as a **man**, is associated with self-esteem and with my capacity to naturally express my innate female side. It may be related to the very fact of being a man and to the unconscious desire to be a woman. It is one aspect that I must balance in my life.

The left side belongs to the affective domain, and the right side, to the rational domain. A **cancer in the left breast** therefore indicates all my affective difficulties and repressed emotions as a woman (it mainly concerns my immediate family) and it is in my interest to accept↓♥ the woman and the mother in me, and the inner feelings I have about each of these two roles. In the **right breast**, **cancer** points at the responsible woman and what is expected of me (what I expect to do with this 'outer' woman). Here, the notion of 'family' can include any grouping or association that I may consider as my family. I note that this also applies to men, although **breast cancer** is rarer in men. For me, as a woman in the physical world, the volume and shape of my breasts may have a certain importance depending on the circumstances. It has been noticed that if my male side is dominant (Yang)[4], I may have smaller **breasts** or I may often consider them as useless or worthless. The body speaks, and so do my **breasts**; It is for me to decide the importance of this female and sexual symbol.

The search for a point of balance is important, and the body will adjust its energy according to the decisions made by the woman (or the man) in the future. Everything depends on one's attitude of **Love** and acceptance↓♥ of oneself. I become **Aware** of the fact that I forget myself and live only for others. I am born biologically, but not yet emotionally. My emotions are repressed, and I can avoid being in contact with them by exaggeratedly taking care of others. I give myself a clear **conscience**. At bottom, I know that I am powerless to live for and by myself. I cling to someone. I fill my emptiness with the emotions of others instead of my own. I accept↓♥ that healing will be found by changing my attitude toward myself and the future. Instead of destroying myself with my negative thoughts, I will reconnect with my inner world. I welcome my emotions, even those that are linked to difficult events of my past. I take a step back and ask myself how, in all of these situations, I could have respected myself more and given myself more **Love**. My grief goes away because I accept↓♥ to see the lessons that life has to teach me. I express everything I have always wanted to hide. It is by respecting myself and believing in my potential that I can create the life I want and recover perfect health.

CANCER of the BRONCHI *See: BRONCHI — BRONCHITIS*

CANCER of the CHEST *See: CANCER OF THE BREASTS*

CANCER of the COLON *See also: INTESTINES / COLON [AILMENTS OF THE...] / CONSTIPATION*

The **colon** is a part of the large intestine where I digest food. It eliminates what my body has found useless or dirty.

It enables me to discard what is no longer beneficial, and turn the page. My fears, especially about material things or money, will affect it. It is said to be one of the most frequent types of **cancer** in North America because of the

---

4. **Yang**: It is the name given in Chinese medicine to the rational or male energy. Affective or female energy is called **Yin**.

excessive consumption of meat, refined grains and sugar. These foods are difficult to digest and assimilate. There are also other reasons: the constant search for material satisfactions, pleasures and desires, added to the various physical, emotional and mental states I may experience every day (attaining excellence, anxiety, anguish, etc.) are the primary causes of a food or digestive disorder. I have little inner joy and I am more or less satisfied with my life as it is. I feel soiled in one aspect of myself. I eat and I repress my emotions: it is easier, and my needs are filled far more quickly. A separation or a divorce can trigger the development of this **cancer** because they induce a great emotional shock where I cannot 'digest' the situation. I choose a form of reward that is within very easy reach for me. I seek a special satisfaction that I find in fatty and heavy foods. A **cancer of the colon** can derive from causes similar to those of **constipation**, but with a more significant and deeper emotional factor: it is probably a need to 'let go'. I must ask myself what is the situation that I haven't 'digested' yet, or won't admit, and makes me experience resentment? For that reason, it is as if I didn't want to assimilate it to my reality. I am extremely annoyed by this. I see this situation as a dirty trick, as a disgusting, ***abominable*** action. I just can't turn the page. It is as if I was 'stuck' there. Generally, when the **ascending colon** is affected, the situation involves my parents or superiors. The **transverse colon** involves my collateral relatives: sisters, brothers or cousins. At work, it is my colleagues who have the same level of responsibility. The **descending colon** is related to my children, or my subordinates at work. In the case of **constipation**, the energies or emotions closer to the surface are involved, whereas in the case of a **cancer of the colon**, the more deeply located energies and emotions are involved. That is why my intestines may function normally or regularly, while I nevertheless develop a **cancer of the colon**. My intestines therefore do everything they can to keep me in good health, and I must respect them by preserving them in good condition for as long as possible.

I accept↓♥ to be **more open** to the joys of life, and I **express** the emotions that are part of my life! I begin to **practice** various forms of **physical and inner relaxation** that help me take the time to live a better-balanced existence.

CANCER of the ESOPHAGUS *See: ESOPHAGUS*

CANCER of the GANGLIA (of the lymphatic system) *See also: ADENITIS, ADENOPATHY, GANGLION — LYMPHATIC NOD*

The **lymphatic system** is located throughout my body in parallel to my vascular system. It transports a whitish opaque fluid, like diluted milk, called the lymph. Because the lymph contains proteins and lymphocytes (white globules), it plays an important role in the organism's immune and defense process.

The **lymphatic system** is related more directly to my emotions, to my affective side. The **ganglions** serve to filter the impurities from the lymph, in much the same way as the kidneys, the liver and the spleen do for the blood system. A **cancer of the ganglions** indicates to me great fears, guilt and desperation in relation to my **Love** and sexual emotions. Even if my current

Love life is harmonious, deep disappointments may surface in this form of **cancer**. I am seeking a place where I can find ***safe shelter***. I believe that the only way to do so is to be in a group, even to the detriment of my couple.

I must accept↓♥ that everything can find its place in me by allowing life to flow, like water in the river, in harmony and in **Love**, by working on my wounded inner child. I find this feeling of security within me. I know that I am protected at all times and that I only need to allow myself to be guided by the flow of life.

CANCER of the INTESTINE (in general) *See also: CANCER OF THE COLON, INTESTINES / COLON [AILMENTS OF THE...] / SMALL [DISORDERS]*

This **cancer** is usually located in the part of the **intestine** called the **colon**. When I develop this disease, I must ask myself the question: What am I not able to digest and is 'going down sideways'? It may be something I was told and that I found nasty, or maybe an action that I find unfair and unacceptable. The piece to swallow is so big that I don't know if I will be able to digest it. I may also experience great fear, and wonder if I will always have 'enough food in the fridge'. I am afraid of dying of hunger for lack of food. I feel deep anguish because I feel helpless in certain situations. I cling to certain persons, ideas or emotions out of a fear of the unknown, but I would like so much to be rid of them!

Whatever the situation, I accept↓♥ to take a more positive attitude, knowing that life intends the best for me and that I accept↓♥ to live in abundance. I also learn to forgive those persons who have told me, or done to me, something that I find intolerable to digest. I take the time to express to that person how I feel, in order to restore harmony in this situation. I eliminate resentment from my life, and replace it with understanding and openness of mind.

CANCER of the JAW *See: JAW AILMENTS*

CANCER of the LARYNX *See also: CIGARETTES, THROAT DISORDERS*

Cancer of the larynx is also called the '**cancer of smokers'**.

When a malignant tumor starts to grow on the walls of the **larynx**, it means that I feel a great need to express my inner grief. I need to scream to the whole world the inner drama I am going through, but I am afraid of expressing my distress. Is there a person or a situation that prevents me from expressing myself, that is ***braking*** me? Maybe I am telling myself: *"I may as well shut up, because speaking up will be futile!"* This makes me shut myself in emotionally; I can't take it any longer! I feel that others are attacking me and I feel like getting angry, but I don't dare do so. I don't feel respected for who I am. I am afraid of my deeper emotions. So I avoid facing myself squarely. I play the victim, letting others control my world, my vital space. I want so much my life to be a private preserve! I find it easy to leave my personal authority in the hands of another person or organization outside of me. Revolt and fury are part of my daily bread.

I accept↓♥ to take my place and tell the truth as I see it. This will help me to better perceive my place in my environment and in the Universe.

CANCER of the LIVER *See: LIVER DISORDERS*

CANCER of the LUNGS *See also: BRONCHI — BRONCHITIS, CIGARETTES, LUNG DISEASES*

As the **lungs** are directly related to my capacity for living (inspiration-expiration), a **cancer of the lungs** indicates to me my **fear of dying**. In fact, there is a situation in my life that is gnawing at me inside and giving me the impression that I am smothering and dying. The **lung** is the organ that is related to sadness, and when grief is not expressed outwardly, it is the **lung** that absorbs it. It may follow a separation or a divorce, the death of a loved one, the loss of a job very important to me. There is a very clear notion of failure. In fact, any situation that consciously or unconsciously represents my reason for living. When my reason for living is gone or I fear it may disappear, this highlights the fact that the alternative available to me is, in a sense, death. I feel ***condemned*** to live a situation for the rest of my life. I am often drastic in my judgments. Everything is black or white, nothing in between. I am afraid however of outwardly expressing my thoughts and opinions. I believe in the notion of evil, in my sexuality as well as in the other areas of my life. I feel great helplessness. Others judge my way of living, and I resent them for it. My life is no longer meaningful, and I am disappointed by others who don't meet my expectations. I am constantly worried about someone close: I have invested so much in this relationship, emotionally as well as materially, and here I risk losing everything. What's the use of living if all these efforts were in vain and this is where I now find myself? Then, what about the relation found between smokers and **lung cancer**? I can ask myself if it is cigarette smoke that causes me to have **lung cancer**, or if it is the fear of dying that makes me smoke cigarettes and, as a consequence, makes me develop **lung cancer**. When I smoke, I pull a veil over emotions that bother me and prevent me from living. As this doesn't resolve the conflict, it may grow in me to the point of making me develop **lung cancer**.

Then, I must accept↓♥ life and think that in each inspiration and expiration, it is life that is flowing in me with the air I breathe. I decide <u>to take my place, to give myself space, and I choose what I want to experience</u> despite my fears, and I decide that life is worth living and that I deserve to live. I accept↓♥ that there is no evil on earth, only experiences. I live and let live, with the eyes of a child. I live life to the full!

CANCER of the MOUTH

Mouth cancer may be located in the floor of the **mouth**, in the lips, the tongue, the gums or the palate.

As the skin is the demarcation line between the outside of me and the inside of me, the **mouth** is the main entrance, the hallway between what comes in (air, food, drink) and what goes out (air, words conveying emotions). I may be a person of whom it is said that "he chews up his neighbor". I may have destructive feelings toward myself or one or more other persons, which makes me say: "That one, I would devour!", meaning that I wish him harm, or death, in a sense. My great inner emptiness increases my difficulty in being myself, as an autonomous being who savors life. I feel far from other people, physically or emotionally. I can no longer stand the coldness of my existence.

I accept↓♥ that I have a great need to let feelings of **Love** come into me, and express the same feelings to the people around me and to myself, saying words of **Love** to myself. I accept↓♥ the pleasures of life.

CANCER of the NEVUS / MOLE *See: SKIN — MELANOMA [MALIGNANT]*

CANCER of the OVARIES *See: OVARIES [DISORDERS OF THE]*

CANCER of the PANCREAS *See: PANCREAS*

CANCER of the PHARYNX *See: THROAT — PHARYNX*

CANCER of the PROSTATE *See: PROSTATE DISEASES*

CANCER of the RECTUM *See: INTESTINES — RECTUM*

CANCER of the SKIN *See: SKIN — MELANOMA [MALIGNANT]*

CANCER of the SMALL INTESTINE *See: INTESTINE — SMALL [DISORDERS]*

CANCER of the STOMACH *See also: STOMACH DISORDERS*

If I have **stomach cancer**, I must become **Aware** of the issue or the situation that I can't digest. This situation 'that just won't go through' is something I feel very intensely and strongly. "*What they did to me and I had to endure is abominable. Worse, I never saw it coming*!" "*I am totally **flabbergasted!***" That may convey what I am experiencing. I have reached the point where I want to give up, as the burden has become too heavy. I tend to blame others, holding them guilty of interfering in my life. As I give all this power to others, I feel powerless to create my own life. I have given up my dreams and ambitions even if deep down, I would like to show others what I am capable of. Frustration overcomes me, anguish gnaws at me, but above all, it is the grief and sadness that are so intense that I no longer find a reason for living.

I accept↓♥ to become **Aware** of the reason for this situation and of the lesson to be drawn from it, in order to 'weather the storm' and make the **cancer** resorb itself. I can only be a winner if I let go of my anger and my resentment and replace them with acceptance↓♥ and forgiveness.

CANCER of the TESTICLES *See also: OVARIES [DISORDERS OF THE]*

It is in the **testicles** that the sperm essential for reproduction is produced.

If I develop a **cancer of the testicles**, I must check whether I am experiencing an intense feeling due to the loss of a ***child***, or something in my life that was almost as important or precious to me as a child. I may have suffered the death of one of my ***children***, from an illness, in an accident or following an abortion. Or it could be, for example, one of my ***children*** who left home 'slamming the door' and whom I never saw again. As he went out of my life suddenly, I may experience this situation as the **loss** of a loved one, as if he had died. Or again, as a businessman who made bad investments, I have lost the company to which I 'gave birth' and that I considered as 'my baby'.

Whatever the situation involved, I have surely felt guilty of some things I have done or 'should have done', words I 'shouldn't have said', etc. I feel I have failed on a test, or badly muffed a project. I examine how this can negatively affect my perception of my sexuality and my virility. Whatever the situation experienced, I accept↓♥ to become **Aware** of the feelings inside of me. I accept↓♥ them in order to heal my wounds and learn to laugh again, and look ahead instead of mulling over the past.

CANCER of the THROAT *See: THROAT — PHARYNX*

CANCER of the TONGUE *See also: ALCOHOLISM, CIGARETTES*

Though it is a known fact that **cancer of the tongue** can be induced by smoking or alcoholism, it comes from a **deep feeling of despair that means I no longer have a taste for living**. Furthermore, I may not even express this pain of living, and I may repress these emotions inside of me. Alcoholism and smoking are but amplifiers of the feelings I have; with alcoholism, I flee my emotions, and with smoking, I blow a smokescreen over these emotions that I don't want to see. As it is with my **tongue** that I catch and position food in order to be able to bite it with my teeth, if I have a **cancer of the tongue**, I must ask myself, figuratively, if I feel I am not able to **catch the 'piece** of food'. I see what I want to catch as vital for me. It may be work, food, or a new relationship. The situation I am in is making me crazy! I feel I am going to explode! I have so many emotions imprisoned inside of me. I need to search outside of myself for a semblance of strength, when that strength is, quite simply, inside of me. I control myself perfectly because I feel great insecurity. I have so much resentment, often toward myself, because I 'closed my trap' too often. If the cancer is located on the edge of the **tongue**, where it comes into contact with the **teeth**, maybe I want to 'tear to pieces' something or someone I just 'can't swallow'.

I accept↓♥ to feel like living again, to increase my self-esteem, and I learn to express my emotions. This way, I will discover everything beautiful life has to offer me. I go into action and I will get whatever I need because I deserve it! I accept↓♥ that I may feel helpless at times, because I have no control over other people, but only over myself. Once I accept↓♥ that, it is easy to resume contact with my inner strength, and that is when I can create my life as I see fit!

CANCER of the UTERUS (cervix and corpus) *See also: UTERUS (IN GENERAL)*

The **uterus** represents femininity, the original womb and the **maternal home**, especially the **corpus of the uterus**. As a woman, I probably repress certain emotions concerning my **home** and my **family**. I may feel guilty, resentful or hate-filled, but I don't talk about it. The home often represents an ideal to attain, in relation to my couple or my family. I ask myself questions, not so much about my relationship as a couple, but about my home and my incapacity to have a child. I feel great sorrow, and my joy in living is affected. This type of **cancer** is deeply rooted in the principles of the home that feeds you, and in my attitudes and behavior linked to it. I may experience great fears, insecurity, ***anger*** or guilt at the idea that this home may not take form as I wished, or it risks falling apart, which would mean a failure for me. There will follow a cheapening of who I am and of what I am able to achieve: I will think that I am nothing! Am I afraid of experiencing again in my own home the judgment of a failure I suffered in the family home where I grew up? A cancer of the **corpus of the uterus** often affects older women past their menopause. A **cancer of the cervix of the uterus** will usually affect younger women. It is the **cervix of the uterus** that comes into contact with the man's member during sexual relations. Am I being dependent on my spouse in an unhealthy way? Do I feel that he is destroying me or killing me through some of his actions or attitudes? I tend ***to be ruled by*** events, feeling I have no power or control. I may also be facing a situation involving my sexuality, where I see it as disgusting and feel compelled to do my marital duty. I feel that I have to **exhibit** myself. I am sexually very frustrated, feeling abandoned by my spouse, or separated from him, even if nothing shows on the outside. I find it difficult, even painful at times, to open up to my partner because there is something amiss in my vision of having a child with him. I may feel **helpless** before life. This feeling is often found if I experienced a situation of sexual abuse early on. The fear and the rejection of my true needs, ***impulses*** and fantasies may also lead me to shut myself off from a part of me of which I feel ashamed. I must ***repress*** my emotions. I am experiencing a duality about the notion of ***abstinence***; to practice it or not, and for what reasons: that is the question! I want to be ***desirable***, but at the same time, I fear the consequences. I feel like wearing a ***scarf*** over my face to hide it from myself and from others.

I accept↓♥ to take a new look at this home that is mine and also at my relationship as a couple. I must harmonize the ways I perceive myself in my roles as a mother and a woman, in all their many respects.

CANDIDA *See also: INFECTIONS, THRUSH*

There are several sorts of **candida**. The most frequent form in humans is **candida albicans**. Though it may be found in both men and women, it is most often mentioned in women. **Candida** is a Latin word meaning **white**. It is a vaginal infection resulting from the proliferation of fungi in the form of yeast. It resembles the white, crusty yeast that manifests itself following a disorder of the vaginal flora. The bacteria of the vagina normally control the **candida**, but in this instance, the situation changes.

This infection is naturally related to my **commitment** to myself or to my partner, involving my sexuality or any undiscussed situations, expressions and emotions following certain previous personal conflicts. I call into question my sexual activity, my sexuality and my willingness to share with my partner the more intimate aspects of myself. The infection risks occurring when, for example, I have a new partner and my relation with him is very intimate. Chances are that I will be more open to **Love**, sharing and giving. This is new for me, and I need a little time to deal with this recent situation, even if **candida** appears. **Candida** may also result from a feeling of having been **humiliated** or having **been, or felt, sexually abused** by someone. It is a form of **physical and sexual protection**, as the **irritation** prevents me from making **Love**. What is irritating me so? I verify what inner aspect of my sexuality is upset, and I find the actual cause of the physical and inner irritation. Where does my frustration come from? Do I have the impression that I allow others to decide about my life? Will I take the risk of opening up to others, especially of the opposite sex, or will I remain enclosed in my shell? Why do I feel left aside, yet sacrifice myself, and still not take my place? I am afraid of losing my naiveté, my innocence, my pure side.

I accept↓♥ to take my place in life by respecting myself. I must become the **candidate** who will carry the victory and win first place. I take the time to see and assess what is going on and I accept↓♥ my **Love**, openness and inner patience as well as those of my partner.

CANDIDIASIS / MONOLIASIS *See: CANDIDA, THRUSH, VAGINITIS*

CAR SICKNESS *See: SEA SICKNESS, TRAVEL SICKNESS*

CARDIAC ATTACK *See: HEART♥ — INFARCTION [MYOCARDIAL]*

CAROTID ARTERY *See: BLOOD — ARTERIES*

CARPAL TUNNEL SYNDROME *See: CRAMP [WRITER'S]*

CATARACT *See: EYES — CATARACTS*

CELLULITIS

Cellulitis is characterized by an inflammation of the sub-cutaneous cell tissue. **Cellulitis** is usually of a female nature (though possible in men) and manifests itself by water retention and an increased irregular distribution of toxins and fats in the buttocks, the legs, the abdomen, the neck, the back, etc.

Cellulitis is related to anxieties, aspects of myself that I hold back, repressed emotions, **regrets** and **resentments** that I hold on to. It is related to my commitment to myself or to someone else. **I am afraid of fully committing myself** to the person I **love** and I refuse to go ahead. The source of this fear may be an event where I suffered **abandonment**. I refuse to see a part of my youth, often because I was hurt and marked by certain **traumatic** experiences that still make me suffer today and impede my creativity and my inner child's **heart♥**. **Cellulitis** is found more often in women than in men because I, as a woman, began very early on to be concerned with my **appearance** and my **figure**, which I want to be perfect according to the norms of society. I feel like a 'pressed orange'. I feel ugly and inferior, and I tend to develop relations of dependence with others. The æsthetic aspect is excessively important. I hold back my creative side, and so I intoxicate myself by imprisoning all this energy ready to express itself through art, communication or sexuality. '**Jodhpur thighs**' show me how I feel compelled to constantly watch over my children (or anyone standing in for my children) to make sure they get what is best. It indicates how much I want to protect my power as a woman (femininity) and how much I fear being abandoned. **Cellulitis** shows me how passively I live my life. I allow others to lead my life instead of being proactive and assertive in my choices and my actions. I am very insecure, as I fear losing my 'haven of peace'.

I accept↓♥ to identify the feelings that prevent me from moving forward and I integrate them gently in my everyday life. I acknowledge my true worth and allow my creativity to manifest itself. In so doing, I allow energy to flow in my body.

CEREBROVASCULAR ACCIDENT (C.V.A.) *See: BRAIN — CEREBROVASCULAR ACCIDENT [C.V.A.]*

CERVIX (cancer of the) *See: CANCER OF THE UTERUS [CERVIX AND CORPUS]*

CHALAZION *See also: EYELIDS (IN GENERAL)*

It is a small inflammatory tumor (a supple red nodule), usually located on the inner edge of the eyelid.

As the tumor is generally linked to an emotional shock, it appears when I feel an intense emotion about what I see, or saw or no longer can see, and I find that bad. Many things are imposed on me, I must change within rigid rules and constraints, and I can't take it any longer. I am frustrated and feeling great anger. I can verify which eyelid or eye is affected: the left eye is linked to the affective domain, and the right eye represents the rational domain and my responsibilities.

I accept↓♥ to remain open to what I see and I am more focused on myself.

CHANCRE — ORAL ULCER (herpes) *See: MOUTH DISEASES*

CHANCRE (in general) *See also: ULCER (IN GENERAL)*

A **chancre** is located at an isolated place on the skin or on a mucous membrane in the form or an ulcer. It is the sign of a contagious disease at its early stage, and is often of venereal origin.

I am feeling anger about my sexual relations. The location where the **chancre** appears indicates more precisely to me what I am experiencing in this situation. Thus, the **chancre** may appear on the genital parts, on the anus, on the face, or on the inner mucous surfaces of the mouth. When a **chancre** is found **in the mouth**, in the form of an ulcer containing pus, it is because I am holding back from saying certain things. I am dissatisfied, I disapprove of certain situations in my life and I don't dare speak about them. I hold in certain words, so they **ferment** and produce pus. I reject and condemn a situation or an individual. I hold others responsible for my pains. I feel like spitting in their faces.

I accept↓♥ to speak and express myself, **although** I may disagree with life and other people. I must do so if I wish to remain open to the active energy of speech and self-expression. I accept↓♥ myself in my sexuality, and I give myself the right to discover the **Love** that will help me to flourish.

CHAP *See: SKIN — CHAPPING*

CHARCOT'S DISEASE OR AMYOTROPHIC LATERAL SCLEROSIS (ALS)

Charcot's[5] **disease**, or **amyotrophic lateral sclerosis**, is a degenerative disease of the nervous system that mostly affects men.

I constantly diminish myself and I come to believe that I can accomplish nothing in life, that I will never get any advancement in my job. I stagnate in old pains that I preserve preciously, that I feed and keep up over the years. I do inner violence to myself, everything worries me, makes me insecure, makes me hyper-tense and nervous. I trust nobody, and especially not myself. I think I am under surveillance, ***pursued*** even, and they want to ***tail*** me. I imprison myself with my negative attitudes toward myself, I am inflexible.

I accept↓♥ to ask for help, to trust a therapist who will be able to help me lighten this **chariot** of suffering that I bear. I accept↓♥ to be able to create my life positively. I acknowledge that I am a unique being and that I have all the necessary potential to reach the goals I set for myself. By rebuilding a positive image of myself, my body will do so as well.

CHEEKS (gnawing one's inner) *See: MOUTH DISORDERS*

5. **Charcot** (Jean-Martin): A French neurologist (1825–1893). He contributed, through his work on hysteria and hypnosis, to the development of neurological pathology and discovered the locations of many cerebral centers responsible.

CHEST

The **chest** is the anterior and external part of the trunk that extends from the shoulders to the abdomen.

The **chest** is linked to my sense of identity and to the inner part of my being. I tend to stick out my **chest** to give myself courage and show I am strong or, on the contrary, I will shrivel up in fear, shyness or despair. This is where my **heart ♥** and my lungs are located. If I feel **discomfort** or **pain** in this area, I can ask myself: "Has my sensitivity about my family relationships been touched or affected lately?", "Am I afraid of committing myself to a person or a situation, which leads me to avoid opportunities for giving and involving myself?", "Have I buried all sorts of negative emotions that intermingle and destroy me?", "Am I disillusioned with my couple?". I experience a situation as a failure and it weighs heavily on me.

I accept↓♥ that it will be very good for me to show my true feelings and my vulnerability: I am always a winner when I am true!

CHICKENPOX *See: CHILDHOOD DISEASES [VARICELLA]*

CHILBLAIN / PERNIO *See: SKIN — CHILBLAIN / PERNIO*

CHILD / BABY (blue)

The arrival of a **blue child (baby)** is related to a malformation of its **heart♥** at the embryonic stage, which has the effect of redirecting the oxygen-poor blood (blue blood) from the veins into the great arterial circulation flow, without first going through the lungs to receive more oxygen (red blood).

If I am a **blue child**, also called a **blue baby**, I may have felt, in my mother's womb, her great fear of opening herself to **Love** from the outside world. That may have come from a great wound or an 'inner withdrawal from **Love**' caused by an event that broke her **heart♥**. I must not hold my mother responsible for my condition. By the law of affinities, I arrived in this family because I had similar challenges to take up about **Love**. I am only showing in a physically more concrete way the step into **consciousness** that I must take, and I and my mother will be able to mutually help each other in this.

I accept↓♥ now that **Love** is life itself and that my growing power to **love** will form a **Love** shield that will protect me in my exchanges with the outside world.

CHILD (stillborn / deadborn) *See: CHILDBIRTH — ABORTION*

CHILDBIRTH — ABORTION / MISCARRIAGE — STILLBORN CHILD

An **abortion**, or a **miscarriage**, is a **termination of pregnancy** before the 180th day (about 6½ months) of gestation. The term **abortion** is generally used in the case of a voluntary termination, or **induced abortion (IA)**. When the

termination is spontaneous, when it is a non-induced loss of the fetus, the term **miscarriage** is used. When the death occurs after 180 days of gestation or during labor, then the fetus (child) is described as **stillborn**.

When I have a **miscarriage**, I ask myself who wanted a child, I or my spouse? Unconsciously, I am afraid that the child to be born will change my life as a couple, my work, my habits. I am afraid I don't have the necessary qualities to become a good mother, and this may go back to moments experienced in my own childhood. Will I ***fail*** in my desire to be a good mother? Am I fully living my life? Am I having doubts because this may not be the right time for having this child? Do I want a child solely to fill my inner void? I feel so insecure that I constantly feel I am 'walking on ***eggs***'. As a mother, I may be living so much in a psychological prison that a child would be 'too much' at this time. I need freedom. I need some escape, to expel everything. I feel stifled, and it may be best, for me and the child, that I wait until I am stronger and better focused on myself before giving birth to a child. It may also be that the **Soul** who was taking body changed its mind or only needed to experience a few months of life on this earth. Life may have appeared to be a prison for it too. In many situations, there is a **gemellary pregnancy** (more than one ovum) and the body rejects one ovum or fetus. The surviving baby, Aware of this, may be eternally in search of the other, of **Love**, with a feeling of guilt over it having survived, but not the other. I may also prevent myself from feeling any pleasure, or therefore any orgasms, because in a sense I am a carrier of death. In the case of an **IA**, I may be in reaction against men and feeling very aggressive. I may often gain weight, which corresponds to the weight of the child who would have been born.

Whatever the situation, I accept↓♥ to remain open in my **heart♥** and mobilize my energy to resolve this 'immature' situation; otherwise, any future pregnancies risk being complex and incomplete. **Love**, responsibility and mutual respect between spouses (if such is the case) are the essential feelings that must be shown if I want my child to arrive **at full term**. I learn to take good care of myself. I commit myself to being happy and to loving myself as I am. I recover my freedom to be who I am. By being capable of taking my own responsibilities and decisions, I will be able to present myself with the gift of having a child and having the inner strength to guide it through life.

CHILDBIRTH / DELIVERY (in general) *See also: BIRTH [HOW MY BIRTH TOOK PLACE], PREGNANCY / DISORDERS / PROLONGED*

Childbirth may be one of the most traumatic transition experiences there are for the child being born. It is a natural phenomenon; I, as a woman, deliver the child I am carrying. The pains of **childbirth** may be linked to several fears, mainly those of suffering and delivering, to the accumulated pain of **my own inner child**. The ailments or sufferings may also originate from the fact that the child to be born will constantly remind me of reality and my responsibility to my inner child. I may feel some concerns about **this part of me made up of my own flesh and blood**, for which I am taking responsibility. In this situation, as in many others, **childbirth** carries several more or less founded beliefs, such as that it is necessary to suffer in order to give birth (as it is to be beautiful!). This is not necessarily true, especially on the higher planes of consciousness. The pains can instead call up in me, mostly unconsciously, the **painful memory of having crossed over from the world of Light into the more limiting one of bodily matter**. Difficulties in **childbirth** often occur when I am afraid of dying during the process, or afraid, consciously or not, that the baby might die. This is especially present if I already lost a baby once or almost died myself. When I am carrying a child, I have a feeling of fullness: the baby to come fills my inner emptiness. I feel so fused with my baby that we are like hand in glove, inseparable. At the moment of **childbirth**, I must again face this void that was outwardly filled for some time, but is always there inside of me. I may therefore experience **childbirth** as a tearing-away, a loss, a painful separation. I may have planned how I will go through my pregnancy: what I eat, what I drink, the right exercises, I go on smoking or I stop. I felt I had some control over the conditions in which I wanted my baby to spend the first 9 months of its life, but now I no longer have any control over how my **childbirth** is going to take place. I feel helpless in this process, and part of me may resist the birth of this child. Several other questions may also come up: What can I expect after the birth of this child? Will I still be as desirable for my spouse? Am I a good mother? Does my child have everything it needs? Can it be that I don't want to give birth because I am in a blessed state, more Loved and fussed over than usual by my spouse?

In any case, **childbirth** is a tremendous experience. It enables me to really show my ability to face any future moments of transition and change. I accept↓♥ to trust myself, knowing I have all the strength and energy needed to give birth to my child and adequately care for it. I take the opportunity to be reborn to myself. I also accept↓♥ to take care of my inner child: by being able to give myself **Love** to fill this emptiness, I will be able to be far more present for my child.

CHILDBIRTH (premature)

A **premature childbirth** is one that takes place between the 29th and the 38th weeks in the absence of menstruations.

When this occurs, it may be that I don't feel sufficiently **mature** to carry this child to term and that unconsciously, I wish to get rid of it before it has reached full term. I may unconsciously want to 'reject' this child, as I myself may feel rejected sometimes. I may have kept this pregnancy a secret, hidden from someone out of fear of that person's reaction. The anxiety, even unconscious, of having to take on a responsibility for which I am not ready, or the fact that I don't feel ready, could make me "ardently desire to **give birth** as soon as possible" in order to make this waiting anxiety stop. In any case, whether I want to make this anxiety stop or whether I reject the child, this state of **Consciousness** is generally denied. I imagine the scenario: who, me – a woman who **consciously** renounces her own child? It is possible, but this situation usually transforms itself into an unconscious rejection of this marvelous experience.

In any case, I accept↓♥ that everything has turned out for the best, for myself and for the child to be born.

CHILDHOOD DISEASES (in general) *See also: DISEASES [IN CHILDREN], MUMPS*

Rubella, the measles, chickenpox, whooping cough, the mumps, scarlet fever, in short, all the **typical childhood diseases** usually coincide with a **child**'s developmental periods. If I am a child, these **diseases** often occur in the midst of difficulties at school or when I am anxious about a situation. If I sense dissension or a war between my parents or other people I **love**, I become more vulnerable and more easily manifest a **disease specific to children**. I am seeking security and affection. When one of these **diseases** appears, I develop my immune system that represents my capacity for adjustment or my capacity for entering into relationships: "I in relation to others". It may be a period of rest that the body requires. If I am a **parent**, giving a child tenderness, **Love** and attention will enable her to become stronger in order to go forward in life more confidently. An **adult** experiencing one of these **diseases** has some unresolved childhood issue, a situation that was poorly managed: "Is the situation I am currently facing linked to an emotional situation that I experienced in my **childhood**?" For example: it may be that I suffered a rejection in school that I wasn't able to manage and today, I am experiencing much the same sort of rejection at work.

I accept↓♥ to resolve the feelings from my **childhood** to grow more fully, and I no longer fixate on such emotions, but free myself of them instead.

CHILDHOOD DISEASES — MEASLES

The **measles** is a contagious, epidemic viral **disease**, producing a feverish eruption of cutaneous and mucous red spots, preceded by rhino-pharyngitis. It can further be complicated by bronchopulmonary and neurological symptoms (encephalitis), which explains why it is one of the prime causes of infant mortality in poor countries.

The **measles** occurs after en event where I experienced an unexpected separation. I am in a state of shock, for it came as a surprise, and this situation 'stinks'. "How *could* he do that to me?" "They went behind my back, that's for sure". I have always tried to satisfy the desires of others (parents, friends, etc.) at the price of my own freedom. **Unaware** of my worth, I feel vulnerable. I easily turn 'angry red'; I blush for the slightest reason. I am afraid of being spontaneous for I am uncertain of my possibilities. My inaction protects me to a degree and of course, people take care of me without any effort on my part. It is not 'my fault' if I am sick. Where is the real power? How can I be guided but not be controlled?

I accept↓♥ to no longer live in anonymity, to be given the needed space for discovering my limits and my capacities. I become a whole, autonomous being. I am a unique being, and I let go of the rigid structures I needed in the past: I am strong enough, and I listen to my inner voice to know what is good for me.

CHILDHOOD DISEASES — RUBELLA / GERMAN MEASLES

Rubella is a contagious, epidemic, viral **disease** that produces a feverish eruption of cutaneous red spots of varied appearance. Its seriousness resides in the risk of a miscarriage or of anomalies or malformations in the fetus when it affects a non-immunized pregnant woman. It is related to the measles.

I experienced an unexpected separation that felt like a real 'slap in the face'! I must now speak through a third party. I am ashamed of having been 'had'. How totally unfair! Still, these things can happen, because I am poorly **Aware** of what goes on inside of me and outside of me. I allow others to take charge of my life.

I accept↓♥ to develop my own immune system and build up my own will so that I can build solid foundations. By being **Aware** of my values and my capacity to take charge of myself, I can stand up and assert who I am.

CHILDHOOD DISEASES — SCARLET FEVER / SCARLATINA

Scarlet fever is an eruptive fever typified by a sudden onset (violent shivers, angina and headaches), an eruption on the oral and pharyngeal mucous surfaces and a generalized scarlet-colored eruption followed by peeling in large flakes.

I am anguished, in a form of uncertainty or insecurity. I am far away from a person whom I especially like. The fact of growing closer to one of my parents makes me uncomfortable about the other, whom I see as more distant and from whom I am afraid of being separated. I am afraid of betraying either one of them. I am afraid of a failure that could result in a punishment, or I anticipate a failure at any moment without being able to identify it. This fever is a constant bated fire inside of me, which surges up suddenly. This makes me stay silent in my corner.

I accept↓♥ to allow my feelings to express themselves, trusting in the fact that my parents will welcome me as who I am and in what I am experiencing. The fact of outwardly expressing my anxieties makes room for more calm and security.

CHILDHOOD DISEASES — VARICELLA / CHICKENPOX *See also: SKIN — SHINGLES / HERPES ZOSTER*

Chickenpox or **varicella** is an infectious, contagious **disease**, usually very benign, characterized by an eruption, in several bouts, of vesicles that wither and dry up within a few days. It generally appears between the ages of 2 and 10.

I am very easily swayed and affected by what happens around me, especially with my mother (or my father, or the person who most plays the role of a parent, which I consider essential for me). As I am very receptive and sensitive to my environment, I react if any changes occur. **Chickenpox** appears if these changes are interpreted as putting more distance between me and this parent, which could even be experienced as a separation. It may only be a change in habits involving meals or bathing (the person is still present, but I still feel left behind).

I accept↓♥ that life involves many changes to which I must adjust, and if my parents feel the need to make such changes, it is for my greater well-being and to prepare me for what my future development holds in store for me. I can express my opinions and frustrations: that is part of the process of becoming autonomous. I assume the right to ask this parent questions to better understand the situation. Without feeling wronged, I can better adjust to any change.

CHILDHOOD DISEASES — WHOOPING COUGH / PERTUSSIS

Whooping cough is an infectious, contagious and epidemic **disease** due to Bordet[6] and Gengou's bacillus. It is characterized by spasmodic fits of coughing in the form of bouts separated by a long wheezing inspiration called a recovery (whoop). It mostly affects children under the age of 5 and its prognosis is serious for infants, because there is then a risk of asphyxiation during a bout of coughing.

If I have **whooping cough**, it seems to me that death is prowling around me (or my parents). I wonder if I will be able to hear the **rooster** whooping another day. This death may manifest itself by a separation, especially if I am in a relationship (or that of my parents) where I have the impression of finding myself only with the leftovers. I groan sporadically (or episodically) about a situation or about life. I realize that I am not the 'idol'; someone else has this title, which disturbs me, and it makes me choke up. Or on the contrary, have I acquired this title because, as a newcomer, I receive all the attention and it makes some people jealous? I may feel myself stifled, imprisoned and powerless. All the attention is focused on me, which makes me feel 'examined under a magnifying glass' and criticized. I play the role of the 'good boy' ('good girl') instead of being myself.

I accept↓♥ to be in contact with my emotions, to be true to myself. The look of others thus no longer affects me, so I can drop my masks. By marking out my vital space, I stop suffocating; I breathe easily and recover my feeling of freedom.

CHLAMYDIA INFECTION *See: VENEREAL DISEASES*

6. **Bordet** (Jules): A Belgian physician and microbiologist (1870–1961). Considered to be one of the founders of serology, he discovered hemolysis and the bacillus of whooping cough in cooperation with Octave Gengou (1875–1957). He received the Nobel Prize in 1919.

CHOKING *See: RESPIRATION — CHOKING*

CHOLERA *See: INTESTINES — DIARRHEA*

CHOLESTEROL *See: BLOOD — CHOLESTEROL*

CHRONIC FATIGUE SYNDROME OR MYALGIC ENCEPHALOMYELITIS *See also: CHRONIC ILLNESS, FIBROMYALGIA*

Chronic fatigue syndrome or **Myalgic Encephalomyelitis** can surface following a viral attack and may last for several years. It may also happen because my body's natural defense system, my immune system, is weakened. It may also be that I am psychologically affected because of depression, stress, burnout, loss of motivation, etc. Mentally, I am drained, and this is reflected in my emotional instability. I use up all my energy in self-pity. I would like so much to be recognized and admired by others. This is difficult however because I make myself up into another personality to respond to the wishes of others, and my true self is completely left aside. My future does not look promising. Physically, I suffer from headaches and little by little my muscular strength diminishes. The least exertion brings on intense **fatigue**. I have lost the will to live. Where have all my dreams and ambitions gone? I had to sacrifice them, at the price of the 'success' and performance that society demands of me or that I impose on myself. I am ***intransigent***, I want to manage alone and I hesitate to ask for help. Yet, I so much want to succeed in what I undertake! I am also very afraid of failure, of life and of any responsibilities. I am incapable of living up to what is expected of me. I have the impression that I have fallen so low that I no longer can climb back up the slope. This illness can appear following an event such as an accident, where I survived while others died. The guilt linked to my survival (why me, and not the others?) can be so great that it saps all my energy. In fact, this illness allows me to withdraw, is my excuse for not taking action, or may be a way to get more attention. I thus feel more secure in my illness than in my 'face-off' with life. What was I undergoing at the time of the viral attack? Did I decide to leave home? Had I just suffered the loss of a loved one or lived through a separation or a rejection? I become **Aware** that all this is connected to **Love**, namely the **Love I have for myself**. I destroy myself by constantly wanting to live my life 'from my head', when I should instead be living it from my **heart♥** and my 'guts'. I am too **head**strong and I use up furious energy in stubbornly resisting, when it would be far easier to go with the flow. I become **Aware** of how easy it is for me to denigrate and belittle myself and compare myself negatively to others. The more I see myself negatively, the more I diminish my vital energy and destroy myself.

I accept↓♥ to learn to **love** myself more. **I am the most important person in my life.** In learning to **love** myself, I do things for myself and I benefit from every moment. I am part of the Universe, where reciprocity is the law. I **love** myself, so I attract **Love** from others in return and I **love** them back. I trust the Universe that helps me to move forward every day. By listening to my inner voice, I avoid useless detours that require much energy. I could also use this saved energy to do things that I like and that help me to renew contact with my deeper qualities and whet my taste for life. I accept↓♥ that any situation is perfect. I replace all my obligations with life choices. I thereby freely create my future.

CHRONIC ILLNESS

The word **chronic** is derived from the Greek word 'chronos' that means 'time'. A **chronic disease** may take months or years to set in. For a **chronic** disease, the term suggests something permanent and irreversible that can only be corrected.

I develop a **chronic disease** when I refuse to change out of fear of what the future has in store for me. Whatever **chronic disease** I have attracted upon myself, I can ask myself what I felt I could not change. On what area of my life do I sense that I am telling myself: "In any case, there's nothing that can be done, or there's nothing that can be changed"? I am like a stick of dynamite on the point of exploding; I am holding back because I need so much to find an alternate solution. What 'gifts' is this **disease** bringing me in the form of attention from the people around me, of confirmation of my finally deciding to change my point of view on life, etc.? The easy solution is no doubt for me to do nothing, because it seems that there is nothing else left to do but to give up.

The challenge I must take up is to accept↓♥ to take charge of myself, to open up my **Consciousness** to the idea that everything is possible. I can document the results obtained by persons who had **chronic diseases** and healed themselves. What approaches did they use? Sometimes, when the conventional methods have produced no results, I can examine alternative therapies, energy-based or others, **with discernment**, to find which one might best help me. By starting from the idea that everything is possible, I will be more able to find solutions that, if they do not heal me completely of my disease, will still help me to improve my physical, mental and emotional health.

CIGARETTES *See also: BUERGER'S DISEASE, CANCER OF THE TONGUE, DEPENDENCE, LUNGS (IN GENERAL)*

Cigarettes are related to the lungs, symbols of life, freedom, autonomy and communication between me and the Universe. They are considered as a form of protection, a 'veil' that enables me to hide certain deep anxieties. I believe that I am protecting myself with this smoke-screen that wraps itself around me and prevents me from seeing the truth. **Cigarettes** also unconsciously fill some unmet needs of childhood: a mother's first suckling warmth, **Love** and affection. I light up a cigarette without thinking; it is a habit, a compulsive mechanical gesture that has become so important to me. I need to balance the degree of my nervousness, my nervous excitability. I live too much in my head, and **cigarettes** become a way out, a superficial way of releasing my stress. I find it difficult to take time for myself and often, the only moment when I stop is when I smoke a **cigarette**. I want to feel again my mother's reassurance and security. Like many others, I may have enjoyed very little of this feeling of security when I was a child. I felt alone, far from everybody, anxious. My mother may have not taken care of me, and I may have the impression that she moved me away from my father. Having grown up too fast, I don't know how to handle all my emotions and I don't dare experience any bodily pleasures. **Cigarettes** then become 'a real pleasure' in themselves. They become my joy in living because I have no such thing in my life. It may be that this joy was present only when my mother was close to me when I was very young, and now that she is no longer as present, I feel that I no longer have anything and I am in a state of withdrawal. Relations with others scare me. If I smoke, **it is because I am escaping** a situation that is too unpleasant, my family, my life. This smoke makes my decisions still murkier. It shows a refusal of others and enables me to keep my distance, mainly with people who don't smoke and are therefore closer to their sensitivities. **Cigarette** smoke becomes a companion who makes me feel less alone. **Cigarettes** increase my **heart♥**beat and act as a stimulant. What are the decisions that I can't seem to make and that make my life dull? I accept↓♥ to identify my real needs.

I become **Aware** that I may be living in the illusion that **cigarettes** protect me from the outside world: sometimes, it becomes an opportunity to open a conversation with a stranger ("You have a **cigarette**; do you have a **light**?") or it gives me something to do when I am bothered by a conversation ("I am going outside for a smoke"). It fills the emptiness or the pauses during a conversation. **Cigarettes** become an integral part of my relationships with people. It is useful during uneasy moments. When the time comes for me to stop smoking, I must rethink my whole way of interacting with people.

I accept↓♥ to communicate more and more easily. If I want to stop smoking, it would be good to start by first finding the emotional cause to which this habit is linked, which will greatly facilitate my stopping. I will then see what I really want in life, and my needs will be filled in harmony with my true being. The limitations disappear and I feel free to develop at my own pace. I taste every moment and I feel secure because I know that I deserve to be loved.

CIRRHOSIS of the LIVER *See: LIVER — CIRRHOSIS [OF THE LIVER]*

CLAUDICATION / LIMPING *See also: SYSTEM [LOCOMOTOR]*

Claudication is characterized by an irregularity in walking. The cause can be muscular, neurological, related to paralysis or stiffness in a foot, a knee or a hip.

It is certain that in my life, everything is not going as I would like it to, especially in my sexuality. Something is amiss. I am 'in hot water' about a certain situation where I must take action or make a decision. I want to go forward, but fears are preventing me from advancing harmoniously. If I **walk**

with my feet turned inwards, I am going in a direction in which I don't feel like going.

I accept↓♥ to identify my fears and I can thereby put more harmony in my life, which will help me recover more regularity in my walk.

CLAUSTROPHOBIA *See also: ANGUISH, ANXIETY*

Claustrophobia comes from the Latin word CLAUSTRA that means *closing* and *bolt*. Derived from this is *claustralis-claustrale* that means '**that closes'**. It is therefore the irrational fear of being smothered or caught in a closed situation or place (elevator, plane, cave or tunnel) where I have no control over what goes on. For this reason, I suffer from **claustrophobia**, the anxiety of living in 'closed' places, alone or with other persons.

This may originate from the moment of my birth, when I had to go through the 'tunnel' of the cervix of the womb. I may have sensed my mother's fear at that time. The fear may also go back to a moment when I found myself in this closed and secure place in my mother's womb and which the contractions forced me to leave, which raised in me a great fear of the unknown, of what might happen. Thus, finding myself in a closed place will call up this great fear that I registered in me. I have the impression of being a **prisoner** and **locked up** in a situation where I am entirely helpless. What must I do? First, I verify if this fear may not come from some thought or mental fixation going back to the earliest periods of my life. Most of the time, this phobia comes from a 'sexual fear' that appeared during childhood. This does not necessarily mean that any improper fondling or sexual abuse took place during childhood, but rather that the fear was registered in my emotional memory and that I felt trapped, or was afraid of feeling trapped, in this sexually meaningful situation. Today, I constantly hold back my sexual impulses, which feeds my feelings of guilt.

I accept↓♥ to take action and to free myself of this guilt in the way that will best suit me. Often, a psychotherapy may be adequate to clean up the guilt in order to change the emotional memory and allow me to live with more inner freedom. I may also ask myself: when I feel trapped and stifled, could I be repressing my emotions and feeling I am their prisoner? Do I need to express my creativity, but I prevent myself from doing so? I need some breathing space, but do I allow myself to exist, to assert myself, and take my rightful place? If I succeed in respecting my needs, if I take my proper place while respecting myself and others, I will no longer need to escape and I will feel comfortable wherever I am. I accept↓♥ to reclaim the place that I let go of. I assert who I am. I regain my vital space. I accept myself in all the emotions that I experience, without any judgments. I express my creative side: it enables me to live from my **heart♥** and to be truly in contact with my divine essence.

CLAVICLE (pain in, fracture of) *See also: BONE — FRACTURE, SHOULDERS (IN GENERAL)*

The **clavicle** is an '**S**'-shaped long bone located between the shoulder and the sternum, above the rib cage.

As the **clavicle** is directly related to the shoulder, a pain in the **clavicle** means my anger regarding the responsibilities I am given and about which I may experience a feeling of submission and obligation. I may sometimes express good ideas, but I can't materialize them. Most often, a **fracture of the clavicle** happens after a fall on the shoulder and indicates that I am being subjected to strong pressures about my responsibilities. The emotion that this generates may lead me to think I am going to 'break' under the weight of my responsibilities, and this revolts me. I feel like running away. I can neither speak nor take action. I feel subjected to decisions that were imposed on me. I question the authority figure. I am in a dead-end, pushed against the wall. Life is not flowing in me: I resist it or reject it!

I accept↓♥ to look at situations objectively and I begin to understand that life cannot give me more responsibilities than I can take. I trust, and I try to find solutions or another viewpoint that will help me to better take on life.

CLAVUS *See: SKIN — FURUNCLES*

CLEFT PALATE / HARE LIP — CONGENITAL CLEFT PALATE

A **cleft palate**, also called a **congenital hare lip**, is a malformation characterized by a cleft in the upper lip (more frequent in boys) and/or the palate (more frequent in girls). It is due to an interruption in the sutures of the embryo's face buds between the 35th and the 40th day of its intra-uterine life. The **cleft palate** results in no handicap except for an æsthetic disadvantage, and impedes eating and the learning of speech.

Already at a very early age, I knew it would be difficult for me to communicate and assert myself, to 'open my mouth'. I feel inferior, and I try to hide and withdraw because the others 'manage my life'. Some things escape me; the pieces seem 'too big to swallow'. I need to develop my self-esteem, to place myself first.

First, I must face this reality of my birth and digest this situation while accepting↓♥ to make room for surpassing myself, and accepting↓♥ my integration in earthly life. I consciously choose to know myself, to recognize myself as a **Soul** in development. By accepting↓♥ my qualities and my inner strengths, I am building a new, far more positive image of myself. I choose to claim the place that is mine by divine right and to embrace life. By being myself, I can make contact with my divine essence and I know exactly what road to take. I can freely express my needs and take action!

CLOT *See: BLOOD / COAGULATED / THROMBOSIS*

COAGULATION (deficient) *See: BLOOD [COAGULATED]*

COCAINE CONSUMPTION *See: DRUGS*

COCCYX *See: BACK DISORDERS — LOWER BACK*

COLD (freezing up)

A **freezing up** occurs when my mind becomes stiff. I feel accused and threatened. **Freezing up** gives me an **excuse to be alone**. I become **Aware** of the fact that I stiffen against the events of my life. What is the reason for my feeling threatened? I verify what caused this tension (person or event) and realize that it is my fears and my need to please others. I need to be loved and appreciated. It is the lack of **Love** that makes me feel **cold**. The **cold** represents solitude, suffering, terror, the dark side of things. Something **chilled me**, froze my **heart♥**. I 'chilled up' upon seeing something, and it 'sent a **freezing shiver** up my back'.

I accept↓♥ to let go and not judge myself. I act more flexibly with myself; the others are only a reflection of myself. In life, everything that happens to me is there to teach me to surpass myself and make me grow.

COLD (head) / CORYZA *See also: ALLERGY TO HAY FEVER*

A **cold**, also called **rhinitis**, is a viral infection that causes coughing and a running nose. The best known is **acute rhinitis** (**coryza**), commonly called a **head cold**. A **cold** also causes stiffness and fatigue, and the nose becomes obstructed. It is very widespread and contagious. As a germ or a virus is affecting my body, this indicates a failure of my immune system.

It may result from a **confusion in my thoughts**, or from the fact that I am frantically busy. It is total disorder, and my sensitivity is greatly affected. There are too many things to manage at the same time. I then wonder where I should start. I am stifling under family or work obligations. I feel cold and therefore I 'catch cold', and a cold appears. The **cold** then brings me a respite during which I can 'protect' myself from people for some time and 'keep my distances' in order to regain contact with myself. As there is a release of secretions, I am probably experiencing a special emotional situation that affects me and calls up many emotions that seek release. Is there something about which I really feel like crying but without admitting it? As my nose is obstructed, is there a person or a situation that 'stinks' and that I want to avoid smelling? As the **cold** can affect the chest (the body) as well as the head (the spirit), there may be an imbalance if I focus all my attention on one of them while ignoring the other. As a cold is often related to the fact that I 'froze up', I must ask myself what is the situation, or what are the words someone told me, that 'cast a chill' on the relation concerned, or so froze my whole body that I felt hurt, disappointed, guilty, etc. Am I 'out in the cold' with someone? Who is speaking behind my back? Or is it that I am becoming cold over my own pain and sorrow? By feeling that I am a victim, I accept↓♥ that others will give me 'viruses'.

I accept↓♥ to need human warmth. I must begin by taking care of myself first, so that others may do the same. I drop all my masks because I feel 'immunized' against any outside attacks. I need some time off to enable me to see more clearly in my life. I need to regain my strength. I adopt new attitudes and new behavior. I clean up my life and stop allowing popular beliefs to affect me ("**Colds** are hitting hard this winter!" or "I always catch a **cold** by December."). I learn to know my limits and not exceed them. Harmony can thus set in, and I become the master of my life. If I need someone to take care of me or to comfort me, I dare to ask for it!

COLD (sensitivity to)

I am a person who is **sensitive to the cold** if I fear the **cold** or if I feel the **cold** very intensely.

Sensitivity to the cold often appears after an event where I experienced a separation from a person, an animal or even an object (a teddy bear for example) that I wanted to hold on to and that I know I will never see again. I feel a great emptiness, a great **cold,** for I have lost the **Love**, the attention or the physical contact with the object of that separation. I am no longer in contact with human warmth and I feel alone. It may often be my relationship with my father that I feel to be empty, distant or absent. My timidity intensifies this feeling of **coldness**. Especially when I am a child, I believe or have been taught that when persons have left (died), they go to heaven. But it is **cold** in the heavens! And I start to be **sensitive to the cold** because, if I am in contact with the **cold**, I am also in contact with the deceased person! Thus, I become **Aware** that I need more 'warmth' in my life, or more **Love**, or to make peace with what had separated me from what represented **Love** for me. It is important for me to become **conscious** of the event that 'triggered' the **sensitivity to the cold** and to truly accept↓♥ (acknowledge) the departure of the person (object, animal) from whom I was separated in order to make peace with myself and with the situation. I accept↓♥ how difficult it is for me to give myself this warmth I so need. I tend to denigrate myself, thereby preventing **Love** from flowing through me. The anxiety I feel makes me curl back into myself. I seek refuge in my thoughts. I should really come out of my shell and express who I am.

By accepting↓♥ **Love**, I make better contact with myself and with the people around me.

COLIC (renal)

Nephritic colic is a violent pain in the lumbar region, radiating into the bladder and the thighs because of an obstruction of the ureter. It is usually due to the migration of a calculus or a foreign body from the kidney to the bladder, through the ureters.

It often manifests itself when I experience a situation where I am struck down by what I saw, learned or heard. This situation ***rattles*** me so much that it makes all my values suddenly ***collapse***. Something is stuck and is hurting me. I question everything, and it often happens that my spouse may be involved. Am I satisfied with my life as a couple? I feel I am losing my vital space, or I feel myself deceived or betrayed. Someone is ***infringing*** on me and my goodness of heart, and that irritates me no end. I am upset and troubled. I take the time to observe what is stuck in my relationship as a couple or in my affective relationships. What is the main irritation I feel and can no longer tolerate? What was my illusion?

I accept↓♥ to take an objective look at my life. I redefine my values and priorities and dare to assert them. I thereby take the place that is rightfully mine to allow myself to occupy my rightful place, the first place!

COLIC / GRIPPING PAIN *See: INTESTINES — COLIC*

COLITIS (hemorrhagic) *See: INTESTINES — COLITIS*

COLITIS (mucosity of the colon) *See: INTESTINES — COLITIS*

COLON (cancer of the) *See: CANCER OF THE COLON*

COLOR BLIND *See: EYES — DALTONISM*

COMA *See also: ACCIDENT, BRAIN — SYNCOPE, FAINTING*

A **coma** can occur as a result of an **accident** and consists in a partial or total alteration of the state of **consciousness**.

It often happens that, just before finding myself in a **coma,** I saw death coming to me, as if 'my last hour had come'. Instead of being 100% conscious of that moment, the **coma** occurs just before. 'Consciousness' disconnects. Often, when I awaken from a **coma**, my memory of the intense trauma that was experienced has been wiped out. It is as if I was placed in safety because I was in danger. What produces an accident is guilt related to my fleeing from a person or a situation. If I find it difficult to take up the challenge of this guilt, I find refuge in a **coma**. I may feel quite powerless to resolve a situation because I feel too unfocused, which makes me ***furious***. I have great changes to make in my life but I feel incapable of making them. Now, I can rest in my cave, where nobody will come to bother me and tell me what to do. I have regained a feeling of freedom where I don't have to account for myself, for the time being. **Coma** comes from the Greek *'koma'* that means *'deep sleep'*. This state is related to an intense desire to **flee** a person or a situation. I have so much **pain** inside of me that I retreat into myself because I am feeling great despair, solitude or frustration. I want to make myself insensitive to the difficulties of life. I protect myself with this deep sleep. It makes me insensitive to what is going on around me. I prefer to exist in this state of total un**consciousness** until my life can become more pleasant. I have a decision to make: to live, or to go. The same decision must be made in the case of **diabetic coma** that is caused by an excess of glucose (blood sugar) in the blood and especially in the brain. My sadness is so great that I feel like escaping this world in which I live. My ***fury*** is just as great. Even if a **coma** can last for long periods (weeks and years), it is very important that the people close to me show me **Love** and affection, and that they tell me that the decision to go or to live is mine to make. My loved ones must feel the necessary detachment to avoid 'holding' me in a **coma** against my will. When I am in a **coma**, my brain may be active to the point where I can hear people speaking or sense their presence and the impressions they make, even though I cannot move or express myself. It may happen that the fear of death will keep me un**conscious**. I must therefore be reassured and told that I can safely go, if such is my desire. If I can see the energies of a person in a **coma**, I will notice a marked break of energy links, depending on the depth of the **coma**. It would thus be appropriate to give energy treatments to regularize the situation in order to return to the HERE AND NOW.

It is important to reassure myself and tell myself that I will get all the help I need, and I accept↓♥ the fact that I have all the capacities and qualities needed to carry out all my projects. I know that the necessary changes in my life will go smoothly and for the good of everyone around me, including myself!

COMEDONS / BLACKHEADS *See: SKIN — BLACKHEADS*

COMPULSION (nervous)

Compulsion is a behavioral disorder defined by an irresistible urge to perform certain acts, which the person can't resist without feeling anxiety. Compulsion can involve sexuality, food, drink, shopping, excessive cleanliness, etc.

Nervous compulsion concerns an aspect of my personality that I judge to be negative and that annoys me so much I refuse to see it. I repress it deep inside of me. As long as I refuse to see it and accept↓♥ it, life will make me experience more and more situations where I will have to face this side of my personality.

When I experience **nervous compulsion**, I examine what bothered me, I accept↓♥ to face it instead of **fleeing**. **I accept↓♥ to be a human being** with strengths, weaknesses, qualities and defects. I become **Aware** of the fact that I am **my most severe judge**, I forgive myself and **I learn to love myself**. The fact of accepting↓♥ myself as I am will enable me to thrive harmoniously and I will no longer need to seek release through **compulsion**.

CONCERN / WORRY

Worrying manifests itself by agitation, anxiety and apprehension. It results from an inner insecurity that I feel and that makes me very emotional. My **worrying** may have its source in my childhood, most especially if I experienced physical or social insecurity, or if I felt I was missing something in my affective experience or in my education, or if I felt abandoned at some point in time. This **worrying** may reappear in adulthood, when I re-live a situation similar to the one I experienced in my childhood and that 'reactivates' that feeling. I also experience **worrying** over a situation when I believe I have no power to change it, or if I perceive myself as a victim of events rather that a creator of events. I then think that I will have to submit, instead of thinking that I can very well be present in action and acceptance↓♥.

I accept↓♥ to learn to trust in life. I also must learn to trust myself. I must be stronger than my anxieties in order to control them, instead of seeing them controlling me and feeding my impression of helplessness in life.

CONCUSSION (brain) *See: BRAIN [CONCUSSION]*

CONGENITAL *See: INFIRMITIES [CONGENITAL], DISEASES [HEREDITARY]*

CONGESTION (brain / liver / nose / lung) *See also: BRAIN — CEREBROVASCULAR ACCIDENT (C.V.A.)*

Congestion is the body's system of defense used to respond to repeated attacks against certain parts of my body. Different parts can be **congested**.

In the liver: it represents repressed criticism or irritation that I accumulate because I can't express it verbally. I may feel dissatisfaction, bitterness or disappointment. **In the nose (sinus)**: what is the situation or the person that I can't stand and that makes me angry? **In the lungs** (**pneumopathy**): I feel stifled by my family relationships, whether it is my parents, my spouse or my children. Are my family relations as harmonious as I wish them to be? Do I worry too much? **In the brain (C.V.A.)**[7]**:** I feel overwhelmed and don't know how to react to certain persons or situations. My brain is no longer working as clearly or as quickly as before. It is advisable to stay far from liquor or drugs. Whatever part of the body is affected, the result is frustration, irritation and rage toward others and myself. I am in a situation of perpetual tension. My emotions are **congested**. I am afraid of myself because I sense that there is something bad inside of me. I therefore avoid being impulsive and living my life spontaneously. Yet, it would be profitable for me to release my creativity, because it is my natural impulses seeking to be free. I tend to focus much attention on my spiritual life and very little on my physical needs. I need some rest and a vacation, but I don't allow myself to take it. I take the time to verify what is currently disturbing me in my life and I take responsibility for it.

I accept↓♥ to take the place that is rightfully mine: **my place**. I realize the importance of **expressing what I feel**, and I do so without attacking others. Because I express my feelings, I accumulate no frustration or hate. When I am open and receptive, others are, too. I once again feel in harmony with myself

7. **C.V.A.**: Cerebrovascular accident.

and with those around me. I thus achieve a new balance, in my spiritual as well as my physical life.

CONJUNCTIVE TISSUES (fragility of)

A tissue is a group of cells that have the same form or carry out the same function. The role of **conjunctive tissues** is to support the other tissues of the body, ensuring nutrition for the muscular, nervous and epithelial[8], tissues as well as filling the interstices (clefts) that are found between these tissues.

I must ask myself: What do I need in order to nourish myself emotionally as well as physically or spiritually? Do I feel supported enough, or do I feel I have to do everything myself, including 'filling gaps' at work or at home, for instance? Because I easily depreciate myself, I must make myself useful and important. I often feel stifled in my freedom, and I tend to place the responsibility for my troubles on others. I tend to be resentful and I find forgiving difficult.

I accept↓♥ to communicate my states of being and my needs: this will help me in discovering myself, in taking charge of my life and in getting the help I need and that I can rightfully ask for.

CONJUNCTIVITIS *See: EYES — CONJUNCTIVITIS*

CONSTIPATION *See: INTESTINES — CONSTIPATION*

CONTUSIONS *See: SKIN — BRUISES*

CORNS ON FEET *See: FEET — CALLUSES AND CORNS*

CORONARY *See: HEART♥ — CORONARY THROMBOSIS*

CORYZA *See: COLD [HEAD]*

COUGH *See also: THROAT / (IN GENERAL) / [AILMENTS OF]*

A **cough** is a state often minimized, if not denied. Yet, it manifests an irritation; whether in the **throat** or in the lungs, I feel a nervous tension that irritates me and of which I want to free myself. I may feel stifled by a situation or a person I can no longer stand. I feel frustrated, I feel like screaming or 'spitting out' my grief, but my education prevents me from doing so. By **coughing**, I get to release my emotions, to reject something that bothers me and that I no longer want. It can be solitude, bitterness, sadness, bewilderment, frustration, boredom, etc. I sometimes need to **cough** and even force myself to, for I feel something stuck in my **throat**. It is usually something I refrain from expressing

8. **Epithelium**: A tissue (skin) that covers the outer surfaces of the organism.

for fear of the reaction of others. A **cough** appears when I see that someone wants to deprive me of something. When I want to keep everything for myself, my body reacts by 'repelling the enemy' with this **cough**. It is a **dry cough** (**irritative**) when I am irritated and critical about what is around me and can't stand it. When I am nervous and tense, I may develop a tic that consists in **coughing** and disguises my discomfort, my tension or my nervousness. If I quarreled with someone and a situation has not been resolved, the **cough** persists. I want attention. Something is caught in my **throat**, but in fact I am the one who feels caught in a situation. I 'revolt' in a subtle manner. I hesitate, and instead of speaking directly and firmly, what I have to say only emerges in bits and pieces. A **wet cough**, which comes with secretions, appears to issue from deeper inside. A **fit of coughing**, characteristic of the whooping cough, expresses my resentments and sometimes my tantrums, which I can only express violently because I am very irritated.

By accepting↓♥ to acknowledge what is irritating me, my **cough** goes away. It may be an aspect of myself that I find difficult to accept↓♥. If it persists, it is because I can't free myself from it. It will do me good to take some time to discover the causes of my irritability and thus be able to correct some irritating situations and feel all right with those I must accept↓♥.

CRAB LICE *See also: VENEREAL DISEASES*

I 'catch' **crab lice**, also called **lice**, usually by venereal or medical contact.

I feel guilty and dirty for having had sexual relations outside of our society's allowed limits, or I may feel that their only purpose was to fill my personal needs, without any commitment on my part to the other person. I am ashamed and I don't want to face my deep feelings about my body and my sexuality. I am afraid of being hurt. I am dependent on others: It is easier for me to be submissive than to stand up, at the risk of being rejected. I feel invaded in my space, my intimacy. A child who has **lice** may react to a parent, often the mother, who can't stand her child's disorder or uncleanliness, which does not meet the parental criteria that are sometimes very high or even unrealistic. As a child, I am very sensitive to my parents' criticism and remarks, which I feel like parasites on me.

I accept↓♥ that any actual situation is an experience, and I learn to recognize my needs and what is good for me. I learn to be proud of what I am.

CRAMP(S)

A **cramp** is the involuntary, painful and momentary contraction of a muscle or a muscle group.

Cramps indicate great tension, a sometimes excessive inner straining. I hold back the divine energy and prevent it from flowing in me because I am stuck and limited. I insist on hanging on to a fear, an inner wound or a stress that are no longer beneficial for me. Some of my mental patterns need to be more integrated. I am currently facing much **pressure** and **tension** that may be accompanied by a feeling of powerlessness over something or a situation. I wonder what I should do and what solution would best suit me. Because of my fear, **I hang on to** set ideas. I experience a degree of submission, having to 'grovel' before certain persons to avoid their wrath. I dread life to the point where I radically block ('lock') energy at one precise location. I want to take refuge at home. My anxiety makes me want to avoid or flee a situation. If this anxiety is experienced at home during the day, I may find myself with **cramps in the night** that awaken me and remind me that I should flee. Depending on the **cramp**'s location, I have an indication of what I must change: a **cramp in a foot**, the direction I am taking; a **cramp in a leg**, my way of advancing in life; a **cramp in a hand**, my actions and my undertakings.

I am **Aware** of the inner pains that overwhelm me, and I realize that I can change this. I accept↓♥ to let go and remain open to the divine energy. I take the time to stop and think. This pause will enable me to start off again more slowly and differently, and to feel better overall.

CRAMP(S) (abdominal) *See also: STOMACH DISORDERS*

The abdomen is related to the chakra of intuition and creativity. Thus, an **abdominal cramp** indicates the fear of following my intuition, my refusal to fully unleash my creativity, by blocking the divine energy at this location, namely close to, or lower than, the navel. I thus stop any process that would enable me to see what could help me to advance normally. I am afraid of discovering that the future could be endlessly profitable for me. I want to control everything because I am afraid of experimenting new things. I expect the worst, namely that abominable things will happen to me.

I accept↓♥ to open myself and to trust life. This way, I can allow myself to be guided more by my intuition, and I can use my creativity to move in the direction that suits me, in harmony with what I am.

CRAMP (writer's) *See also: FINGERS (IN GENERAL), HANDS (IN GENERAL), WRISTS*

It is a sensation of numbness or tingling in the fingers, caused by a compression of the median nerve in the carpal tunnel, located in the anterior zone of the wrist.

I am affected by a great **inner tension**, so when I write, I put enormous effort into it. Whom do I want to **impress**? Whom do I want to convince? Me, or the others? I am **pretentious**, and my ideas of grandiosity make me a person who is **too ambitious**. It is possible that I wear a mask, thus hiding my true personality, which protects me against the judgment of other people. This results from the fact that I have little confidence in myself and that I believe myself incapable of accomplishing great things. I ask myself questions about marriage and how I take a position about it. The doubts I have about my capacity to express my creativity lead me to abdicate and abandon my goals. I will only 'try', but a part of me has already 'thrown in the towel'[9]. As the pain can manifest itself more at night or upon waking up in the morning, while I am still connected to the inner worlds, this pain reminds me of the inner adjustments I must make to be more flexible.

From now on, I do things naturally, by taking the time to be truly myself. I have nothing to prove to anyone. I accept↓♥ to **love** myself as I am, without any artifice and remaining totally free in my attitudes. It is the first step toward a great achievement, self-achievement.

CROHN'S DISEASE *See: INTESTINES — CROHN'S DISEASE*

CROUP *See: THROAT — LARYNGITIS*

CRYING

Tears are a streaming of the eyes, a releasing of emotions. Whether related to joy, **Love**, fear, or disappointment, **crying** releases me from an overflow of very strong feelings and thoughts. Or my eyes may have been fascinated by viewing a scene that was unbearable and horrifying, but that I was moved to watch, as if to catch every last detail. I may also **cry** because I feel incapable of communicating what I feel. People ignore me: it is as though I were invisible. I have little contact with my inner world. I become too attached to people and things for fear of losing them. I am anxious, feeling fragile because I have little confidence in myself. I endure dependence. My **tears** are an evacuation of sadness, of disappointment. I therefore have a reaction that lowers the pressure. I may also use my tears to attract attention and sympathy so that others will take care of me. That is futile however, for I can simply show all the good qualities I have and I will get the same result. I may have the impression that I am always struggling, and I am exhausted. I always **feel like crying** because what I am going through is just too much! I need help and don't ask for it. The fact of **crying** may sometimes give another person the impression that they are stronger, have made me 'break down' and have a certain power over me. By being unable to **cry**, I avoid seeming weaker. The **blocked tear ducts** indicate to me that there is a resistance to my free expression, maybe linked to the belief that **crying** 'is just for babies'. In a previous situation, I wanted to not show my suffering with my tears, and I **blocked my tear ducts**. I want to show that I exist, but it doesn't work. If a baby has an **inflammation of the tear ducts**, it is vulnerable if someone touches it. It is afraid of being hurt or injured. My tears, by flowing from my eyes, carry with them things that they prevent me from seeing, maybe for fear of not seeing them become realities.

I accept↓♥ to let myself move ahead freely, which releases me from disruptive emotions and accumulated toxins and thereby promotes healing and renewal. I accept↓♥ to respect myself and to live in joy.

---

9. **Throw in the towel**: To give up, to surrender.

CUSHING'S[10] SYNDROME *See also: GLAND — CAPSULE [SUPRARENAL]*

Caused by the overproduction of a hormone (corticoid) of the surrenal glands, the main symptoms of **Cushing's syndrome** are obesity located in the face, the neck and the trunk (bison's hump), arterial hypertension, stretch marks, excessive pilosity, muscular atrophy with asthenia (weakness), etc.

Then there exists a mental and physical disorder, an imbalance that brings on the feeling of **being invaded** by others because I have gradually lost all contact with my own power. A feeling of helplessness is experienced, 'drowning' me in an overflow of ideas that invades me. I am lost, not knowing what direction to take. Thus, by reaction, consciously or not, I tend to want to crush the people around me. When these glands function abnormally, a series of symptoms appears, known as **Cushing's syndrome**. I notice that certain parts of the body are transforming themselves: the face, the neck, the trunk; and I also notice that the lower limbs are becoming thin. I am experiencing a physical and mental imbalance. My helplessness makes me no longer **Aware** of the power I have within me. It is as if "anybody can attack me at any time". I am in a state of survival and I carry a very heavy past.

It is important for me to get in closer contact with reality by taking actions that help me. I use this power to improve my quality of life. I learn to trust myself and I accept↓♥ to take my place and live according to what I feel and what I am.

CUT *See also: ACCIDENT*

A **cut** indicates an emotional disorder, a deep mental pain that manifests itself in the physical body and may hide great guilt. It makes me become **Aware** of an inner wound and of the fact that I may unconsciously wish to destroy myself. It is a warning, a sign that I must reassess the direction in which I am going. I want to go too fast and do things too quickly. It is the sign of a deep inner conflict. I push my limits a little too far! I locate where I cut myself and note the activity I was doing at that moment, which enables me to identify the aspect I must integrate. For example, a **cut** on a hand may indicate that I feel guilty of expressing my creativity in everyday situations, or that I am irritated because I am doing something I don't like; I hurry up, and I become ripe for a **cut**. At the moment of the **cut**, there is often an emotion that I can't control. Do I feel that I am defenseless and that someone wants to take advantage of me or injure me? The depth and the severity of the **cut** indicate the reason for this affliction: **little cuts** manifest mild guilt that often concerns some everyday details on which I focus too much attention, or on the contrary, I let things ride, and my carelessness makes me omit some details that are important. A **deeper, wider cut** shows me that this guilt is much more important: I feel '**cut off**' from my deeper nature or from the rest of the world, divided over a decision

10. **Cushing** (Harvey William): An American neurosurgeon (1869–1939) who, in 1832, described certain disorders linked to the surrenal glands.

to make, torn about a person or a situation. I then feel vulnerable and unable to act. My level of stress and anxiety is high because I feel I must constantly be on guard. I may feel imprisoned in the image I want to give, in the ideals that were imposed upon me, either by myself or by society. I feel my freedom stifled and I feel like revolting. I feel '**cut off**' from my true self, from my unlimited potential.

I accept↓♥ what I must understand, I stand by my choices and I make the necessary changes. I take the time to stop and assess my life and my goals. I have the power to achieve all my dreams: I only have to accept↓♥ my true nature, my inner strengths, and everything becomes possible. I renew contact with myself and the people helping me in my progress.

CUTICLES *See: FINGERS — CUTICLES*

C.V.A. *See: BRAIN — CEREBROVASCULAR ACCIDENT (C.V.A.)*

CYPHOSIS *See: SPINAL DEVIATION — CYPHOSIS*

CYST *See also: OVARIES — [DISORDERS OF THE...], TUMORS*

A **cyst** is a cavity located in an organ or a tissue. It contains a liquid, soft or sometimes solid substance, and is limited by its own envelope.

A **cyst** forms when I feel remorse about a project or a desire I was unable to achieve. I 'pumped' myself up, I collected information and data of all sorts for a project that I was never able to complete: they have remained prisoners of my body and my mind and they become a 'ball that blocks my vital energy'. I remain hooked to certain past experiences. A pain follows me everywhere. It is a refusal to forgive. The **cyst** may also correspond to a solidification of attitudes and 'mental patterns' that unconsciously accumulated over a certain period of time. These may serve me as protective barriers, holding me imprisoned in a well-delimited framework and allowing me to avoid facing certain persons or situations. This also has the effect of slowing me down or preventing me from going forward, because I have difficulty in opening myself to other opinions or other ways of thinking. My ego may be deeply hurt, and my resentment solidifies to become a **cyst**. It is my feeling of powerlessness that makes me immerse myself in all this pain, this hate, sometimes even with the feeling that I want to take revenge on someone. I seek the acknowledgement of my full potential, but it is late in coming. I played the victim for a long time, but I am now becoming Aware that only I can create my life as I want it. I am searching for my creative power. I tend to withdraw and repress everything inside of me until there is too much, and it transforms itself into a **cyst**. I flee a conflict instead of facing it. When I also see a vital fear or a mortal danger, it becomes cancerous.

I accept↓♥ to allow energy to flow freely throughout me, I have confidence in the fact that I can make my projects go forward, and I ask to see the solutions for everything to flow better in my life. I forgive myself, I **love** myself, I turn to the future, and I am therefore at peace. I dare to say the real things. I free myself of all these encysted emotions. By my negative thoughts, I attracted negative events; so now, I sow only good thoughts and good words around me so that I can at last create the life I dream of. I am the creator of my life and move confidently ahead.

CYSTIC FIBROSIS (CF) / MUCOVISCIDOSIS *See also: LUNGS (IN GENERAL), PANCREAS*

Mucoviscidosis, also called **cystic fibrosis** (of the **pancreas**) is the most frequent of the hereditary mortal diseases in children. It is defined by an enzymic defect. It mainly affects the lungs and the digestive system. There is an abnormal viscosity of the mucus secreted by the glands of the bronchi and the pancreas.

My rigid way of thinking and my mental patterns are such that I have refused to move forward in life. I have clung to so many old ideas that I haven't followed the flow of life. The pains I feel paralyze me. I am discouraged, and nothing is working in my life. I may have the impression that I have always held back from doing or saying things for fear of the consequences. That is why my legs and my arms are often affected, because they symbolize my fear of embracing the situations of life (arms) and my fear of moving forward in life (legs). I complain and feel sorry for myself and I would want others to do the same. I think that life has nothing to offer me. I feel the need to **overprotect** myself. I may find myself at the **heart♥** of certain quarrels despite myself, and I want to get out of them. There is something I must absolutely prevent my physical body from absorbing (a noxious substance), or I must avoid being in contact with certain persons or situations that might 'enter my bubble' and could endanger me. I control my emotions and my environment and resist them so much that I must constantly eat to fill the emptiness that is never filled up.

I accept↓♥ to open myself more to life and I let go of my old ideas. This way, I enter a new period of growth in life and in my rightful place in the Universe. I live spontaneously by listening to my wisdom that expresses itself in my inner voice. I have the necessary strength to assert my needs. Energy flows within me and helps me to recover my balance.

CYSTITIS *See: BLADDER — CYSTITIS*

CYSTOCELE *See: PROLAPSE OF THE UTERUS*

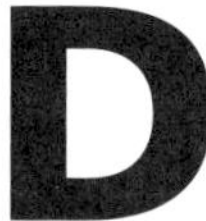

DANDRUFF / SCURF / PELLICLES *See also: HAIR DISEASE*

Dandruff is the hard, dry layer of the **skin.** It has the appearance of white flakes and is generally found on the scalp.

As there is an accumulation of dead skin, there is also an accumulation of dead attitudes and 'dead patterns' that I no longer need. My scalp is related to the mind, the abstract; these are mental thought schemes that I must let go of to make place for more openness and more flexibility. Whether I am intellectually very active or, on the contrary, very inactive (for example, if I let others think in my place), both may produce **dandruff**, because in both cases there is an imbalance in my rational and mental functioning. I feel under attack, and I need to release this anger in a healthy way. I feel controlled by others, but it is only my own emotions that are haunting me and I don't know what to do with them. I am cut off from reality and I invent scenarios to help me deal with situations where I felt hurt. I still don't understand some situations where I experienced a difficult separation. I scatter my energy in all directions. Various social, religious or moral situations present themselves to me, and I must reposition myself with respect to my new beliefs or convictions. Great uncertainties arise, and I must experience myself and discard what no longer suits me. I am afraid of being unmasked in my new reality.

I accept↓♥ to open myself more and more to the new ways of functioning in life and I feel increasingly flexible, letting myself be guided by the flow of life. I make contact with my emotions and I become **conscious** of my true worth. By allowing the flow of life and all my creativity to circulate freely, I am increasingly in contact with my whole potential and I become the master of my life.

DEAF *See: EARS — DEAFNESS*

DEAF MUTE / DEAF AND DUMB *See also: EARS — DEAFNESS*

If I am **deaf** for a congenital reason or if I lost my hearing in early childhood and was unable to learn to speak, then I will be described as a **deaf mute**[1] . My degree of hearing however can vary from 0% to 30%.

In the course of my life, there are surely some things I didn't want to hear, which led me to experience this situation. To clarify what I didn't want to hear, I can look to my parents, and more especially my mother, to find out what she

1. **Deaf mute:** Especially in North America, the term '**deaf**' is preferred to '**deaf mute**' for, though the person does not hear, they are nevertheless capable of producing sounds, or even words, with orthophonic training.

didn't want to hear. It may be a situation where she told herself: "I don't want to hear it any more", while she was pregnant with me. I am responsible for what happens to me and, if it did affect me, it was because I, too, had something to understand. As a baby, I may have found it difficult to become autonomous and independent, or just develop my individuality (especially after enjoying 9 months of fusion with Mom). I may have wished to protect myself from the outside world.

I accept↓♥ to become **Aware** of this situation and I increasingly develop my inner hearing that enables me to benefit from the joys of life and flourish with the people around me.

DEAFNESS *See: EARS — DEAFNESS*

DEATH *See also: AGORAPHOBIA, ANXIETY, EUTHANASIA*

Death is not a disease, but a state. It occurs when my body's vital functions, such as **heart♥**beat, respiration, or cerebral activity, stop: my body can no longer pursue its functions, unless mechanical or other means are used to reactivate some of them.

It sometimes happens, in cased of serious illnesses such as certain cancers, AIDS, some incurable diseases, etc., that I will heal just before the moment called **death**. In fact, while integrating in my **heart♥** and in **Love** the **consciousness** I must achieve, I may be released from all physical and psychological suffering. If I am too advanced in the disease, my brain may disconnect me once I have reached the relevant level of **consciousness**. That is why it is so important for me to understand and accept↓♥ in my **heart ♥** the reason for my experiencing this illness. The more I accept↓♥ what life teaches me, the more I will be able to depart[2] in harmony, in **Light** and in **Love**. My loved ones have a great role to play in this healing process by accepting↓♥, in their **hearts♥**, my departure so that I can freely pursue my journey. The more situations I integrate before leaving my physical body, the more advanced I will be in the work still to be done after my departure. As life goes on (for those who believe it!), I would prefer that people spoke of me as having 'departed', as having 'left my physical body' or as having 'passed on to the other worlds'. Using these expressions sounds more real to me than to say that I am '**dead'**. In the cases of **clinical or apparent death**, there is usually a cardiac and respiratory arrest and a suspension of **consciousness**. It is an initial phase that is reversible, for there may be a cardio respiratory reanimation (it is different, however, from a deep coma). I ask myself what deep conflict I am involved in is making me wonder if I should live or not. I may live a situation with no means of escape. I feel in prison. I can no longer move forward and the pain has become unbearable. I must be very vigilant: if I send off thoughts such as: I "no longer want to live on this earth", or life "isn't worth living", I

---

2. **Departing:** This term is preferred to 'dying'.

am calling up a situation where I will really die. I may feel very vulnerable, and the whole world of emotions is so unfamiliar to me that I prefer to flee rather than face it.

I accept↓♥ to take my life in charge, and I know that by sowing positive thoughts I will only attract beautiful experiences. I must trust myself! I embrace life and celebrate it in each instant!

DECALCIFICATION *See also: BONES — OSTEOPOROSIS*

Decalcification is a substantial decrease of the **calcium** content of a tissue, an organ or an organism, generally in the form of a demineralization of the skeleton.

I feel fragile and I have the impression that bad luck is dogging me. I feel beaten up, worn down in my intimacy, broken inside by certain situations or persons. I begin to depreciate and diminish myself, sensing that I am losing my power little by little. I become dependent on others, not knowing what direction to take. I feel I am missing something, 'missing the boat', losing somehow. As bones are the structure of the body, I must re-examine the overall composition of my life, my mode of functioning and my reactions to the various situations I am currently experiencing.

I accept↓♥ to trust myself and to acknowledge my qualities and my inner strength. I choose to live by my deeper values. I learn to take my place and take charge of my life, knowing I can't be struck. I am always protected and guided.

DECAY (tooth) *See: TEETH — TOOTH DECAY*

DEHYDRATION of the BODY

Cellular **dehydration** is a deficit of water and sodium. It is often associated with demineralization.

There is a loss somewhere, a dryness. How has my body come to lack water and salt? Water cleans, purifies and circulates: without water, I die. What part of me feels like dying, what are the emotions I want to get rid of? What is the obsession that takes up all my energy? I distance myself from my creativity and my inner potential. I no longer see any way out, and it is as if I was withdrawing from life because the pain is too intense. I allow myself to be emptied of my energy and let myself be 'dried out' by others because I focus my attention too much on them.

I accept↓♥ to **love** myself more, to nourish my cells with healthful food and water. I allow all my emotions to express themselves through my creativity. I take care of myself because nobody can do it in my place.

DEMENTIA *See: ALZEIMER'S DISEASE, SENILITY*

DEMINERALIZATION (general) *See also: DECALCIFICATION*

This term is used to designate the loss, by the skeleton, of mineral elements that the body needs, such as phosphorus, calcium, sodium, iron, silicon, magnesium, etc. **Demineralization** can cause anemia. It manifests itself by fatigue, a deficiency in the bones and lack of sleep. White spots on the fingernails are a sign of demineralization.

My body lacks vitality and liveliness. I 'lose' minerals and my tone is poor. Do I tend to think that life is escaping from me, or that I am missing something? Am I settling into old patterns to the point of sinking into them? My negativism and my defeatist and victim's attitude create an 'energy leakage' in me.

I accept↓♥ to trust my inner guide and I learn to restructure myself. I take the necessary decisions to make the needed changes in order to reorganize certain things that had become harmful for me and to taste the 'salt of life'. I accept↓♥ to focus my attention only on the positive aspects of my life.

DEPENDENCE *See also: ALCOHOLISM, CIGARETTES, DRUGS*

A **dependence** is related to a deep **inner emptiness**, to an outside attempt to fill what is mainly a lack of self-**Love** or an affective deficiency linked to one of my parents. By a **dependence** (alcohol, drugs, food, cigarettes, sports, sex, work), I want to fill this gap, this despair and this sadness. My life is devoid of meaning, it no longer satisfies my deepest desires. I feel revolt against the outside world and I have difficulty in preserving my ego. I can't get to **love** myself as I am, and this temporary incapacity manifests itself by anger and resentment against the whole world. I live in a psychological prison where I feel I am the slave of a substance or a type of behavior. A **dependence** is therefore a sort of **substitute** that helps me to live temporarily in a world without problems. While alcohol gives me a degree of ecstasy and numbness in relation to what I am going through, the 'nonprescription' drugs (cocaine, hashish, heroin, LSD, PCP, marijuana, etc.) propel me toward new sensations with the desire to reach unknown summits of **consciousness**. I have the impression that I feel secure in a pleasant world, but sooner or later I find myself facing my insecurities and fears. **Cigarettes** allow me to 'fog up' my emotions, which become enshrouded in all this smoke. **Food** serves to fill a lack of tenderness and **Love**. **Sugar dependence** especially is a sign that I sense a hollowness lacking human warmth and gentleness and that I reject my desires. Any **dependence** thus leads to more or less familiar reactions by the human body. These forms of abuse are basically negative, and various types of uncontrolled fears (neuroses) may appear if the **dependence** is strong (drugs, for example). Lastly, **dependence** can manifest itself through a tendency (sexual, for example) that is difficult to control. The first important step to take is to become **Aware** of my situation. This requires much **Love** and courage to take on and break this slavery that is disrupting my life. I identify the deficiency I am experiencing in my life. This is what I am trying to run away from, by 'losing' myself in something else (drugs, for example) or someone else. My desire to live is great, but I feel I am not succeeding. I feel like a 'loser'. I have no place that is rightfully mine in my own life or in society. I base my level of happiness on the success of others. This **dependence** makes me live from failure to failure, which confirms my sense of helplessness. I must put aside the part of me that feels guilty and ashamed of this **dependence**. Judging myself or whipping myself, knowing that I must change my behavior, will only increase my anger and the difficulty of freeing myself from it. I am afraid of failing, I am afraid of my past.

I accept↓♥ to be open to the unknown and to the road that will lead me to my goals of self-fulfillment. Unconditional **Love** is the beginning of my healing. I ask others, search, check and take the first steps. I become familiar with the emotions inside of me because they are part of my true personality. I seek out what method of natural healing can help me to focus and harmonize myself and increase my inner strengths to enable me to lovingly integrate the different deficiencies endured during my youth. I gradually take on my responsibilities and resume contact with the divine being that I am. I can thus take leave of my **dependence** and become independent and autonomous, because I deserve to be loved and I fully accept↓♥ my worth and my qualities that make me an exceptional being.

DEPIGMENTATION *See: SKIN — LEUKODERMA*

DEPOSITS (calcium)

Calcium is a mineral that corresponds to the most 'rigid' energy of the human body, namely the bones.

Calcium is therefore related to my mental energy, to the mental structure of my being. The **deposit** forms when the energy sets and 'crystallizes' at a given location (similar to calculi in the liver), causing pain and inflammation. Why is it so? Because the **calcium deposits** generally come from rigid thoughts, from the **lack of flexibility about authority** that I refuse to accept↓♥. I consider that bending to this extra demand in my life prevents me from being totally free. A way to change these **calcium deposits** into **Love** is to keep an open mind and focus on communicating, moving and doing sports.

I accept↓♥ that by being open to others, I come less under the control of authority and I experience much more a sharing instead. This way, I remain autonomous and free and I acquire wisdom!

DEPRESSION *See also: NEURASTHENIA*

A **nervous depression**, commonly called a **depression**, is a pathological state marked by **deep sadness**, with psychological pain, loss of self-esteem and psychomotor retardation.

A **depression** takes the form of **self-depreciation** and **guilt** that eat me up inside. Both of these elements must be present for there to be a **depression**.

As soon as I have resolved one of them, whether it is the self-depreciation or the guilt, I have come out of the **depression.** If I am **depressive**, I feel miserable, less than nothing. I may even feel guilty of who I am. I constantly live in the past and I find it difficult to come out of it. The present doesn't exist and the future scares me. It is impossible for me to live in the '**here and now**'. I prefer to live constantly in the past, always looking rearward. The ***current news*** leaves me indifferent. I ***feel like*** doing nothing. To avoid being frustrated, especially sexually, I cut myself off from all my desires. I don't feel like taking myself in charge. It is important for me to make a change now in my way of seeing things because it is not like before. A **depression** is often a decisive stage in my life (adolescence, for example) because it forces me to question myself[3]. I want to have a different life at all costs. I am turned upside down between my ideals (my dreams) and reality (what actually goes on), between what I am and what I want to be. It is an inner imbalance (possibly chemical or hormonal) and my individuality is unrecognizable. I feel constricted in my space and I slowly lose my taste for living, the essence of my existence. I feel useless, miserable, ***lazy***, a burden for others. I tend to be easily resigned, and I feel like abdicating, ***resigning***, giving up. I put great **pressure** on myself to contain my emotions and bury them deep inside of me. When this **pressure** becomes too high, **depression** sets in: others are then forced to suspend some of my responsibilities. This **pressure** may also come from my parents, my spouse, my boss, or simply society. The obligation to succeed, to have a good reputation, to project the image of having a successful marriage and family life, all this contributes to increase my stress, to demand more and more of me, to set the bar much too high, and as soon as an event occurs that 'pops the cork'[4], **depression** sets in. I feel stuck, helpless and inferior. In other terms, **depression** has its source in a situation involving my territory, namely what belongs to my vital space, including persons (my parents, my children, etc.), animals (my dog, my fish, etc.), or things (my work, my house, my furniture, etc.). The conflict I am experiencing may be linked to an element of my territory that I am afraid of **losing**, or to a **dispute** taking place on my territory and that bothers me (the ***classic*** quarrels between brothers and sisters, for example) or to something I already lost and about which I blame myself for certain words or acts. Here are some expressions that show how I may be feeling: *"You smother me!"; "You're sucking out my air!"; "Make yourself scarce!"* Sometimes I also find it difficult to delimit or mark out my space, my territory. What is exclusively mine and what belongs to others? I am permanently dissatisfied with a situation that often involves a member of my family. **Depressive persons** are often very receptive to their entourage. I sense everything going on around me and this increases my sensitivity tenfold, hence my feeling of constriction

3. Children too can suffer from **depression.** It is more difficult to identify, or the parents do not pay attention to it, but it is common. If I am a child who easily feels guilty, if I think I am the cause of the problems in my family or in my parents' relationship as a couple, then **depression** may threaten me.

4. **The cork popped**: An expression meaning that the **pressure** in the champagne bottle got too high, like the 'last straw that broke the camel's back'.

and my sense of being invaded by the people around me. Instead of having a certain detachment, I experience everything 'from close up', which takes up a lot of my energy to no avail. Even if I fought, I know I would lose. I therefore tend to not finish what I have started. I find it very ***oppressive*** to always assume that anything I do is never good enough. I may even lean toward self-destruction. I am ***nostalgic***, huddling up inside, ***submissive*** like a dog to not bother anyone. I have the impression of ***bearing*** and dying. Laughing is no longer part of my life. I have allowed others to invade me. I may also have a 'need for attention' to help me discover my own worth, and a **depression** then becomes an unconscious means to 'manipulate' the people around me. I may expend lots of energy on a project or something that I **heart♥**ily want to do but that may not be the best thing for me. Life will therefore make something else happen that may even be better for me, but I am so focused on 'the' thing that I desire that I won't see all the good happening to me. I must develop the habit of taking an overall view of events, and see how this may be even better than what I had wished for. **Postnatal depression** appears a few weeks after childbirth, or even a few months later. I feel discouraged, I am afraid I won't get there and I don't know how to get it over with. The baby may have filled a gap temporarily. I am now facing myself, this solitude and emptiness inside of me. As I don't believe in my own possibilities and strengths, I don't see "how I am going to make it". All this may be amplified by my own painful childhood or childbirth memories. Whatever the reason for my **depression**, I check out right now the underlying causes of my **depressive** state. Did I experience being pressured when I was young? What are the major events I underwent in my childhood that are making my life so insignificant today? What is this drama of my life that is still gnawing at me from inside? Is it the loss of a loved one, my reason for living, or the direction of my life that I am no longer able to see? Fleeing reality and my responsibilities is futile (suicide, for example) even if it seems to be the easiest way. It is important for me to see the responsibilities in my life, because it will take more than antidepressants to make the **depression** disappear: I must go to the source and heal the ***sickness*** of the **Soul**.

By contrast, a '**down**' is a depressive disorder, a passing state: a period of despondency, disgust, lassitude, dejection and discouragement. This '**down**' is usually of short duration (for one or a few days). A '**down**' is also called **seasonal depression** or **winter depression**. It refers to a depressive state that occurs in the fall and the winter. At that time of the year, the amount of daylight diminishes due to the shorter days. I feel an immoderate need to eat and sleep, in addition to having the symptoms of a **depression**. The increased presence of darkness reminds me of the dark sides of my personality and the conflicted situations where I "can't see the **Light** at the end of the tunnel", where no solutions seem to exist. I look negatively at everything that happens to me. I feel I am a helpless victim. I withdraw into myself and cease all communication, even with myself, to avoid being questioned and held responsible for myself.

I accept↓♥ to stand back and examine my life. I take a detached look at what happens to me and I accept↓♥ to see what lessons I must learn. I focus my attention on my priorities and realize that life has been providing me with many gifts. I allow myself to have a good time, to rest and pull myself together in order to regain my energy and my ideas. I thus regain control over my life and find the energy needed to complete all my projects. I accept↓♥ that I am unique. I have all I need to change my destiny, and I can consciously choose to let the caterpillar transform itself into a butterfly. I can choose between 'dropping' or 'fighting'. I stop resisting and forcing things to go my way, I discipline myself, starting ***one thing at a time*** and taking care to finish it. By acting responsibly, I gain more freedom and my efforts are rewarded. I begin to do projects again, to dream and create my life as I want it, in a way that ***respects*** who I am! I no longer need others to approve me. I let them lead their lives and I give myself the right and the necessary space to thrive. I drop the burdens I only bore for the sake of looking good. I am simply myself: by ceasing to put futile pressure on myself, the **depression** will disappear.

DERMATITIS *See: SKIN — DERMATITIS*

DERMITIS (seborrheic) *See: SKIN — ECZEMA*

DESIRE (absence of) *See: SEXUAL FRUSTRATIONS*

DIABETES *See: BLOOD — DIABETES*

DIAPHRAGM

The **diaphragm** is the great muscular wall that separates the upper part (lungs and **heart♥**) from the lower part (liver, stomach, intestines, etc.) of my being. It represents respiration, the **capacity to let go** completely by breathing deeply.

When the **diaphragm** is compressed, I have the feeling of withdrawing into myself. I need to be relaxed to be able to breathe life fully. The **diaphragm** is effective when I abandon myself to life instead of trying to control everything. If some tensions appear, it is because I **hold in**, **repress** or **block** liberating energies that are beneficial for me. I may experience situations that prevent me from freely expressing my deepest feelings and thoughts. Maybe my way of life prevents me from really being who I am, which makes me breathe in a superficial and limited way. I feel stuck, closed in. A fragment of my personality is kept 'under lock'. The **diaphragm** is related to the period of my first movements as a fetus, when I discovered that something else existed besides me. Since becoming an adult, this region blocks when exchanges between my inside and outside worlds become conflicted, for example if I do many empty and superficial things without any depth.

I accept↓♥ that life brings me a lot of good. From now on, I don't have to hold in uselessly, I trust myself, I give myself the space I need and I allow myself to embrace life more. The **diaphragm** is a very important muscle that, when I breathe fully, enables me to contact my inner self and reach the energy of the Universe. I now see my life quite differently. **Here and now**, I freely express my deeper thoughts, feelings, and emotions. My life is full of ***frenzy*** and excitement!

DIARRHEA *See: INTESTINES — DIARRHEA*

DIGESTION DISORDERS *See: INDIGESTION*

DIPHTHERIA *See also: THROAT— LARYNX*

Diphtheria is an infectious disease that first causes false-membrane angina and later develops lesions with its toxin in the nervous system (paralysis), the kidneys or the **heart♥**. **Diphtheria** is typified by the formation of membranes in the larynx and the pharynx (throat), causing swelling. I have difficulty in swallowing.

As the throat enables me to speak, communicate and exchange, it indicates to me that I **hold back** in my exchanges with others. I can't express what I feel and I **choke back** my emotions and my needs. I am afraid of drowning in these repressed emotions. I choke on everything I don't express. I feel ridiculous to be living with so much anxiety. I am, or was, afraid of not being able to call out for help when in danger, and I may have this fear in my dreams. I **fear rejection** and I **presume** the reaction of others. I am hard on myself, as I expect the same treatment from others. I silently and helplessly allow others to control my life. I find it difficult to accept↓♥ my body. I fear what I am and I am afraid of dying. However I must become **Aware** that I am already dead in several areas of my life, for I don't let the natural flow of life course in me and express itself through me.

I accept↓♥ that it is essential for me to make my needs and my feelings known to others instead of choking them back. I must change. I must accept↓♥ myself as I am and learn to **love** myself. Singing is an excellent way to make my **throat** work, and celebrate life. If I **love** and respect myself, others will **love** me and respect me in return.

DISC (displaced) *See: DISC [HERNIATED DISC]*

DISC (herniated disc) *See also: BACK DISORDERS, LUXATION*

An intervertebral disc is a round and flat structure located between each pair of vertebræ in the spine, with a jelly-like core (like gelatin) that serves as a cushion that can absorb shocks. In a **herniated disc** (or **slipped disc**), the pressure of the vertebræ provokes a backward protrusion of this core into the spinal canal, reducing the shock-absorbing effect and painfully compressing the roots of the nerves in this area.

In a **disc herniation**, beyond the general meaning of **hernias**, there is an abnormal release of fluids, which involves, from a metaphysical viewpoint, the emotions. There is also pain in the nerves, involving mental energy and guilt. All of this indicates a deep conflict that affects all the aspects of my being. In the situation of a **disc herniation**, there is necessarily a conflict with **pressure**. I can feel it in my family and financial responsibilities, at work, etc. It is as if I was exerting pressure on myself by exceeding my limits, by taking myself for someone else because I want to go too fast. This pressure may come from me, from others or from somewhere else. I take everybody's burdens on my back. I feel that I am alone in life, I lack affection, I am not supported and I hesitate to admit it to others and especially to myself. This gives me the feeling of being a prisoner and indecisive. I don't feel up to scratch and I am lacking in self-confidence. I tend to live for others. I allow myself no mistakes. I am collapsing under the weight of my responsibilities. Instead of treating myself gently, I am very rigid with myself. I live my life like an automaton instead of allowing my child's **heart♥** to have fun and be spontaneous. As everything is automatic, very rational and thus devoid of emotions, it brings difficulties in my interpersonal relations. My emotions are trapped in my body and lead me to be very rigid. I revolt against a situation that I consider a dead end. It is important that I refer to the affected part of the spine to better understand what is going on in me. I am learning to become more flexible with myself and I now feel supported by life. I free myself of all guilt and all pressures. I **love** myself as I am. I do my best, and I leave the rest to God.

I learn to trust myself and accept↓♥ to be able to support myself. I leave to each person their responsibilities; I am thus freer to live my life according to my own existential values. I no longer have to be on the 'front line'. I can be a spectator. I become **Aware** of the fact that each time I sought an answer or some support, I found confirmation of what I already knew or felt. I **accept↓♥ to listen to my inner voice** that is always there to support me and guide me. **I learn to trust myself**, and I discover all the strength that is in me and the happiness it gives me to stand free and confidently.

DISC (intervertebral) *See also: BACK DISORDERS — LOWER BACK*

An **intervertebral disc** is a pliable cartilage that joins the vertebræ and plays the role of a shock absorber. Following a trauma, the displacement of the protuberance of the **intervertebral** disc provokes intense pain at the location of the expulsion. It generally provokes a compression of the roots of the sciatic nerve and persistent neuralgia in this nerve.

I experience a situation that destabilizes me, that 'throws me'. I feel caught between two persons, having to play the role of a mediator, of a 'buffer'. I must cushion the blows, and that makes a lot for me to bear. All the more so that at work, I may not feel competent to carry out the tasks I am asked to perform. The fact of criticizing myself and being so severe with myself may lead to a **disc degeneration** (**discarthrosis**). I am stuck like my discs, but I am doing nothing to change the situation. If there is any inflammation (**discitis**), it means I react exaggeratedly to a situation, like a fire that explodes or a bomb that detonates, when I am thwarted. I am direct, sometimes scathing, in my remarks or criticism, which air some of the anger I am experiencing.

I accept↓♥ that I am responsible for myself and my reactions. I question myself, I learn to cushion my reactions to life, others and situations, by admitting my wrongs. I settle my differences with myself and I take the place that is rightfully mine while respecting the opinions of others. I thus acknowledge my worth and I am more objective about the help I must give others.

DISCARTHROSIS *See: DISC [INTERVERTEBRAL]*

DISCONTENT, DISSATISFACTION

I am not satisfied with what is going on in my life. Still, I could be more satisfied, but there is always a 'but'.

Maybe I am too much the perfectionist. I hold back pressure and I have a desire for vengeance that is not expressed in words. **Dissatisfaction** can often be seen in my facial expression. I need to make changes in my life, change my structures and framework for living, but I am afraid of the consequences that might follow. I therefore prefer to ruminate and complain instead of taking action. For if I made myself happy, what would happen?

I accept↓♥ to seek the cause of this **dissatisfaction** and thereby enable myself to achieve positive changes by taking appropriate means to get there. I will then be the first to benefit from more joy in my life, which will then reflect itself in my entourage.

DISEASE (Addison's) *See: ADDISON'S DISEASE*

DISEASE (Alzheimer's) *See: ALZHEIMER'S DISEASE*

DISEASE (Bechterews') / ANKYLOSING SPONDYLITIS

Bechterews'[5] **disease** is a rheumatic pain that occurs after a trauma.

It results from rigidity and lack of flexibility in my way of thinking. I put aside my ego, which is taking up too much place.

I must accept↓♥, for the sake of **Love**, to be more flexible with myself, to trust the situations of life.

DISEASE (Bouillaud's) *See: RHEUMATISM*

DISEASE (Bright's) *See: BRIGHT'S DISEASE*

DISEASE (chronic) *See: CHRONIC [ILLNESS]*

---

5. **Bechterews** (Vladimir Mikaïlovitch): Russian neurologist (1857–1927). He was one of the collaborators of I. Pavlov. In 1893, he described the disease that would bear his name. In 1904, he proposed his 'tarsopharyngeal reflex' marking an alteration of the pyramidal tract. We also know '**Bechterews**' nucleus' in the upper acoustic vestibule of the ear. He wrote a treatise on conduction in the brain and in the spinal cord.

DISEASE (Crohn's) *See: INTESTINES — CROHN'S DISEASE*

DISEASE (Dupuytren's) *See: HANDS — DUPUYTREN'S DISEASE*

DISEASE (Friedreich's) *See: ATAXIA [FRIEDREICH'S]*

DISEASE (hamburger / ground meat / BBQ syndrome)

Hamburger disease is an inflammation of the colon caused by the bacterium E. coli naturally present in the digestive tracts of animals. Certain carriers include cattle, pigs and sheep. Infected persons are also carriers of the disease. The bacterium E. coli 0157:H7 can infiltrate the blood system and cause disorders there and also in the kidneys. When **hamburger** meat cooked on a barbecue is not fully done to a turn, there is a risk of exposure to food poisoning caused by the bacterium E. coli 0157. This infection is known as the **hemolytic** and **uremic syndrome** (HUS). There are other strains of the bacterium E. coli that can cause infections. The strain 0157:H7 is well known for having been involved in recent flare-ups of infection. I persist in remaining in a situation where I no longer have any reason for staying, but I hang on. I am angry and boiling inside, and I poison myself with 'mad cow'.

I take the time to consider what is irritating me so, and I accept↓♥ to review my behavior and my attitudes. I stop attacking others with my sarcasm and violent behavior. I accept↓♥ to be more responsible and take charge of my life. I become a bearer of **Light** rather than allow myself to be destroyed. I taste life.

DISEASE (Hansen's) *See: LEPROSY*

DISEASE (Hodgkin's) *See: HODGKIN'S DISEASE*

DISEASE (imaginary) *See also: HYPOCHONDRIA*

If I have an **imaginary disease**, I believe that I am sick without actually being so. I feel anxiety and I need **Love** and attention. I tell myself that nobody takes care of me, so I am worthless. How can I change this situation? Invent myself a **sickness**! I believe it so much that it becomes real in my eyes. If I keep on telling myself that I am sick, then sooner or later I actually will develop the disease. I verify if I bought the old recordings of one of my parents who used the same cassette against their fears, or if it is a pattern coming back to haunt me so that I can resolve it now.

I accept↓♥ to see that this so-called disease manifests a sickness of the **Soul**, a poorly managed emotional injury. Instead of living in my imagination, I resume contact with the physical world. I can thus make the changes I need for my well-being. I trust my body and thank my spirit, and I celebrate life because I am in perfect health.

DISEASE (immune) *See: SYSTEM [IMMUNE]*

DISEASE (mad cow's) *See: BRAIN — CREUTZFELD — JAKOB'S DISEASE*

DISEASE (Ménière's) *See: MÉNIÈRE'S DISEASE*

DISEASE (Parkinson's) *See: BRAIN — PARKINSON'S DISEASE*

DISEASE (psychosomatic)

The word **psychosomatic** indicates the relation that can exist between the spirit (*psyche*) and the body (*soma*). It was originally believed that the spirit had an influence on the body and conversely, that the body had an influence on the spirit. However, this influence attributed to the body on the spirit was gradually discarded, so in medical language the term **psychosomatic** now mainly signifies the relation between the spirit and the body.

Furthermore, when I am told that 'my' **illness** is **psychosomatic**, it is a little as if I had an **imaginary disease** and that it was all happening solely in my head. From the **metaphysical** viewpoint, all **diseases** have their origin beyond the physical, and I could therefore state that they are all **psychosomatic**. I must treat my body to the best of my knowledge by using the knowledge and know-how of health-care professionals, while finding out the true cause that brought about the onset of the ailment or the **disease**. The subconscious has an enormous power to regenerate tissues and the capacity to produce physical effects according to the interpretation it forms. Here are a few examples. A person is found dead in the refrigeration car of a train, where the person had been locked in by accident. The autopsy revealed that the person died of freezing, although the refrigerating system was turned off, which the victim was probably unaware of. People can walk bare feet on burning coals without developing burns or blisters on their feet because their subconscious, influenced by suggestion, has registered no danger; and so on.

ALL ILLNESSES APPEAR FOLLOWING A CONFLICT, AN EMOTIONAL SHOCK OR A CONSCIOUS OR UNCONSCIOUS TRAUMA. The brain then sets off a biological survival mechanism directed to the conflict or the trauma experienced. Restoring health is then a matter of being able to decode the message and modify the program sent by the brain.

Knowing this, I accept↓♥ to take care of my physical body in order to restore it to a more healthy state.

DISEASE (Raynaud's) *See: RAYNAUD'S DISEASE*

DISEASE / SICKNESS / ILLNESS / AILMENT / DISORDER

Humans are made to be healthy, but are endlessly faced with their bodies' functioning difficulties, emotions and thoughts. One's spirit and body, however, are inseparable. When a living being's health is affected, it is faced with **illness**.

There is a disharmony (a conflicted state) that the body is trying to express. When a dysfunctioning sets in, it is necessary to interpret ***'what the sickness is saying'***, because a **sickness** implies a cause, symptoms, clinical signs, a clinical development and a treatment. Being sick is not a random effect: it is a sign my body is sending me to inform me of a conflict or a trauma that I am experiencing, in relation to myself and/or to my environment.

Accepting↓♥ to decode the message, understand it and what is required to reharmonize myself will help me recover my health more quickly. I must change my way of living or thinking, because true healing is to be found chiefly in Me.

DISEASES (auto-immune) *See also: SYSTEM [IMMUNE]*

An **auto-immune disease** is characterized by the fact that my **immune** system is attacking my organism.

If such is the case, then my life is empty and 'isn't worth living'. I depreciate myself by feeling guilty over certain 'mistakes' made in the past. I detest some of my personality or physical traits that I can't stand. I make decisions according to others and their expectations. I don't believe I deserve any happiness or that I am able to change anything in my life. My own thoughts, emotions, states of feeling or negative beliefs are what is attacking my body: I am destroying myself.

I accept↓♥ to welcome each part of my being in the openness and the unconditional **Love** of who I am and in my own divinity. I detach myself from the expectations and values of society in order to build my own frame and terms of reference. I immediately stop all aggressions against the Being that I am. I thus connect myself to my powers of creation and healing that nourish and reinforce my natural immunity.

DISEASES (hereditary) *See also: INFIRMITIES [CONGENITAL]*

In the medical sense of the term, **hereditary diseases** are transmitted by the genes in the reproductive cells of one or both parents. It is **diathesis**, which is a predisposition to contract **diseases**. In fact, if I want to speak of **heredity**, it consists, rather, of the unresolved thoughts, emotions or inner conflicts of my parents or grandparents. For example, if I say that diabetes is **hereditary** in my family because my grandfather was diabetic, my father was diabetic and I am diabetic, it is rather because my grandfather experienced **deep sadness** (deep sadness can be considered as one of the metaphysical causes of diabetes), because my father experienced deep sadness and because I am experiencing deep sadness. So, instead of thinking that this **disease** is **hereditary** and that there is nothing I can change about it, I can then begin to find out how I can change my thoughts and emotions or resolve the inner conflict that made me develop this **disease**. As a child, I may not accept the environment in which I must develop, and this leads to a permanent stress that, if poorly managed, will transform itself into **so-called congenital physical anomalies** or **diseases**, whatever my age. By keeping in mind that any **illness** must favor a gain in personal **Awareness**, I know however that the metaphysical reason for the **illness**, with respect to my thoughts and emotions, is to be found in either one or in both of my parents, even if they are not necessarily those who originally developed the **illness**. From the moment of my conception, I begin to accumulate experiences and feelings. If I soon perceive myself negatively or have the impression that I deserve little, this frame of mind will be openly revealed by a **disease** or a **physical anomaly**. If I was born blind for example, it is because, as a baby, I had difficulty in seeing and accepting↓♥ the life that offered itself to me.

I accept↓♥ the responsibility for my own emotions. I examine in what respects they may be related to those of my parents. By opening the door to a physical healing following an emotional healing, I become **Aware** that all is possible!

DISEASES (in children) *See also: CHILDHOOD DISEASES (IN GENERAL)*

These generally refer to ailments or **diseases** described in this dictionary. Also, if I am a child who has an ailment or a **disease**, chances are strong that the expression of the **disease** is manifesting the inner malaise of one or both of my parents. My parents may not develop a **disease**, but my great sensitivity connects me to the inner reality of my parents. I am then in resonance with my parents' inner child.

I accept↓♥ that the **disease** I am currently experiencing will highlight only the state of **Awareness** I must **also** reach. My parents are not guilty of what I am experiencing.

DISEASES (incurable)

Incurable means "that which cannot be healed by any form of medicine".

I must ask myself if it suits me somehow to have a **disease** that is said to be **incurable**. In what sense can it suit me? Must I agree with this '**incurable**' label that means that nothing can be done any longer to remedy it? I must look inside of myself to find the deeper cause of this illness: fear, anger, jealousy or despair may be the cause. I sense that, beyond the **disease** itself, there is a situation in my life that I believe is impossible to change. It is a 'problem' with no solution.

I must accept↓♥ that **Love** flows freely in me, as only **Love** can heal everything.

DISEASES (infantile) *See: CHILDHOOD DISEASES (IN GENERAL)*

DISEASES (karmic)

I come on this earth to pursue an unfolding. I have experiences to live through in order to complete an inner transformation. If I enter this world with an infirmity, it will often be because some issues were not resolved in some other life or lives (for those who believe this).

Becoming **Conscious** and accepting↓♥ to live through the experience are the first steps toward healing, physically as well as emotionally. At that point, everything is possible, for the inner transformation leads to physical healing.

DISEASES (sexually transmitted) / (STD) *See: VENEREAL DISEASES*

DISEASE (sleep) *See: NARCOLEPSY*

DISEASES (venereal) *See: VENEREAL DISEASES*

DISLOCATION *See: BONES — DISLOCATION*

DIVERTICULITIS *See: INTESTINES — DIVERTICULITIS*

DIZZINESS *See: BRAIN — BALANCE [LOSS OF]*

DOUBT

Doubt is directly related to the mind. It is an obsessional state that prevents me from clearly connecting with my physical side. **Doubt** may result from questions such as: "Did I do it or not?" I ask myself very down-to-earth questions or, on the contrary, in a metaphysical form, bearing on the value of life, religion, duty, truth, etc. I constantly query my decisions, wondering if I made the right choices about the situations in my life. **Doubt** can trouble and poison my existence.

I accept↓♥ to listen to my inner voice and trust more in life. By reassuring my inner self, I accept↓♥ to stand free from the mental ties that impede my spiritual development. When it concerns my relations with the persons around me, instead of poisoning my existence with **doubt, I learn to verify** my needs, my impressions and my intuitions with these people.

'DOWN' (experiencing a) *See: DEPRESSION*

DOWN'S SYNDROME *See: MONGOLISM*

DRUG ADDICTION / DRUG ABUSE / TOXICOMANIA *See also: ALCOHOLISM, CIGARETTES, COMPULSION [NERVOUS], DEPENDENCE, DRUGS, LUNGS (IN GENERAL)*

Drug addiction is characterized by the abusive consumption of different toxic products, regulated by law or not, among which are found tobacco, medications, alcohol and **drugs** in all their forms.

I thus develop a psychological or physical dependency. This irresistible need to consume shows a great fear of seeing myself as I am. I prefer escape and unawareness. Not knowing how to love myself, I can't imagine the people around me loving me and appreciating me. I am afraid of failure. I need so much to be recognized and loved that I am ready to consume toxic products, even if death can result from them, in order to obtain them. I have difficulty in entering into contact with others, expressing my frustrations or my despair. I decide in advance that they won't be able to help me because "nobody understands me". In a sense, it suits me quite well to think in such terms. I hide in a fantasy world where I believe that nothing can ever reach me. I don't feel like making any efforts and becoming responsible for my life. I quietly go to sleep by repressing my injuries deep inside of me. I am hurting, even I can't see it any longer.

I accept↓♥ to see how **toxic** this habit is for me. By giving myself a chance to be myself, I can discover the wonderful being I am and open myself up to **Love**.

DRUGS *See also: DEPENDENCE*

A veritable scourge of humanity, **drugs** constitute one of human beings' worst **escapes** for their survival. As substances extracted from plants or synthetically manufactured, **drugs** described as **'soft'** (marijuana, hashish, etc.) or **'hard'** (PCP, cocaine, heroin, etc.) are often used for one or several of the following motives: despair, shame, extreme escape, fear of the unknown and of taking on one's responsibilities. **Drugs** are my refuge, to **protect me against myself**. As I refuse to live and be responsible, my inner weaknesses risk leading me to **drugs**. I am afraid of facing reality and having to make efforts. My will goes to sleep and I tend less and less to make decisions. I 'let myself live'. Several **drugs** often bring about great dependencies that only reflect my 'own inner dependencies': delinquency, absent parents, introversion, neuroses, emotional or sexual compulsions that I try to repress by doping my mind. The impression of being separated, or even 'torn away' either from a loved one (parent, brother, sister, animal, etc.) or from a place or a situation that brought me much happiness, may lead me to experience an inner emptiness that I want to escape through **drugs**. I may suffer from a relationship with one of my parents, often my mother, who was dry of any emotion. These **drugs**, which are stimulants, allow me to 'soar', to reach certain heights and have an experience that gives me the illusion of being 'happy' at last by escaping. I can't do without it any longer, and my dependency intensifies and becomes aggravated as time goes by. The first step is to become **conscious**, frankly and doffing all masks: Why am I using these substances? I become **Aware** that there is always a reason. Whatever its nature, I accept↓♥ to discover the true reason.

I accept↓♥ myself as I am and I learn to express my needs. To stop using **drugs** will demand considerable courage on my part, but the quest for inner peace is my motivation. To succeed in being myself under any and all circumstances will enable me to experience and achieve true inner peace and to feel myself in my own place in this great Universe.

Some of these **drugs** are:

Hashish – **Marijuana**: I am searching for a world without problems, so I am running away.

Amphetamines – **Cocaine**: These stimulate productivity, so I seek success, **Love**, recognition.

LSD – **Mescaline**, **Magic Mushrooms**, **Heroin**: I am seeking sensations and expanded **Consciousness**. In the case of **heroin**, I ask myself how far I idealized my mother or an influential woman in my life whom I considered as a **heroine**; do I still have this opinion, or did she disappoint me or betray me?

Opium: It brings lazy enjoyment and gives a false appearance of inner peace.

DRUNKENNESS / INEBRIATION *See: ALCOHOLISM*

DRY MOUTH *See: MOUTH DISEASE*

DRYNESS (vaginal) *See: VAGINA (IN GENERAL)*

DUCTS (biliary) *See: GALLBLADDER*

DUODENUM *See also: INTESTINAL AILMENTS*

The **duodenum** is the initial and shortest part of the small intestine, following the pylorus and continuing through the jejunum to the ileon. Most of the digestion and absorption is carried out by the small intestine. The **duodenum** thus represents the synthesis of reception and integration. There is a balancing relation between giving and receiving. When there is a dysfunction in the **duodenum**, I feel confronted by new ideas. I doubt myself unconsciously. I lack confidence in my ability to properly manage any adjustment. It may involve affective relations, or it may be in my family where I feel thwarted or am suffering from an injustice. Someone or something is thwarting me and I can't tolerate it. There is a dispute that must be resolved, and I need some help in this. I feel torn: I feel I have to sacrifice myself for the few friends I have and who are often not very nice. A **duodenal ulcer** is caused by great insecurity and distrust toward others. I become **Aware** of the fact that this word is formed from the word '**duo**'. There is therefore a link with interpersonal exchanges. I feel worn down inside, it is burning me up inside. I can't absorb this situation, it irritates me and I persist in wanting to control everything in my relations. Do I feel dominated by someone or something? Am I afraid of not having everything I need to be loved as I am? I become **Aware** of these fears and let go of those old ideas.

I accept↓♥ to become **conscious** of my capacity for allowing energy to flow without resisting life, and that among my strengths are my capacities for trusting and adjusting. By regaining my inner peace, this fire that was eating me up inside abates, and my **duodenum** is faring all for the better.

DUODENUM (ulcer in the) *See: STOMACH DISORDERS*

DUPUYTREN'S DISEASE *See: HANDS — DUPUYTREN'S DISEASE*

DWARFISM / NANISM — GIGANTISM *See also: BONES — ACROMEGALIA*

Nanism is an anomaly in humans characterized by smallness in size as compared to the average size for individuals of the same age, sex and race, with no sexual or intellectual insufficiency, which distinguishes it from infantilism. **Gigantism** has the same definition, except for the size being abnormally large. Growth takes place rapidly and my bone and glandular systems have deficiencies.

Nanism shows me that unconsciously, I want to remain a child as long as possible. It is as if I remained curled up into myself. I am different from everyone else and I don't meet the standards. I distrust others and people in general and I usually maintain a 'smallness' complex in all respects. I want to hide behind others and thus feel safer. I tend to withdraw into myself and live in accordance with very strict rules: I thus feel more in charge of my life if I live in a structured fashion. The fact of growing taller implies that I am also becoming an adult, and if this represents a danger for me (for example, having to take on more responsibilities that scare me), my body will refuse to grow. I may also be forbidden to grow up, or it may be dangerous for me (for example if I am afraid of incest with a parent if I grow too much).

I accept↓♥ to grow, physically and emotionally, in my spiritual development. Each developmental stage brings different challenges, and the **Soul** that I am has everything it needs to face these challenges. Maturity brings greater wisdom and inner strength. My being can fully flourish and display its inner freedom. By freeing myself of my false beliefs, I realize I am consciously choosing to face the situation while being guided and protected by the Source. I take a new step every day by giving myself unconditional **Love**.

Gigantism indicates to me that I feel a prisoner of my body and my emotions and that I want to get out of it at all costs! I am smothering and I don't want to have to bend myself to any authority. Being taller than the others gives me a false impression of power and control over myself and others. I feel overtaken by the events of life in general. I want to enter too quickly into the life cycle, and I don't follow the natural movements.

I accept↓♥ to take charge of my life. I learn to slow down and not force anything, for I recognize my inner feelings and learn to channel them, so the energy in me is positive and brings me more **Love** and freedom. I give special attention to my life goals. I make peace with the **Soul** that I am and I stop pushing to go faster than the others. The only authority is that of my inner voice, which is the road to the total freeing of all my limits. I trust it totally and I flourish ever more each day.

DYSENTERY *See: INTESTINES / DIARRHEA / DYSENTERY*

DYSLEXIA

Dyslexia is a learning difficulty in reading and proper spelling, independent of any intellectual or sensory deficiency or any psychiatric disorder. After easily reading a few words, I am incapable of understanding what follows, I stop, and I can only resume reading after a few seconds of rest.

I want to go too fast in my life. My thought goes faster than my words, and everything is jumbled at the exit. Whether I am living in a disturbed family environment or was over-protected, in both cases I want to satisfy one of my parents (or one of the people close to me) and I am afraid of not being up to their expectations or not meeting their requirements. I feel vulnerable for I am lacking in self-esteem and I stumble over the difficulties. It is the result of an upsetting situation that I am experiencing, especially if I am a **child**. My difficulties with **writing** remind me of '**the crying**' that I hear at home or at school and that I can't tolerate any longer. I don't know how to get out of this situation; I wish it would stop at any costs! If it is a difficulty in **reading** instead, I look at the situation in which I was forced to read, for example before a roomful of many people, or I was ridiculed; and every time I read, it reactivates the stress I experienced in that specific situation. I also feel that the structures in which I live (rules at home or at school) are too strict. I feel like a little soldier who must obey orders or else I will be punished. My parents protect me so much that I see this as a punishment. If I am the **parent of this child**, I look at how I can convey my needs more calmly and with more understanding, instead of screaming my dismay, if such is the case, and using a certain form of non-beneficial violence.

I accept↓♥ to give myself time to do things, one step at a time, without trembling, without getting everything jumbled. I take the time to breathe and calm myself. I know I am an intelligent being and I develop my will by going one step at a time. I accept↓♥ to recognize the **Love** that is in me. I give myself the possibility of loving myself and accepting↓♥ that this state is temporary. I know that I will reach my goals. As a child, I also accept↓♥ to have the power to decide what is good for me. I learn to trust myself and regain my learning capacity, for I know that deep inside, I can get there by dint of courage, will and tenacity. From now on, I will use reading as a tool to open doors onto the world. I risk telling the people concerned what no longer suits me, as I want to live in peace and harmony. I thus feel more freedom and I become **Aware** of the fact that the rules exist to supervise me, support me and guide me.

DYSMENORRHEA *See: MENSTRUATION DISORDERS*

DYSTROPHY (muscular) *See: MUSCLES — DYSTROPHY [MUSCULAR]*

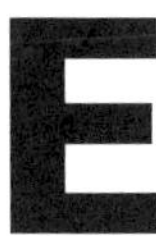

EARS (in general) *See also: EARS — DEAFNESS*

Sight and hearing allow me to locate myself in the environment. I can see things without there being any sound, and I can hear things without necessarily seeing where those sounds are coming from. Taken jointly together, these two senses provide a sort of 'three-dimensional take' on my environment.

Thus, the **ears** enable me to hear all the sounds that surround me, whether harmonious or disharmonious, and warn me of danger. Total or partial **deafness** may occur when I can't deal with or accept↓♥ what I hear. I thereby cut off contact between me and others. If I am **deaf**, it is because a selective information process has set in, for I want to hear only what suits me and I cut myself off from anything that doesn't suit me in the midst of everything that is being said. This selective process is very effective, for it enables me to 'recognize', for example, the voice of my child whom I am searching for in a crowd. Similarly, this process acts in reverse for whatever I don't want to hear. Indirectly, the **ears** make it possible to maintain a body-spirit balance making its way about in the Universe. This balance holds me standing erect and on alert, and allows me to be centered and to follow my way. The **ear** is also a symbol of my inner listening. The fact of listening to my inner wisdom manifests itself through my **ears**. The state of my **ears** shows how open I am to my deepest emotions, and how flexible and accepting↓♥ I am toward them.

I accept↓♥ to remain flexible with respect to my life structures that are constantly evolving. By building solid bases with the help of my inner voice, my **ears** remain in perfect health!

EAR DISORDERS *See also: EARS / BUZZING / OTITIS / TINNITUS*

Ear disorders occur when I feel sorrow, when I am irritated or feel hurt by things I have heard. I may also have the impression that nobody listens to what I have to say, or I am disappointed about what I would like to hear people tell me, but that nobody ever tells me (compliments, thanks, etc.). It is as if I wanted to lock myself in and no longer be in contact with what surrounds me. Maybe I am the one being obstinate and refusing to hear what others have to say. What I am **hear**ing goes beyond my **understand**ing. If I am annoyed because there are words or information that I was unable to receive or hear, for example because of noise or a hubbub around me, and these were of capital importance to me, for instance to make a decision or follow a direction, my anger or my frustration will cause an **ailment** in my **ears**. There is a ***communications*** breakdown and ***noise***. There is often a conflict related to the mother, which manifests itself by an **ear ailment**. An **ear ache** occurs following criticism that **came to my ears** and was aimed at me or at someone else. What

I hear makes me anxious and hurts me, physically and emotionally. I am locked up in my dark past that I hang on to. I resent myself and I feel guilty. I hurt myself and maybe I am the one who allows others to hurt me. If it is an **ear infection**, I probably heard words that caused me to feel irritation, an emotional upheaval, conflict or disharmony. My **ears** react strongly when I hear people I **love** who can't ***get along together***, who can't come to an ***agreement***. If it is an **otitis**, I feel very helpless about what I heard. It is as though my **ears** were ***smashed*** by violence-filled words. If a **child** experiences an **ear** ailment, this may express a conflict related to the family or the school environment. **Ear aches** are frequent **in children** who hear everything adults are saying, their parents' quarrels, without being able to give their own point of view. I may hear different versions of the same story, and this greatly troubles me because I don't know who to believe. Usually, one of my two parents emotionally experiences the same situation as I do. I may be a mirror indicating to that parent that she, or he, should listen more to themselves. **Ear aches** may also manifest themselves in **adults** who have difficulty with oral communication, especially if I feel disgust about using a telephone. I may have difficulty in closing conversations that I find dull, or dealing with the same issues endlessly repeated. I develop a 'telephone phobia', which, if poorly managed, may express itself by an **ear ache**. My body may also tell me that I should listen more to my inner wisdom. I may also be confused over messages or signals that are sent to me and, in a sense, I no longer want to hear what is going on, "I don't believe my **ears**"! My **ears** may become **blocked** if I want to hide and seek refuge inside of me, and I no longer want to hear anything because it hurts too much or is too disturbing. This is the case if I have a **plug or ear wax**: I no longer want to hear any quarrels or hurtful words. I hold in, and ruminate over, everything instead of letting go.

I accept↓♥ to discipline myself and '**lend an ear**' to everything around me and especially inside of me. I learn to keep my **ears** 'open' at all times, while developing my capacity for detaching myself from what I hear. My **heart♥** can thus remain constantly open.

EAR FINGER / FIFTH FINGER *See: FINGERS — ATRIAL / AURICULAR / LITTLE FINGER*

EARS — BUZZING *See also: EARS — TINNITUS*

Buzzing is related to the **refusal to listen to** my inner voice, the inner signs that guide my life. I 'do as I please' and I refuse to hear certain words that I find unpleasant. I may even be obstinate. I resist because I am afraid to **learn the truth**, to be **Aware** of a situation or even to eventually make a decision. It can even throw me in disarray, and I will set off a **buzzing in my ears** to not hear it. I have the impression that a person is thinking about me, whereas in fact it is often the contrary. I may be tense because of the ideas 'trotting about' in my head. I feed on negative thoughts. My anxieties prevent me from listening to my inner wisdom. I create a whole world in my head and I live in illusion. I am too self-centered.

By accepting↓♥ to remain open in my **heart♥**, I can hear words with more detachment. I let go of the preconceived ideas, prejudice and false gods on which I previously built my life. I discover the richness of my **heart♥** and learn to trust my inner voice. I am no longer forced to lend a **deaf ear**. The sages say: *"Listen to what you do not tell yourself"*. I recognize the **Light** that inhabits me and I drink it in. It is thus easier to see the beauty in others.

EARS — DEAFNESS

Hypoacusis is a diminishing of auditory acuity. When this acuity diminishes very substantially or completely, we then speak of **deafness**. *"Better to be **deaf** than to hear that!"* I choose to no longer hear, I decide to isolate myself from others. As I easily feel rejected I 'plug my **ears**', no longer wishing to be bothered. Not knowing how to answer sometimes, I lend a **deaf ear**. I am afraid of being manipulated and I don't accept↓♥ criticism, I don't want to 'hear' the voice of reason; by creating this barrier, I therefore increasingly isolate myself and I persist in not hearing. I prefer to hide inside of myself and 'retreat into my shell' like an injured animal. I am ***deafened*** by what I hear or by what I discover about myself or about other persons. I have the impression that people always keep ***harping on*** about the same things. I am very sensitive to ***what people may say***. I feel assaulted by all the 'racket' around me. Still, whether I want it or not, time will have the effect that the unresolved problems in my life will all come back one day, and I will have to face them in the end. In fact, I tend to want to fix everything by myself instead of asking for help. I am closed to others. I can ask myself if I listen to my emotions, my frustrations and ultimately, my inner voice. Anger is growing in me and I am afraid to allow it to express itself. I prefer to retreat into myself, not knowing very well how my anger could express itself. I don't know very well in what direction I should go. I can be very obstinate and 'lend a **deaf ear**' because I want to do only as I wish, and I don't accept↓♥ anyone telling me what to do or giving me advice. I become **Aware** of the specific situations where I have greater difficulty in hearing: is it with high-pitched sounds or with low-pitched sounds? Does my percentage of hearing acuity improve during certain periods and then diminish later on? Is it with persons of the male or the female gender? With adults or with children? With persons who have a special ***accent***? It is interesting to note that **deafness** shows variations instead of being always constant, and that it varies from one person to the next. I therefore tend to 'block' certain sounds before they reach the brain and begin to disturb my inner tranquility. I can stop these sounds with the presence of **water in my ears**. This water may represent emotions that have accumulated about what I heard and prevent me from communicating to spare others from hearing what they might hear from my mouth. These different forms and intensities of **deafness** make me feel alone and isolated. I prefer to be far from people because in any case I am afraid of making the wrong choices. If I am a **child**, the quarrels, the reprimands, the screams and the noise I hear may become too much for me at some point and I need to cut myself off from all that racket. If I am always afraid that an ***alarm*** will ring, in the proper as well as the figurative sense, it makes my eyes tear and I prefer not to hear it, for it is an omen of danger.

I accept↓♥ to 'lend an **ear**' and listen to my inner voice that is the best advisor in my life. The most beautiful act of **Love** I can do is to open my **heart♥**. I accept↓♥ to hear the messages and I open myself to others. I find peace inside of me. I come out of the shade to live at last in the **Light** of my inner wisdom.

EARS — OTITIS

Otitis is an inflammation of one or both **ears**, and it originates in the discomfort I experience about something I am hearing or have recently heard. **Otitis** is frequent when I am a child, especially about what my parents may say to each other or about what I may be told, as I am often not capable of expressing my dissatisfaction and my frustration. I am very sensitive to my environment and to what I consider as dangerous. Whether I am an adult or a child, even if this sorrow comes from what I hear, it may also come from what I don't hear, such as, for instance: "I **love** you", "Congratulations for what you've just done", etc. When I have an **otitis**, some liquid generally appears behind the eardrum. What I hear must therefore pass through this fluid before being heard. This situation is similar to when I was a baby in my mother's womb. With an **otitis**, I am therefore trying, even unconsciously, to find this special environment again. I may prefer to '**lend a deaf ear'** or '**block my ears**' to not have to hear any longer. I withdraw into myself, with only sadness, lassitude and misunderstanding for companions. I want to be close to my mother, but I want to protect myself from her fears and insecurities. For my parents, it is a signal that tells them that I, their child, who has an **otitis**, am experiencing an inner conflict and that it is important for them to help me to express what I am experiencing in order to foster rapid healing. I seek harmony at home and I flee disagreements. I may be **Aware** of a separation and I don't want to hear about the changes that will result from it. As an adult, an **otitis** allows me to ask myself questions about my inner voice: *"Do I listen to this one?", "Am I receiving messages that disturb me and make me angry about what I must do or about what I am asked to do?", "Do I feel that I am always the one who lends an* ***ear*** *to the others, but when the time comes for me to be listened to, nobody seems to be there to help me?"* **Otitis** is a way to escape my problems. I feel imprisoned and restricted. I prefer to remain in an imaginary world. I thus avoid facing the earthly world in the present moment. I am revolted. I don't want to hear about the suffering or the wrong I may have caused for someone.

I accept↓♥ that it is by listening, inner as well as outer, that I can move forward in life, for listening enables me to focus and to avoid useless obstacles. I accept↓♥ my past, I let go of any feelings of death or painful memories. Whatever my age, I listen to my inner wisdom. I live in the spontaneity of the moment.

EARS — TINNITUS *See also: EARS — BUZZING*

Tinnitus is the phenomenon that makes me hear sounds such as whistling, buzzing or sizzling without any actual relation to my environment. It can be temporary or permanent and can occur with different intensities of sound.

Tinnitus is often found in persons who experience very high performance stress. It often appears following an event where an emotional shock was sustained and the stress level increased significantly: a divorce, the loss of a job, a burglary, etc. I need to be recognized and for people to respect my identity and my rights. I am afraid however of losing my job or a certain social status (at work or in my personal life) and I don't want to face it. I may sometimes find it difficult to question some of my ideas, and I may even become obstinate. I persist in remaining in an unsatisfactory situation. I resist changes that I have not chosen and over which I have no control. Unconsciously, I know that if nothing changes, there may be a separation, in my personal life as well as at work. When this happens to me, I must take the time to ask myself if I have been listening to my inner voice. It is as if I was not perfectly tuned on my 'inner radio set'. When I tune in to a station that is on the air and is not broadcasting music or voices, I can 'hear the silence'. On the other hand, if I move the receiver to a frequency where there is no station broadcasting, I hear a sizzling or a whistling, as if I was using a shortwave set. Are there any emotions that I repressed for fear of disturbing my inner balance? Life thus reminds me to listen to my inner voice, my needs and my desires. I must take myself in charge so as to diminish the 'noise level' or the 'interferences' that may exist in my thoughts and my emotions. The fact of hearing these whistlings or buzzings may also tell me that there is something I no longer want to hear and that these sounds will be 'smothered' to avoid reaching my **ears**. **Tinnitus** indicates to me that my body is under tension. Things are going so fast in my head that I have the impression everything is going to 'blow up'. I am very ***attentive*** to everything going on around me. When I have **tinnitus**, often I am feeling far from a person I **love**. I feel separated from her because we have difficulty in communicating. Experiencing silence scares me and I find it intolerable. I need reassurance, explanations and nice words, but none of that exists. I thus feel attacked in this non-communication. I have no other choice but to retreat into my shell to protect myself from this wall of silence. I am facing a sort of duality: I need solitude, but only when I choose it, and not when it is imposed on me or happens out of my control! This sound that I am hearing can also allow me to stay in contact with a past suffering that I don't want to forget. Does this sound or noise allow me to be soothed, because that is what would happen if I really heard it physically? Sometimes, silence brings on the notion of death and, if I am afraid of it, my brain 'makes noise' to distract me from thinking about it. It is important for me to identify exactly what I hear (whistling, sizzling, buzzing, bells, horns, etc.) in order to identify what I am experiencing. I may hear the following sounds: like the sound of a stream, the roaring of a torrent, bells, the buzzing of bees, a single flute note, the sound of bagpipes, the wind in the trees, thousands of violins, a deep roaring. When this happens, it is because I am in contact with one of the sounds that exist in the inner planes and is representative of one plane of **Consciousness** in particular[1]. In this case, I am not experiencing **tinnitus**; it is a natural sound. My inner, spiritual ear is more open. I should be **thankful** for hearing this sound, for it indicates that I am in more **conscious** contact with one of the inner worlds of creation. I remain calm and my attitude is that of someone who lives right next to a stream and hears that sound normally. The brain registers this sound as normal and I feel comfortable functioning in my everyday life with **this natural sound**.

I accept↓♥ to open up my inner **ears** (located at 8 to 10 cm behind my physical **ears**) more, to be able to receive my inner voice. I can also ask to hear more **consciously** the sounds of nature and the celestial melodies in order to benefit from more peace and rest within myself. Any holistic approach such as yoga, guided relaxation, acupuncture, osteopathy, vitaminotherapy, energy, etc., can help diminish the level of stress and regain inner tranquility. I may also hear something like the sound of a stream, a torrent, the chiming of bells (small, medium or large), bagpipes, wind in the trees, the high-pitched buzzing of bees, or thousands of violins. These sounds correspond to sounds that I can hear on different planes of inner realities and can enable me to determine on which plane I am tuning in. This means, then, that my inner ear is open to hearing more clearly the reality of these worlds.

ECCHYMOSIS / BRUISE *See: SKIN — BRUISES*

ECLAMPSIA *See: PREGNANCY — ECLAMPSIA*

ECTROPION *See: EYELIDS (IN GENERAL)*

ECZEMA *See: SKIN — ECZEMA*

EDEMA

Edema is a swelling caused by water retention. It causes swelling and is very frequent in the ankles and the feet. It can also be found in the other joints and the conjunctive tissues.

The fluids in the body represent my emotions, and I may be holding in, or repressing, my inner feelings. I may also be denying my impulses, or **feeling limitations and barriers to the things I desire**, inviting discouragement and disappointment. I may also want to hold on to someone or something in my past or in my present, and I cling to it like a life preserver. It may also be painful memories. I am in conflict with the passing of time, which is going too fast. Otherwise, I am going to drown in my sorrow, my disappointment

1. Source: "Le carnet de notes spirituelles" de Paul Twitchell.

and my bitterness over events. I feel 'blocked'. Even my thought mechanism is 'frozen'. I take the feelings of others so much into consideration that I neglect my own. I seek harmony and try with all my might to connect and bring together people who have disagreements. I am afraid of expressing what I feel. I feel **powerless** and I feel **melancholy**, **sadness** and a **great lassitude**. I believe I am marked for failure, which prevents me from moving ahead. I have developed an inferiority complex and I am very fearful. I may feel life is very unfair and I sense a great inner emptiness. I can't act for myself, so I show great authority over others and try to make decisions in their place. As I hide from everyone whatever disturbs me, I become **Aware** of the urgency of expressing my needs. **Edema** shows me I need protection for fear of being hurt in my emotions. This fear makes me flee and build myself various personalities that enable me to avoid making contact with my deeper self. Seduction is a tool I use to get the attention and the **Love** of others. The function of the body part affected by **edema** adds further information. In the legs, ankles and feet, I may feel a great desire to move in a different direction, but I feel emotionally stuck in my current direction, unable to assert myself and free myself from it. There are some unclear situations in my life, involving certain persons in particular, that make me feel confused. When **edema** forms after a blow or an injury, or a part of my body is trying to rebuild itself, this is called the **edema of healing**. In some cases, my body draws in this fluid as if to reduce friction and help the immediate environment of the affected part to rebuild itself. **Edema** brings the need to recognize and discover the expression of my **bottled-up** and **contained** emotions.

I also learn to let go in order to allow myself to move forward and make positive changes in my life. I accept↓♥ to be loved for myself, whatever the emotions that are inside of me. I accept↓♥ to learn how to communicate my needs and I realize that it is possible to do so without the other person feeling attacked. By allowing myself to be me, I recover the joy of living and, at the same time, a new surge of energy. My understanding of others increases because I express myself and because I understand myself better.

EFFUSION of SYNOVIA *See: BURSITIS*

EGOCENTRISM

When I am **egocentric**, I tend to relate everything around me to myself. I then consider myself as the center of the world. By contrast with a selfish, egoistic person, I may think of others and help them, as long as it fits with my own interest. I live this way because I need to balance my inner insecurity to avoid having to experience submission.

I accept↓♥ to become **Aware** of the fact that beyond myself, there are others too. While holding my rightful place in life, I can consider the viewpoints of others. I open myself up to my sensitivity. I stop gazing at my navel and open myself to sharing, friendship and **Love**. Therefore I give, and I receive.

EJACULATION (premature)

Premature ejaculation can be related to my first sexual experiences.

When I masturbate, I feel **guilty** because I feel it as being 'bad' or 'forbidden'. I therefore hurry to achieve **ejaculation**. The fact of experiencing sexuality while thinking that I have no right to be doing so urges me to 'go fast': what I am doing is wrong and I am disobeying certain rules. Forbidden pleasure has always held a very strong attraction for me and, even unconsciously, I try to live it over again. In my **desire to perform**, I may also impose **pressures** and **nervousness** on myself. I want to prove to myself and to my partner "what I am capable of", with vexing and often unexpected results. I may have such a great feeling of desire and possession toward my partner that I can't control it. Contact with my partner may revive my fear of losing their **Love** and being abandoned or rejected, and so I "lose my grip on myself". Or could this be an unconscious way to settle my account with him/her?

I accept↓♥ to relax and learn anew the sexual pleasure related to masturbation, in a climate free of restrictions and guilt. Alone or with my partner, I rediscover the pleasure of masturbation, delaying the moment of **ejaculation** as long as possible. This becomes a game in which I find much pleasure. I may also undertake a psychotherapy that will help me to reduce this guilt that I may have experienced in my childhood, or will diminish my anxiety over wanting to improve myself by developing more self-confidence.

ELBOWS (in general) *See also: JOINTS*

The **elbows** represent freedom of movement, flexibility, the capacity to easily change directions in new situations or life experiences. They refer to ambition, possession, work and laziness. It is the supple and flexible arm joint that allows the creativity and the gracious expression of my everyday gestures, and makes it possible to move from a desire to its achievement. My **elbows** enable me to embrace new ideas, to draw guidance from outside of myself in order to choose the most appropriate directions for me. If my **elbows** are strong and flexible, I can accomplish great tasks. **Pain** or **rigidity** in an **elbow** means a lack of flexibility, the fear of feeling 'caught' or stuck in an unpleasant situation. As my **elbows** are related to action, I may be rigid and judge people who have a different way of doing things than mine and who can question my own habits. I need to be well-ordered, and when my routine is affected and 'disjointed', my **elbows** will react. I may fear being incompetent in a field that is important to me and therefore not being able to support my family. I resist taking a new direction by unconsciously blocking the energy of the **heart♥** that leads to this joint. I feel compelled to do things against my will and I '**elbow** my way'. I withdraw into myself because I distrust the world around me. I rest on my positions instead of opening up to new ideas. I cling to what I have because I am afraid of the new and the unknown. Even if I am sometimes afraid to let myself go, I feel myself being '**elbowed** ahead' by another person and I must 'hold in my **elbows**' to protect myself. Two healthy **elbows** allow me to hug someone in my arms.

I accept↓♥ to put in more energy doing everything I want, and I dare to express my emotions more. I then find it easier to accept↓♥ life and its many changes. I abandon myself more easily, and it takes care of me as I deserve. I remain open to **Love**, which helps me negotiate more easily my everyday experiences with no aggressiveness, but with flexibility and openness of mind. I accept↓♥ to draw from inside of me to find all the answers to my questions, and I accept↓♥ the new directions of my life as challenges to be taken up, knowing that the gifts are as great as the efforts expended.

ELBOWS — EPICONDYLITIS

Better known by the name of ***tennis-elbow*** in sports medicine, **epicondylitis** is an inflammation in the **elbow** joint.

My **elbows** give me the necessary flexibility for changes of direction. In the case of an inflammation, I must become **Aware** of why, or to what, I am opposing so much resistance. I may be developing frustration following repetitive events that occur in my life and I feel that I must constantly **cushion the blows**. I may have the impression that I am putting in more efforts than the others to accomplish certain tasks or produce certain results, and I am not receiving my due credit for it. I am very impulsive in my actions. I tend to forget the lessons learned in the past, and so I tend to make the same mistakes over again. **Epicondylitis** may be an indication that there is something I am not achieving, or something I am being forced to do but don't feel like doing. I am feeling great anger about a situation and I feel like punching someone, but am holding it back.

I accept↓♥ to let go of my old ideas and my old patterns to engage in the best direction for my development. I also accept↓♥ to allow **Love** to flow in the events that present themselves to me.

EMBOLISM *See: BLOOD / BLOOD CIRCULATION / COAGULATION*

EMBOLISM (arterial) *See: BLOOD — ARTERIES*

EMBOLISM (cerebral) *See: BRAIN DISORDERS*

EMBOLISM (pulmonary) *See: LUNG DISEASES*

EMOTIONALITY

Emotionality, or rather **hyperemotionality** is the fact that all my emotions are intensely experienced in a raw state. The slightest thing upsets me. When I am in this state, I feel paralyzed, my sight blurs and I can even lose my balance. I feel **insecurity**, **fear** and **anxiety**, I become mentally hyperactive and I tend to dramatize everything. I also tend to be less engaged in action, to accomplish tasks less, to carry out very few projects because fear paralyzes me. I become emotionally and physically fragile. I then reflexively isolate myself from the world to protect myself. The physical symptoms related to **hyperemotionality** are: accelerated heart♥beat, constricted throat, difficult digestion (even to the point of developing stomach ulcers), constipation, diarrhea and muscular stiffness. As I fear the unfamiliar, I therefore develop habits to diminish the anxiety linked to this unknown. Where does this agitation come from? It may result from an affective trauma, repeated conflicts, a usual mood of living based on insecurity (affective or material), etc.

I accept↓♥ to resume contact with my own essence and to consider my **emotionality** as a mode of communication with others. Meditation, relaxation or any other technique that can help me to calm down and bring me back to the **here and now** can help me to regain contact with my inner being and re-balance my emotions. This way, I can rediscover my true needs and learn to trust myself, for I know that everything that comes to me is perfectly suitable for my development.

EMPHYSEMA (pulmonary) *See: LUNGS — EMPHYSEMA [PULMONARY]*

EMPYEMA *See: ABSCESS*

ENCEPHALITIS *See: BRAIN — ENCEPHALITIS*

ENCEPHALOMYELITIS (fibromyalgic) *See: CHRONIC FATIGUE SYNDROME*

ENDOMETRIOSIS

Endometriosis is the formation of fragments of mucous tissues outside of the uterine wall.

It is related to an unconscious refusal of maternity. It often happens that the relationship I have, or had, with my mother or the heritage she left me (physical as well as emotional) is in conflict with what I am and the place I want to hold in this world. I don't know how to position myself before this ***lady*** who was so influential in my life. I am afraid that, by expressing myself, I might antagonize her. Is it possible that my parents loved each other but I deny this fact? If I come from a so-called 'broken' family, I may fear that the family I will offer my child won't be perfect, won't be good enough. It is as if this child's nest was somewhere else, and I can't suitably welcome it in my own home. Do I have any doubts about my couple? Am I afraid that I or my spouse may "go and see elsewhere"? Do my aspirations and my life as a couple make me fear that a child will change everything in my life? I doubt my capacity for being a good mother. Maybe I fear or sense that the ***home*** of this future child will be outside of my house. For example, if I know that my child will have to be cared for in a day-care center for most of the time, I may fear that my child will associate its real home with this place, or this person with whom it spends the greater part of its days. It may also happen that I don't accept↓♥ the world in which I live, or that I don't dare to be part of it. If I don't accept↓♥ this world, how can I bring another being into it? Yet, even before my birth, I chose to come into this world. I wonder why I have difficulty in accepting↓♥ myself as I am and channeling my creativity. I allow people to walk all over me and I swallow everything without saying a word. I feel I don't have the strength to stand up and assert myself, and I constantly experience failures. I become aggressive, for I know I am preventing myself from achieving things, because I have difficulty in ***focusing*** on my goals.

I accept↓♥ to become **Aware** of the relation between my fears, my doubts, my uncertainty and the situation I am experiencing, and I accept↓♥ to openly express what I feel. I assert myself as an individual. I recognize who I am and I no longer allow anyone to abuse me. Everyone will respect me, and I can thus flourish and let my creativity express itself.

ENTERITIS *See: INTESTINES — GASTROENTERITIS*

ENURESIS / BED-WETTING *See: BED-WETTING, INCONTINENCE (FECAL, URINARY)*

EPICONDYLITIS *See: ELBOWS — EPICONDYLITIS*

EPIDEMIC

An **epidemic** is the propagation of a contagious disease. Most often, it involves a disease of infectious origin.

It can be easy for me to think that if I contract the disease at the same time as many other persons, it is not because of the emotions I am experiencing but, rather, because "the **epidemic** spares nobody". In fact, the difference between the fact that I contract the disease alone or along with others is quite simply because there are several of us experiencing similar situations[2]. Similarly, I may experience insecurity personally and collectively concerning politics, the economy or the environment, as I may experience personal anger at the same time as other persons. The nature of the disease will indicate to me what I must become **Aware** of in my life.

I accept↓♥ to give **Love** to the part of me that is pressing for it in order to find more peace and harmony in my life.

EPIGLOTTIS *See also: THROAT / DISORDERS / LARYNX*

The epiglottis is a large piece of cartilage flattened in the form of a leaf, overhanging the glottis and located behind the root of the tongue. It protects the larynx and is free to swing upwards or downwards; it acts as a trap door that closes during swallowing, which allows food to enter the esophagus.

2. It is a group thought-form called EGREGORE; it can be negative or positive.

When the membrane becomes inflamed (**epiglottitis inflammation**) and swells (**swelling**), it secretes a great amount of mucus and choking may occur. It is important to rapidly clear the respiratory tract. I will find it difficult to swallow, there is something I am holding back, a situation I find difficult to swallow. When **epiglottitis** occurs, the fire of anger, or even accumulated rage, rises in me. I swallow and 'take it' without defending myself. There is a power struggle between two persons, often my parents, and it affects me. I hide my emotions, trailing my past experiences behind me.

I accept↓♥ to study myself and decode what I feel like expressing and "why I willingly shut my trap". I must reconsider my way of functioning, learn to clarify my thoughts and change my way of communicating. By choosing new directions in my life, I release my sorrow and negative thoughts, and at last I can focus my attention on more positive things.

EPILEPSY *See: BRAIN — EPILEPSY*

EPIPHYSIS *See: GLAND [PINEAL]*

EPISTAXIS / NOSEBLEED *See: NOSE BLEEDING*

ERECTION — ERECTILE DYSFUNCTION *See: IMPOTENCE*

ERUCTATION / BELCHING *See also: STOMACH (IN GENERAL)*

Eructation is a loud venting through the mouth of gas coming from the stomach.

Though it is considered to be very impolite according to our customs, Orientals see it as a sign of appreciation and thanks for an enjoyable meal. **Eructation** is related to my desire to go too fast. I don't take the time to interiorize and assimilate each step in a process, whether it is personal or work-related. This way, I avoid facing my fears. The tension rises because I have to digest new ideas, and I feel the need to relieve this tension. I am invaded by something or someone and the piece is too big for me to swallow all at once. A relationship is weighing heavily on me, and I feel that I am gasping for air and freedom. I am unconsciously pushing back or rejecting someone, especially if a bad odor is also present. I feel unstable and I am afraid of losing control. A **belch** can make me recall all these impressions, positive as well as negative, that are beyond me. I don't know how to integrate them in my life. If I go too fast and if I am anguished, the **belching** becomes more frequent and powerful.

I accept↓♥ to slow down and take the time required for my meals. I become **Aware** that by going too fast, I pass up so many beautiful things that make life pleasant. I accept↓♥ to take the time to live, I feel less out of breath in the hectic pace of life, and I feel all the better for it.

ERUPTION OF SPOTS *See: SKIN — ERUPTION OF PIMPLES*

ESOPHAGUS

The **esophagus** is the passageway for food on its way to be digested. It connects the pharynx to the stomach.

It makes it possible to let in new experiences, which provides me with an opening on the world and helps me develop. Generally, if I have emotions or ideas that 'go down the wrong way', the **esophagus** tenses and the passage is more difficult and can even provoke irritation, which manifests my inner irritation over something or someone I have difficulty tolerating. I show a lot of intransigence. There are things that don't suit me, but I am passive and I do nothing to change them. My apprehensions, my anxiety and my sorrow will make my **esophagus** contract, even to the point of completely **obstructing** the passageway. I compel myself to do things for others instead of doing what I really feel like doing. I let everything pass in order to avoid any confrontations. My emotions paralyze me and prevent me from 'swallowing' new experiences. There are some situations or ways of thinking that I force myself to swallow and accept↓♥ as being part of me, but I know that deep down inside of me, I don't want them to be incorporated in me or in my life. I may '***swallow the wrong way***' because I fear outside authority or because "the pill just won't pass". I prevent myself from moving forward and growing. Maybe I want to swallow too fast out of gluttony, for fear of lacking **Love** and affection later on. I prefer 'shutting my **trap**'. I have the impression that I depend on someone else to 'put bread on the table[3]'. I am too attached to the past. I thus take a limp, passive attitude. As the **esophagus** is the passageway from my mouth, which represents the entry of new ideas, to my stomach, where I must digest them, if I feel strong anger or hate about something in my life that 'just won't pass', I may develop a **cancer of the esophagus**. It happens when I am experiencing a situation from which I see no way out; whatever happens in my life, I tell myself that there is no longer anything that could happen that could enable me to ever find hope again. **The lower part of the esophagus** refers to my desire to take and swallow everything and waste nothing. I "bite off more than I can chew". I am afraid someone will steal something that belongs to me and at the same time, I have difficulty in really enjoying what I do have. **The upper part of the esophagus** throws **Light** on a situation that I refuse to 'swallow' even if I am forced to. Something or someone is "going down my throat the wrong way".

I accept↓♥ to let go of any bitterness and to see each experience in my life as an opportunity to grow, so that the joys of life will nourish me. I accept↓♥ to be a pioneer, a leader! I am engaged in action: I seek new opportunities for flourishing. By forgiving any act or word that injured me, I release these dark clouds that floated above my head and prevented me from moving forward. I open myself to the lessons that life will show me and I thus gain greater freedom and inner peace.

3. **To put bread on the table**: To earn my living, to earn money in order to provide for my needs.

EUTHANASIA *See also: DEATH*

Euthanasia is not an illness, but an act by which someone wants to spare an incurably sick person from suffering pain judged to be intolerable.

This act thus makes possible a departure, a death without suffering. I may experience a moral malaise if I am in the position of having to decide for another person whether that person's days should be shortened. It is important that I remain anchored in my conviction that life exists even beyond what is called death, if this is part of my beliefs. If such is not the case, I can ask myself if the person who is before me is truly manifesting life. I become **Conscious** of the fact that this is part of an individual choice. I can inform my close relatives, verbally or in writing, of the decision they may have to make for me in the event that I am not conscious.

I accept↓♥ to express my will or my wishes, in the hope that this will facilitate the decision-making of others as the case may be, and they will be more in harmony with the choices to be made.

EWING'S SARCOMA *See: BONE [CANCER OF THE] — EWING'S SARCOMA*

EXCESSIVE APPETITE *See: APPETITE [EXCESS]*

EXCESSIVE WEIGHT *See: WEIGHT [EXCESS]*

EXHAUSTION *See: BURNOUT*

EXHIBITIONISM

Exhibitionism involves the exhibition of the genital organs.

Exhibitionism is directly related to the education I received and to the way I live **sexuality**. Indeed, if I was taught that sexuality was bestial, dirty and degrading, I surely tried to repress it and, if I didn't do so, I act according to what I learned. Thus, I feel the need to free myself of this constraint I am experiencing regarding my sexuality. The fact that I devote myself to **exhibitionism** is for me a way to push back my own limits to make myself accepted↓♥, a way of provoking. As I am not in contact with my inner self, **Love** appears to be something that is not for me. I can't enter into an intimate relationship with someone because I am afraid of being hurt. I prefer to 'have' experiences with certain persons, but with a distance separating us. I can thus run away when I want. I seek excitement outside of myself because I feel empty inside. **Exhibiting** myself gives me a certain power. My impulses and unconscious desires control me. I may be unconsciously seeking revenge against someone who did me wrong when I was younger. I feel sexually powerless and unrecognized. I become **Aware** that humans were created with sexual needs, but that these must be experienced in **Love**.

I accept↓♥ that sexuality is something beautiful and healthy, in which I can flourish. Sexuality is also part of my physical development. I accept↓♥ to open myself to **Love** with a capital 'L'. By respecting myself, I gain the necessary strength that enables me to express my vulnerability. By daring to be true, others will follow suit and a beautiful relationship of coziness and sharing can take form.

EXOPHTALMOS *See: EYE DISEASES*

EXPOSURE TO COLD *See: COLD [EXPOSURE TO]*

EYE BALL *See: EYES (IN GENERAL)*

EYELIDS (in general) *See also: FACIAL FEATURES [SAGGING]*

My **eyelids** cover and protect my eyes.

Swollen, irritated or baggy **eyelids** are the sign that I am experiencing sadness that may be due to a situation such that there is a person I won't be seeing again, and that expresses itself by tears, but I want to hold it in and keep my pain inside of me. "I close my eyes on obvious facts that are difficult for me to admit". I am experiencing a separation from someone, but it could also be from my country. I must deliberately close my eyes when I want to rest or sleep. But if my **eyelids** are **permanently half-closed**, there is something or someone in my life that I want to flee or that I don't have the courage to look at straight on. It may be someone or something I mustn't see. I refuse the look and the judgment of others because it is easier for me to denigrate and reject who I am. I am on the defensive and I feel pressured. If I also experience great tension, my **eyelids** tend to blink more rapidly. **Drooping eyelids (ptosis)** indicate deep sadness and resignation over events that I no longer want to see. It is as though the curtain were falling on a part of my life. What I see is far from my ideal. I witnessed an event ***worse*** than anything I'd ever seen before. **In a woman**, this manifests itself most often in the left eye and reveals a matrimonial situation where there is a deadlock and great disappointment. When the **eyelids** (most often the lower **eyelid**) turn **outward** (**ectropion**), I am feeling great insecurity: because my life is all confused, I am anguished by the unknown and by death. If the **eyelids** turn **inward** (**entropion**), I am not receiving the attention and tenderness that I need from others. **Blepharitis** (inflammation) expresses my duality between telling the truth or 'closing my eyes' and remaining silent. I can also try to hide my tears.

I accept↓♥ to see that I close my eyes to better center and interiorize myself, but it is also important for me to open them wide to see all the beauties of the Universe and see all the possibilities that present themselves to me.

EYELIDS (blinking)

My **eyelids** tend to blink faster when I am experiencing stress or tension greater than usual. I am over-excited about what I am seeing. Is there a situation in my life that I'd rather not see?

I accept↓♥ the moments of calm and relaxation in my life and I learn to 'see' the positive side of everything.

EYE(S) (in general)

My **eyes** are the mirrors of my **Soul**. They enable me to see outside and, through them, I express all the emotions and feelings that I experience inside of me. According to their depth, it is possible to discover my relations with the outside world. The functioning of **my eyes** reflects the way I see life and my relation with it. They also represent the fact of seeing clearly in my own life and inside of me. They reflect the look I cast on things. They indicate how information external to me is transmitted inside of me. If there is any interference, rejection or resistance in relation to the information in contact with my **eyes**, the latter react strongly. If I have difficulty seeing clearly in a situation or if the truth seems hidden, my **eyes** cloud up. If I have difficulty with what I am seeing, my understanding is poor and my **eyes** react. My **eyes** are affected if I experience any special difficulty in dealing with the truth, reality or the future. Each **eye** represents a special aspect of my being. The **left eye** represents the inner emotional and intuitive aspect, my feminine side and the relation with my mother. It acts as my lookout, enabling me to keep watching out for anything that might constitute a danger and to react promptly. A difficulty in my **left eye** shows how attached I am to something or someone. I feel distrust toward who I really am, and I may want to hide or veil what I see. I want to feel safe and I prefer to rely on others. I am emotionally dependent. I feel that I can't control my emotions, which ask only to show themselves! The **right eye** deals rationally with the world and outside situations. It is the **eye** of recognition that enables me to fashion my identity. It refers to my masculine side and the relation with my father. If my **right eye** is afflicted with a certain ailment, this indicates that I must firmly anchor my roots and make contact with my own authority. I must be my own pillar. I no longer have to cling to someone and feel helpless. I find a way to take on my responsibilities and effect control over the direction of my life. Lying clouds up my **eye**. **Eye problems** are an indication that there exist some things that I refuse to see and that often bring into question my fundamental principles and my notions of justice. It is very important to mention that the quality of the images that the retina sends to the brain depends on the way my nervous system reacts to the images that are sent by those nervous impulses: in addition to what I see physically and is real, there is also all the 'coloration' with which I infuse each image on the basis of all my past experiences and all my emotional baggage, personal as well as family or social. In addition to my **eyesight** as a sense involved, there is another sense that is intimately related to it, which is my inner **perception**. I may develop an **ailment in the eyes** without having the **impression** that I saw or experienced any great traumas or stressful situations. It is more a matter of **seeing** how much I accepted↓♥ a situation that I saw, outwardly as well as inwardly: the stress experienced is therefore more related to the emotion I feel about what I see than to the event itself.

I accept↓♥ to live in laughter and joy. I reinforce my structures by trusting my inner wisdom. Opening my third **eye** (chakra) enables me to have an accurate vision of myself, things, people and situations and leads me to discernment. By turning my look deep inside myself before directing it at the outer world, I thus find a new overall view and a new insight on the road of my existence. My gaze is true and without judgment.

EYE DISEASES

Eye diseases, including blindness, are a way for me to close myself off from what I see. I choose to ignore what is going on around me and I renounce the visual impressions that impugn me. Rather than accept↓♥ a reality that could prove painful, repugnant or confused, I prefer to **close my eyes**. I deform my perception of people to help me face my everyday reality. For instance, I may want "to see my children grow up in my mind's **eye**" and, in my head, I imagine them staying young. I prefer to ***glance at*** things rather than to see everything clearly, for that might be very disturbing. There may be an undisclosed secret or my mother's silence about a situation that affects me, even unconsciously. I consciously decide to 'close my **eyes**'. I have a difficulty in locating a danger that I dread. **Blindness** may be caused by diabetes (*see* this disease) or by an accumulation of things I refuse to accept↓♥, inducing confusion and a feeling of no longer knowing where to go. Often injured by shocks, traumas or a great inner fear, my eyesight withdraws and so does the energy of my visual organs too. I thus keep in the dark the memories, the recollections and the past emotions that I prefer to hide. It may also involve the fear of losing someone or something that is dear to me. I am ***frightened*** and I prefer to not see what is in store for me. Still, the outer darkness generally seems to provide an inner openness, a private world, secret and colorful. I therefore open myself up more to my inner spirit. I may damage my **eyes** by my own negative attitude. If I use them to abuse others, to manipulate or seduce for selfish reasons and to control others, my **eyes** let this reality show through, and they become darker and bleary. **Red eyes** express my inner fatigue from struggling against my emotions that I repress. My **eyes prickle** when I am annoyed by what I see and what I experience. My **eyes** are constantly searching for things or persons that I want to 'acquire'. **Dry eyes** indicate to me that I am experiencing a situation where I am losing, or have *lost* my dignity and I want to stay impassive. It is as if my **eyes** congealed, preventing their lubrication. I hold back from crying in front of people. **Baggy eyes** indicate that I am in a situation where I either caught someone red-handed or I was so caught myself, unless I am afraid of something bursting out into the open. It may involve secret acts or thoughts that I don't want to see revealed. A **deformation of the eye** (astigmatism, myopia, presbyopia) indicates that I am trying too much to find answers outwardly, rather than within myself. The more I seek outside of myself, the more I move away from my inner core. **Veiled vision** (cataract, glaucoma) denotes that my version of reality is contrary to the one I see. This tells me that I find it difficult to concentrate on the main things and that I refuse what I see. My look is ***furtive***, to avoid being noticed or simply to not clearly see everything that goes on around me. I become **Aware** of the fact that if I need **eyeglasses** to correct my eyesight, they will give me a way to protect myself from outside attacks. While preventing intruders from entering my world, I can also hide behind my **eyeglasses**, thereby not having to display my 'true colors'. If I develop **an excessive sensitivity to Light**, I see my life all in black and see only the dark part of my being. A '**black eye**' is the externalization of my inner violence. My negative attitude attracted someone or something to strike me as I would have felt like doing myself. If my **eye balls come out of their orbits** (**exophtalmos**), I am constantly on the lookout. There is a distortion between what I see and reality, which causes me enormous stress. Sensing myself in danger with a tendency to paranoia, my eye balls are pressed out forward to better see what is around me.

I accept↓♥ the beauty that is around me and I give myself time to look around. I focus my **eyes** on what is beautiful around me and within me.

EYE DISORDERS (in children)

An **eye problem** in a **young child** allows one to predict stress in the family and a refusal to see what is going on there. I see or feel all my parents' sadness and pain, and I prefer to hide my **eyes** to not see it. When it develops at school, it shows that I am experiencing anxiety about the unknown and I don't know what road to take. I want to escape from the world that surrounds me. An **eye problem** that occurs in adolescence may denote a fear of sexuality. It is important for me as a parent to bring my child to communicate her fears in order to reassure her and help her to overcome them.

EYES — ASTIGMATISM

Astigmatism is a defect in the sphericity[4] of the cornea or the lens. The vertical curvature of the cornea is more pronounced than its horizontal curvature, or vice versa. It is as if I was looking through a deforming mirror.

This malformation generally denotes a fear of looking at myself in the face, as I am. **Bad eye coordination** can mean that my way of acting and my thoughts are in disagreement with my entourage, thus causing inner conflicts. I want to create a different reality for myself and try to free myself from the influence of my parents or of other persons I consider abusive. Often confronted with rage, anger or fears during my youth, **my eyes** have kept this expression of **fright** and the muscles surrounding the **eye** have remained in a constant state of shock. My **eyes** become irritated if what I see outwardly or inwardly irritates me. My definition of an ideal world is very far from the reality, and I prefer not to see and know all the details. For example, if I idealized my father and then realize that the reality is quite different, I refuse to look like him. I then have an attitude of "I will organize myself all alone". I feel ***contempt*** for myself and others. I easily ***label*** people. This makes my relations with others difficult, especially with my partner because I remain aloof from him. I feel ***scorned*** but

---

4. **Sphericity**: A characteristic related to 3-dimensional curvature.

I want to keep everything to myself, not letting my inner suffering show. I prefer to endure it, but this is very difficult and I must deform reality for it to be tolerable. I want to remain silent about my emotional scars. **Astigmatism** also results from great curiosity. My insatiable need to see everything has 'worn out' **my eyes**. My body thus tells me to take the time I need to appreciate things. It can also mean I should recognize my own beauty, the magnificent being that I am.

I accept↓♥ the fact that I am capable of fully standing by who I am and being in contact with my deeper feelings. I accept↓♥ **Love** by being open with myself and I manifest this **Love** to others. I ask to see the truth by being able to receive in an ordered way the messages given by my inner voice. I can thus take stock of my life in an enlightened fashion.

EYES — BLIND

I am considered to be **blind** if I have 10% vision or less.

If I experience this situation, I ask myself what I don't want to see or what I am afraid of seeing in my life, whether it is a person or a situation. I want to protect myself by curling up in my world, which I can create to suit myself: I thus feel safer, and my new reality is far more pleasant than anything I could see in real life. That helps me to deal with this danger that I sense constantly behind me and want to get rid of. If it happened to me after an accident or an illness, I search for the cause that could be linked to this loss of vision. I then work to integrate this cause into the state of **Awareness** I must achieve and I accept↓♥ to 'see' again, by allowing my inner vision to develop more and more in **Love** and understanding. If I have been **blind since birth**, I ask myself just how afraid I was of the outer world, even at a very early age, as if I was in danger and the only way for me to feel safe was to cut myself off from the world. Did I really want **to be born**? Did they want to hide me, even when I was in my mother's womb? The fact of not seeing around me dispenses me from comparing myself with others. If I feel ugly or limited, I don't have to constantly face it. It is sometimes easier to not see human misery than to face it. It is the reflection of my inner poverty and by accepting↓♥ to focus my attention solely on the treasures inside of me, my **eyesight** improves and I am then capable of seeing the beauty in everything. At whatever age I became totally or partially **blind**, there is a refusal to be born, first to myself, but also to the world around me. I want to close my **eyes** to memories that hurt me, especially if I am an orphan and my parents never saw me or looked at me. I am dependent upon a person because of my special situation. I curtail my own freedom. I conform to the outer world whereas I could live according to my personal needs and my deeper truth. I may possibly recover my **eyesight** completely: I must accept↓♥ who I am but also the world that surrounds me, with all its beauties but also all the negativity and the inequalities that exist.

I accept↓♥ **here and now** to face all my fears, but also all my potential. I accept↓♥ to cast away my role as a victim and I accept↓♥ to become the creator of my life. I look myself in the **eye**, as I am. I accept↓♥ to be born to myself and not for others. By becoming master of my life and accepting↓♥ that the world is as it is and that the only power I have is over myself, the outer and inner realities will be clear, and I may recover my **eyesight**. And the person to congratulate is me!

EYES — BLINDNESS

By refusing to **open my eyes** and see the outer world, I have no other choice but to look inside of me and become **Aware** of my inner Universe. "Is there a person in my life that I allow to **blind** me to the point of no longer trusting myself?" What is clouding my judgment?

I accept↓♥ to see the wealth that inhabits me and the **Light** that is in me.

EYES — CATARACTS

A **cataract** is a disease where the lens (the **eye**'s biconvex lens) gradually becomes opaque to the point where eyesight becomes clouded and deformed, resulting in blindness sooner or later.

This form of physical disability occurs in my life at a time when I no longer want to see what is going on under my **eyes**, what is going to happen, or what risks influencing my life and the decisions I may have to take. What I have seen or what I expect in the future leads me to say: "I don't believe my **eyes**!" "I wish so much that things would remain as they are now!" My eyesight is declining because the energy no longer goes there. It becomes dull and darkens, and I view the future with a dark and veiled **eye**, with no joy or **heart♥**iness. I may possibly have an egocentric attitude and I want to see life only my way, without taking into account the realities of others. This is a selfish attitude that may even make me believe that I am superior to others. I refuse to see certain events or individuals transparently. This **cataract** moves me away from the present and removes me from the world around me. This displeases me on certain levels, and I must become **Aware** of the outer and inner aspects of things. I see the world around me as a threat. A constant danger is present. I feel isolated, alone in my corner. I need the others, I would like to be able to experience my emotions in the presence of others, but I am afraid of their reaction. By 'veiling' their faces, I distance myself and I thereby feel more protected. It is interesting to note that a **cataract** is an opaque membrane that prevents **Light** rays from reaching my retina. As the sun symbolizes the father, I can ask myself if I am afraid of him and feel a need to protect myself. Or do I fear the gaze of the heavenly Father, God, He who will pronounce the Last Judgment? **Cataracts** usually appear toward the end of the life cycle, at a time when the fear of aging and becoming disabled or impotent sets in. I have the impression that doors are closing before me. I use the **cataract** as protection, because "I don't want to see the future image of myself even if it is not here yet, for fear of finding it too unpleasant". I refuse to see what is happening or will happen and, because it seems unavoidable, I want to slow down, or prevent, the event or the 'aggression' from getting closer to me. If I have children, I find them 'ungrateful' about a situation. Being rigid prevents me from seeing 'the reverse side of the medal'. By no longer being able to see what is happening today, I force myself to remember the past, which I consider to be 'the good old days' and don't want to lose. I lose my flexibility of mind and action, I become less tolerant and I often forget events that have just happened to me. I therefore have no interest in seeing the future, which can appear very gloomy (**cataracts** are frequent in the developing countries). I no longer can use my imagination to envision my future. It is as though my **eyes** were constantly full of emotions, which cloud my vision. However, I can raise this curtain that prevents me from seeing my true reality by concentrating my attention on my inner **Light**. This is especially true if I am younger and have **cataracts**: for then I must decide that life will provide me with everything I need, physically and emotionally as well as spiritually.

I accept↓♥ to make the effort to look inside of me, and I see all the **Light** and beauty around me. I leap into life!

EYES — CONJUNCTIVITIS

Conjunctivitis is an inflammation of the transparent membrane covering the inside of the eyelid and of the **eye** ball. There is a direct relation between **conjunctivitis** and what I see. Unconsciously, **I refuse to see a situation or an event** with which I disagree or that hurts me. My way of seeing is painful because I refuse to have a new understanding of a situation or the viewpoints of others. I am incapable of putting myself in the other person's place, hence an impossibility of forgiveness. This leads me to experience frustration, irritation and revolt. "I can't stand what I am seeing! It burns me to see such a thing!" It is as if my **eyes** were always trying to wash out the **dirt** I see in the situation that makes me **angry**. It may be something despicable and I absolutely must 'whitewash the family' from any judgment or scandal. The result causes swelling and mental numbness as well as an emotional overflow similar to the action of crying. Life, joy and enthusiasm are absent in me. My memories hurt me, and I escape into an unreal world of romantic dreams. I resist life, and reality is intolerable for me. My sadness and despair regularly make me think about death, because I want my pain to end. I prefer to be temporarily blind, because what I see makes me suffer. I want to get rid of the link that exists in the look that the other directs at me. I am experiencing a situation with a person and I would like to use my gaze to initiate a relation with that person. A situation with my spouse, likely to lead to a separation, can bring about the onset of **conjunctivitis**.

I take the time to stop and **accept↓♥ to see this situation that bothers me and I ask myself why it bothers me so**. I give myself permission to cry, and thus externalize my sorrow and my despair. I remain open and receptive: I thus avoid experiencing **conjunctivitis** again. I resume contact with my reality. I let go of the past. I take charge of my life. I accept↓♥ my sorrow so that it can transform itself into inner peace. I am thereby **Aware** of all the possibilities available to me, and I now create my life as I desire.

EYES — DALTONISM / COLOR BLINDNESS

To be **color blind** is to see the world without its **colors**, grayish and undifferentiated. It may also be a case of certain specific **colors** that I am unable to see, or a visual confusion between certain specific **colors** (most often red and green).

I must therefore ask myself in what situation of my life I experienced an enormous stress linked to this, or these, **color**(s) that I can't distinguish. For example, if I can't see red, I may have narrowly escaped death, as a youngster, when a red train was coming my way. As red is now associated with a high level of stress and symbolizes the threat of death, then unconsciously I will no longer want to see that color. If it is the full **color** spectrum that I can't distinguish, the same principle can apply. There is often a lot of violence in my life, I was treated very roughly when I was younger, and I want to cut myself off from the world, for I no longer trust anyone else. My life structures are not in harmony with my values. I may also have decided one day to stop ambitiously 'dreaming in **color'** in order to avoid being disappointed and seeing life only in shades of ***gray***. As our dreams of today create the realities of tomorrow, I will stop seeing **colors** in my everyday life. I choose my **colors** right now, and decide to make place for my imagination. I imagine pink, green or blue. As an artist, I choose my mix of **colors**. I immerse myself in this unity that the world offers me. I give free rein to my fantasy and express my joy in living in countless ways.

I accept↓♥ the fact that I have power only over myself, and I broaden my horizons in order to have a new vision of things. This enables me to see my life in a new **Light**, including the lessons that I have to learn.

EYES — DEGENERATION (macular) of the RETINA

Macular degeneration is the most frequent and most serious form of **degeneration of the retina**. It consists in a progressive destruction of the **macula** (the central zone of the retina where visual acuity is at its maximum). It is more frequent in persons above age 70.

I am faced with situations where there is a point of no return. This is often the case when I see a loved one transcend their physical body. I feel helpless about my pain, for I have no power over death, whether it is mine or that of others. This vision that I find difficult to tolerate leads me to disconnect myself from the world, for I no longer want to see it. I even ask myself what I am still doing here.

I accept↓♥ to still have a role to play on this earth. By my presence, I manifest **Light** and **Love**, which radiate over my entourage, especially the people I **love**. I decide to realize my dreams, thus allowing life to flow in me. My body, especially my **eyes**, regenerates itself and I have all the energy necessary to live my life to the full!

EYES — DETACHMENT of the RETINA

The **detachment of the retina** is an affection of the **eye** caused by the separation of the **retina** from the underlying layer as a result of the passage of vitreous liquid behind the **retina**.

A **detachment of the retina** follows from a situation where I saw something happen in front of me that provoked an enormous stress or even a shock, which I hold in, even unconsciously. I have the impression that this image of an event that I found horrible and ***appalling*** will **stay impregnated in my memory for all my life**! I was unable to 'detach my **eyes**' from the person or the situation. The first great stress in the **eyes** often occurs when I am a young child, for I don't yet have the reflex, as an adult has, to protect my **eyes** when I see something traumatizing. My **eyes** instead are riveted or '**stuck**' to what is going on before me. Later on, any great stress in the **eyes** may transform itself into a **detachment of the retina**. What has imprinted itself in me can no longer '**detach**' itself. I can also ask myself if I desire, in a sense, to separate myself from the world in which I live. I have lost trust in life in general and I no longer feel like involving myself because I distrust everything. I turn down the people around me because I no longer want to suffer. I no longer want to 'touch others with my look'. I distrust others. The wrong that was done to me makes me retreat into myself. My sad memories follow me everywhere. I feel cut off from the **Light**. I must face this image instead of wanting to hide it at the bottom of a chest or denying it. I can ask a therapist to help me find out why I had to see that troubling event and identify the life lesson that I must draw from it. Once I have experienced this process, I will avoid any other situations where I might develop another **detachment of the retina**.

I accept↓♥ that I may have created my life with my negative thoughts toward myself and others. I accept↓♥ to resume contact with my dreams and aspirations. I accept↓♥ to get closer to people and share my experiences from the **heart♥**. By being closer to my emotions, I get closer to my divine essence and my **eyes** can thus begin a process of healing.

EYES (dry) *See: EYE DISEASES*

EYES — GLAUCOMA

Glaucoma involves a blocking of the **eye**'s drainage canal, thereby preventing the inner fluid from being released and causing a build-up of internal pressure.

This liquid represents all the tears that should have flowed throughout my whole life and which, having accumulated, bring increased pressure to bear on the retina, thus causing my eyesight to deteriorate. It affects more frequently people over age 60, who often feel that they **have seen enough**. It may be the sign of old resentments and a refusal to forgive. I may feel overwhelmed and **submerged** by life and I fear the future. As I feel easily fatigued, life becomes different and more difficult to accept↓♥ emotionally. I refuse to see myself get older; I can't see any images of the future, and that suits me perfectly. As an **eye** affected by **glaucoma** reacts like a magnifying glass, there is something or someone in my life that I want to get closer to as fast as possible, **toward** whom I want to move. It may be in terms of time or space. It is as if I was late. The goal is so close, but I sense a danger pursuing me. **Glaucoma** compels me to look only forward, and not laterally, as if I was wearing horse blinders. I have the impression that I missed or passed up certain things in my life and I feel resentful about them. It is as if opportunities are slipping through my fingers just when I am about to obtain or accomplish something. I feel myself as in a tunnel, with life passing through at full speed: there are so many things going on inside and outside of me that I feel in a sort of vacuum; my previously familiar points of reference are changing, and I am very sad about losing what I wanted so much to keep. My life is ***gloomy***, full of melancholy and misery. "What does the future hold in store for me? Do I really want to know anyway?" I don't see any possibilities, or any way out, for me to be able to make my life a success. Opportunities present themselves to me but I constantly **bungle** them, and I restrain my freedom. I would want so much to hold on to my past and for things to remain as they were. I feel extreme tension and I feel I am going to crack!

I accept↓♥ to remove the veil and to see with **Love** and tenderness. I stop clinging to others and live the present moment intensely. I forgive, and I accept↓♥ to see life more tolerantly.

EYES: HYPERMETROPIA and PRESBYOPIA (farsightedness)

In the case of **hypermetropia** and **presbyopia**, near vision is hampered. **Hypermetropia** is more frequent among young children and is due to an anomaly of ocular refraction. In the case of **presbyopia**, there is a progressive decrease of ocular accommodation, which generally affects persons beyond the age of 40.

Both denote a fear of the present. What is it in my life, close to me, that I refuse to see? It may involve my incapacity to focus and see clearly what is accessible and close to me. I allow myself to be more interested by others, by my personal relations and by outside events, rather than look inside of myself and increasingly develop my inner self. This condition may have been caused by a shock or a trauma that made me believe that this present was not for me. By becoming extraverted and looking far away, I choose to ignore what is going on closer to me, and my dreams are turned toward the future. My **eyes** become like a lookout who constantly watches from afar what in going on. I can take a step back from certain aspects of my current life and I therefore peer far into the distance to see what the future has in store for me. I have difficulty in being close and intimate with the people around me. I flee who I really am. I don't even dare look at myself in the face. I don't like what I see and I avoid being too closely concerned with upsetting situations. There is something that escapes me. I want to foresee everything ahead of time. Even the roof under which I live seems dangerous. With respect to **presbyopia** more especially, I feel concerned because what I am currently seeing makes me worried: I am getting older, the children are leaving home and I am becoming sadder. I am more sensitive to gossip and criticism. My eyesight thus transforms itself according to what I want, and don't want, to see. I stand back to take a more detached view of things, and I therefore move away from my current life. I am more **conscious** of death and I feel vulnerable about what is to come for me and my family. This death may be symbolic of the moment when I go into retirement. I must prepare myself and have projects, and I ask myself if I will have sufficient financial resources to do everything. **Presbyopia** may appear earlier in life if I had to face death at an early age. I already feel 'old' despite my young age. I have the impression that I have been through so many ordeals in my life that it is as if I have led two lives at once. My body feels worn out and bruised. If only one of my two **eyes** is affected, it is important for me to consider the situations related to the side of the body that is affected (left: intuitive; right: rational). I accept↓♥ to see life today with all its manifestations of beauty, and I know that I am safe, **HERE AND NOW.**

I accept↓♥ to look straight on at my emotional world and the situations in which I find myself and am uncomfortable in. I look at my anxieties and my insecurities. It is only by accepting↓♥ to look at the present that I can create the future, for I must become **Aware** of what I want to change and apply all my energy to create a new world adjusted to my needs. I accept↓♥ to listen to my inner wisdom that speaks through my intuition.

EYES — KERATITIS *See also: INFLAMMATION, ULCER*

Keratitis is a severely painful corneal inflammation that can form into ulcers.

It happens when I feel sad and helpless about something or someone I see that makes me angry. It affects me so much that I could even strike a person physically or, symbolically, I could wish "a calamity to hit the persons or the situations concerned" for me to feel some satisfaction. It may derive from my jealousy. It may also be because I want to quickly hide myself from something or someone to avoid being seen, or to hide something other than myself. I may find myself in a situation where I lose visual contact with a person, and a contact with something or someone else is imposed on me. As the **cornea** is the 'glass' of the **eye**, I must make it opaque so that it will be replaced by a protective 'wall'.

I accept↓♥ that my body is simply telling me that **I must learn to look at life with other eyes, with a new attitude of openness and understanding**. I can see things that don't suit me, that don't agree with me, and I must detach myself from what I see. I must learn to let go of the control I want to have over the things, the persons or the situations around me over which I have no power.

EYES — MYOPIA

Myopia makes my far vision difficult.

My insecurity about the future makes me see events as greater, or more worrisome, than they actually are. It seems that I am not ready to face them.

I see what is close to me, but my far vision is blurred because of contracted and tense ocular muscles. A ***fog*** is preventing me from seeing the danger in the distance. I can deal with my life on a day-to-day basis quite easily. On the other hand, I find it difficult to create my own vision of the future and see the possibilities before me, or face my fears and insecurities and move beyond them. Or I may be deeply disturbed by a ***mystery*** that may never be resolved, for which I may never find the solution. My inner perception of the truth is ***blurred***. There is a distortion between what I feel and what I see. The fact that I see quite well from up close underlies a difficulty in finding my maneuvering space in some situations. I find myself in situations where I come very close to being involved, for instance, in a car accident. If I am **myopic**, I tend to be shy and introverted, which may result from childhood incidents that I experienced as terrifying or abusive (such as the hostile or enraged look of a parent). For example, if a teacher or an uncle used to beat me, I became **myopic** because I was afraid of him and didn't want to see him because as soon as I saw him, I would become all nervous and worried, knowing what was in store for me. I felt that I was being ***hounded*** and I wished it would stop. I felt the ***necessity*** of protecting my world with **myopia**, somewhat as in autism. Usually, unless I have experienced another conflict, my near vision will be better than average because I know, even unconsciously, that it is important for me to see clearly what is happening close to me in order to be able to defend myself or take the right actions once this threat is close to me, so that it won't hurt me. **Myopia** generally indicates an excessive subjectivity. The expression "to not see beyond the end of one's nose" aptly describes this state of being. I may also not want to see far away, out of weariness or laziness or life's disappointments. "I don't believe my **eyes**" aptly illustrates how I feel. Indulging in self-pity is sometimes easier than doing something. Is my spouse spending much time abroad? I may ask myself if the saying "Out of **sight**, out of **mind**" applies to my situation. Or maybe I miss my father's presence. I have great misgivings about outside reality and about my future because I don't see my own inner strength and wisdom. As I feel hurt by others, I no longer feel like interacting with them. I feel powerless and unsupported, and this prevents me from moving forward.

Accepting↓♥ to see the outside world enables me to learn about myself. My vision broadens by developing my inner space. I choose new roads and I trust myself. I accept↓♥ that each person is responsible for their own life and that, by envisioning the future in beautiful and positive terms, that is exactly what will manifest itself in my life.

EYES — NYSTAGMUS

Nystagmus is a series of rapid, jerky, involuntary movements of the **eye** balls, often symptomatic of an affection of the nerve center. If my **eyes** suffer from **nystagmus**, it means that they are constantly in a scanning movement.

I must ask myself when the **nystagmus** appeared in my life. This will usually coincide with a period when I was experiencing a situation in which a danger existed and I searched endlessly, 'scanning' all the possibilities available for me to be able to get out of it. I have the impression that I can make good only by constantly monitoring my environment in search of elements that will make me appreciate life. I don't know where to point my **eyes**. It is important for me to trace back this event in order to become **Aware** of the source of this disease and thereby heal it. I also sense that there are images constantly streaming past, even in my head, and this makes me dizzy. I feel like closing my **eyes** for it all to stop.

I accept↓♥ to be **Aware** that, while the danger to me was real in the past, it no longer exists, and I am constantly guided and protected.

EYES — PTERYGIUM

Pterygium is a thickening of the conjunctiva, triangular in form, extending from the cornea to the inner angle of the **eye**.

If I have **pterygium**, I feel exposed to the storms of life and vulnerable to everything that surrounds me; nobody protects me from what I see. I get along badly with the outside world because my child's **heart♥** doesn't know how to react and protect itself from all these assaults. I feel unable to face what I see, and some things in my entourage elude me.

I accept↓♥ to make contact with my inner power. I watch what goes on around me without passing judgment. I become **Aware** of the fact that what bothers me or saddens me leads me back to my own inner injuries. I can be the master of my own life only, and I know that each individual possesses this same power; it is a matter of accepting↓♥ it.

EYES — PUPILS

The **pupil** is the central opening of the iris, through which **Light** rays pass. It doses the quantity of **Light** that enters the eye. **Mydriasis** is an abnormal dilation of the **pupil** with an immobilization of the iris.

When this problem occurs, I ask myself what is fundamental for me; I can't grasp the center of my life. What is the meaning of my life, the goals I want to reach? I can't see this, because I am looking outside for answers I can only find inside of me, in my center, in the **heart♥** of my **heart♥**. A **pupil that is too dilated** (**uveitis**) indicates a situation that must be urgently resolved (see also: Inflammation). If there is a **difference in size between the two pupils** (**anisocoria**), there is a situation or an aspect, a facet of my life that I can't tolerate to see. Things are not clear, everything is dark. I can no longer stand the images reflected in my **eyes**. I feel alone like an orphan who has no dad or mom to turn to for help and protection. There is a duality deep inside of me. I try to stay balanced despite my great pervading pain.

I accept↓♥ to throw **Light** on unclear situations and I take the time to think about what I need to clarify. I listen to my inner voice and I adjust situations according to my own needs. This way, I can see the **Light** at the end of the tunnel and move ahead in life with confidence and determination.

EYES — RETINITIS PIGMENTOSA / RETINOPATHY (primary pigmentary)

Retinitis pigmentosa, also called **primary pigmentary retinopathy**, is considered to be a hereditary disease that causes the **Light** receiving visual cells to degenerate. It usually affects children. The **eye** cannot adapt to darkness and the visual field diminishes as time goes by. I therefore no longer see the **Light**.

This disease develops if I am **ashamed** of myself, of who I am, physically as well as intellectually. I feel ***ridiculous***. It is as if I was never born, part of me is **on standby**. This shame may also result from a situation that I witnessed and that I find despicable. My vision as a child was soiled. This mustn't be known or seen! It must remain in the dark. I want to resist this horrible vision of calamity. I want others to look anywhere else but at me. I may be a perfectionist, and the fact of 'seeing far and wide' before me causes me to feel great stress. I may be afraid of not overcoming everything life has in store for me, or I refuse to see myself getting older because death scares me. A situation where I endured abandonment has the result of removing me from someone I **love** and whom I no longer can see as before.

My body responds to this stress by diminishing my visual field, hoping to thus diminish my stress. I have to learn to accept↓♥ myself as I am and cast a positive **eye** on myself, for I am a unique and exceptional person.

EYES — RINGS (under the eyes)

Eyes strongly underscored by dark rings are generally a sign of fatigue, often caused by an allergy, resulting in turn from a dependence on a product. It may also be anemia, indicating a lack of iron. I feel limited in my life, which is dull. I feel watched, surrounded, threatened even, and I don't know how to get out of it.

I accept↓♥ to be more independent and the fact that my happiness must depend only on me. The approval of others then becomes a 'plus', and not a condition for my well-being.

EYES — STRABISMUS (in general)

If I am affected by **strabismus**, I am usually described as being **cross-eyed**. The visual axes of my **eyes** are not parallel.

Strabismus denotes contradictions, dualities and uncertainties about my relations with my entourage, a perpetual struggle between a need for solitude and a need to be admired, a desire for independence and a fear of being alone. The mildness of silence is in constant contradiction with this need to question. I have difficulty in ***concentrating*** on one issue at a time. I am apprehensive about persons and situations; I find them 'shady'.

I accept↓♥ to learn how to identify my true needs and feel comfortable in any situation.

EYES — STRABISMUS (convergent)

Convergent strabismus (**to be cross-eyed** or **squint**) is a deviation of the **eyes** toward the nose.

It generally means that I refuse to see things as they really are, often because of the insecurity they represent for me. I may hope that this way, I will evade some individuals I consider threatening to me and whom I see as ***predators***. I prefer to wear blinders. My **eyes** therefore constantly scan the vicinity to detect any possible dangers. I fear what may, or will, happen to me. Depending on which **eye** is squinting, I can discover certain aspects of my personality. If it is my **left eye that is deviating inwardly**, I am a timid person suffering from a strong inferiority complex. If on the contrary, **it is my right eye**, I am probably very touchy and resentful. It is a way of centering all my attention and intelligence on myself or on a thing or a person that I must constantly monitor. The **left eye deviated completely upward** denotes that I am dreamy, irrational and devoid of the notion of time. If it is **my right eye**, I am an undisciplined person with an irrational intelligence. Another effect of **strabismus** is to only allow me to see in two dimensions. If I am **cross-eyed**, I have difficulty with the directions to take. My insecurity and my anxieties lead me to seek a reassuring presence. I "have **eyes** only for that person". When I am young, it is usually one or both of my parents, but it may also be a group or a teacher. If it is a physical person, it is as though one or both of my **eyes** were constantly searching for the ocular presence of this person who represents security and also a certain authority. My **eyes** search in various directions. **Eyes** that are **crossed** tell me there is a situation where I am confused and alone. I am torn between two persons and don't know how to position myself. In order to unify my perception, I should observe things from all angles and accept↓♥ their reality. I pay attention to all the messages my body sends me, and discover the pleasures of a view of life grasped in its entirety.

Instead of finding my security around me, I accept↓♥ to enter inside of me. I leave everything that may have influenced my life and I build myself a life on the basis of my needs, my aspirations and my inner strengths. I thereby find stability within myself. The more I am in harmony, the more my **eyes** will resume their normal position. My viewpoints may differ from those of others. The important issue is to be faithful to myself.

EYES — STRABISMUS (divergent)

Like convergent **strabismus**, **divergent strabismus** is also a **deviation of the eyes** but, in this case, **turned outward**.

It also denotes a fear of looking at the present straight on. When **my right eye** is affected, this shows that an intellectual effort is undertaken to facilitate the relation between my intelligence and the situation. I have the impression that my intelligence is running in circles, which may turn me into a potential case of depression. If it is **my left eye**, I am a person of great sensitivity. The actions I take are based on this sensitivity. I see myself as an easy ***prey*** because

I feel very fragile. **Divergent strabismus** indicates to me that I am in the position of a helpless victim. I need a panoramic view to see as many things as possible and thereby protect myself. It may be in my affective life, where I see potential spouses approaching, and I want to avoid being hurt again.

I accept↓♥ to live in the present moment and to face each situation head on. My sensitivity now enables me to take enlightened decisions, knowing that I am constantly guided and protected.

EYES — TRAUMATIC EDEMA of the RETINA *See also: BRAIN [CONCUSSION]*

Physically, a **concussion** occurs following a violent shock (direct or indirect) on some part of my organism, causing hidden lesions that need to be more thoroughly examined.

In the case of a **retinal concussion**, I refuse to see what is staring me in the **eyes** because I have difficulty in changing my view of things and letting go. I resist and I persist.

I accept↓♥ to let go of my old thoughts or old ways of seeing things, and I make room for new thoughts that are already here. Now, I am ready to listen and let myself be guided by my intuition and feelings. I feel far more free and serene.

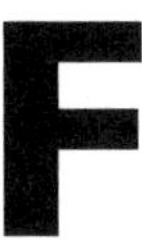

FACE / FACIES *See also: SKIN / ACNE / BLACKHEADS / PIMPLES*

My **face** is the first part of my being that meets or welcomes the world. It is my 'identification card' or my 'business card'. Usually, a single glance will give me an impression of someone, depending on whether the person's **face** is radiant, luminous, smiling or, on the contrary, somber, irritated or sad. It projects my inner world. My **face** is thus related to my image, my identity and my ego. If I want to hide a facet of my personality or am hiding something from myself, my **face** also wears this mask by becoming tense and grimacing. Similarly, if I depreciate or criticize myself, if I feel incompetent or feel that nobody **loves** me, my inner discomfort will express itself in the appearance of my **facial** skin, which becomes pimply or dries out. A mental irritation makes my skin imperfect. My inner injuries express themselves by 'injuries' on my **face**: scars, wrinkles, pimples, spots, etc. I experience stress if I constantly live according to the image I want to project, if I am ashamed of my appearance. Is the 'eye' of others more important than mine? Do I hover over the surface of things to avoid coming into contact with my deeper self? As a result, I may be 'double-**faced**'. Do I have a pervasive fear of 'losing **face**'? Maybe I want to protect myself by letting only my negative side show. If I am involved in a **car accident** and my **face** is affected, this indicates my need to question my personal image, my priorities and the way I manage my life. A **trauma to my face**, such as a **nose fracture**, occurs when my feelings lead me to depreciate myself: a situation becomes intolerable, such as pursuing an extramarital relation that no longer satisfies me. I am no longer able to ***face*** a person or a situation. I allow others to transgress my ***borders***.

For the features and the skin of my **face** to clear up, soften and clean themselves, I accept↓♥ to first clean up my inner world and get rid of the negative feelings and thoughts that I have held on to. I make room for more **Love**, more understanding, more acceptance↓♥ and more openness. My **face** lightens up more, and I no longer need to wear a mask.

FACIAL FEATURES (sagging, slack)

My **features** are **sagging and slack** when I feel that everything and everyone is 'letting me drop' or that I am 'dropping' myself. My skin becomes slack and lifeless. My drooping **eyelids** allow the sadness in my eyes to show. I let myself go. I resent life. I cultivate resentment. I lack 'firmness' in my decisions.

I accept↓♥ my need to 'raise my spirits' and rediscover my taste for living. I allow myself to enjoy each instant of my life, and I make room for the child in me.

FAINTING / LOSS of CONSCIOUSNESS *See also: BRAIN — SYNCOPE, COMA*

Fainting is a temporary **loss of consciousness** of variable duration, ranging from a brief instant to half an hour. If I sustain a complete, brutal and brief **loss of consciousness**, it is called **syncope**. If the **loss of consciousness** lasts for a longer period of time, it is a **coma**.

In any case, a **loss of consciousness** allows me to **escape reality**. I withdraw momentarily because I am so tired and my endurance is run down. I am incapable of facing the situations of my life or taking them in charge. I alternate between states of **fear**, **anguish**, **discouragement** and **helplessness**. I often fear losing power and not being 'up to' certain persons or situations. I am here, but ***elsewhere*** at the same time. I tend to do things ***mechanically***. I feel beaten in advance. I no longer feel nourished and supported by life. When I hold on, I block all the energies and strengths within me. I need my life to change.

I accept↓♥ to stop clinging to the past and to my old ideas. I allow life to follow its course. I accept↓♥ to trust the world, because everything is here for my development.

FALLING BLOOD PRESSURE *See: TENSION [ARTERIAL] — HYPOTENSION [TOO LOW]*

FALLOPIAN TUBES / OVIDUCTS *See: SALPINGITIS*

FALSE CROUP *See: THROAT — LARYNGITIS*

FASCIITIS (necrotizing) *See: BACTERIUM (FLESH-EATING) INFECTION*

FAT, OVERWEIGHT, OBESITY *See also: WEIGHT [EXCESS]*

Fat symbolizes energy, power and the 'little sweets' we give ourselves. The more active and free-flowing my energy is, the less it will tend to congeal in **fat**. The heavier I am, the more difficult I find it to move, and therefore to use my energy, which corresponds to my emotions and my creativity. Then, if I am a **corpulent** person, I am someone who is hypersensitive and I feel the need to protect myself. This need to protect myself is felt mainly in the second chakra[1], the chakra of sexuality, and the third chakra[2], the chakra of emotions. Emotions and ideas accumulate and add on to each other, as pounds accumulate in my body. Men appear to have a greater need to protect themselves in those areas. **Obesity** is often an expression of affective insecurity or deprivation: I expect something that doesn't come and I search for it in the wrong places, which brings dissatisfaction or frustration that makes me swell. I need **Love**, and at the same time, I distrust it. I may have been ***assaulted***

1. **Second chakra:** Located between the navel and the pubis.
2. **Third chakra:** Located at the level of the solar plexus, at the base of the sternum or the rib cage.

(physically or psychologically) and this makes me experience aggressiveness. I prefer to count only on myself. I feel constricted in my life, and the fact of sensing emptiness around me makes me feel abandoned. As I want to be perceived as a strong person, I may unconsciously show this strength by being a 'hefty', corpulent person.

To reduce **weight**, I accept↓♥ to change my attitude in my human relations. I stop waiting and calmly eject everything that is useless or harmful. I learn to trust myself and life, to enable this protective **fat** to go away. I express my emotions freely and learn to **love** myself as I am. I accept↓♥ to move ahead in my life, by no longer worrying about what others will say or think about me. By living on the basis of who I am, I increase my self-confidence, my worth, my self-esteem. As I recover my inner beauty a little more, my physical body will naturally shape itself to the mould of my new self-image. I show more joy and ***exuberance***.

FATIGUE (in general)

Fatigue gives me the impression of being prostrate.

I feel drained inside. The source of my **fatigue** is my lack of **Love** for the life I am leading. Where has my motivation gone? My worries, my fears, my sorrows and inner injuries lead me to struggle, resist and refuse certain situations. Instead of focusing my energy to find the common point of my difficulties, I dissipate it in too many directions at once. I even despair of finding a solution. I experience a weariness with life, an inner **fatigue**, because I have to struggle to continue moving ahead. Even depression is possible. I feel ***dejected***. I have a feeling of incompetence, of deficiency, of disinterest and even ***impotence***. I no longer know how to orient myself in life, for I have lost my joy in living. I am **bored**, I live in **the night**. I can ask myself questions about the aberrations of life. I have many questions, and no one to help me find answers to them. I may have experienced difficulties with the models provided for me by my parents. If I had a very masculine mother or a very feminine father, as a child I may have used up much energy in understanding whom I should resemble. Whatever the cause of this **fatigue**, I feel a moral as well as a physical **weakening**.

I accept↓♥ my need for a pause and rest to take stock and replenish my energy. I stop clinging to the past and accept↓♥ to live in the present moment, because each instant brings me the energy I need. By doing things that I like and especially enjoy, my energy returns naturally!

FATNESS / OVERWEIGHT *See: WEIGHT [EXCESS]*

FEAR *See also: KIDNEYS [RENAL PROBLEMS]*

Fear is an anxiety or an apprehension that I feel about a **real or imaginary** danger. When I am **afraid**, my **heart♥** pounds and I become tense.

Fear rises in me when I feel worried, unsure of **myself**, discouraged or very emotional. The object of my **fear** may be the **fear** of failure, abandonment or rejection, the **fear** of being injured, etc.; it becomes so real in my eyes that my whole body will react to it, and especially my **kidneys**. My **fear** only increases the likelihood that everything I apprehend will occur. **The very fear of a sickness can be a determining factor in making it appear**. It is important here that I become **Aware** of the fact that my **fears** are what control my life, not people or situations. The six basic **fears** are:

the **fear** of dying

the **fear** of illness

the **fear** of poverty

the **fear** of losing the **Love** of a loved one

the **fear** of old age

the **fear** of criticism.[3]

The fact of being **afraid** shows me that I have let go of my power. Should anything happen, this thing or this other person may control my life. When my **fears** have come to control my reason, I may have **panic attacks**. I am no longer capable of being neutral and detached from what I am experiencing. I am in an inner state of constant imbalance and vulnerability. I am more focused on what others expect from me than on my own needs. I no longer have any points of reference, and I sometimes feel that I am going crazy.

I accept↓♥ right now, to replace **fear** with trust. I have full power over my life. I always ask to be guided and protected in the actions I must take or the words I must say, for the well-being of all. The same applies for my family and all the persons I **love**.

FEET (in general)

My **feet** represent my contact with the earth of nourishing energy. They are connected to my relations with my **mother** and to my conflicts with her, which may go back to my conception. My **feet** give me stability in my movements toward a goal, a desire or a direction. They help me to feel safe in my relation to the Universe. They represent the position I take toward the situations I encounter as well as my social position. The fact that my **left foot** is stronger than my **right foot** (or vice versa) can inform me about the different tendencies I must favor in my movements and contacts with the ground, physically and mentally as well as spiritually. Also, if I walk with my **feet turned outward**, I may feel confused about the direction I have taken or I may dissipate my energy in different projects, whereas if my **feet** are **turned inward**, I experience a closing or a resistance about the directions to choose in my life.

3. **Fear** indicates to me in what area of my life I must put more **Love**. **Fear** points out to me the road I must take to become more **Aware** of the emotional conflict I must resolve or integrate in order to enjoy more **Love**, Wisdom and Freedom.

FEET — FOOT AILMENTS

It is with my **feet** that I move ahead on the road of life. My brain is the command center of my **feet**. The science of reflexology teaches us that our entire body is mapped over the whole surface of our **feet**. Therefore, all the problems I can relate to my **feet** enable me to know what part of my body is speaking to me. A problem related to my **feet** shows a conflict between the direction and the movement I am taking, my trouble in moving toward a goal, and reveals my need for more stability and security in my life. The future, in all its unexpectedness, scares me. I also find it difficult to let go of the past. I can ask myself what conflicted situation I am experiencing with my mother (whether she is still alive or has departed): as the Earth represents the mother in the broad sense of the term, and my **feet** are almost constantly in contact with 'her', what sort of situation am I facing where I feel uncomfortable about my sense of fusion with my mother: either I wish to put a little distance between us and I find it difficult, or I have always dreamed of being close to my mother but conditions have made this closeness impossible. Am I finding it difficult to detach myself from the family nest? Do I easily allow people to 'tread on my **feet'**? My **feet** may react if a member of my family is about to leave his physical body: I know unconsciously that he will be 'buried in the ground', and I refuse this reality. I would do anything to help him. When my **feet hurt**, I must slow down my pace. Is it out of boredom or discouragement over all my responsibilities and everything I have to do that seems impossible to get done? Or on the contrary, am I rushing at 200 miles an hour and my body is telling me to slow down before I 'have an accident'? I am carrying heavy responsibilities and I find it hard to follow the normal flow of things. I want to rush and ***expedite*** things, but rely on others instead of counting on my own inner resources. I fear I won't be able to set up a project or an undertaking. A **cramp** in the left **foot** or the right **foot** tells me how intensely I am hesitating or refusing to advance, or what direction I am afraid of taking. Is the block inside of me or outside of me? I must take a position in a given situation, and I may fear 'losing my **foot**ing' or "**I don't know where I stand**". If I **twist my foot**, I feel like leaving and distancing myself from a person, but I am forced to stay. If I only **bump my foot**, something or someone is impeding my life. If there is a **fracture**, I am persisting in going in one direction and life is asking me to stop and reconsider my life and the decisions I have to take. A **flat foot** indicates a very straight, very rigid spine, and therefore a very inflexible structure. The absence of space between my whole **foot** and the ground I walk on shows that my personal boundaries are poorly demarcated. I give up my identity. I therefore feel vulnerable and to protect myself, I will 'skim' the surface of things instead of making deeper contact and solidly 'taking root', whether in an affective relationship, a job or any other area. Another result is that I will mix my work with my private life, as both very often overlap in any case, to the detriment of my other relationships. As the earth represents the mother, the fact that my **feet** are almost constantly 'glued' to the 'mother' denotes a need for proximity or fusion, **conscious** or not, with my mother or the person playing that role in my life. I want to stay 'glued' to her. By contrast, if my **plantar arch is high**, this tells me of a heavier displacement such as a very heavily loaded spine. It also denotes that I have clearly separated my public life from my private life. This makes me be silently standoffish, uncomfortable in initiating conversations and being outgoing with others. Regarding the relationship with my mother, in this case I rather tend to avoid her. I want to be autonomous and different from her. Holding back my emotions about the direction to take in my life will take the form of **swollen feet**, and the excess of these released emotions takes the form of **perspiration**. Something in my life is dragging (**dragging my feet**), and I want it to go faster! I may fear being 'sent home on **foot**'. **Cold feet** lead me to ask myself questions on my relationship with my mother and about why I have **cold**, even **frozen**, **feet**. It may simply be that I find my relations with her distant and 'cold'. There may also be a situation involving death, which chills me. If I **walk on tiptoes**, why do I feel a need to hide or go unnoticed? It is as if I constantly had to run away from something (just as having a **club foot** symbolizes my need to escape from something). My spiritual aspirations are very high, and being in contact with the physical world is difficult for me.

I accept↓♥ to **love** my **feet** because they are what transports my whole being on the road of life. The more I **love** and accept↓♥ them, the easier they can go about their work. I choose to follow the road of joy, the road that is in harmony with my deepest aspirations. By making contact with my roots, I can flourish and advance with grace and determination.

FEET — CALLUSES and CORNS *See also: SKIN — CALLUSES*

Calluses and **corns** are localized cutaneous thickenings related to repeated rubbing. A **corn** forms a painful yellowish cone and gives a soaked appearance (**soft corn**). It is found on the backs of the toe joints or between them, or on the soles of the feet. A **callus** is a localized thickening of the cutaneous layer of the epidermis on a friction zone of the **foot**. It is rounded and preserves on its surface the normal pattern of cutaneous lines, contrary to the wart.

I go forward with my **feet**, but something tells me that it is snagging a little. It is the **callus**, this little swelling that indicates an attitude of apprehension in my current life. I don't see all the positive aspects of my life, which leads me to not fully benefit from it. If it is a **corn**, the difference is found in the pain that is far more present and intense, which indicates to me a deep feeling of guilt. It is a fear of confidently advancing toward the unknown, for I can't manage to remain 'natural' and do things simply. I let others decide in my place. Moving forward is difficult for me: life is difficult materially and it requires great efforts to move ahead. I want to rush into the future, but I hesitate and I push too hard or maybe not hard enough. What worries me so much? I find it impossible to live the present moment. I may want to take revenge on someone. I harden myself. I avoid expressing my inner pain. It therefore eventually comes to manifest itself in my physical body. I want to move forward and reach my goals, but my emotions are so knotted up that they prevent me from doing so. I may feel that my mother is preventing me from living. What person is a 'thorn' in my life? What situation do I experience repeatedly, or am I experiencing pressure or great friction? I look for the cause of this difficulty in experiencing my present or in facing my future. Is it because of my sadness and sorrow, or the fear of not succeeding? Of course, I can surgically reduce the size of my **callosities**, but this isn't enough, because I am not working on the real cause.

I accept↓♥ to see what is disturbing me so much and preventing me from moving ahead. I accept↓♥ to chase away all these dark thoughts and this guilt. I am thus more in agreement with life. My trust in the future will be all the greater.

FEET — MYCOSIS (between toes) / ATHLETE'S FOOT *See also: SKIN / (IN GENERAL) / DISEASES, SYSTEM [IMMUNE]*

Mycosis is an infection caused by a microscopic fungus. **Athlete's foot** is one of the many forms of **mycosis**. It is located between the toes and is characterized by more or less deeply split or crevassed skin.

This indicates that my mind is irritated or thwarted, that I feel constricted or incapable of moving forward as I want to, now as well as in the future. I have difficulty in accepting↓♥ myself as I am; I would like to enjoy the acceptance↓♥ and the adoration of the people around me, as a successful **athlete** is adulated. On the contrary, I feel ***banished***. Do I have to **go into *exile*** to find peace? This produces stress and inner pain. I am experiencing a deep duality: I appreciate being able to live safely under the 'wings' of others. At the same time, I feel like a prisoner. I wear a mask of hardness to avoid showing my true face. The irritation in the toes is related to the details and directions of my future life, to abstractness and to the energy concepts. It involves fears and a lack of understanding.

I accept↓♥ to envision myself on a road where it is pleasant to move ahead and where I feel fully confident. This will help me to let go of my fears and will bring more harmony in my life. I learn to live according to my needs and desires. I remove my mask and I experience my emotions simply and naturally.

FEET — SPUR (calcaneal / Lenoir's) *See also: HEEL*

Lenoir's spur, or the **calcaneal spur**, is a bony outgrowth located in the lower face of the calcaneum, which is the bone that forms the protuberance of the heel and is the posterior support of the **foot**'s plantar arch.

I don't know very well where I am coming from and I have no clear notion of where I am headed for. One thing is certain: I am not anchored, and I have no inner foundation or stability. I am like in a black hole. Which direction should I take? What meaning should I give to my life? It seems that my life was so difficult at times that I have forgotten some parts of it. I need to become rooted somewhere and find some stability, some balance. What is askew in my life? Is it in my life as a couple, in my affective relations, or in my work?

I accept↓♥ to go into myself, connect with my deepest aspirations and choose new purposes for myself. I hold my attention focused on the present while trusting that the future can only bring me good things. By listening to what my inner voice tells me to do, doors open up for me, bringing me great inner satisfaction and infinite joy.

FEET — WARTS (plantar) *See also: FEET — WARTS*

A **plantar wart** is usually noticed by the appearance of a small translucid particle under the **foot**, around which a callosity forms, provoking pain when subjected to pressure.

A **wart on the foot** indicates that I am experiencing fear about my future and about my responsibilities. It is a way of crying for help. The pain it provokes wants to make me understand that I feel anger in my way of understanding life. What is the direction in which I must go but that hurts me or frustrates me? I probably allow myself to be easily stopped by the small pitfalls that appear before me. I may also give priority to the needs of others before my own needs. I may also be feeling depreciated over my physical capacities or abilities in sports. I may be very good and above average in sports and still experience depreciation because I always force myself to be the best and to always perform just as well under all circumstances. I may have the impression that "my **feet** aren't doing as well as the **feet** of others". I also have the impression that I play hockey badly, which means that I compare myself to others and I feel very inferior as compared to their physical capacities. I play a role to make others accept↓♥ me. I accumulate frustrations. I feel vulnerable and I rely for support, as my **feet** do on the ground, on persons or things outside of me.

My body tells me that it is useless to make myself suffer so, and that I can move forward in life quite confidently. I must accept↓♥ my strengths along with my weaknesses, and by persevering, I too can succeed.

FEMALE DISORDERS

Female disorders indicate to me that I am experiencing difficulties in accepting↓♥ to be a woman. I don't even know how to express my femininity. Acting to meet the expectations of what a woman is supposed to be scares me. I am afraid of being submissive. Yet, I grew up in proximity to women who had to be 'strong', who made decisions, etc.; in fact, they wore the trousers[4]. Or did I live in an environment where women were submissive and had abdicated their own personality?

I accept↓♥ to become **Aware** of the fact that because of the education I received, I developed more prominently my masculine side, or I swore to be the opposite of submissive and to be myself, favoring my masculine side to the detriment of my **femininity**. I accept↓♥ to be a woman because as a woman,

---

4. **Wearing the trousers**: Describes the person who directs or holds authority, for example at home. Thus, when it is the woman who ***wears the trousers*** at home, it means that she is the one who runs the home and makes the main decisions in the household.

I am whole and I express my feelings. I can be strong and know how to give gentleness, **Love**, understanding, etc. Each woman has her own unique way to express her **femininity**, and it is for me to choose my own. I will realize just how happy I am to be a woman.

FEMALE PRINCIPLE *See also: MALE PRINCIPLE*

Whether I am a man or a woman, the right brain and the left side of the body represent the **female principle** (the *yin*), the seat of **creativity**, **artistic gifts**, **compassion**, **receptivity**, **emotions** and **intuition**; it involves my inner nature. It also manifests itself through tenderness, sensitivity, gentleness, harmony, beauty, purity. It links me to my **female** nature and to that of others. It is my maternal side. It is represented by the moon. The main difficulties experienced are related to the expression of feelings. Do I feel all right when I comfort someone? Am I able to say *"I **love** you"*, *"I feel sad"*? I don't feel comfortable when I am the one who is receiving, especially when it involves **Love**. Whether I want it or not, the **female principle** is part of me. The attitude I have developed toward my **female nature** is directly linked to the relations I had with the women in my life: mother, daughter, friend, wife, etc. The way in which I express my **femininity** (easily or with difficulty) will depend in great part on the parental model and on my identification with one or both of my parents. If I am a **man**, I have difficulty with my emotions, whether to express them, to free myself from them or to receive them from other persons. If I am a **woman**, there is an aspect of my **femininity** that I deny or repress. It is by following my intuition that the left side of my physical body and my **female polarity** will be healthy. If my **female side** is overly developed, I question myself about my level of self-confidence and self-assurance and I allow my emotions to gain too much the upper hand over my logical and rational side.

I accept↓♥ that the **female principle** is part of me and I open myself more to it, knowing that this process is essential for balancing my twin principles (**female** and male). Each one completes the other in order to bring about the spiritual, emotional and physical balance of my whole being.

FEMUR *See: LEG — UPPER PART*

FERMENTATION *See: STOMACH DISORDERS*

FEVER (in general) *See also: HEATSTROKE / HEAT EXHAUSTION*

When my body temperature reaches 100.4° F (or 38° C) or higher, I have a **fever**.

A **fever** is symptomatic of **emotions that are burning me up**. These emotions transform themselves into **anger** against myself and others or against an event. It invades my entire body. Why do I need to go to that extreme? Is it my way of compensating in order to get some rest and receive more **Love** and attention? Do I need this pause to adjust to a rapidly changing reality? What irritates me in my life? It generally involves a 'burning' emotion that erupts, or life becoming 'too hot' to handle, or a challenge to take on in the form of intense anger, indignation, disappointment or worries. I take care of everything around me except the most important one: my inner well-being. I want people to be proud of me, but how do I see myself? If I am a **child**, a sudden **fever** may be linked to inner conflicts, rage, or a repressed injury. As a child, I express my emotions through my body because I am not yet able to do it verbally.

In any case, I accept↓♥ to identify the cause of this **fever** and I find an accumulation of irritation and anger, which often appears when I ruminate over the misfortunes of the past. Instead of constraining myself, I become **Aware** of my needs and accept↓♥ to learn how to communicate so I can express how I feel. From now on, I will no longer accumulate: I know that the solution is dialogue.

FEVER (hay) *See: ALLERGY — HAY FEVER*

FEVER (swamp) *See: MALARIA*

FEVER BLISTERS / COLD SORES *See also: HERPES (IN GENERAL)*

Eruptions of **fever blisters** are directly related to my need for **Awareness**. I ask myself many questions about myself and my life in general. I am in conflict between my own identity and my relations with others. The only way my body has found to externalize my emotional conflict and free myself from it is to produce these **blisters** accompanied by **fever**. What is preventing me from being myself? My fear of rejection!

When this happens, I accept↓♥ to find out the reason why I am not in harmony with myself. I become **Aware** of my need to be myself under all circumstances. I also accept↓♥ to express myself, because the people around me can't simply guess what is troubling me. As I accept↓♥ others as they are, I therefore attract understanding. By becoming myself once again, harmony reclaims its place in my life.

FIBRILLATION (ventricular) *See: HEART♥ — CARDIAC ARRHYTHMIA*

FIBROMAS (uterine) and OVARIAN CYSTS *See also: CYST*

A **fibroma** is a benign tumor formed with fibrous tissues.

Most often, **fibromas** appear in the uterus[5], the seat of **maternity**, my **femininity** and my **sexuality**, therefore of everything that involves my home and my family, and concerning which I may have experienced an emotional shock (a past injury or abuse). Could it be that I felt hurt by my partner, that I received a hard knock or an insult that I was unable to manage or express in order to restore harmony? Could it be that long-repressed feelings of **guilt**,

5. These are uterine fibromyomas (in the fibrous and muscular tissues of the uterus).

shame or **inner confusion** present in me have formed this mass of soft tissues? These feelings may result from an emotional shock linked to my first sexual experiences or to an interrupted pregnancy that upset me. I feel an inner emptiness that I want to fill at all costs: I live superficially, fleeing my needs and my desires. I prefer to do like the others. I can entertain resentment toward someone who has hurt me. I may have misgivings about the fact of having a child. Do I have the impression of supporting others and feeding them because I feel indispensable? I may have a taste for renewal and change in my life, but I refuse to give free rein to my creative side and my appetite for adventure. It is interesting to note that historically, a married woman became a 'wife' when she gave birth to a child from her husband. She then bore the '**fiber** of the man'. **Uterine fibromas** often appear in the forties, at the time when I, as a woman, become **Aware** that soon, I will no longer be physiologically capable of bearing children. I may have already made the decision to not have any children, or no more children, but my body knows that it is 'my last chance', the survival of the human species depends on it! Then, if I feel or have felt guilty over the number of children I have, or don't have, this may manifest itself in the form of a **fibroma**. It may also be a baby I created in my imagination, that I wanted so much to have with a certain spouse, but it didn't happen. Symbolically, it may be my company – my 'baby'- that I invested so much time in creating (fertilizing) and at the last minute, did not materialize, for whatever reason. This 'baby' takes physical form as a **fibroma**, a 'baby' that was never born. Feelings of powerlessness and 'It is too late' haunt me and may transform themselves into resentment. I am **Aware** that **soft tissues** represent unconscious mental patterns. There is therefore an accumulation of these negative mental patterns and attitudes that have now taken solid form. It is time for me to communicate with my spouse or any other member of my family and express what I feel. I must stop hushing up what I have known but have never wanted to reveal.

As far as shame, guilt and confusion are concerned, I accept↓♥ that I acted to the best of my knowledge and my development at that time. I forgive myself and I free myself of this burden. I am feeling much lighter, and each day that goes by makes me understand that I accept↓♥ myself and that I am more and more happy as a woman. I take charge of my life and I go wherever is good for me. I stop brooding over the past. I turn to the future, knowing that I am guided. I use my creativity to give life to my passions and my dreams.

FIBROMATOSIS *See: MUSCLES — FIBROMATOSIS*

FIBROMYALGIA *See also: CHRONIC FATIGUE SYNDROME*

Fibromyalgia is a musculoskeletal disorder characterized by constant pain, sensitiveness, burning muscular pains, disturbed sleep, extreme fatigue (loss of energy) and acute morning stiffness. There are 18 especially painful points distributed over the whole body: muscles and tendons located in the shoulders and the neck, between the scapula, in the lower back, the sciatic nerve, the knees, the elbows, the wrists and the chest. Persisting pain in at least 11 of these points is sufficient for the diagnosis. Seven women for every man are affected. Some causes are a chronic imbalance of the nervous system following an emotional shock or an accident, an immune system working in overdrive (it continues to act against a non-existent virus or a virus no longer there, following a bout of the flu for example) or a disturbance of deep sleep. This leads me to think that "I am worth nothing" and to feel incapable of making changes in my life.

This syndrome (a set of symptoms that manifest themselves at the same time) is linked to perfectionism, anxiety, and making high demands on myself beyond my limits. I have a great inner emotional pain that follows me constantly. It may originate from an event experienced at an early age but was a source of great guilt. I feel unwanted and I find it very difficult to assert myself. I don't feel that I am up to the mark. I feel I have been taken aback. I feel a lot of pressure from my entourage but in fact, I am the one pushing myself too hard. I feel anger because I have the impression that I am not receiving any **Love** from the people around me. I don't want to move forward. I prefer to cut myself off from my emotions because I feel no gentleness in my life. Where does this constant pain come from? It often appears when I am doing repetitive and monotonous gestures. It reminds me of my emotional suffering from indefinitely taking on responsibilities that I haven't really chosen. I wanted to dutifully follow certain principles that were in opposition to my deeper needs. I am living a life for which I have no inclination.

I accept↓♥ to learn to take care of myself, to give myself the gentleness I so need. I allow the child who inhabits me, and grew up too fast, to live its child's life. I no longer have to be a superwoman (or a superman): I only have to be me. I have the right to be happy and live joyfully. I allow my creativity to express itself through play, the arts, sports or any other activity that brings me greater well-being. And so I thrive, and a great inner peace settles in.

FIBROSIS *See: SCLEROSIS*

FIBROSIS (cystic) *See: CYSTIC FIBROSIS / MUCOVISCIDOSIS*

FIBULA *See: LEG — LOWER PART*

FILLING (tooth) *See: TEETH — TOOTH DECAY*

FINGERS (in general)

My **fingers** are the extensions of my hands and the tools I use to manifest my actions in my everyday life. They represent action in the **present moment**, the **details of everyday life**, dexterity and knowledge. By touching, I can **love**, caress, scold, build and create. My **fingers** are the concrete manifestation of my thoughts and feelings. An injury in a **finger** indicates to me that I may be trying to do too much, that I waste time on details or that I am going too far or too fast. I give my attention to too many things at the same time and my energy is scattered. I am impatient or bothered about certain gestures or movements that I must carry out. My sense of duty is being sorely tested. I am too worried about things that need to be done. I forget how each small detail or moment of my life is precious. My guilt makes me fear that I may "have my **knuckles** rapped" or that I may kick myself for something I said. I am impatient about some small details, which throws **Light** on my perfectionist side. Whatever the nature of the **injury** (cut, scrape, bruise, etc.), I worry about my current actions. Usually, the level of the injury and the type of tissue involved (skin or bones) are important. For example, a cut to the bone indicates a deeper injury than a simple scrape. I verify the **fingers** involved and the answer to my questions will be clearer. If I **crush a finger**, I must ask myself in what area of my life I am feeling **crushed**, and by whom. I am feeling insecure because I am afraid of losing what I have. If I have one or several **crooked fingers**, it is very important to pay attention to how the **fingers** are bent and to the directions they are telling me to take. If the **fingers** are **intermingled**, do I feel mixed up in all the activities I have to do or in all these everyday details? If they are **widely spaced from each other**, is there a disharmony or a conflict that makes me find it difficult to unite my affective life, my work, and my family and sexual life (according to the **fingers** affected, go and see the definition that applies)? **Fingers that curl up** may indicate that I am withdrawing into myself or that my hands are closing to form a fist, as a sign of my anger and that I feel like punching someone or something. **Stiffness in the fingers** indicates my inflexibility about the details of everyday life. If they are **blocked**, I feel paralyzed in what I have to say or do. I kick myself as punishment for not being able to carry out a job, which is contrary to my ethics.

From now on, I accept↓♥ to take the time to do one thing at a time, for I accept↓♥ my human limitations and I **cut** my impatience that pushes me to move ahead too fast.

FINGERS — THUMB

The **thumb** is related to **pressure**, the one I place on my own shoulders as well as the one I exert on others! It is a powerful **finger** that symbolizes strength, my capacity for taking, my need for power, and which I use to **push**, to judge, to press as well as to appreciate the actions of others (the **thumb** pointed up or down) as well as my own interventions. It is linked to the mouth and to the sense of taste. When I show my **thumb** pointed upward with my hand closed, I am giving my approval, my **thumbs-up**; with the **thumb** turned downward, I am disagreeing or rejecting. The **thumb** is related to my **intellect**, my interpersonal exchanges and my sensitivity. A 'healthy' **thumb** manifests a balance between my thoughts and my feelings. If I am anxious and always worried, my **thumb** will be affected. If I feel '**pushed**' by others or by life, I will tend to easily injure my **thumbs**. I may feel **pushed** into doing things, but also compelled to adopt certain ways of doing things, certain doctrines or religions, with no opposition possible, which may affect my way of interacting with others, even becoming aggressive and in reaction against the others because I am not acting in accordance with my deeper values. What I really want to do remains in my mind instead of me physically doing it. The **thumb** therefore determines the sorts of contacts I have with others and with myself. Difficulties in this area may be linked to my difficulty in letting go of my worries of the past, my old thoughts. As a child sucks its **thumb** in situations where it feels vulnerable, the **thumb** therefore represents security and protection. All injuries to the **thumb** are linked to an over-investment in mental effort and an over-accumulation of ideas and **worries**, often about a child, and a tendency to be defeatist. Are my exchanges with others healthy? Am I **pushing** the others too much, or do I feel myself **shoved** by an overly frantic life? Am I afraid of losing control? Do I always ***push*** myself ***to the limit***? When I have had enough of a situation, my **thumb** will hurt. If I **fracture** my **thumb,** my life must change radically. I may feel backed against the wall. This raises great inner anxiety in me because I must change ingrained habits that have negative consequences for me. The **thumb** also symbolizes life and survival, the desire to live my life and not to die (if I keep my **thumb** in a closed fist, I am an introverted person who may feel like dying, or I feel the need to withdraw into myself to protect myself from the outer world). I try to see if I am afraid of dying or no longer controlling myself. The **thumb** reminds me of my inner strength, my worth, the original forces that inhabit me. It manifests my ability to transform these inner riches and all my desires and needs into physical action.

From now on, I do everything to be in peace with myself. I observe the signs related to my **thumbs** and I remain vigilant when something happens to me. I let my inner sadness rise. I accept↓♥ life and situations without being too dramatic, for I know that the Universe is taking care of me! I stop being negative and I accept↓♥ to rely on my own bases and values: it helps me to detach myself from my family influences that I still cling to. I free myself of my overflowing thoughts and I accept↓♥ to be the master of my life.

FINGERS — INDEX

The **index** is the **finger** of **judgment** and **knowledge** and corresponds to the sense of smell. It represents the **ego** in all its aspects: **authority**, **pride**, **conceit** and so on. In my nonverbal behavior, when I move my **index** by pointing it often, when I ***show*** 'the **finger**' or 'with the **finger**', it indicates a **rejection of authority**, parental or otherwise. I try to express authority 'reactively', namely in reaction to the different forms of authority present. My fear of authority may even cause me to experience digestive disorders. I am afraid of being trapped or of not being recognized at my true worth. I am afraid of authority and I don't accept↓♥ the fact that it is present in my life. I want to make my point at all costs! When I use my **index** to impose my ideas in a rather authoritarian manner, it is my way of asserting my 'personal power' and hiding my feeling of powerlessness. I become **Aware** of the fact that often, it is my fears that make me act in this way. I am emotionally very sensitive and I need to feel safe in life. I am afraid of the judgment of others, afraid that they may reconsider their friendship, business or **Love** relationships with me. I realize that accusing someone else or wanting to win every argument, even over the most insignificant issue, leads nowhere. I save my energy for more important matters. Is it in fact authority that truly bothers me? It may be a feeling of powerlessness or insecurity toward parental authority, going back to my childhood. If I depreciate myself, I may have the impression that others ignore me or want to dominate me. I would therefore want to hold the first place, but this is not happening. I am ***disappointed*** in myself but also in the others. A **fracture of the index** indicates to me that I am clinging too much to certain persons or situations: if I am no longer capable of controlling myself, what will probably happen? I am anxious, and panicked even, because instead of using my true inner power, I prefer to use other tricks in order to get what I want.

From now on, I accept↓♥ the forms of authority that bother me, for I know that they are there to make me develop positively. Instead of experiencing frustration with this authority, I seek my true inner power. Instead of living in my head, I accept↓♥ to live in my **heart♥**, accepting↓♥ the different emotions inside of me. I open my spirit and, instead of pointing a **finger** at others, I dare to look at myself in the mirror and take myself in charge.

FINGERS — MIDDLE FINGER / THIRD FINGER

The **middle finger**, the hand's longest **finger**, represents **creativity**, **sexuality, strength and anger**. It symbolizes the sense of touch, work, productivity and fertility. An **injury** or a **pain** in this **finger** means that my sexual life is not going as I wish, or that I bow too easily before fate. I am experiencing sorrow or tension linked to dissatisfaction, and anger gradually sets in. This reaction prevents me from achieving my secret desires. My creative side is constricted by a lack of self-confidence. I worry too much and dream a lot instead of building my life on a real and permanent basis. My frustrations prevent me from advancing. My feeling of inferiority brings me difficulties in my sexuality, which is one area where I express my creativity. My deeper impulses are not expressed. I tend to live with an extreme attitude: either I flee my responsibilities and stay in place, or I become very oriented to the strict application of laws or to obtaining what I want at any cost. I still have an infantile attitude, as if I have not yet become a mature adult. Right now, I identify what aspect of my sexuality or my creativity is involved. What part of me wants to grow and develop while accepting↓♥ the associated responsibilities? A **fracture of the middle finger** indicates a resistance and a rigidity, especially toward touching, which generates great aggressiveness in me. It may involve my career or my performances (sexual as well as personal or intellectual).

I accept↓♥ to express my needs rather than allow my anger to rise. I realize that only my fears (pride) prevent me from expressing myself. My sexual experiences become enriching, instead of being just a way to fill a vacuum. I learn to create my life every day. Instead of chasing images and trivialities, I base my life on my inner values and priorities.

FINGERS — RING FINGER / FOURTH FINGER

The **ring finger** is the **symbol** of **alliance** or **union** and represents my affective relationships. It represents the sense of vision and also the way in which I am in relation with myself. My **ring finger** is affected if I hide behind others instead of taking my place, if my life is full of disorder or contradictions. It therefore represents the **freedom** I allow myself and the way I **ally** myself with others. Any injury to this **finger** comes from a **sorrow** or a difficulty in my affective relations: it may be with my husband, my wife, my children and, in certain cases, even with my parents. It may even be an associate or someone with whom I signed a contract and with whom I have a privileged relationship. This injury is the outward manifestation of an inner injury about which I have probably not spoken to anyone. It is difficult for me to form a **union** with myself and live with this sorrow that overwhelms me. Maybe I tend to exaggerate the situation. What is bothering me? Am I experiencing some form of injustice about a person or a situation? As I don't control myself, I try to hold power over others, when I should instead accept↓♥ to let go and thus release myself. I am still living according to what others say and think about me, and that affects me. I can feel myself in danger and I may tend to cling to others. I sense a coldness in my relations with my entourage and treat myself in a very cold and inhuman fashion. A **fracture in the ring finger** means I forget myself too much in the interest of others, and at the expense of my own needs. A situation has become intolerable because I don't give myself the necessary space to flourish and be myself.

I accept↓♥ to detach myself in order to better view the situation. What is preventing me from expressing myself? Do I **presume** what the other's reaction will be? I learn to check, and find there is a huge difference between **presuming** and **knowing**. Verifying enables me to enjoy much more harmonious relations and also teaches me how to engage in dialogue. I accept↓♥ to bare my **Soul**, to flourish and be happy, while being in harmony with my entourage.

FINGERS — ATRIAL / AURICULAR / LITTLE FINGER

The little finger is directly related to the **heart♥**. It represents the **family** and all the family-related aspects of my life, especially **Love** and family harmony, but also the secrets and the lies. It is related to hearing (ears) and intuition, and it is not without reason that we say: "My **little finger** told me..." It symbolizes wisdom, integrity, truth, openness and communication. It may also represent my sly and pretentious side, used to satisfy my personal needs. When I inflict an injury on this **finger**, it indicates emotions I am experiencing about my **family**, which I should express outwardly, or a lack of harmony in my couple, or simply a lack of **Love** for myself. I 'turn a deaf ear' and don't always listen to the messages sent to me by my intuition, my '**little finger**'. I need a change in my relations with others so that they will be in harmony with my new ideologies, beliefs and aspirations. Any damage to a **little finger** (a scrape, a burn, etc.) surely denotes an excessive emotionality. I certainly have the unfortunate habit of worrying for trifles, and my emotionality gets the upper hand. I become pretentious, and this puts me off-balance and prevents me from understanding the people and the events in my life. Instead of acting on my inner wisdom, I tend to live according to others. This makes me indecisive and insecure. I ignore my intuition and give full way to my incessant thoughts and ruminations. If I **fracture my little finger**, I have a pressing need to free myself in an area of my life that may be tied to authority. It may also be a secret I have kept for a very long time and is gnawing at me inside.

I accept↓♥ to look at events and situations with the simplicity of a child. By ceasing to dramatize issues and showing some openness of mind, I learn to assert myself and communicate. I move forward far more cheerfully. I need much more inner calm. Instead of playing a role and living in a world where appearances trump actual 'being', I should return to simple things and to myself.

FINGERS (arthritic) *See also: ARTHRITIS (IN GENERAL)*

Arthritis is an inflammation of the joints that causes suffering and symbolizes **criticism**, self-punishment, disapproval, a deep lack of **Love** and even a feeling of powerlessness. **Arthritic fingers** (the details of everyday life) therefore indicate the feeling of being badly loved and of being the victim of events in my everyday life. I relinquish power to others.

I accept↓♥ to **love** myself and forgive myself, because if I don't **love** myself, how can others **love** me?

FINGERS — CUTICLES

The **cuticle** is a very thin layer of skin, like a film forming at the base of the nails.

The thicker the **cuticle** is and the faster it grows, the more I tend to be hard on myself. **I criticize myself** constantly for trifles because I am a perfectionist.

I accept↓♥ to see that I am a developing human being and that I always do the best I can. I stop judging myself so severely, and I accept↓♥ myself as I am in order to be able to continue moving forward harmoniously.

FISTULA

A **fistula** is the formation of a channel connecting directly, and abnormally, two viscera together (**internal fistula**) or a viscus with the skin (**external fistula**).

For such a channel to take form, there must be a significant block in that area, and it must have lasted for some time. Unconsciously, I was so **anxious** that I **held myself in** and I **blocked** the normal evacuation duct. What lies hidden behind my anxiety? I am afraid of being rejected or abandoned, of being ridiculed or making a mistake. I am reluctant to let myself go. I withdraw within myself for protection. Because I am afraid of suffering, I hold everything in, beginning with my emotions. I may even have buried an urge for revenge or to kill someone, often a man, although in fact, I don't have that type of personality.

I accept↓♥ the fact that behind any emotion, there is pride, and the more pride there is, the greater is my fear. I need to refocus myself in the present moment and listen to my intuition. Life is a school where I learn. If I block my learning, I also block my development.

FISTULÆ (anal) *See: ANUS — ANAL FISTULÆ*

FLATULENCE *See: GAS*

FLESH-EATING BACTERIUM INFECTION *See: BACTERIUM (FLESH EATING) INFECTION*

FLU (avian) *See also: INFLUENZA / FLU*

The **avian flu**, also called the **chicken flu**, is an **influenza** virus that is extremely contagious for certain birds and can be transmissible to humans **(A (H5N1))**. Its symptoms are similar to those of the classic **flu**, but more severe.

If I catch this **flu**, I find myself in a situation where I am stuck and confined in an environment that 'stinks'. I must 'cool off' and close myself in so as not to feel all the sorrow and the pain I am experiencing. I prefer to do like the ostrich and hide 'under my mother's wings'. I am as 'proud as a rooster', and chickens will have teeth before I apologize or before I forgive what someone said or did to me. I live in a society I don't agree with, that smothers me and makes me aggressive. I have become unpleasant and uncompromising and I 'easily **take a dislike**' to persons who curtail my freedom or invade my vital space. I don't feel strong enough to fight the situation in which I find myself and I have been 'crying inside of me' for several months, or even for years.

I accept↓♥ to let go of all my preconceived ideas. I heal my old injuries, I stop crying over my lot and I accept↓♥ to share the beautiful things of life. I open myself up to the world with discernment, without judgment. I set my own limits, respecting myself and others. I thus recover the place that is rightfully mine.

FOLLICULITIS *See: HAIR DISEASE*

FOOT — (athlete's) *See also: FEET — MYCOSIS*

FOOT — SPUR (calcaneal) / LENOIR'S *See: FEET — SPUR [CALCANEAL]*

FOREARMS *See: ARM AILMENTS*

FOREHEAD

My **forehead** is located at the level of the brain and, as it is part of my head, it represents my **individuality** and the way I face my life and events, rationally rather than emotionally. It also refers to my will and my eyesight. I can say that the form of my **forehead** and its special features indicate to me how I **face up to** my responsibilities. My openness of mind is revealed by the width of my **forehead**: the narrower it is, the more rigid I am and the more I need to open myself up to new ideas. Any **injury** or **affection** in my **forehead** reveals fear or guilt over my own ideas or opinions, which are different from those of others and that I find difficult to fully acknowledge, knowing that I risk upsetting my entourage[6]. I often face contempt or insults from others. I am always thinking, and I tend to disparage my intellectual capacities. I like to oppose others in order to resolve major problems: this way, I build up my self-esteem, however superficially. I want to project my image as someone who is 'headstrong'.

I accept↓♥ that my personal integrity is very important, and it is vital for me to respect myself in who I am, while remaining open to the opinions of others and knowing that I have the right to hold a different opinion. I affirm my ***boundaries*** in order to keep the space that is mine.

FORGETTING (losing things) *See also: ACCIDENT*

Forgetting manifests itself by a momentary or permanent failure of memory.

It may be a sign that I am clinging to certain events or persons, often from my past, and from whom I must detach myself, for I am living in the past instead of enjoying the present moment. I may also be concerned about one or several situations in my life, which prevents me from being completely present. If I **forget** or **lose** my **keys**, my **wallet** or my **purse**, then it is quite possible that I am **in search of my identity**. I may feel guilty of taking some rest, of enjoying sweets, or wanting attention (because it is 'not reasonable') and thus, I punish myself by losing things. Being 'in the moon' means that I am not in the **here and now**, that I would prefer to be somewhere else (in the past or in the future). I like change and I dissipate myself, I rush to do things instead of taking my time.

I accept↓♥ to let go of things and persons, I leave the past in peace and I open myself up to all the beauty of life in the **here and now**.

FRACTURE *See: BONE — FRACTURE*

FRECKLES *See: SKIN DISEASES*

6. It often happens during puberty that acne manifests itself mainly on the **forehead**. It is the child who rebels and wants to contradict or confront their parents.

FRIGIDITY *See also: FEMALE DISORDERS*

Frigidity consists in a sexual dissatisfaction experienced by a woman during sexual intercourse.

There is generally a deep trauma or an inner conflict. **Fear** is at the center of this state: fear of my sexual impulses and of the pleasure that could make me seem 'indecent', fear of letting go and losing control. I am afraid of 'losing something' by 'submitting' to sexuality. I feel invaded and I have the impression of being defenseless. I need to have control and, as it is nonexistent at the moment of orgasm, I can avoid experiencing it in order to escape from this state where I feel myself at the mercy of the other. I therefore prefer to control my emotions and the events in order to avoid placing myself in a precarious situation. At that point, I feel I have power over myself, but also on the other person. This behavior is reinforced if my sexual education was hidden or if my parents viewed sexuality as bad or repugnant, or practiced it in a fashion that overstepped the norms permitted by society. In fact, it is the fear of facing what I am hiding inside of myself. When this fear is present, I often believe that I am ugly and worthless. I am ashamed and feel deeply guilty. The education I received has a very great impact on my **frigidity**. Was sexuality considered degrading and as representing the basest instincts of human beings? Did I hear talk of resignation and submission before sexual relations, with the tacit understanding that no pleasure was to be found there? Was I sexually abused in my childhood? If so, I unconsciously reject my sexuality, and it is difficult for me to let myself be touched without feeling fear and disgust. I become **Aware** that there is nothing indecent in sexuality. On the contrary, when it is expressed between consenting partners living a relationship of acceptance↓♥ and deep **Love, it is beautiful and healthy**. I accept↓♥ to open myself to my partner and express my fears. I also accept↓♥ to tell this person about my needs. I realize that sexuality is part of my physical dimension and that it is a source of fulfillment for my development. It is important to note that for certain persons (women as well as men), who are engaged in a growth process, their sexual needs may happen to be hardly present or even entirely absent for a certain period. In these moments, I have learned to fully use all my creative energies, and sexual energy no longer holds a preponderant place in my life. Pleasure is experienced through the fullness that I discover at each instant within myself, and in a joy and happiness with which I can connect, even outside the context of sexual relations.

Whatever stage I may have reached, I accept↓♥ that the important thing is to respect my own needs and open myself to sexuality as a source of pleasure and a healthy way to communicate with my partner. If I feel I am being abused or that sex is becoming for me or for the other person a way to compensate for an inner void, it is my responsibility to share this insight with the other person. Then, there are no power games, just an exchange in **Love**.

FUNGI *See: FEET — MYCOSIS*

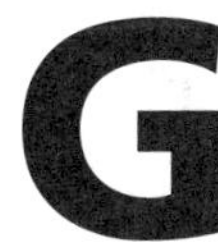

GALLBLADDER *See also: BILIARY CALCULI, LIVER DISORDERS*

The **gallbladder** is a membranous reservoir located under the liver and in which the ***bile*** secreted by the liver accumulates. This bile eliminates toxic substances from the intestine.

Bile symbolizes the elimination of emotions and experiences that are negative for me. It represents my power to assimilate and digest my emotions in order to be able to fully flourish. Difficulties in this area are related to emotional and mental patterns that are full of bitterness and irritation about my life or about others. If these patterns congeal and harden, they will transform themselves into **biliary calculi**. If my **gallbladder** does not function properly, this may derive from my insecurity or my worries about someone I **love** and is dear to me. The fact of experiencing an attachment to this person leads me to feel emotions that I find difficult to manage and take on. The departure (death) of a person becomes very difficult for me and is a source of ***rancor***: it often results in heated discussions over the dividing of an inheritance. Situations that involve confrontations upset my **gallbladder**, for I am afraid of 'losing the game' and having to give up things or persons that are dear to me or that risk being taken away from me. I am experiencing confusion and ambivalence over my emotions. I find it difficult to discern or see clearly in my emotions and my responsibilities and to take proper actions. I have the impression that I always have to justify my acts, and often perceive the situations in my life as 'unfair', which makes me feel very angry. I become ***bitter*** – even ***furious*** – about certain persons, situations or ***gestures***. I even reach the point of ***detesting*** them and seeking ***revenge***. I have the impression that someone is ***encroaching*** on my vital space. My mostly silent anger and my sorrow lead me to retreat from the world. I feel a lot of ***animosity***. I feel like expressing myself and showing the world what I can do, but I remain closed in my shell. This leads me to despair.

I accept↓♥ to free myself of these bitter, irritating feelings. I must consider each experience as an opportunity to know myself better and use my sensitivity positively and creatively instead of controlling and manipulating others. It is only by expressing my inner feelings and letting go of past experiences that marked me that I can free myself of them and live in peace.

GALLSTONES / CALCULI (biliary) *See: BILIARY CALCULI*

GANGLION (lymphatic) INFECTIONS, INFLAMMATION, EDEMA

See: LYMPH [LYMPHATIC DISORDERS]

GANGLION / LYMPHATIC NODE *See also: ADENITIS, ADENOPATHY, CANCER OF THE GANGLIA, LYMPH [LYMPHATIC DISORDERS]*

A **ganglion** is a rounded cellular mass located on the trajectory of a lymphatic vessel.

If I am having difficulty in facing a situation and, instead of speaking about it and asking for help, I keep it all inside of me, **I keep** my discouragement and my despair **a secret**, I feel like dropping everything, and after some time my nostalgia over my life will manifest itself in one or several **ganglions**. My self-esteem has diminished and my fear for the future will make me feel anguish. I am living on the defensive and in inaction. I am in a situation where I have the impression that someone wants to attack me. I am backed against the wall and can no longer move. I may also have communication difficulties with others, and this affects me emotionally or causes me to be fearful in my relations with others. I would like to be part of a group, feel that I belong to an organization, be closer to my friends rather than live in solitude. It is important to go and see in what part of the body **ganglions** appear, because this gives me a clue to find the reason for this manifestation. For example, if I am worried about something that I want to express but that I keep inside, chances are that one or several **ganglions** will appear in the region of the **throat**. I am submerged by emotions that I flee. If there are things that I don't want to hear, then the **ganglions** near my **ears** may impede my hearing. **Ganglions** in general show me that I am ambivalent about a situation. I worry a lot. I feel stuck, jammed. I feel under attack and must constantly ***defend*** and ***protect*** myself, but I see no place or ***nook*** where I can find ***shelter***. Unconsciously I would want my father to defend me. I feel bound to keep the family tied together and on good terms. I also wonder if I am ready to take on full responsibility for my life or if I prefer to be 'up in the clouds'. I am afraid of my emotional world; the whole sexual aspect feels like a threat to me. By cutting myself off from my own emotions and covering myself with a ***shell***, how can I be in contact with my entourage? When there is a **swelling of the ganglions**, there is an overload in my organism and toxins must be eliminated. It may be generalized or localized (in the groin for example) and it is related to the central nervous system. The burden of responsibilities that I take on is probably excessive. I don't talk about it and I keep this frustration inside of me. I observe my attitudes toward a person close to me and I find that it would be better for me to disengage myself from a role that I took on, but which is now too heavy a burden for me.

I accept↓♥ to communicate my needs at all levels, so that my despair will go away and make place for hope and the joy of living. I must let go of my problems and have trust: a higher force is helping me in my progress. I accept↓♥ to feel everything that inhabits me. The more I integrate my physical body and my inner feelings, the more I am restoring a body-mind balance for my greater well-being. I learn to **love** and respect myself by setting certain limits, to be expressed when I have 'taken more than enough', and my relations thus become more authentic.

GANGRENE *See: BLOOD — GANGRENE*

GAS (pains caused by) / FLATULENCE / METEORISM *See also: SWELLING / BLOATING [OF THE ABDOMEN]*

Flatulence (also called **meteorism**) is a production of intestinal **gas** with ballooning. The emission of **gas** can take place either through the mouth or through the anus. The **gases** accumulate in the digestive tube.

When I cling to, or want to hold on to, a person or a situation, it is as if I was keeping things for myself that are undesirable and not beneficial for me and that manifest themselves in the form of **gas**. **I am afraid and I cling fast** because I am anxious and I feel that I am going to lose something or someone important, emotionally, intellectually, materially or spiritually. I may also be ruminating over the same feelings and the same insecurities, which ferment inside of me and are evacuated when I least expect it and make themselves 'felt'. I may also try to 'swallow' (figuratively) a situation, a person or an emotion that goes against my principles and my **conscience**. The consequence: I swell up. I want to resolve the problems of the whole world and it is becoming heavy to bear. Could there also be some 'parasites' in my life that are harming my development? There is a war on that is breaking my inner peace. If the **gases** are nauseating, then there are some things in my life that 'don't smell right' and that I want to eliminate to recover my freedom and my space.

I accept↓♥ to give myself permission to feel what is going on inside of me, and to let go. I learn to trust and to let go, knowing that I always have what I need.

GASTRIC ACIDITY *See: STOMACH — HEARTBURN*

GASTRITIS *See: STOMACH — GASTRITIS*

GASTRO-ENTERITIS *See: INTESTINES — GASTROENTERITIS*

GÉLINEAU'S SYNDROME *See: NARCOLEPSY*

GENITAL ORGANS (in general)

The **genital organs** differentiate men from women. They are related to the **male principle**[1] and the **female principle**[2] in each of us. They are also related to the seat of sexual energy, the gonads and the basic chakra[3]. This center is related to the pleasures of life and creativity. If I experience difficulties with respect to my sexuality, it is usually my **genital organs** that will be affected.

---

1. **Male principle**: *See*: Male Principle.
2. **Female principle**: *See*: Female Principle.
3. **Basic chakra**: Related to the energy center at the level of the coccyx.

GENITAL ORGAN DISORDERS *See also: FRIGIDITY, IMPOTENCE, VENEREAL DISEASES*

The difficulties I experience with my **genital organs** indicate to me **fear**, **guilt**, shame, distrust, regrets and **anger** over my sexuality, which risk taking the form of **venereal diseases**, **frigidity**, **impotence**, etc. This region is related to my gonads (testicles in men, ovaries in women), and the sexual energy related to sexuality is very powerful because its primary purpose is to perpetuate the human species. However, it may be that I am using this energy inappropriately. The notion of **pleasure** related to sexuality puts me in contact with one of my basic needs, pleasure, and connects me with **my wounded inner child**. My sexuality can thus lead me to highlight these fears, injuries or rejections that are part of me. I may not accept↓♥ myself in this body (sex) that I am; I may experience an inner conflict between my physical desires and those of a religious or spiritual nature; if I am afraid of saying no and I have sexual relations to avoid being rejected, for fear of losing a person's **Love**, or just for a selfish purpose, etc., all these situations can lead me to experience difficulties in this area. There is an inner confusion or conflict, a difficulty in communicating and sharing. I don't always feel respected and considered, and I find it difficult to trust people. Also, if my parents wanted a daughter and I am a boy or vice versa, or if I myself wanted to be of the other sex, this can lead me to experience **genital problems** because I reject one part of my sexuality and I may even feel guilty of being who I am. The whole notion of evil related to sexuality and pleasure and conveyed by society and by moral and religious instruction can lead me to experience great guilt. I have the impression that I am 'not all right' or not good enough. I poorly integrate my femininity or my masculinity in each area of my life.

I accept↓♥ to remove all this guilt, so that my sexuality can become the expression of my loving qualities and of the attention I give others. It is important that **Love** be present in my sexual experiences and also each time I look at myself in a mirror, so that I will accept↓♥ myself more and more as I am.

GILLES DE LA TOURETTE'S SYNDROME *See also: BRAIN — TICS, NERVOUSNESS, OBSESSION*

Gilles de la Tourette[4]'s syndrome is also called the '**tic disease**'. It is a rather rare disease, often running in families, beginning in childhood (usually between the ages of 2 and 10) and of scientifically unknown causes. It is typified by multiple tics (including a voiced tic), obsessive-compulsive symptoms and attention disorder with hyperactivity. There is an issuing of obscene words and a repetition of fragments of words or sentences.

4. **De la Tourette** (Gilles): A neurologist (1857–1904) at the Salpètrière Hospital in Paris, who described the symptoms of the disease in 1885 in the case of the Marquise de Dampierre and nine other cases presenting the same clinical picture.

The history of my genetic heritage at once precedes me and follows me throughout my life. When I carry inside of me this background of doubts, perfectionism and rigid education, my cellular memories are coded accordingly. I am *irritated, annoyed* and ***infuriated*** and I don't know where it comes from. I am seeking out my place. I sense danger coming from all sides, I feel I am boxed in and nobody can come to my rescue. It is a ***dead end***. I have often lost face and I have been told to 'shut up'. My body reacts by unconsciously expressing my inner frustrations. Everything I would have wanted to express in my gestures or words, but haven't, wants to express itself. My repressed desires are expressing themselves. I perceive myself negatively, and so I repress my strengths and my talents. I am afraid of being myself and of expressing my deeper emotions. As I feel impure and diabolical, it is this image that others will reflect back to me, especially my parents. I am a mirror for them, and they too must become **Aware** of the fact that I am different and have my own personality. They have their own frustrations and anxieties.

I accept↓♥ to find links with the baggage of my past, to clean up and to let go of some family patterns in order to find my own identity.I allow my spontaneity and my emotions to express themselves. I acknowledge my inner power and strengths. This brings me a greater feeling of security and freedom.

GINGIVITIS *See: GUMS — GINGIVITIS [ACUTE]*

GLAND(S) (in general)

A **gland** is an organ, the functioning of which is characterized by the synthesis and secretion of a substance. These substances are specific and essential for the harmony of the body. There are two main types of **glands**: the **endocrine glands** and the **exocrine glands**. The **endocrine glands** (with no canals) secrete their **hormones** (which are messengers) inside of the body, in the blood as for example the thyroid, the liver, the surrenals, etc.; they have an interior function and their name means "I separate". These **hormones** are necessary for maintaining the body's equilibrium (homeostasis). The **exocrine glands** secrete their products outside of the body through a canal that opens onto the surface of the skin, a mucous membrane or in the digestive tube (for example: the salivary, sudoriparous and lacrymal **glands**, the liver or the pancreas).

The **glands** are the mirrors of the SELF and each of them is linked to an energy center (chakra). A bad functioning of my endocrine **glands** manifests an imbalance or a disharmony among my energy centers. The **glands**, whatever their type, inject into my body certain products that are like fuels my body needs to be able to function and set other organs in action. The intercommunication between the **glands** is what brings about harmony or disharmony and a proper equilibrium or an imbalance. The fact of becoming increasingly conscious and creating my own life instead of living like an automaton ensures a proper functioning of my **glands**.

GLAND DISORDERS *See also: ADENOMA*

A bad functioning in one or several **glands** indicates that I am having difficulty in finding the motivation or the 'fuel' for starting up a new project or for taking action about a situation (I tend to put things off). It may also involve rational matters, where I am experiencing confusion and having difficulty in getting a clear view of what must be done. This denotes my inner insecurity. I am as disorganized and untidy in my life as in my thoughts. **Glandular** dysfunctioning can also result from unfulfilled desires or overly strong emotions. As the mirrors of the SELF, the **glands** reflect the expression of my inner life. They are affected if I live passively with the attitude of a victim or choose to live unconsciously and in my head instead of being in my **heart♥**. If there is a **glandular inflammation**, I am resenting those who hurt me or humiliated me. I am only protecting myself.

I accept↓♥ to trust myself again, for I have all the necessary qualities to move ahead and take action.

GLAND — CAPSULE (suprarenal) *See also: ADDISON'S DISEASE, CUSHING'S SYNDROME, FEAR, STRESS*

The primary function of the **surrenal**[5] **glands** is to produce the stress hormone called adrenaline, along with cortisol and cortisone. The function of these **glands** is to regulate the pulse and blood pressure and to enable the body to sense dangerous situations (fear, confrontation, survival, etc.). They are linked to the solid parts of my body that keep me in contact with Mother Earth, therefore with the material world, with my basic needs and the acceptance↓♥ of the bodily part of my personality.

When this center is in **disharmony**, I am endlessly concerned with my material possessions, I distrust others and I am never satisfied. When I am feeling fear, stress or worries (real or imaginary), my behavior will be aggressive, angry and impatient, especially when my **surrenals** are **overworking**. When they are **in default**, I easily become discouraged, I put things off until later and I don't want to face my problems, preferring escape. I lack the courage and the will to face life. When I feel ***panicked***, in danger or am really in danger, my perception may be different, but my body will immediately respond to any stressful and tense situation that it senses as threatening, whether this situation actually materializes or not. Thus, we can see that the body responds seriously to the warnings that stress can provoke. It will lack ***coordination***. I can relate this danger to a situation in my life where I am afraid of losing time, money, a reward, a spouse, etc., because I made a 'bad decision' or took a 'bad direction' in my life. "Am I on the right track?" I want to go very fast and very far in one of the areas of my life, but that requires great determination and judicious choices, and I won't allow myself the right to make any mistakes, although this is in fact just another experience in my life.

5. They are related to what is called the base energy center or the base chakra, called the coccygeal center.

Hence, an intense level of stress. I sometimes have the impression of '**losing my bearings**'. I may be living in fear of ***losing myself***, in the proper sense of searching to find my direction and my way in a given situation or in my life in general. I may also feel that I am ***lost*** or that I am losing myself by not following my basic values and trying too much to please others. I risk feeling ***dejected***. I feel like the sheep left far from its herd: I feel ***isolated***, a little lost, on the fringes of society, ***disoriented***, without any ***bearings***. I ***wander*** here and there, not knowing very clearly what direction to choose, like a ***vagabond***. I feel on the ***fringes*** of society. I sometimes have the impression that I am ***hallucinating***. I may be experiencing an impossible **Love**, because I am mistaken about my feelings or because the person is inaccessible. I can't take my place; I mustn't be seen or known. The **surrenals** are located above the kidneys, which are considered to be the seat of fear and sorrow. The adrenalin that is released when I am in a state of excitation can have the effect of stimulating me and making me creative or, on the contrary, can cause me harm or even destroy me. Too great an accumulation of stress can lead to total exhaustion. The 'go for broke' syndrome may then manifest itself regularly. There are several situations in my life or in society in general that I find ***abnormal***. I always look elsewhere for what may be right under my nose. I have an insatiable need to have the best, in any area.

When the **surrenals** are in **harmony**, I feel in symbiosis with all of earth's creatures. I accept↓♥ to get rid of my defeatist attitude and I decide to set myself a goal in life. I adopt a simple lifestyle and become more open, and I find my balance. I have confidence in what the material world can bring me (safety and protection). I get up full of energy in the morning, I feel like living and I am able to take action. I become **Aware** of what I truly ***desire***. I ***stroll*** through life **all over the place**, with faith and confidence.

GLAND (pancreatic) *See: PANCREAS*

GLAND (pineal) / EPIPHYSIS CEREBRI

The **pineal gland**[6] is the main mirror of the Self and blends the energies of the six other centers. It is linked to the **I Am** and the highest planes of **consciousness**. The **pineal gland** is linked to my inner voice, my spiritual quest. It manages everything that involves my existential questioning. It collects anything concerning the perceptions of the earth and puts them into contact with my inner experiences. I can thus get an overall view of my existence. When it is in **disharmony**, it means I am not integrated, and I pity myself, which prevents me from fulfilling myself. I feel confronted and in duality with myself. I do violence to myself. I thus lose my capacity for wonderment and I have difficulty in carrying out my mission on earth. As I don't know what structures to base my life on, I reject my living environment, if not life itself! I am afraid of making a mistake and being judged, especially in my career choice. I find it difficult to integrate in my life the subtle

6. The **pineal gland** is related to what is called the coronal energy center or the crown chakra.

information I receive, and my relation with time leads to an inner struggle. I am living spiritually, but I feel cut off from my physical body and the earth. I become anxious, which makes me see negativity everywhere. I set limits on myself and I live artificially and impersonally. When it is in **harmony**, this **gland** brings calm, serenity and openness of mind. I then feel the divine presence and my energies are in harmony with the WHOLE. I am happy about being on earth. The Ego makes way for the universal **Consciousness**, and duality no longer exists, for I am in the present moment (neither in the future nor in the past) and I can adapt myself to all situations. As it is the bridge between the planes of **Consciousness** and the earthly world, it is through this energy center that I integrate myself and am **Aware** of my understanding of God.

I accept↓♥ to stride forward in life and take appropriate decisions in order to truly fulfill myself.

GLAND (pituitary) / HYPOPHYSIS

The **pituitary gland**[7] is an endocrine **gland** located between the eyebrows, behind the root of the nose, under the brain on which it totally depends, under the **hypothalamus**. It is related to the face, the eyes, the ears, the nose, the sinuses, the cerebellum and the central nervous system. It also secretes stimulins that act on the other **endocrine glands** and it plays a major role in the regulation of hormonal secretions. It therefore acts as the **master gland** with respect to the other **glands** of the body. It plays the role of the orchestra conductor. It receives messages from the brain and redistributes them to the other **glands**. It therefore has a very important role, for it receives oxygen and vital energy (*prana*) and redistributes them to all my cells. This **gland** controls the secretions of the endocrines, the thyroid, the corticosurrenals and the gonads[8]. It also regulates the periodicity of sleep.

The **hypophysis** constantly seeks balance. It processes all new experiences and data in relation to the data accumulated throughout my existence. It makes possible great inner transformations, as long as I remain open instead of resisting change for fear of the unknown. Its proper functioning helps to balance my rational and intuitive sides (Yang and Yin). When it is in disharmony, this energy center is related to a disorder in my thoughts. I remain at the level of my intellect, of cold reason and egocentrism, and I thus prevent myself from having an overall view of the great Totality. I become arrogant and scornful of others, which creates problems of confusion in my thoughts and in my relationships. A slowing of the **hypophysis** generally results in laziness and lack of interest. If an imbalance appears, either because my rational side is 'overheating' and I am leaving no space for my intuitive, creative and emotional sides, or because my intuitive side or my psychic gifts are 'overheating' in turn because I want to go too fast: by taking study courses, reading all sorts of books, trying out all sorts of techniques, etc., I am creating

7. It is also linked to what is called the energy center or chakra of the 3rd eye.

8. The gonads correspond to the testicles in men and the ovaries in women.

an imbalance because my physical body can't stand all the inner changes taking place. I will be disorganized and panic will easily take hold of me, for I don't know very well how to react in different situations. It is as if I no longer have any control over what is going on in my life; I listen more to others than to my own inner voice. I have lost my phlegmatic behaviour[9]. When the **hypophysis** is in harmony, it makes me become **Aware** of my mental codings and of the relation between me and my thoughts. It is through this energy center that I can determine what I wish for myself and for others with respect to abundance, and that I can achieve my desires. The accurate view of things is related to this center, and it is through it that I can find solutions. As the **pituitary gland** controls the proper functioning of my organism, I make sure that my body and spirit are in balance by avoiding excesses, and I undertake to master my thoughts and my emotions. If my **hypophysis** is affected by a **tumor**, I may experience a deep feeling of **powerlessness**, with the impression of not being able to reach the objectives I had set for myself. Figuratively speaking, it is as if I was stretching my arm out as far as possible to reach the apple in the tree but can't quite make it. The obstacle may be physical or emotional. I have the impression that I am 'too small' (in both the proper and the figurative sense) to reach the goal and I may be afraid of the means I must use to achieve my ends. How can I reach the summit? How can I be taller? I want to grow fast. I may also want to ***increase*** my power, my self-esteem, my worthiness in the eyes of others, but this seems ***inaccessible*** to me. I don't feel up to it (I who am often a perfectionist). I often have the impression that I am ***out of touch***, upset in my natural rhythm without knowing very well why, and I tend to wonder what is wrong with me. I remain in my prison, repressing everything and refusing to ask for help.

I accept↓♥ that the goals I have set for myself may be too high. I am learning to be very understanding and patient with myself, knowing that I always do my best and that I want the best for myself and for others. By being true, I will always be proud of myself, whatever my achievements. Life takes care of me, and all my wishes will be ***granted***! I accept↓♥ to live my life intensely in the present moment.

GLAND (thymus) *See also: AIDS, SYSTEM [IMMUNE]*

The **thymus** is a small **gland** located in the thorax at the **heart♥** [10] level and that produces a type of white globules (T lymphocytes) that play an essential role in the organism's immune response. It is linked to the immune system, the upper back, the lower lungs, the **heart ♥**, the skin, the blood, the vagus nerve and the circulatory system.

It symbolizes altruism, forgiveness, empathy, my perception of **Love**, divine power, the will of the **Soul** and the unity of universal **Consciousness**. It is the center of **Love** and exerts its action on the immune system that produces the

9. **Phlegmatic**: Calm, imperturbable.
10. The **thymus** is the endocrine **gland** that is directly related to the energy center of the **heart♥**, also called the **heart♥** chakra.

lymphocytes. It is influenced by the hypothalamus and integrity. It is a YIN-YANG center, at once male and female. It is related to the capacity for being touched and feeling things, and is related to unconditional **Love**. It is a relay, a link between the **Love** of my parents and how I position myself toward that **Love**. It is responsible for the immunity of the newborn child. Its activity decreases with age. When this center is in **disharmony**, it means **a non-acceptance of oneself**. I will find it difficult to give and receive and I will feel uneasy with **Love**. I will be afraid of rejection or ridicule. I will retreat into silence to protect myself. When there is resentment, my energy is centered on hate and is used for revenge instead of forgiveness, which causes a decrease in energy because the lack of **Love** leads to a decrease of immunity.

A difficulty in the **thymus** also tells me that I feel that something that belongs to me has been taken from me, that I have been dispossessed of something vital to my life. It may be my job, my spouse, a material object, etc. "The food was snatched right out of my mouth!" For a moment, I therefore felt 'defenseless', not knowing how to react: this is how it goes in my struggles with others. My reflex is to ask my mother for help in extricating myself. I seek autonomy, but I doubt myself. My insecurity leads me to want to cling to others. I refuse to take care of myself with **Love** and acceptance↓♥ of who I am. I live in sacrifice. The fact of holding on to my past prevents me from living the present moment. A **tumor** in my **thymus** (**thymoma**) indicates to me a questioning of who I am in relation to my family, of how I position myself with respect to my roots.

When the **thymus** is in **harmony**, it helps me to be **Conscious of my identity**. It is a channel of divine **Love**. I am capable of inner healing and unconditional **Love**. I do things from the **heart♥**, I give and receive with **Love** and I find the strength to not be manipulated. I accept↓♥ that forgiveness is necessary for my development and inner harmony. The joy of living increases my immunity. I realize how protected I am in my everyday life. I appreciate what I have here and now, for life is but movement, and what I will have tomorrow may be different from today. The more I detach myself from the material world, the greater is my feeling of freedom! I let go of hate and the duality in me and I replace it with the truth.

GLAND (thyroid) (in general)

The **thyroid gland** is located at the base of the neck, under the larynx. It is directly related to the throat[11]. It is linked to the respiratory system, the throat, the back of the neck, the jaws, the ears, the voice, the trachea, the bronchi, the upper parts of the lungs and the arms.

The **thyroid** is the center of speech, verbal expression and creativity. It also acts on the neuromuscular system. This **gland** is related to self-expression and communication. Through this energy center, I express my tears, my joys, my anxieties and my feelings. Essentially a producer of energy, the role of this

11. It is also related to the energy center called the throat chakra.

gland is to secrete two very important hormones, thyroxine and triothyronine, both of which have the distinctive feature of containing iodine, known as a powerful antiseptic and necessary for the proper functioning of the entire body. These hormones activate the metabolism of cells and cellular growth and functions. Without them, I could not live. Because the **thyroid regulates** the body's temperature, it also acts like a thermostat and makes what goes on inside of me adjust to outside conditions. My body can thus harmoniously express my emotions and my thoughts.

The **thyroid** also symbolizes my capacity for expressing my divinity and outwardly displaying my creativity. It shows me how to take my place instead of letting myself be limited by others. My **thyroid** reacts when I am 'left breathless'. I am helpless because I can only remain silent in a given situation. "Do I agree with the **rules** I impose on myself?" When this energy center is in **disharmony**, it indicates a non-expression of myself. I often have the impression of having a lump in my throat, I rationalize, I become rigid and refuse my own right to exist. My words will be abrupt and my communications will become conflicted. I don't take my place. I smother and feel a prisoner. I am like a butterfly with its wings cut off. The normal hormone level determines self-control: **hyperthyroidia**, heat and exhaustion; and **hypothyroidia**, cold and slowing down.

Because this energy center is also linked to self-expression, a case of a **hyper- or hypo-functioning thyroid** may present itself if I feel I am always choking on insults or that life is unfair with me. Obligingly playing this role, I even reach the point where I provoke problematic situations around me in order to increasingly be a 'poor victim'. I feel like dropping everything, ***getting out*** far away from my problems or shipping them off to the other end of the world. I'd like them to ***disappear***. Also, when I am having a conflict with time and I feel forced or urged to go faster or slower, the **thyroid** will react. I may feel unable to create for lack of time, or feel that I had to grow up too fast or had to become an adult too early, or that I am not quick enough to catch something, etc.

The neck, connecting my head to my body, enables me to sign YES or NO and makes of this region the link between the body and the spirit. If my pride is overpowering and closes my **heart♥**, I bypass my true needs. The throat's energy center represents my creativity. I may feel in a submissive position before an outside authority. I idealize others, but it makes me feel inferior. This attitude can make my body react with a **thyroid cancer:** others become tools to fill my inner void. I fear power because I deny mine, which leads me to live passively.

When the **thyroid** is in **harmony,** I feel open to others and ready to listen, but I am not easily influenced. I can say no when it is warranted. I remain open-minded and I become creative. I am able to tell the truth, without judging myself or others. This center of creativity (speech) enables me to have a balanced **Love** relationship when expressing my **Love**. Instead of wanting power over others, I should trust my inner voice.

Right now, I accept↓♥ to express myself freely and I use all my resources. I develop my creative spirit. I accept↓♥ to live in Truth.

GLAND (thyroid) — BASEDOW'S DISEASE / EXOPHTALMIC GOITER

Basedow's[12] **disease** is a pathological state caused by a hyper-secretion of **thyroid** hormones, and characterized by an abnormal protuberance of the ocular globes and an increase of the **thyroid**'s volume. This disease affects women more often than men. The persons affected undergo an increase in their whole metabolism and are filled with 'nervous energy'. The nervous system is irritable and always in a 'hyper' state due to the incapacity to bind iodine. They present sleep disorder, hand tremors, weight loss, nervousness and heavy sweating.

With this hyperactivity, what am I trying to show others? What am I unable to express? I may want to prove who I AM without being able to stop. I am always doing more than what is asked of me. I am constantly in a whirl and continually putting a strain on my thyroid gland. I repress my true feelings, I don't express them, I choke them back but I want to show them, or even 'get revenge'. To whom do I need to prove something? I punish myself because I wasn't able to save someone or a situation in time. My guilt is great. I have become distrustful and I feel forced to do everything myself, which gives me the impression of no longer having any control over events.

I learn to express things as I go along, I choose to do my best without constantly being 'performing', and I thus let go of self-destruction. I notice that I need to give (even something I haven't been asked for) in order to feel loved, while finding it difficult to receive things. I choose to take care of myself, I accept↓♥ to recognize my needs and take stock of who I really am. I stop going in circles and I understand that I don't need to do so much in order to be appreciated. I take the time to express myself, respect myself and choose myself. I learn to **love** and accept↓♥ myself as I am: I thus find stability in my health and balance in my everyday life.

GLAND (thyroid) — EXOPHTALMIC GOITER *See: GLAND [THYROID] — BASEDOW'S DISEASE*

GLAND (thyroid) — GOITER

A **goiter** is a swelling of the anterior part of the neck. A **goiter** usually shows that my **thyroid gland** is overactive.

This results from an acceleration of several bodily and mental processes. This **gland** is responsible, notably, for regulating the respiratory process. It is closely related to my desire to live, to my involvement in life. **Hyperthyroidia**

---

12. **Basedow** (Karl von): A German physician (1799–1854). We owe him the description of hyperthyroidia (**Basedow's** disease).

is a stressful response that denotes my anguish, my sorrow and other intense but unexpressed emotions that make my **thyroid gland** (throat) swell. **I have the impression everything is going too fast!** For lack of organization or because of a very low energy level, I feel in an endless whirl of events that overwhelm me. It can also result from a feeling of being smothered by life and my responsibilities. My **thyroid gland** asks itself: "Should I continue maintaining life or not?" I should express my needs, desires and emotions instead of repressing them, in order to allow my **thyroid gland** to function normally. If a **goiter** results from **hypothyroidia**, because the **thyroid gland** has worked insufficiently over a long period of time, as if it was vanishing, this manifestation displays my defeatist personality and my tendency to despair, for I have little taste for accomplishing things and I take the attitude of a 'victim' about what happens to me. I thus endure much annoyance and bitterness and feel that the whole world resents me. A **goiter** shows me how much I can feel abandoned by others. I need **Love** and attention, but I prefer to live in withdrawal. I escape my anxieties by shutting out my emotions. I want to hold everything inside of me.

I accept↓♥ to develop a more positive attitude and take myself in charge to be able to reach my goals.

GLAND (thyroid) — HYPERTHYROIDIA

It denotes hyperactivity, excessive activity in the **thyroid gland**. My metabolism increases, I get hot and I sweat.

I am greatly disappointed over not being able to accomplish what I really want to do, or unable to express what I have to say, for I respond to the expectations of others instead of my own. I feel bypassed by events. I accumulate unexpressed thoughts and I crush my own personality. I feel compelled to respond to the expectations of others. I then experience resentment, frustration and hate toward everything that doesn't fully meet my expectations. I reach the point where I focus my attention only on negative things. Or I may always listen to the advice of others without listening to my own inner voice. I build myself my own prison that I can't easily get rid of because I turn down those who could help me. I feel powerless to change things in my life. I also set very short deadlines for myself, which makes me always rush to finish current projects on time. **I always have to go faster**! I must ***dash things off*** in a wink (especially in business), which subjects me to great stress. I have the impression that things are very ***fleeting*** and quickly disappear and that I don't really have the time to enjoy it. As when the children grow up too fast, or when I worry too much about them. I have countless unfulfilled desires. When my **thyroid** is **hyperactive**, I often have difficulty in dealing with time and the fact of being late. I try to see if the fact of focusing so much attention on certain things in particular allows me to neglect other responsibilities. I become a little like a child living innocent and carefree, trusting that others will take care of the things for which I don't want to be responsible. My body then sends me a message. I have lost contact with my deeper self. I prefer to stay on the surface of things and my emotions rather than go deeper and risk making unexpected discoveries.

I accept↓♥ that life is not a sprint[13] but a ***marathon***. I take over my power at last. I thus take my decisions and I create my actions according to my inner discernment. I am the co-creator of my life.

GLAND (thyroid) — HYPOTHYROIDIA

Hypothyroidia is an under-functioning of the **thyroid gland**, a **thyroid** failure. The physical causes are: a breakdown of the immune system, a destruction of the **thyroid** by **thyroiditis** with or without the formation of antibodies, and an iodine deficiency, which result in an increased cholesterol level, fatigue, tingling and coldness in the extremities, constipation and a lowering of the reflexes, an increase in the volume of the tongue, etc.

Discouragement can even appear, making me morose and defeatist, with a feeling of being misunderstood. My body is sending me a SOS. The metaphysical causes are important also. The throat chakra is linked to my communications and my creativity. How are my communications with myself, my close relatives and others? How do I exercise my creativity in what I do? What is the resentment I carry that is 'eating me up inside'? Where does this absence of desire for my life come from? **Hypothyroidia** may also come from my incapacity for facing a situation that has reappeared several times in my life and to which I don't know how to react. I should be going slow, but I find this is asking me a lot, either at work or in my interpersonal relations, for example: I 'rush things too much' and I should slow down and give myself some time and the other person too. I want to flee my responsibilities. I prefer to live in an unreal world. I create an artificial security for myself. I find it ***hard*** to have to be resigned to the fact that I am overwhelmed by events.

I accept↓♥ to remain in contact with my emotional and physical body. I am safe and I have everything I need to face my responsibilities. I am the creator of my life. I communicate harmony all around me. Confident, I see life with a new outlook. I let myself be supported by life, as a ***kite*** is lifted off by the wind.

GLAND (thyroid) — THYROIDITIS

Thyroiditis is an inflammation of the **thyroid gland**. The most common form is **Hashimoto's**[14] **thyroiditis**.

I am experiencing a situation that often involves the family and where I feel stuck because I can't express my frustrations and my anger. I end up living in slow motion because my negative emotions are gnawing at me inside. I feel like spitting fire, but I don't want to reveal certain secrets that could risk

---

13. **Sprint**: The fastest speed a runner can achieve during a race.

14. Also known as **Hashimoto**'s disease, **Hashimoto**'s thyroiditis is named after the Japanese physician **Hashimoto** Hakaru (1881–1934) of the medical school at Kyushu University, who first described the symptoms in 1912 in a German publication.

breaking up the family unit. I prefer to remain silent and feel stuck rather than to open the door of my **heart♥** and dare to express myself.

I accept↓♥ to recognize and welcome the emotions I have inside of me. I choose to verbalize them in order to free myself of them. The **Love** and the **Light** that I carry form a shield that protects me in every instant.

GLANDS (lacrimal) *See: CRYING*

GLANDS (salivary) *See also: MUMPS, SALIVA*

The **salivary glands**, the largest of which is the **parotid**, are symbols of **Love** and sweetness. As these **glands** are part of the digestive apparatus, a bad functioning of my **salivary glands**, producing too little or too much saliva, indicates that I am feeling insecure about finding the food necessary for my survival. Maybe I don't have the money to buy food, or I have the money but don't know how best to use it. I may also fear poisoning myself. So food is available, but either I can't buy it, it is out of reach or I don't trust it. My mouth will water and I will experience a feeling of deprivation. I want to stock up as much as I can in case there is a food shortage and I am deprived of food. In a broader sense, I may be a person who likes to collect things: here, I have an unconscious need to stock up on certain objects, for fear of not being able to obtain them someday. However, this has the effect of intoxicating and soiling my vital space. If I am prevented from doing it, I may depreciate myself and **parotiditis**[15] may ensue. An **inflammation of the salivary glands** reveals my dissatisfaction with one of my parents. I may also wonder if I feel like baring my teeth. Am I in rivalry with someone? Do I feel the truth has been soiled? Was I in contact with another person's saliva and it upset me? I feel coerced to denature things. Where does my impatience come from?

I accept↓♥ the anger in me and allow it to express itself in order to restore peace and harmony. I accept↓♥ the situations I experience by becoming **Aware** that I too have the right to feed myself well and life gives me all I need.

GLANDS (sublingual) *See: GLAND [SALIVARY]*

GLAUCOMA *See: EYES — GLAUCOMA*

GOITER *See: GLAND [THYROID] — GOITER*

GONADS *See also: OVARIES, TESTICLES*

The **gonads** produce gametes (spermatozoa in men and ova in women) and sexual hormones that fight mental anorexia, asthenia and promote physical and affective energy. This center is linked to creativity and reproduction.

When this center is in **disharmony,** my sexuality is focused on selfish pleasure and possessive **Love**. I am losing contact with the innocence of my

15. **Parotiditis**: An inflammation of the **parotid** gland, which is the main **salivary gland**.

inner child. I lack maturity and spontaneity, I distrust the opposite sex and I refuse the tenderness that is offered to me. I lack self-confidence. I blow a fuse very easily and fly in a rage for trifles. I must ask myself what I have lost and is causing me such great sorrow: it may be a child who has left or has died (a person dear to me), a material possession or a symbolic loss such as a loss of my self-esteem or my pride, etc. I no longer feel that I am the creator of my life, and I adopt a defeatist attitude to life.

When I am in harmony, I feel spontaneous and open to relations with persons of the opposite sex. Life flows fully in me and this center is linked to all forms of pleasure. When this center is in balance, I know how to adjust to situations and life makes me passionate and enthusiastic. I am comfortable in the bustle of life, without any resistance. I communicate confidently without any biases and I accept↓♥ myself in my entirety as a man or a woman. I accept↓♥ to let go of my fears and I build up my trust in myself and in life.

GOUT *See also: ACIDOSIS, GALLSTONES / RENAL CALCULI*

Gout is a metabolic disease characterized by an accumulation of uric acid in the organism, affecting the joints, especially in the big toe, and sometimes taking the form of renal lithiasis (renal calculi). It also frequently affects the hands, the wrists, the fingers, the knees, the ankles and sometimes the elbows.

The accumulation of uric acid means that I am holding back negative emotions that should normally be released in the urine. I need to have my vital space and some solitude, but I allow my entourage to invade me. I feel pushed from behind. The way in which certain animal species mark out their territory is to urinate all around it to set down their boundaries, as a sort of barrier (cats, for example, do this). It is their way of showing the rest of the world the place that belongs to them. If we follow the analogy with humans, I know that urine (fluid) represents my emotions. If I can't express them, an overflow of emotions will result, as an excess of fluid inside the body. The emotions involved here refer to my frustrations, my disappointments, my incapacity to assert my limits, my zone of intolerance, for I want to be the 'good boy' or the 'good girl' in the eyes of others. I want to avoid being scolded, judged or criticized; so I remain silent, but this disgusts me. **Gout** is a starting point of a hesitation between pleasure and duty: by becoming bedridden, there are no more choices left to make. I feel 'stuck in the past' and looking to the future is difficult. My body becomes as rigid as my thoughts and as my attitude toward myself and others. Clinging to my past prevents me from advancing, and I feel stuck because I don't know what direction to take. I am '**drowning** in my sorrow'. I can act very impatiently when things aren't going as I want. I need to completely **dominate** and **control** my life, which can sometimes prove very difficult. I can go to the opposite extreme and be impatient and angry and try to dominate the others, thinking that this will restore some balance in my life. **Gout** thus appears in someone who is very ambitious and rigid or, on the contrary, in a person who has no goals and no enthusiasm about the future. My ambitions are very limited and people shouldn't ask too much of me.

Otherwise, it is 'the last straw that broke the camel's back'! Despair then takes hold of me. **Gout** indicates that I want to hide my emotionality and my sensitivity by showing myself to be strong. My insecurity leads me to be possessive, as I feel left aside and not integrated, in my family or in my community. I want to hold on to everything. I have such a need to prove my worthiness and what I am capable of! I feel vulnerable with my own emotions and I am intransigent about what I judge to be negative, bad or evil. The **big toe** is affected when I collapse upon hearing news that vitally affects my life. As **gout** often presents itself in men beyond middle age, I may have to learn to let others be, instead of dominating them; to trust in life instead of controlling; and to be more flexible with myself and others instead of being rigid. I no longer have to endure an inner conflict between the pleasures of life and my duties: I now find myself 'forced' to be inactive and to enjoy a 'well-deserved rest'!

I must allow more **Love** to enter me to balance and release the negative, painful, hurtful and angry emotions so that I can recover my movement, my freedom and my well-being. I accept↓♥ that all my inner emotions are part of who I am and I must accept↓♥ them to help me understand why they live in me. By expressing them, I discover who I really am, I am in contact with my inner power and I can detach myself from the persons I clung to before.

GRAND MAL SEIZURE *See: BRAIN — EPILEPSY*

GRIEF / SORROW *See also: MELANCHOLY*

Grief is related to a form of anxiety, a worry or a sadness that manifest themselves by crying, sounds of pain, solitude or the gritting of teeth.

My **heart♥** is wounded and sick following a regrettable and painful past experience. My **grief** may be long-lasting or short-lived. I look for the real cause, often deep or unconscious. After many years, several childhood injuries can resurface, along with certain gains in **Awareness**.

I accept↓♥ to remain open to what I am experiencing and quickly identify the true source of my **grief** to be able to change it. I accept↓♥ what I have become **Aware** of and I integrate it. I recover my joy in living and I have 'grown taller'.

GROIN *See also: GANGLION [LYMPHATIC NODES], HERNIA*

The **groin** is the region joining the abdomen and the thigh by forming a fold.

When this region is affected by an **abscess**, a **pain** or a **lymphatic engorgement**, it indicates a gap between my desires (most often sexual) and my actions. I retreat into myself and don't express my dissatisfaction. Feeling in a prison, I reach the point where I feel hate. I live more in my head than in my emotions, and I am always in a rush. I resist my deep needs for calm and rest. I refuse to allow my creative urges to express themselves. I thus curtail my freedom and my dynamic is affected. Do I agree with what I feel and what I do? A **hernia** in this area shows me that I have had enough of living for others.

I cling to the past, though the way I have lived so far no longer satisfies me. I have forced myself to stay in certain situations (affectively as well as at work) for fear of expressing my creativity. Outwardly, my life seems calm and under control, but I am destroying myself inside. A **swelling of the lymph ganglions** in the **groin** indicates that I am rejecting my true nature. I am creating obstacles for myself that will become 'good reasons' for not carrying out my true desires and passions.

I accept↓♥ to open myself to my emotions and to let the energy flow. This is how I can know true freedom, by being in contact with everything that is inside of me, which I can thus integrate and surpass.

GUILLAIN-BARRÉ'S SYNDROME *See: SYNDROME [GUILLAIN-BARRÉ'S]*

GUILT FEELINGS *See: ACCIDENT*

GUM DISORDERS *See also: ABSCESS, MOUTH (IN GENERAL), TEETH (IN GENERAL)*

The **gums** serve to support the solidity of the teeth, and the state of the teeth greatly depends on the state of the **gums**. The **upper gums** are related to male energy and the father, while the **lower gums** are related to female energy and the mother.

Gum disorders indicate that I feel stuck with a person or a situation because I persist in remaining in the past. Instead of climbing up the next step, I rather feel like backing down. Indecision is very present in my life. I have doubts because I wonder if I will be able to support my decisions and their consequences in my life. A **pain in the gums** may be related either to a decision I should have made a long time ago and have been putting off, for fear of the consequences this decision may have on my life; or to a decision I have already made but haven't yet carried out. I am in a passive state of fear, insecurity and uncertainty about my future. The words I say carry no weight. I am often angry with myself. I feel left to my own devices, and I find it difficult to define my tolerance zones and my limits. It is like a small volcano erupting and letting long-repressed negative emotions burst out. I may be feeling intense inner pain about the emotional nourishment that I need and feel I am lacking. If I feel **emotionally estranged**, especially from my mother or my children, and I am collecting sorrow and disappointment while feeling guilt over what is happening, an **abscess** will appear. I want to get rid of my inner suffering and expel it at all costs, to be rid of it forever. If my **gums** are also **bleeding**, I am experiencing a loss of joy over decisions about which I feel torn and tormented. Sensitive **gums** that will sometimes even swell reveal my great emotional sensitivity and my vulnerability, for I need much **Love**, and I feel I am not receiving any, or afraid of losing it. I feel vulnerable about the limits I have imposed on myself and about my capacity for discerning what is good for me and what isn't. I feel resourceless and left to my own devices. I resent myself for some of my words or gestures, and my **gums** will be affected.

I accept↓♥ to assert myself and to have more self-confidence because the **gums** support the teeth, which in turn are linked to decisions. I learn to trust myself in the decisions I make, and I also trust in life that brings me everything I need. I thus become more truly myself, and I learn to assert myself freely. I am consistent in my actions. I look at reality face on, letting go of my past and confident about what the future holds for me.

GUMS (bleeding) *See also: BLOOD — BLEEDING*

Bleeding gums show my insecurity and doubts about a decision I must take in my life, and show a loss of joy in my self-expression. Am I right to be having doubts or regrets? I find it difficult to hold my positions and to be firm in my decisions. I feel that my freedom is under attack. I feel helpless and hold others responsible for my discomfort.

I take my responsibilities and I calmly accept↓♥ the changes that occur in my life. I trust myself because I know that the choices I make are there to make me grow further and enable me to pursue my development.

GUMS — GINGIVITIS (acute)

An infection in the **gums** indicates that I am feeling fear; it may be about myself or a decision I made and now regret, or a decision I have made that I am calling into question; or it may be about my indecisiveness in coming to a decision. This fear may also concern another person (my boss, my spouse, my religion, for example) whose decisions may directly affect me and over which I have no control. Someone has acted too fast, and this irritates me. I feel frustration and dissatisfaction, which could lead to confrontations that may not be necessary. The **upper gums** refer to my work or my role in society. The **lower gums** refer to my whole emotional side. When the **gums** become inflamed, they express distress and poor self-defense accompanied by lassitude, melancholy and fear. I learn to channel this fear and express it in order to avoid inflammation in my **gums**. **Gingivitis** usually involves **bleeding** in the **gums**, which indicates sadness or loss of joy over not being able to express myself, either because I am not allowed to or because I am the one preventing myself from saying certain things: I may feel that what I am saying is not important and I won't be listened to. As the **gums** are the foundations upon which my teeth rest, I may also experience anger and sadness, with the impression that my foundations are collapsing and leaving me with a feeling of powerlessness over life's events or in relation to others. I stamp around and criticize instead of seeing how I could move ahead in my life, by leaving the past behind. A feeling of powerlessness is gripping a person affected by **expulsive gingivitis**, which is characterized by **receding gums**. Reality is no longer holding fast, and my inner strength is affected by this. My **gums** are awash in the tears of my teeth — my emotions. I always ask myself if I have made the right decisions and I have difficulty in maintaining my choices. I am experiencing an extreme duality because I doubt myself. I want so much to be accepted↓♥ by others that I will be extremely flexible and understanding, but meanwhile I am putting aside my own personal needs.

I can take a moment of silence with myself to recover my strength. I become **Aware** of the fact that each event of my life is there to make me grow and that any important change is necessary for me to achieve the goals I have set for myself. I accept↓♥ my true worth and I move ahead in life with determination.

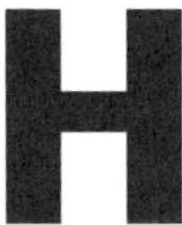

HABITS *See: DEPENDENCE*

HAIR (in general)

Protecting the cutaneous part of the head, the **hair** symbolizes strength, vitality, freedom, beauty and power (think of Samson in the Bible). **For women**, it represents their power of attraction and seduction; and **for men**, their virility. It is directly related to the dignity of a being, to the essence of power, to my self-image. It puts me in contact with the spiritual, cosmic and supra-cosmic energies. It also represents my relation to the father or his equivalent. My **hair** grows near the seventh chakra or energy center, the crown chakra. It is called an 'antenna' because it links the physical to the spiritual. The rootedness of **hair** (and **hairs** in general) physically symbolizes the rootedness of the spiritual world in the physical world. By describing the state of my **hair**, I describe the relation that my spiritual side maintains with my rational and physical side. To some extent, my **hair** symbolizes my female strength, my creativity, my intuition. As it constantly grows, it reminds me how I too, as a human being, must act responsibly about my personal growth or the fact that I have the power to change old ways of thinking, my old notions that slow me down in my development. As **hair** refers to intuition and is a symbol of femininity, it is interesting to note that men who let their **hair** grow are often artists in their Souls, or will more often be young men who are in reaction against the authority that prevails in society and want to reclaim their own power within themselves, where its seat is in their **hearts♥** and their inner voices. The state of one's **hair** is also a representation of one's sexual, genital and reproductive potency. The **hair** is associated with the surrenal glands (energy of fear or confidence) that are related to the ancestral legacy (2nd chakra). Several myths exist about **hair** (blonds, brunettes, the bald). It is important to know that my **hair** is an image of the power I have to direct my own life. What do I really want in life? Do I feel that others are directing my life? My strength and my courage in taking the reins of my life in hand will increase my sense of freedom and the vigor of my **hair**. Their **hair** reflects people's joy in living and its neatness indicates their interest in taking care of themselves and in being here.

I observe the different states of my **hair**, which correspond to certain inner states (**hair** that is split, dull, thin or brittle, thick, etc.). I accept↓♥ to remain open to this glorious power from heaven that is present in my **hair**!

HAIR DISEASE

Several causes may bring about the onset of **hair diseases**: a great emotional shock (such as a fright), an excessive reaction of helplessness before a situation, a latent conflict or several repressed feelings such as despair, worries or boredom. Nervousness sets in, emotional instability grows, and inner strengths and resources are exhausted. I am experiencing an inner disorder. This insecurity may result from my fear of death or the fact that nothing is permanent, that everything can change, suddenly and without warning. Doubt has set in about spirituality, and I am asking myself many questions. I am seeking God or His manifestation in my life and I need 'That' to touch me in the deepest reaches of my being, but at the same time I am afraid of it because I feel vulnerable. I close myself off from the vital energies, and my **hair** changes its appearance. It falls out, becomes oily or dry, whitens (white **hair**), or loses its sheen. **Dandruff** appears, resulting from an inner conflict between me and my social role. I feel that I can't exert any influence around me or leave my mark on the world (a feeling that is present in most diseases affecting my **hair**). I would like to go higher and be the 'Chief', but I don't make it. I feel separated from the world and I don't understand why I remain in the dark, the others being incapable of giving me any reasons or arguments for their actions or words. My stress level is constantly high and I easily become exhausted. I aspire to autonomy, to be recognized by others, to true and clear communications. **Folliculitis** (an inflammation of the follicles) indicates that I don't feel protected. I am like a porcupine, feeling 'cut to the quick'[1]. **Brittle hair** indicates that I feel divided between taking the 'reins' of my life back in hand or leaving that power to someone else because that would suit me somehow. Do I listen to my intuition or to my rational side? I feel powerless and I resist change. I may experience a situation where my **heart♥** is split and divided, and I must make peace with this situation. I need oxygen! It is the first thing to do to bring back strength and vitality to my **hair**.

I accept↓♥ that I need to change my thoughts and my attitude toward the situations of life. I accept↓♥ to remain open and observe what is now taking place, especially how I go about facing the different situations of my life, and I stop **tearing out my hair**! I accept↓♥ to enjoy life and I am more tolerant for myself.

HAIR — ALOPECIA AREATA / PELADA

Alopecia areata is a skin disease characterized by the **loss of hair** in rounded patches.

It may result from an emotional shock, anger or a loss of self-esteem leading me to feel shame and give up the spiritual part of myself or whatever connects me to my highest values. I sometimes feel like a piece of **trash**, I feel my degree of intelligence is low as compared to others, and this is causing difficulties for me in my relations. I was ***exasperated*** by something or someone. It is as if my bodily security was affected and I had lost my protection. I may have experienced a separation, often with my mother, and I am now very worried. I tend to be as 'smart as a fox'[2] to escape embarrassing situations, but

1. **Cut to the quick**: To be affected or touched at one's most sensitive point.
2. **As smart as a fox**: A person who is quick-witted, cunning and subtle.

I thus avoid taking some of my responsibilities. I often feel I have to 'plead my case'[3] for others to listen to me and believe me. My insecurity leads me to feel deep fear that appears repeatedly. The fact of losing my **hair** may return to me the image of my father who had lost his. If he is dead or very old, it is a constant reminder that I will have to separate myself from him, if it is not already done. When I look in the mirror, it is as if I see my father, and this bothers me. I may even want to deny the link that ties us together.

I accept↓♥ to make peace with myself and consider solutions that will enable me to better live in harmony with my highest goals.

HAIR — BALDNESS

Baldness is the partial or total loss of **hair**. Though it is mostly associated with men, more and more women are afflicted with **baldness**.

The **hair** is the mirror of a certain inner strength and of my roots. Samson (in the Old Testament scriptures) lost his strength when his **hair** was cut. The **hair** represents the link between the physical and the spiritual, which links me to the cosmos and spiritual energy. It is often compared to a form of antenna attuned to the beyond. It is said that heredity is the main factor in **baldness**, more frequent among males. However, among the different types of **baldness**, we find the **bald bearded** type, which is associated with individuals who use their intellectual faculties more than their emotional faculties. **Loss of hair** (also called **alopecia**) means that I have moved away from the divine in me. I am a person oriented to the material rather than to the spiritual. I may have a lot of intuition, but I prefer to count mainly on the more material and rational aspects. Often, if I am losing my **hair**, I am experiencing one or several situations where **the tension is so great** that I feel like 'tearing out my **hair**'. Several stressful or even traumatic experiences may accelerate the **baldness** process: a childbirth inducing fear or worrying, a serious emotional shock, a separation, great tension at work or at home, a taste for surpassing myself materially or a depreciation of my intellectual capacities. When I have a lot of worries and great fears, I lose contact with my divine inner power. When I **lose** my **hair**, what do I feel I am losing in my life, or what am I **afraid of losing** in the future (which may be something or someone)? I can revolt: I want to free myself from this pressure that is stifling me. I want to be me, and stop living according to outside obligations. By losing my **hair**, I am freeing myself from what imprisoned me. I probably received little kindness, especially from my father, and I tend to revolt against authority. I am rather materialistic, and spirituality is not very much a part of my life. I try to control everything as much as I can because I am afraid of opening myself up and losing control. I imprison myself in rigid structures and obligations that are no longer needed. I am scattered, and my thoughts are tangled and confused. I am so exasperated over a situation that I am 'tearing my **hair** out'. I am experiencing an inner heartbreak like an ***ordeal***. I don't want my children to miss me and thereby

---

3. **Plead my case**: To have to defend myself and produce arguments.

lose their **Love**. I tend to depreciate myself intellectually and I am experiencing an injustice. If I was gifted for a certain activity in which I excelled and my performance has started to change and decline, my **hair** will fall too. I refuse the basic functioning of life, alleging that I can do better than it. Any inner fear leads to the incapacity to take action, along with despair and tensions that take me unawares. It is an illusion to believe that I can do better than life itself. There is no reason for me to fight life, because it is **always with me** to support me, and it will help me if I listen to it and remain open.

To stop the process of **hair loss** and allow it to grow back, I accept↓♥ to make appropriate changes in my life, which will free me from this additional burden I accepted↓♥ to take on but no longer need. I accept↓♥ to trust in life, with the attitude that everything will be for the best. Instead of seeking my power outside of myself (symbolized by my **hair**), I accept↓♥ to go deep inside of me and draw on all the strength and courage that are there, in order to move ahead and enter a new stage in my life. I learn to harmoniously integrate laws into my life, knowing that they exist for my good, personally as well as collectively. I accept↓♥ to quietly ask, and life will give me what I deserve. This is the start; I must trust in life and in my inner being and see the solutions everywhere, because they do exist! The world is there to help me. What else do I need?

HAIR (Gray)

Gray hair symbolizes wisdom. However, the sudden appearance of **gray hair** is related to stress, to a situation where I experienced an intense emotional shock. When this happens in one's twenties, it represents great worries (tension or stress), **conscious** or unconscious, about allowing oneself to be spiritually guided. Do I believe I need to live under pressure and that the pressures in my life are necessary for my 'own good'? It may be a pattern related to performance in this life. Usually, **gray hair** appears with age, which means a diminishing of vigor and vital strength. It appears at the time when it is important for me to become **Aware** of how I may have come to live for others and not for myself. I am pressured by society, my family, my friends and the obligations related to my work. I live at a pace set by others instead of living at the pace of my personal needs. When was the last time I laughed out loud? As my **hair** represents my power, I must ask myself to whom I am letting it go, because otherwise, my **hair** would keep its natural color.

I revise my general attitudes and accept↓♥ that life continues as it is, no more no less, and I free myself of the burden of being competitive. I discover the treasures buried inside of me. I accept↓♥ that this **gray hair** is the heralding sign of a rebirth to my true self, to a new life filled with joy. I am taking a new direction. I take care of myself. I accept↓♥ all the emotions that are inside of me and that make me an exceptional being. I stop being a slave to time and obligations. I may be disturbed by the new image I project, but it is time for me to live at the level of 'being' instead of 'appearance'.

HAIR LOSS *See: HAIR — BALDNESS*

HAIR — TINEA *See also: HAIR /ALOPECIA AREATA / BALDNESS / LOSS*

Tinea is a parasitic and contagious fungus that affects the surface of my skin, my **hair**, my scalp and my fingernails.

I let myself be affected, 'attacked', 'destroyed' and bothered by others, because I have little self-confidence and I am vulnerable. I feel ugly, dirty and turned off. I may feel I am losing control of certain situations. Thus, my head's hat (my **hair**) will be affected. I may feel very disturbed by the words of others and also affected by the idea they have that 'if the hat fits, then wear it!' I let others decide for me. I was separated from my family or someone I especially liked, and I find this situation despicable.

I accept↓♥ to take my place and trust myself. Only I have power over my life.

HALITOSIS *See: MOUTH — BREATH [BAD]*

HALLUCINATIONS *See also: ALCOHOLISM, DEPENDENCE, DRUG ADDICTION, DRUGS*

When I am physically or emotionally exhausted, I can stack up a mountain of dark thoughts, often false. I can thus be out of my depth in reality without being **Aware** of it, and become disconnected from reality; my body, and the **Soul** that I am, become disconnected. Confronted with a reality that I don't want to see, I invent one for myself, though it may be false, and thus isolate myself from the rest of the world. I can then feel that I am right and 'prove' my own interpretation of this reality that I can't accept↓♥. These interpretations, these imaginary worlds, entirely made up by me, can also highlight my own fears. I may fear my dark and negative side, and I feel that I must defend myself so that it won't appear out in the open.

The **hallucinations** that I see and that scare me only represent the parts of my personality that I deny and refuse to see. Sooner or later, I will need to become **Aware** of them to be able to change them. By denying who I am, I am moving away from my essence and no longer in contact with my inner reality. I feel that life must punish me because I am not perfect. I have the impression that I have a double personality: the person that everyone **loves**, and the negative one I want to escape from. I feel powerless over the negative one. I may have **hallucinations** when I experience a very high level of stress, and I tend to shoulder heavy burdens.

For instance, if I am searching for a document that I absolutely need, and the loss of which would involve millions of dollars, my brain may create an image of this document (a hologram) that will seem quite real and will lower my level of stress for a few moments. Later on, upon realizing that it was a **hallucination**, I can now think more clearly and ask for help in my search, or explore other places where the document is likely to be found. Without this **hallucination**, I would have continued to be a 'prisoner' of my state of stress. As far as **drugs** are concerned, they create a state of expanded consciousness. The person can thus experience dimensions that are ordinarily inaccessible to them. Why am I taking **drugs**? Is it to escape my inner sufferings that I am unable to face without help? ***I may become dependent on drugs***, whatever they are. They can provide me with a temporary state of well-being. But once I am 'straight' again, back to normal, the tune isn't the same any longer. Where to search, then? Inside of me. I only enter there with **Love** and with my personal and spiritual development.

I seek a spirituality that frees me from the chains of the past and gives me back my freedom and my autonomy. It is also possible that following an accident, intense stress or simply my personal and spiritual development, my third eye will open increasingly wider, enabling me to see colors around persons, currents of energy in space or translucent (immaterial) presences in my entourage. I may thus feel that I am having **hallucinations** mainly because my sensitivity is usually greater when I experience this sort of perception.

I accept↓♥ to refocus myself and re-balance my body and the **Soul** that I am. I then trust myself and feel surrounded by white and golden **Light**, knowing that I am constantly guided and protected. I increasingly like to discover and experience my true reality, the 'I AM'. I accept↓♥ all the emotions that are part of who I am, I look at them head-on and I make peace with them: they can thus help me to discover what I want to change in my life and take the appropriate actions in order to concretely achieve my desires.

HANDS (in general)

The **hands** represent my capacity for taking, giving or receiving. They symbolize the performance of the act and execution of work. They are the intimate expression of myself in the Universe, and the power of **touch** is so great that I feel helpless when my **hands** are damaged. They enable me to exchange with others, but also to command. Their character is unique: like my fingerprints, they represent my past, my present and my future. My **left hand** is that of the **heart♥**, the one that receives and catches. My **right hand** represents my will, my power. It represents action and assertion. I hold in my **hands** the situations of my everyday life, and the state of my **hands** shows to what extent I grasp my reality, how far I express **Love** as well as hate (in the form of a fist), how I '**hand**le' events or people. The quality of my contacts with others is reflected in my **hands**, notably those who are involved in my work. If my **hands** are **cold**, I withdraw emotionally from a situation or a relationship in which I am involved. I may also refuse to take care of my basic needs and enjoy myself. I may feel that my relationship with my father is a cold one. A situation involving death disturbs me. **Sweaty hands** betray an excessive level of anxiety and nervousness. I am overwhelmed by emotions, feeling maybe too involved or too active in a certain situation of my everyday life. I want to fix everything and 'put out the fires' myself with my **hands**. Maybe I fear a contact where I will be hurt. If I feel **pain** or **cramps**, it is because I refuse to be flexible in some current situations. I must ask myself what is bothering me, or what it is that I don't want to achieve. I may have a feeling of impotence or a great fear of failure. This makes me want to bring everything under control with my **hands**, or want to possess everything in case something or someone should 'slip through my **fingers**'. Do I feel I am losing control over a situation or a person? Has some **gesture** or action done with my **hands** had the result of causing an injury, physical or emotional? Am I capable of 'taking things in **hand**' and rendering my ideas concretely? If my **hands** are also **bleeding** (e.g.: dry **hands**, eczema, etc.), there is surely a situation in my life, a dream or a project that I feel I can't achieve, and that makes me feel sad. I outdid myself and it didn't work. Then my joy in living goes away. If my **hands** become **paralyzed**, I may feel 'paralyzed' over the means for carrying out a certain task or action, and I feel helpless about it. Paralysis in the **hands** can also occur after a very intense mental activity where I feel overexcited or thwarted and pressure is boiling up inside of me. I may even feel like 'wringing someone's neck' with my **hands**. My **hands** will be **stiff** if I show rigidity in the way I carry out certain tasks or express what I feel. They will even **block** when I feel under the sway of parental authority. If I **injure my hands**, maybe I am resisting being touched, avoiding a certain intimacy, or the touch I can give or receive from another person. This fear of making contact may be linked to a special current event that reminds me of an abuse experienced in the past. It may have been an event where I felt **manipulated**, and I am re-living the same feeling in my current life. It is also a good thing to ask myself: "What am I incapable of doing, or what am I forced to do now, for me to feel **pain** in one or both of my **hands**? Who or what do I want to hold back with my **hands**, and that I should instead release and let go of? Who do I feel like 'punching'?" If my **hands** are affected, I ask myself what part of me I want to dismissively 'flick away with the back of my **hand**'. I tend to be uncompromising with myself or with others. This may be in reaction to the fact that I was always very accommodating in the past, without always being supported in my actions, hence a possible **fracture**. I force myself to follow a certain route, when I might well take another one more beneficial for me. Do I lead my life by reason or by my intuition? What do I feel I must ***maintain*** at all costs in my life? Is it my social status, my lifestyle, my popularity? An injury in the ***palm of my hand*** indicates a fear of losing myself, of ***straying***, or 'being left **stranded**', emotionally or socially. The **back of the hand** is affected when I feel rejected, when I have been cast aside or given a 'back-**hand**ed blow'.

I accept↓♥ to let go and 'reach my **hands** to the sky', by becoming **Aware** that the only power I have is over myself and not over others. I take my life 'in **hand**' by accepting↓♥ all the facets of my being.

HANDS (arthrosis in) *See: ARTHRITIS — ARTHROSIS*

HANDS — DUPUYTREN'S DISEASE *See also: FINGERS / ATRIAL [AURICULAR] / RING FINGER*

Dupuytren's[4] disease affects the **hand** by a permanent flexion of certain fingers toward the palm, especially the ring finger and the little finger.

This disease shows a 'contraction' in my attitudes, denoting a withdrawal into myself, shutting out my spouse or my children. I feel like someone is holding my reins, I am being 'held by my ***bridle***', someone is trying to put the ***brakes*** on a project. Or maybe it is I who wants to have everything, is reluctant to let go and won't 'let go of the reins'. I wanted to get better control over my life, but everything is escaping me and I lack the strength. With my **hands** closed and contracted, what am I trying to keep for myself at all costs? Or what do I no longer want to take?

I accept↓♥ to be more flexible and openly express my emotions. I accept↓♥ to see the deeper meaning of my life.

HARE LIP *See: CLEFT PALATE*

HASHISH CONSUMPTION *See: DRUGS*

HATE

Hate is the cause of many diseases. Maintaining **hate** makes me detest other persons, makes me nasty, impels me to hurl biting words with rage in my **heart♥**. The feeling of **hate** leads to self-destruction: it destroys the person who still maintains it even more than the person or the situation concerned. When I experience **hate** or **rage**, I feel something burning in me, in different systems: the digestive, the pulmonary, and also the gallbladder and the liver.

Increasingly serious 'dis-eases' are portended in this progression of signs displayed by the body. I may even attract a cancer. **Hate** appears when I feel that others are preventing me from living my life. I want to have my own way, and when things are not going my way, I strongly react. Instead of remaining open and trying to understand the other person's point of view, I persist in staying on my position. I thus refuse all responsibility for my life.

I accept↓♥ that **Love** is the basis of all life. I learn to forgive myself and forgive others. I accept↓♥ to understand people and situations differently, with **Love**. It is only in openness to others that I can change my view of things and free myself of these judgments and this **hate** of which I was a prisoner.

HAY FEVER *see: ALLERGY — HAY FEVER*

---

4. **Dupuytren**, (Guillaume, Baron): A French surgeon (1777 – 1835). Considered as one of the founders of pathological anatomy, became in 1815 the chief surgeon of the Hôtel-Dieu de Paris Hospital. In 1829 he wrote *Leçons orales de clinique chirurgicale* in which he gave, among other things, a description of the bimalleolar fracture and the retraction of the palmar aponeurosis, a disease that bears his name.

HEAD (in general)

My **head** is my communications center, **it is related to my individuality and my autonomy**. It is often called the 'control center'. It is through it that all my emotions and all my communications pass, by means of my five senses. It is my **head** that governs.

If I am experiencing difficulties or ailments in my **head**, I must ask myself if I am experiencing a conflict involving my thoughts, my spiritual life, my personal growth, or some reality that I don't want to deal with. This can be explained by the fact that the **head** is made up of bones, which are made up of a hard tissue and symbolize my spiritual energy, and these bones surround the soft tissues and the fluids, which symbolize my mental and emotional energies. If both aspects are in harmony, there will be a fusion of my body and spirit. However, if the blood in my **head** is not circulating well or is exerting pressure, this indicates that I have difficulty in expressing or receiving **Love** and any feeling that inhabits me (for the blood transports my feelings throughout my body). My incapacity, or my too great desire, to control induces a discomfort in my **head**. I don't feel that I measure up, which prevents me from fully playing my role as a leader.

As my **head** receives and expresses various aspects of my communications, with the body's outwardly displayed sensations and impressions, I accept↓♥ to learn how to remain open to my entourage, and accept↓♥ the messages entering my senses throughout my body, to learn the lessons of life that bring me greater spiritual awakening.

HEAD — MIGRAINES

Migraines are characterized by an intense pain that usually affects only one side of the **head**. They occur in the form of attacks and are accompanied by nausea.

They diminish my vital strength. I tend to withdraw into my corner instead of fully taking part in life. **Migraines** are also often associated with eyesight and digestive disorders: I no longer want to see, and no longer want to digest, what is going on in my life. They involve anxieties and frustration over a situation where I am unable to make a decision. I may have a sense of something that must be done or achieved or is required of me. A **migraine** often appears after having experienced an annoyance. A change in my pace of life, involving a difficulty in adjusting on my part, may also generate a **migraine** (like a **weekend migraine** for example). It reveals my resistance related to my incapacity for carrying out what is asked of me. My **head** 'overheats' and hurts at the mere idea of the goal to be reached, which seems inaccessible. My **head** resembles a pressure cooker[5], and the pressure is so high that I don't always know what solution or what attitude to adopt. The pressure may come from

5. **Pressure cooker**: A cooking vessel that is hermetically sealed, equipped with a steam control, and used to cook food under steam pressure.

my desire to be hyper-responsible and/or performing, especially at work. I can be passionate about a subject and find it difficult to stop myself. There is a conflict between my thoughts, my overloaded intellect and my personal needs and desires. Do I feel up to standard of do I feel incompetent, especially in the intellectual sphere? Why do I resent myself or experience so much hate? I feel under constant surveillance: when it is not the others, it is I who am monitoring everything and wanting to control everything in my life. They poke fun at me and I lose my **head** over it. By constantly turning my problems over in my **head**, I end up forgetting that I exist, that I have emotions that demand to be expressed. I tend to deny reality, which greatly increases my level of stress. I must become **Aware** of the fact that I am running away from what bothers me, or I feel some misunderstanding and a lack of **Love** on someone's part. It is important for me to identify what emotion I want so much to repress, or what situation I want so much to forget, that is creating a constant acute tension inside of me, provoking a **migraine**. **Migraines** can also be linked to sexual problems, such as its repression since childhood, resurfacing. It is like a struggle going on inside of me between my thoughts and my sexuality, and it goes to my **head**. I may have the impression that my **head** is about to explode. I may also ask myself questions about my father's identity, either consciously or unconsciously. My life structures need to be adjusted to my current situation, but it is hard to let go of the familiar to move toward the unknown. When a **migraine** is located in the **forehead**, I ask myself with respect to what situation I feel diminished and helpless. I need to perform better and find a solution, but I feel limited in my capacities, especially my intellectual capacities. I must understand that when I have a **migraine**, there is something I must become **Aware** of, there are things I must change and I must be able to change them, by taking action. And a **migraine** gives me a pause, which can also be a way to obtain more **Love** and attention.

I accept↓♥ to face reality head on. I allow events to flow freely in my life, and in return I receive joy, peace and harmony. By being more flexible and tolerant with myself, I feel lighter and can fly off like a hot-***air balloon***.

HEADACHES

Headaches can have several causes. For example: stress and tension, when I try as best I can to 'be' in a certain way or to 'do' such and such a thing. A **headache** often appears when I try too hard mentally to accomplish something, or I am obsessed by what is in store for me and I worry about what the future holds for me. I then feel much hesitation, anxiety and concern. I may also react to strong pressures exerted by nearby situations or events. A **headache on the left side** generally points out a problem involving my relation with the feminine, the mother or the daughter. On the **right side**, it reveals difficulties with my masculine side, the father, the son. I may endure an intense feeling of failure, of doubt or self-hate that gives rise to criticism, especially self-criticism. My feeling of loyalty is being questioned. I am stuck, 'boxed' inside my **head**, not liking what I see and judging myself severely, giving myself '**knocks on the head**'. A **headache** can also come from the negation of my emotions and thoughts, which I find inappropriate or not in agreement with my values. Either I don't have the courage to express them, or I simply don't listen to them, because I rationalize and intellectualize everything I experience. "It is right, or it is wrong!" Maybe I want too much to understand, or go too fast, to know or have answers to my questions right now. I 'rack my brains' without finding any solutions, it is a real puzzle. I am fed up, but maybe the time isn't ripe yet and I must develop my patience, my sense of humor and my confidence that everything will come in its own time. A **headache** also often expresses negative emotions that are 'trapped' in my **head**, such as insecurity, torment, excessive ambitions, or an obsession with being perfect, which cause the blood to dilate. Finally, if I am afraid of facing a certain reality, I may seek another place on which to refocus my attention and escape: the **headache**. I call my social identity into question. My need for control and perfection makes me want to define in advance what goes on at each moment of my life. I like to just have my way. I refuse my spontaneity, which is an expression of my **heart♥**'s desires, and I replace it with my inflexibility, feeling compelled to plan everything in advance: instead of listening to my **heart♥**, I listen to my **head** that is overheating. I resist change and novelty. Because of my insecurity, I **stubbornly persist** and stand by what is familiar to me instead of daring to do something new. The expression: '**to head up a business**' aptly shows me that, in my own life, I may feel powerless to manage certain situations as I wish. A **headache** in the **forehead** most often involves a situation at work or in my social role, whereas in the **side of the head** (near the temples), my emotional side (family, couple) will be involved.

Whatever the cause, a **headache** is directly related to my individuality and I must learn to be more patient and more flexible with myself and others. I accept↓♥ to keep a distance from what I experience and this way, my ideas are more and more clear. I learn to find the right place for my intellect as well as my emotions in order to reach a proper balance. I will then be more in harmony with myself, and my head will feel freer and lighter.

HEARING DISORDERS *See: EARS — DEAFNESS*

HEART♥ (in general) *See also: BLOOD (IN GENERAL)*

The **heart♥** is connected to the fourth chakra or energy center: this chakra is Yin-Yang, male as well as female, and mental as well as emotional. It symbolizes the home and represents **Love** (my emotions and my capacity to **Love**), joy, vitality and security. Symbolically, the **right side** of the **heart♥** represents the father and the **left side**, the mother. Energy from the **heart♥** radiates throughout the body, especially between the neck and the solar plexus. The **heart♥** is a sort of energy pump that circulates life (blood) throughout the body. The blood circulation distributes the vital energy essential for happiness, well-being, **Love** of life and inner peace. It is therefore essential for me to show my **Love** by guiding my **heart♥**'s energy toward the best spiritual energy available for me. If I am in a situation where I have the impression that 'my heart♥ has been torn out', that my whole being is engaged, that I am not being nourished by **Love** from those around me, that I am taking life too seriously, my **heart♥** is going to react to this. A **heart♥** ailment reminds me of a fundamental aspect of ***Love***, which is that either I don't **love** myself enough or I don't receive **Love** from others, from life or from God. This leads me to ask myself if I feel guilty and if this makes me feel unable to live up to, and be worthy of, being loved. The more I focus on ***Love***, compassion and forgiveness, the more my **heart♥** will work toward joy, peace and jubilation. My **heart♥** will be emotionally balanced and protected from disappointments. A **heart♥** with a gentle, harmonious beat indicates a person's inner peace. My heart♥beat varies when I am unbalanced, upset in **Love** or sensitive to my feelings.

I agree↓♥ to open myself to **Love**, I return all feelings of blame to the care of the Universe, I stop making myself sick by criticizing myself; above all, I accept↓♥ to forgive myself. By forgiving myself I can fully accept↓♥ **Love** from others.

HEART♥ — ANGINA PECTORIS / ANGOR *See: ANGINA PECTORIS*

HEART♥ ATTACK *See: HEART♥ — INFARCTION [MYOCARDIAL]*

HEART♥ — CARDIAC ARRHYTHMIA

Cardiac arrhythmia is a disorder of the **heart♥**beat rhythm.

The **heart♥** represents **Love,** and **palpitation problems** are a sort of alarm signal for me, a call for help involving **Love**. My deep fear of losing or not having the **Love** I need so much is such that my **palpitation problems** are like a cry for help about **Love**. My **heart♥** beats as fast as I live my life. I feel that I don't have control and I don't feel safe. I need to find more calm in my life. I search in all directions but find no answers to my questions. My **heart ♥** beats for several different things at once: it may be persons (in **Love**) but also things I passionately like to do (work, hobbies) and I feel I must make some choices. I know I must let go of someone or something, but it is very difficult. I feel unable to do it, as I am very dependent. I am experiencing a duality: I or the others: to whom do I assign priority? Who must I first take care of? The choices are hard to make. I feel divided, maybe over the meaning of life itself. I may become ***infatuated*** with people because I feel such a need to be loved! Like my **heart♥**, I am unstable in my life with respect to my emotional reactions. There are things I am asked to do and that I do **half-heart♥edly**. Instead of living at my own pace, I follow the frenetic pace of society. An **anomaly in my pulse**[6] shows me how much my **heart♥** vacillates between two choices, how difficult it is to make a decision with all its implications. When the **heart♥**'s ventricles contract irregularly and inefficiently, it is a case of **ventricular fibrillation**. This can originate from an injury to the cardiac muscle, an electrocution, a moment of panic in the case of a fetus (at birth). If this state is not resolved within the

6. The normal average pulse varies from 50 to 80 beats per minute (bpm).

few following minutes, sudden death will ensue. This denotes an important decision I must take involving **Love,** and that is vital. I feel helpless. I begin by giving myself all the **Love** I need in order to replace my worries by more inner security, and I trust in life. **Auricular fibrillation** shows me that it is not legitimate for me to **love** whom I want and the way I want. I feel constraints related to the fact of showing my **Love** for people. **Tachycardia** is characterized by a rapid rhythmic contraction of the **heart♥**. Its **heart♥** beat accelerates to more than 90 beats per minute and this state is often due to intense exertions or emotions. An anguishing situation, a physical or mental exertion and fear provoke an imbalance that momentarily affects my **heart♥**, which sends me a SOS. Episodes of **tachycardia** are perceived as painful in cases of anguish, with adrenaline inducing very high heartbeats, or when an abnormal rhythm appears. I always thought I had to do more and faster to be loved, or even to have the right to live. I may also have the impression that I must make up for the time lost in a certain situation. **Bradycardia** is a slowing down of **heart♥** beats. It is initially developed by the practice of endurance sports; but the **heart♥** may abnormally slow down suddenly and cause faintness, which sometimes justifies implanting a pacemaker. An accumulation of deep griefs, especially related to my father, may bring on this faintness, as if my **heart♥** could no longer stand the suffering and decided to stop beating. I withdraw to protect myself because I no longer feel like struggling. I prefer to savor each instant of happiness and **Love,** for it seems to me that they are rare. **Extrasystole** (premature contraction) shows me how much I miss the **Love** of my parents, especially my father. **Love** comes to me with interruptions, often after frequent separations and reunions that tear up my **heart♥**. In any one of these situations, I become **Aware** that **Love** is involved. I breathe calmly and deeply and I listen to my **heart♥**.

I let go of everything that is no longer good for me. With determination, I choose the road I want to follow. I accept↓♥ that harmony will come back into my life, emotionally as well as socially.

HEART♥ / CARDIAC FAILURE, CONGESTIVE CARDIAC FAILURE (CCF) *See: HEART♥ — CARDIAC PROBLEMS*

HEART♥ — CARDIAC PROBLEMS

As the **heart♥** symbolizes **Love**, peace and the **Love** of life, **heart♥ problems** often originate from a loss of **Love**, from sadness, or from a resurgence of deep emotions, even after several years. All secret, impossible **Loves**, family **Love** cheapened by conflicts, will 'attack' my **heart♥**. My **heart♥** has been hardened by my previous wounds. I really and truly believe that life is difficult and stressful and that I have to fight every inch of the way. I often feel as though I were in a position of self survival, a state where I believe that only my own efforts will bring me any reward. I have to adjust myself to the pace of others, and this creates great stress. I am worried, over-excited and anxious; I have difficulty in setting my limits, or I feel too fragile to be able to keep my emotional balance. I unconsciously smother my inner child and prevent it from expressing this marvelous joy in living. A **heart♥ pain** shows me that I am hanging on and depending on someone or something; my insecurity makes me experience an intense inner tension. The **heart♥** is associated with the thymus gland, which is responsible for the production of T cells in the immune system, which weaken and become less resistant to invasions of anger, hate, frustration or self-rejection. **Heart♥ failure** shows to what extent I judge myself incompetent, and I see certain situations of my life as failures. Instead of following the impulses of my **heart♥**, I prefer to listen to others, which puts a brake on my development. The **heart♥** needs **Love** and peace. Life is made to be lived with a child's attitude of openness, joy, curiosity and enthusiasm. Even if I have emotional needs to be met, I try to remain well balanced and with enough openness of **heart♥** to allow me to appreciate every gesture of my existence. If I must undergo '**open heart♥ surgery**', have I always spoken to the people concerned with an **open heart♥** about my difficulties and sorrows?

I accept↓♥ to **love** myself better, to remain open to **Love** for myself and others. I enjoy myself, I relax and I take the time to be myself. I stop 'taking myself seriously'. I feel free to **love** without any obligation, knowing that I am still happy. There are many ways of describing the **heart♥** and its different states: to be '**heart♥**less', to be 'good–**heart♥**ed', to 'listen to one's **heart♥**'. If someone says to me "you have no **heart♥**", I check this message that life is sending me. It could be a sign that it would be better for me to change something. Am I experiencing an imbalance? Is my **heart♥** racing? Am I emotionally disturbed? Whatever the answer, I don't wait to be sick before I understand and accept↓♥ the necessity for changes in my life. I remain **Aware**, and open my **heart♥** to all that is beneficial for me. I listen to my **heart♥**.

HEART♥ — CORONARY THROMBOSIS

A **coronary thrombosis** is the formation of a blood clot in a coronary artery (at the **heart♥** level). This blocked blood circulation causes the onset of a myocardial infarction within the first 15 minutes of obstruction in almost all cases.

This clot affects the **heart♥**, which is the main organ that represents **Love**. I must check, in my life, what is preventing me from loving freely. It may be anger or a violent resentment I may have felt toward someone I **love**. Why do I feel attacked in my self-esteem? Did I receive news that appeared to dispossess me of my reason for living, of what enabled me to manifest my **Love**? I tend to isolate myself. I don't feel up to facing what comes my way. I don't dare put forward any proposals, for fear of being taken aback.

I accept↓♥ to make peace with myself and others. To resolve this situation, I become **Aware** of the forces of **Love** inside of me, I abandon myself and I discover that the Universe provides me with the support I need.

HEART♥ — INFARCTION (myocardial) *See also: INFARCTION (IN GENERAL)*

When I hear about someone who had an **infarct**, in popular parlance this usually means that the person sustained a **myocardial infarction**. It is also called a '**heart♥ attack**' or a '**cardiac attack**'. The organ most frequently affected by an **infarct** is the **heart♥**, the center of **Love** inside of me, the core of my emotions.

A **heart♥ attack** is a desperate way for my body to show me that I am going too far, that I am giving far too much attention to unimportant details. I cherish and protect my social status instead of coming back to the core of my life, which is my **heart♥**'s joy of living in my family, in expressing **Love,** loving oneself and savoring each moment with intensity. It is as though I were breaking the law of 'well-being and self-**Love**'. I am very afraid of not succeeding. I am so attached to everything that is part of my 'territory' (my wife, my work, my friends, my house, my ***stronghold***) that if I feel that I ***have lost*** or am about to lose something or someone in my territory, I may resist what is happening and I will suffer a **heart♥ attack**. I feel that I am about to have to ***abdicate*** and ***resign***. I risk seeing my whole life topple over. I would want 'with all my **heart♥'** to remain the boss, the master on board. I don't want to ***resign*** and give up so easily. I look at everything I was able to ***acquire*** over the years and I try to see if I now have the impression that I have been ***dispossessed*** or am about to be. It may consist of objects, persons, my pride, or my physical, intellectual or emotional capacities. My level of ***greed*** and ***envy*** is excessive. I may even have the impression that they want to ***expropriate me***, for I am no longer welcome. Am I being prevented from running things my way? **Heart♥ attacks** are also related to my own feelings and what I am experiencing about them. To what extent am I capable of feeling **Love** and expressing it to others? How far am I capable of loving and accepting↓♥ myself as I am? Do I force myself to 'be someone else' and try to do too much to prove to others what I am and what I am worth? The fact that I underrate myself to such a degree prevents me from allowing anyone to enter my world and my **heart♥**. Because I have the impression that I am weak, I project a hard image to others. I have an ocean of emotions pressed inside and if I accept↓♥ plunge into them, I feel I am going to drown, so much have I accumulated for so long! That is why ***commitment*** is becoming something difficult to experience for me. It is my anger, my frustration, my aggressiveness, my ***hate*** that, repressed for too long, can't stand it any longer and explode. The discovery of the most important and significant aspects of life cannot be reduced to the amount of money I have earned or the degree of success I have achieved. As much as the **heart♥** can be associated with compassion and **Love**, so can it be associated with its opposites of hostility, hate and rejection. A **heart♥ attack** often occurs in a period of my life when either competition is too strong or I am experiencing financial pressure, combined with the growing disaffection of the family and my close loved ones. Life becomes a ***battle***. I experience ***clashes*** that bring me a high level of stress. It is all or nothing, and my life loses its meaning if I fail. I run myself dizzy with scores of projects to avoid being in contact with my inner life and with the persons around me. I feel ***scorned***. What atrophies my **heart♥** is the separation between my feelings, my involvement, my relationships and the Universe with its natural rhythms. I no longer enjoy myself, and my **heart♥** is no longer in my work. Instead of heeding my body and my **heart♥**, I totally restrain myself. Everything is programmed and compartmentalized. I think I am rejecting the others but in fact, I am rejecting myself. I end up alone and **unloved**. I don't believe I have the right to stop: I can only live in work. I think that I am ***despised***, but in fact I am the one ***despising*** myself. I want to 'muddle through on my own'. I sometimes feel like ***running away***, leaving everything behind, because this is too much. I no longer have the ***fiber*** of a fighter. The more I distance myself from others, the closer I get somehow to my emotional death. I feel I am falling in ***ruins***. I believe I have to fight. I must push back my self-imposed limits that are now preventing me from reaching a new level of **Love** and acceptance↓♥. If I take refuge in my rational side and confine my body to prevent it from feeling the various emotions of my everyday life, it will harden, and I wipe out any chances of being able to understand and forgive myself as well as others, and so be able to heal my inner wounds.

I accept↓♥ to go with the flow and take the time to accept↓♥ everything that life has to give me and teach me, in order to recover inner peace and feel in my whole body the tenderness, gentleness and **Love** that inhabit me and only ask to nourish my **heart♥** and keep it in health. It is an ideal opportunity to re-think my priorities and see what is truly important. I accept↓♥ that there are some facets of my personality that I refused to see, and I know I have all the necessary strength to look at myself in the mirror and accept↓♥ myself as I am. I welcome my emotions to at last resume contact with my affective side that enables me to live life to the maximum. I accept↓♥ that I ***deserve*** to be loved and to be helped.

HEART♥ — MYOCARDITIS

Myocarditis is an inflammation of the cardiac muscle (myocardium). It is one of the causes of sudden death in young people during violent exertions. In adults, it takes the form of acute (and often mortal) cardiac failure.

I don't feel in full control of my capabilities. I am afraid 'my **heart♥** will give out' or that 'my **heart♥** isn't solid enough', properly as well as figuratively understood. I have a very strong mind and I don't know how to manage my emotions. I feel I am in a duality between two situations, between my **heart♥** and my head. My emotional weakness carries over into my work, 'my **heart♥** is no longer in my work' and I find it increasingly difficult to carry out the tasks required of me. My self-esteem is affected and I wonder how I can get out of this predicament. I feel in prison and if I see no solutions, I may unconsciously bring on a **myocarditis** that will put my life in danger.

I accept↓♥ to stop and contact the emotions that ask only to be expressed. I make peace with the unresolved situations of the past and I live the present moment. I am in top shape when my rational and emotional sides are in balance and each side has its appropriate place. I rediscover **Love** in me and thereby, my stability: this is what is called the 'intelligence of the **heart♥**'.

HEART♥ — PERICARDITIS

Pericarditis is an often infectious (viral) inflammation of the **pericardium**, the membrane covering the **heart♥**.

As the **pericardium** serves to protect the **heart♥**, **pericarditis** will occur if I feel that my **heart♥** will be under attack, in both the proper and the figurative senses. I am afraid for my **heart♥** and for someone else's too. The bad news that a person I **love** has a **heart♥** problem automatically raises my own fear that something may happen to me. Do I sense that the inherent features of my territory are in danger? Do I feel I am being '**burned alive**'? Do I feel constantly dissatisfied with myself and with life? Am I in a situation where I feel ***torn***? Do I feel anger toward my father who stays far away from me and from my life?

Instead of showing anger, I accept↓♥ to stay calm, I am learning to ease my anxieties and I ask to be protected at all times, knowing that everything that happens is for the best.

HEART♥ — TACHYCARDIA *See: HEART♥ — CARDIAC ARRHYTHMIA*

HEARTBURN *See: STOMACH — HEARTBURN*

HEAT RASH *See: SUN STROKE / INSOLATION*

HEAT STROKE / HEAT EXHAUSTION *See also: SUNSTROKE / INSOLATION, FEVER (IN GENERAL)*

Heat strokes can occur following prolonged exposure to the sun, at the beach or doing other outdoor sports, following intensive heating in the winter or if I find myself in a very small, poorly aired room. I may then present general muscular weakness, burning and dry skin, my face grayish and circles under my eyes.

On the metaphysical level, heat can be associated either with **Love**, when it is a matter of healing because more energy is circulating or with **anger** when fever or burns are involved. Here, a **heat stroke** represents guilt about **Love**, related to a feeling of lack of self-esteem. I need to **love** and be loved, and I haven't found how to do it, to fill this inner void in me and neutralize my dissatisfaction. I feel cut off from the affection that is available but doesn't reach me. It may be my parents who live nearby but give me no marks of affection. I may compensate for example with a prolonged exposure to the sun, which gives me some temporary comfort. My whole body indicates to me the urgent need to find **Love**.

I accept↓♥ to see how I can increase my self-esteem, or how to integrate a situation that affected me in my childhood and is now re-surfacing. I **love** life, and life fully returns the compliment.

HEEL

The **heel** symbolizes the past on which I rely, my foundation. Suffering from a **heel pain** indicates that I am experiencing anguish and feeling misunderstood, **not supported in the things I have to do**. As the **heel** is the support point of my body, a pain at this location shows that I am feeling uncertainty about my future. I feel hesitant and dissatisfied with myself or with my life, and I feel that I am losing control over my body. As it is on my **heels** that my whole body stands, I may feel the need to have a solid support in life to be able to continue advancing safely. Maybe I allow someone to drain my energy, and 'he/she is always on my **heels**'. I feel constantly hounded by my supervisor. I cling to the past. I feel I am less than nothing. My existence is very unsatisfying and I often feel 'my stomach in my **heels** from hunger' because there are many things that don't suit me and that I have trouble digesting. I carry the burdens of others on my shoulders, not knowing how to express my limits and feeling disconnected from my inner power. I feel forced to constantly put on the brakes. If the **calcaneum** (the voluminous bone that forms the **heel**) is affected, I feel myself intensely called into question about my reason for being here and who I am. Do I live my own life or do I want to imitate someone else's? What is the situation to which I am **recalcitrant**[7], and that I want to flee, from which I want to extricate[8] myself?

I accept↓♥ to trust myself and move ahead safely. I take my rightful place. I let go of the past and turn toward the future, heeding my inner authority, my little voice that knows exactly what I need.

HEMATOMA *See: BLOOD — HEMATOMA*

HEMATURIA *See: BLOOD — HEMATURIA*

HEMIPLEGIA *See: BRAIN — HEMIPLEGIA*

HEMISPHERES (right / left) *See: BRAIN (IN GENERAL)*

HEMORRHAGE *See: BLOOD — HEMORRHAGE*

HEMORRHAGE (intracerebral) *See: BRAIN — CEREBROVASCULAR ACCIDENT (C.V.A.)*

HEMORRHOIDS / PILES *See also: ANUS, BLISTERS, BLOOD / BLEEDING / VARICES, INFLAMMATION, INTESTINES — CONSTIPATION, PREGNANCY DISORDERS, TENSION [ARTERIAL] — HYPERTENSION*

Hemorrhoids are varices, wider dilations of veins, a sort of blister. They are found in the anal and rectal region.

Given that **hemorrhoids** can occur in cases of **constipation** and **pregnancy**, I am going to check in these texts to see if I am experiencing one or several

7. **Recalcitrant**: Who resists stubbornly.

8. **Extricate myself**: To extract myself from.

situations that are linked to it. When there is **pain**, it is related to stress; when there is **bleeding**, it is related to a loss of joy. **Hemorrhoids** often appear when I am having difficulty with my mother: it may be an unfinished bereavement or the desire to not see her leave. I may have a great need of her, of her opinion, and new conditions have made me feel abandoned by her. **Hemorrhoids** indicate tension and an inner desire to force elimination, as if I was trying to make something come out very strongly; and at the same time, the action of holding in appears. The conflict between pushing and holding in creates an imbalance. The veins suggest a situation indicating an emotional conflict between the action of ejecting and pushing out and the action of wanting to hold in and block the emotion inside of oneself. For example, this conflict can appear in children who feel emotionally abused by their parents (and want to reject them) and who **love** them nevertheless and want them to stay with them by holding them back. There is therefore a certain inner conflict between my feeling of loss and my notions about **Love**. I call into question my ***identity*** and my family ***affiliations***, especially my father, my work and society in general. I feel that I am just an '***umpteenth***' individual (of no determined rank), when I know deep down that I am a marvelous being with a unique place in the Universe. Do I want to live ***anonymously*** for some time? Do I feel like an ***impostor***? Would I like to ***substitute*** myself for someone else and take their place? Or on the contrary, I may want to attach myself too much to my family blood ties, especially my mother. I don't know how to deal with criticism directed at me, especially when it comes from my spouse. Other causes are related to **hemorrhoids**: an intense feeling of guilt or an old tension, poorly or not expressed, which I often prefer to keep for myself and that I am feeling about a person or a situation that irritates and angers me. My body is sending me an alarm signal. Something in my life needs to be cleared up, for I am very **disturbed**. Something is trying to erupt, like a volcano. I am surely feeling stress and pressure overload, about which I feel guilty. I may have deadlines to meet and I find it very hard to let go and to trust, and I may feel compelled to meet my obligations and responsibilities even if what I want to do is to speak and express my needs in order to rectify or adjust certain situations. Do I feel I am in control or do I have to give in? I must force myself in a foul situation and I can't get free of it. There is a constraint and some resentment that I should rid myself of. I am only half alive, and I want to run away from home. The social pressure is enormous! Furthermore, I am bearing this burden alone, because my pride will demand that I not ask for help from anyone. I may also be experiencing a feeling of submission to a person or a situation where I feel diminished, as though I were an 'asshole'. I am unable to take my place by showing my sensitivity and my creativity, and I yield my place to someone else. I live a lot in **obligingness**[9] because even though I try to find my identity and to be different, I also want others to **love** me.

Once I have found the metaphysical cause of my malaise, I become **Aware** of it and accept↓♥ this temporary situation that will allow me to find help to

---

9. **Obligingness:** A tendency to always agree with the requests of others in order to please them.

release myself from it. My thoughts and actions are sustained by **Love**. Everything harmonizes in me and the **hemorrhoids** disappear. I accept↓♥ to let go, and I dare to express what disturbs me. I regain control over my life and I let go of these negative emotions that fed me. I build new foundations where I feel well and free. The feeling of helplessness disappears and I fully control my destiny.

HEPATITIS *See: LIVER — HEPATITIS*

HERNIA

A **hernia** is a tumefaction (swelling) of soft tissues or an organ protuding through the muscle wall at a weak point that allows this protusion. It may be a tumor formed by a viscus that has extruded through a natural or accidental orifice out of the cavity that normally contains it. The **hernia** is caused by a pressure of soft tissue under the muscle at a point where it is weak and under-used. **Hernias** can appear at various locations.

The location indicates its nature and its message. They are more frequent along the **abdominal wall** (**hernia of the abdominal wall**) such as the **inguinal hernia** for instance, which refers to a secret I carry inside and don't reveal to others, and my difficulty in expressing my creativity. I ask myself: "Am I sexually satisfied? Do I try to respond to my partner's needs by forgetting myself?" Around the **diaphragm**, it is called a **diaphragmatic hernia** (such as the **hiatal hernia**). It is related to anger or even a rage where I feel helpless. "I am blowing a fuse". An **umbilical hernia**, which also affects babies, is usually related to a poor cicatrization of the umbilical cord after its section. This swelling can express my refusal as a baby to leave my mother's cozy bed or my refusal to be born. As an adult, I am afraid of being controlled, under the sway of, or simply influenced by, my new life environment. A **hernia** may represent a great unexpressed desire to break with a situation or a person who is unpleasant and to whom I feel committed. I want to get out of it and extricate myself from a situation that has become intolerable for me. It may involve the break-up of my couple, initiated by me or my spouse, and that I have difficulty accepting↓♥. Am I finding life heavy to bear? Why work so hard? I feel so weak. I need to be supported, but I am not ready to ask for help. A **hernia** can also express self-punishment because I resent myself for feeling helpless or incapable of achieving certain things. I am thus feeling much frustration with myself because I know that I live too much according to others and not enough according to my own needs. I respond to the expectations of others: parents, friends, spouse and boss. How about me in all that? Through the control of my constraint, I reach a level where everything explodes, or rather 'implodes', in me. As I haven't outwardly released my distress, it must find a way to get out. The abdominal wall protects my internal organs and keeps them in place. Therefore, the **hernia in the muscle** may be linked to the desire to keep my world in its place by not allowing the release of aggressiveness or of stronger expressions. Will I allow myself to free it? I may feel guilty of being in this state, and I feel pushed and forced to go too far, or I try to achieve my goal in an excessive manner. There is a 'mental urge' (stress) that is trying to burst out. I want to get out of a state or a situation that is unpleasant and in which I feel compelled to stay. It is a certain form of self-punishment. The time has come for a new departure.

I accept↓♥ to express my creativity. Now, I dare to be me by expressing myself more freely. I feel more **Love** for myself and others, for I know who 'I am'. I take the time to go inside myself and be alone to see clearly in my life and know where I am going.

HERNIATED DISC *See: DISC [HERNIATED DISC]*

HEROIN CONSUMPTION *See: DRUGS*

HERPES (in general), ORAL, LABIAL — HERPES LABIALIS

See also: MOUTH DISEASE

Herpes, a grouped cutaneous eruption of inflammatory vesicles, is commonly called a **cold sore** or a **fever blister**. This very contagious virus affects a high percentage of our population and also persists in the body for life.

There is something 'poisoning my existence', a link between the skin and the nervous system that is hurting itself: "That's why it hurts". It can reappear even after several years of 'sleep'. The eruptions of the ***herpes simplex* virus (HSV)** produce ulcers that mainly affect the mouth, the lips or the genital parts. Several causes are related to **herpes**. It may be frustration because I haven't been able to achieve certain desires and I feel somewhat 'helpless' and 'impotent'. I may want to push someone away to not let myself be kissed, either because I judge him or because I want to punish him. I need to withdraw (in both the proper and the figurative senses!) for some time because the pressure is too much; it may involve my sexual life, my work or my family. I may regret having said certain hurtful words, and I now tend to crawl. I had to defend myself and I may regret some of the words I said. I may pass a severe judgment on a person of the opposite sex and then generalize it to the whole category. ("Men are all…"). These are all different ways for me to stay at a distance from others, for the regions where **herpes** develops are usually the lips and the genital parts, the basic places for verbal or affective personal communication with other persons. The ulcers can indicate that I am enduring emotional and mental grief (as the soft tissues and fluids are involved), and suffering great inner pain that wants to emerge openly. As it is with the lips that I kiss my loved ones (spouse, children, parents, etc.), **oral herpes** means that I am in a situation where I am undergoing a separation from a person I used to kiss. The contact with the skin of the lips was withdrawn for some reason, and **herpes** appeared. I had projects but can no longer carry them out. Sharing my beliefs is difficult for me. I therefore have the impression that others are directing my life, and that does not suit me. On my nose (rarer), **herpes** indicates that I may be feeling rage because some people around me think that

I 'stick my nose everywhere'. Eruptions seem closely linked to stress and conflicted situations, especially when I do something half-**heart♥**edly or when I act contrary to my inner feelings (for example: when I have a sexual experience with a person I don't want to be with). **Herpes** may also send me the message that I am experiencing grief, a lassitude with life or a lack of self-esteem. This virus puts on the table all the issues of shame, guilt, compromise and self-denial related to sexuality (by observing the body part that is affected, I can find the cause). I must question myself about the intimacy I am sharing with my partner and see what frustrations, fears or disappointments I am experiencing about it. Do I feel ashamed of my sexuality? Is it satisfying, or has it become merely a sensual pleasure devoid of the deep meaning that it should embody?

I accept↓♥ to stop severely judging myself and others. I am learning to open myself to others. I trust myself more and more in my intimate relationships. I **love** myself more, and my life is sunny once again. I am proud of who I am.

HERPES (genital / vaginal) *See also: SKIN — ITCHING, VAGINA — VAGINITIS*

Vaginal herpes, following popular belief, derives from sexual guilt and the unconscious desire to punish oneself. **Genital herpes** can appear if one senses an absence of sexual contact. I may have had a partner and we separated, which makes me feel frustrations. Or we may have been physically separated, as when one of the partners has gone on a business trip for a period of time. Having no physical contact with the skin of my sexual organs and finding this 'separation' very difficult, I show my uneasiness through **vaginal herpes**. My frustration may also be intensely linked to my sexual relations, either because they are not satisfying or on the contrary, because while being fully satisfying, they bring up unhappy memories. In other words, I may wonder why I have endured so many years of dissatisfaction when today it is going so well, so why didn't I experience this earlier? Common religious teachings even asserted that this was willed by God to punish us. The feeling of shame even leads me to deny, to not accept↓♥ my genital organs. Genital parts have been scapegoats for many religions.

I accept↓♥ to become **Aware** of the fact that I want to escape my deeper nature. I am vulnerable; am I ready to engage myself totally? I **love** my body and I rejoice in my sexuality. God has created me in His own image. I am amazed by the beauty that I embody. I must totally accept↓♥ myself and give myself completely to myself in order to then do the same with my partner.

HERPES LABIALIS *See: HERPES (IN GENERAL)*

HICCUPS

Hiccups are sudden and involuntary spasmodic contractions of the diaphragm.

I may be feeling inner revolt, guilt or self-judgment. This disturbs my organism. Always **hiccups**? They may be frequent and durable. It is a very bothersome and unpleasant experience for the person who has it. Is there something bothersome and unpleasant in what I am experiencing or would rather experience, but is not manifesting itself and is causing me frustration? Are there any noises or thoughts that I can't stop? Am I consistent in what I think, say and do? Are the **hiccups** programmed (for instance: "Each time I have a soda drink, I have the **hiccups**"?) Is there a situation in my life that I can't tolerate, over which I have no control and that I would want to change and stop, just as with my **hiccups**? On what issues am I in disagreement and about which I feel that I can't make myself heard? Do I always heed my inner voice and its approvals? I may feel an emotion about a person in authority and I feel like telling them: "That's enough!" I am afraid of something or someone and the **hiccups** remind me that I must free myself of that. My impatience and impulsiveness over an event can also cause **hiccups**.

I accept↓♥ to take life more calmly. I am learning to fully taste and appreciate my life. I accept↓♥ that everything is in place in the divine plan, that everything is OK, and the **hiccups** will disappear. I accept↓♥ to have full control over myself and to take charge of myself.

HIGH BLOOD PRESSURE *See: TENSION [ARTERIAL] — HYPERTENSION*

HIP(S) (in general) *See also: PELVIS*

They hold my body in perfect balance and are located between the pelvis and the femur[10]. I lean on my **hips**. My **hips** enable my legs to move in order to make my body move forward.

They determine whether I move forward or not. They represent my basic beliefs about what my relations with the world are, or should be. The **hips** contain my positioning about living, either based on myself or based on others and how they perceive me. As the pelvis and the **hips** form a whole, they represent **my striding forth in life**. The **hips** therefore also represent my level of determination for advancing in life.

I accept↓♥ to move forward in life joyfully and confidently, knowing that everything is an experience to help me discover my inner riches.

HIP DISORDERS

It is from the **hips** that the legs' movements, and therefore walking, are initiated. The legs serve to advance freely; there is therefore a link with **autonomy**. I may be holding back from moving forward and making important decisions in my life. When I start engaging in a period of personal change, I often begin to ask myself questions on the 'whys' and 'hows' of things, and pains will appear in my **hips**: Hence my indecisiveness about advancing in life

10. **Femur**: The long bone that runs along the inside of the thigh and forms its skeleton.

or what new directions to take. I ask myself if I have the right to live for myself or if I must sacrifice myself for others as I have always done. Therefore an enormous duality is preventing me from advancing, and if I continue to live under pressure, following a road I detest, I may well **fracture a hip**. I may feel that I must give in, against my will, to something or someone that is stronger than me. By the **problems in my hips**, my body is indicating a certain stiffness, resistance and rigidity; I am therefore experiencing inflexibility about a situation or a person. This may originate from a situation where I felt betrayed or **abandoned** by someone, which affected me so much that I have been calling into question all my relations with others. I also feel like setting new rules to protect myself and avoid being hurt again. I may have some concerns about the future; I am therefore anxious when I have an important decision to make, for I may feel that I am going nowhere, that I will never achieve anything or that I simply perceive myself as 'good for nothing'. Am I able to fulfill the dreams that are dear to my **heart♥**? When my **hips hurt** (with **arthritis** for example), my body sends me a message: there is an imbalance in me. I can't impose my ideas and my personality, so I turn to submission. I am angry because others don't see my needs. I wish they would respond to my needs without having to ask for it. When I feel **pain**, some sort of guilt is involved. A **pain in the hips** or **hips that no longer want to move** can indicate that I am blocking my sexual pleasure out of fear or guilt. I consider myself a poor sexual partner for I find it difficult to welcome the other. I may fear intimacy, and it is sometimes easier to move away from the person I **love** than to face my apprehensions. I may even use a weight gain in this regard to help create a physical space between me and the other person. I may feel impotent, sexually and in my capacity for accepting↓♥ myself as I am, with my tastes, my desires, my pleasures. I will be sexually and emotionally troubled, thus preventing my **hips** from working normally. This helplessness can also be experienced in the fact that I don't, or no longer, feel capable of taking my place and **opposing** someone or something. I don't give myself the right to **go forward** in a situation or a place that could give me some sexual pleasure, because of the taboos I have set for myself or have accepted↓♥ from society. This situation forces me to think about the limits I have given myself. I examine to what extent I have prevented myself from moving forward, for instead of living my life with my emotions, I live it in my head. **Degeneration** or **decalcification of the hip** indicates that my security is shaken; I feel helpless and no longer dare to move. I feel empty because I feel I have given a lot: I feel worn out.

I accept↓♥ to no longer be 'everybody's mother' and allow myself to receive **Love** and be nourished by it. My body helps me to develop my **conscience** in order to move forward in life with confidence and security and shows me that I must be more flexible in the way I make decisions, thus ensuring myself a better future. I am balanced and I move forward in life with confidence and serenity. I thank life for everything it makes me experience in each instant. I learn to live in balance with these experiences. I let go of the burden of responsibilities that I no longer need: this facilitates my decision-making.

HIV (Human Immunodeficiency Virus) *See: AIDS*

HOARSENESS *See also: APHONIA*

When my tone of voice becomes dull, husky or rasping, my voice is said to be **hoarse.**

Hoarseness means that I am suffering from mental and physical exhaustion. Something is preventing my 'wheels' from turning without snagging. I am experiencing an emotional block, an intense emotion, and holding back my aggressiveness. As the throat is linked to the energy center of truth, communication and self-expression (the throat chakra), I may feel trapped by the truth, that I find hard to assimilate, and by my personal convictions. I use certain stopgaps or stimulants such as coffee, alcohol, cigarettes, etc. And when the effects have disappeared, the **hoarseness** reappears. The fatigue I feel amplifies the concerns and worries I didn't want to face. There is a very strong duality inside of me: "To tell, or not to tell? Will I tell the truth or not?" If I am concerned about how others will receive what I say or if I am unsure of what I am advancing, my fear or my uncertainty will show through my voice, which is becoming **hoarse.** Instead of truly communicating what I think and feel, I say instead what I think others expect me to say, which in a sense is close to a lie. Instead of relying on my inner strength, I therefore rely on others, which is very fragile (like my voice) and makes me feel insecure.

I am **Aware** that I need time for a pause and accept↓♥ to give myself the rest and time I need to regenerate myself. Once I have rested, situations and events resume their true proportions and I am far more objective and lucid in making the necessary decisions. I allow myself to express my emotions. I become **Aware** that if I speak from my **heart♥**, I am in full control of myself and feel at ease to express myself freely. My voice too can fully express itself, for I now trust what I am saying and I know that others listen with their **hearts♥** to what I am saying.

HODGKIN'S DISEASE *See also: BLOOD — LEUKOPENIA, CANCER OF THE GANGLIA [OF THE LYMPHATIC SYSTEM]*

Hodgkin's[11] **disease** is a cancerous development affecting the lymphatic ganglions, the spleen and the liver. It manifests itself by a loss of strength caused by a diminishing of the white globules.

It is strongly related to a **great guilt** that I feel. I don't find I am good enough and my self-esteem is at its lowest point, where I even refuse that people give me compliments. I fear being attacked and disapproved and I feel very discouraged, I have lost the taste for living (blood means joy) and lost my defenses (white globules) because it is as if I had no right to live or didn't

11. **Hodgkin**: British physician (1798–1866). **Hodgkin's disease** is a type of lymphoma discovered in 1832, and characterized by the presence of large atypical cells, Reed-Sternberg's cells. STERNBERG's cell is essential for the diagnosis. Its actual nature is still little known but it appears that it is of lymphoid B clonal origin.

deserve to live. I can't fulfill the expectations of others, especially those of my parents. I feel I am in a frenzied race: I feel the need to demonstrate to others or to myself that I am somebody and that I can accomplish great things. I can harbor feelings of hate and resentment against someone or a situation, which ***undermines*** my mental and physical health. Maybe I am resenting myself, because I am 'fed up' with living according to others. I wonder who I am, and I wear masks to please others. I am like a chameleon in its corner, changing colors to **protect** itself from outside authority. I see myself as a monster, I am a prisoner.

I accept↓♥ that my great joy will be to **love** myself for who I am. I trust myself and go at my pace. My body regenerates, for I am connected to **The Source** that is in me. I am taking charge of my life. I become **Aware** of the fact that others can truly **love** me only if I am myself. I rediscover the riches in me and live by my own inner truth.

HOMICIDE

I may have a desire to kill someone. If I feed this desire with resentment and hate, I expose myself to the egregore[12] of negative energy involving this form of thought, which may push me to take action. **What do I want to kill in myself**? My **suffering**, my **bad temper**, my **hate**? I resent myself for losing someone or something; I hold others responsible for my grief and dismay. My inner wound is intolerable. My inner suffering demands courage. The courage to ask for help, to trust a person who receives me unconditionally and in whom I can confide.

I accept↓♥ to free myself of the past, to forgive, and I recover the strength to take myself in charge.

HOT FLUSHES / FLASHES *See: MENOPAUSE*

HUMP (Buffalo) *See: CUSHING'S SYNDROME*

HUMP / LUMP (in general) *See also: CYST*

A **lump**, also called a **growth**, is a tissue alteration that is palpable on a part of the body or in an organ.

It is like an explosion of the body crying out in me, which needs to express itself outwardly. Like an egg ready to hatch, I can no longer hold back what needs to express itself, to clarify itself, to have its say. Do I feel that I allow myself to be 'slammed into'? That I am doing far too much for few results? Am I experiencing a conflicted situation with my boss? I am experiencing a duality between what exists and what I express: everything I hold back can explode in the form of a **hump**. This can give rise to confrontations with my entourage.

---

12. **Egregore**: It is a **conscious** form of energy, formed by the shared thoughts of several, or a multitude of, persons.

I wonder about a situation where I couldn't express my needs and that I may have amplified by trying to hold everything deep down.

I accept↓♥ to freely express my ideas and emotions. I can also inwardly write what I need to clarify about what is going on in me, before sharing it with others. This exercise allows me to release what was in excess, return to the **heart♥** and find peace. I thus recover my inner calm and harmony with what I am, as with my entourage. I now can clearly express my thoughts, confidently and in unconditional **Love**.

HUMPBACK / HUNCHBACK *See: ROUNDED SHOULDERS*

HUNTINGTON'S DISEASE *See: BRAIN — HUNTINGTON'S DISEASE*

HYDROPHOBIA *See: RAGE*

HYGROMA *See: BURSITIS, KNEE AILMENTS*

HYPERACTIVE CHILD *See: HYPERACTIVITY*

HYPERACTIVITY *See also: AGITATION*

Hyperactivity mainly affects children whose activities are intense and constant. It is important to distinguish between dynamic and **hyperactive** behavior.

If I am a **hyperactive child**, my behavior is turbulent and disrupting or even strange. It is my usual way of ignoring the situations and circumstances around me, by becoming so involved in what I am doing that I don't need to focus my attention on 'my' immediate reality, maybe because this reality isn't pleasing and comforting. I am revolted by certain situations or behaviors of my entourage. The nervousness I express throws **Light** on some inner states, some unstated thoughts, some fears that I or others are experiencing. It may also be a rebellion against authority, a way to avoid facing a certain reality that I find intolerable. We know that **hyperactivity** is caused by artificial additives: excess sugar, dyes and fast food. This type of food is often the symbol of the parent trying to provide me with the **Love** I may be lacking: for example, giving me chocolate when I am in greater need of a hug. When I am a **hyperactive child**, it is often because I need to be more focused on my inner self and my **heart♥**. As a parent, before thinking of putting my child on medication, it would be greatly to my advantage to try treatments that act on the energy level, such as relaxation, acupuncture, homeopathy, etc. It would be important to check the context of the child's birth: the circumstances, whether it was premature, if there was any trauma, etc., for birth has an influence on the child's coming years, because its emotional memory registers everything (consciously or not). The SELF adjusts to constraints by setting up an internal filter in order to **avoid what bothers it in reality**. In this specific case, the parents can explain to the child the story of her birth in order to make the situation less dramatic, or speak to her **Soul** while she sleeps. There are also cases where a child will feel guilty, as for example when the mother experienced a difficult delivery: it must be explained to the child that it was not his fault, and that he is loved, whatever happened. There are also situations where the mother, while the child was in her womb, had the impression that it was no longer moving. The fact of not moving was thus taken as a sign of danger, that the child may have been dead. Once the child is growing up, she feels the need to move in order to show, even unconsciously, that she is alive. It is as if she had the impression of being alive only when she moved. Explaining this to the child will have the effect of removing great stress. The same thing applies to a child who has become an adult and is still **hyperactive**. It may be that the **child** is **hyperactive** because he is in resonance, or in inner contact, with what is called the parent's 'inner child' who is experiencing great tension or great insecurity. In some cases, the child is over-protected by the parents. They may have insisted at home on the idea that rest is not allowed; otherwise you are lazy and slack. The body will then automatically want to move. If we as parents are not energetically centered ourselves, how can we ask our child to be?

I accept↓♥ to take myself in charge for myself, first, as well as for my child's well-being.

HYPERCHOLESTEROLEMIA *See: BLOOD — CHOLESTEROL*

HYPEREMOTIVITY *See: EMOTIVITY*

HYPERGLYCEMIA *See: BLOOD — DIABETES*

HYPERMETROPIA *See: EYES — HYPERMETROPIA*

HYPEROREXIA *See: BULIMIA*

HYPERSALIVATION *See: SALIVA — HYPER- AND HYPOSALIVATION*

HYPERSOMNIA *See: NARCOLEPSY*

HYPERTENSION *See: TENSION [ARTERIAL] — HYPERTENSION*

HYPERTHERMIA *See: FEVER*

HYPERTHYROIDIA *See: GLAND [THYROID] — HYPERTHYROIDIA*

HYPERTROPHY

Hypertrophy is the increase in volume of an organ or a tissue. The reader must refer to the affected body part in order to find more information.

Hypertrophy indicates a special and greater need regarding the emotional aspect concerned. For example, if there is a **hypertrophy of the heart♥**, I am experiencing an important deficiency with respect to **Love**. If I am a **baby**, it is the **Love** of one or both of my parents that I need so much, but which I apparently cannot receive. Whatever my age, I am feeling an immense emptiness and solitude that makes me experience insecurity.

I accept↓♥ to acknowledge my needs and I give myself the means to fulfill them. Instead of waiting for them to be fulfilled from outside, I take care of myself. I give myself all the **Love**, the gentleness and the tenderness that I need. I choose to fully open myself up to life and accept to be someone who is flourishing and fulfilled.

HYPERVENTILATION *See also: ACIDOSIS, ANXIETY, FEVER*

Hyperventilation consists in rapid inspiration and short expiration, bringing excess oxygen into the organism.

The causes can be acidosis, anxiety or even panic, fever or intense physical exercise. I am suffering from **hyperventilation** because I don't accept↓♥ change. I therefore experience a feeling of worry about newness and I hesitate to trust the current situation; I refuse to abandon myself. I may even challenge what is happening in my life. As my respiration is unbalanced, what area of my life displays this same imbalance, often to excess? Do I totally accept↓♥ the gifts of life (inspiration)? Do I quickly give what I have, notably my **Love** (expiration) in order to avoid totally involving myself? I am emotionally overexcited because I no longer know where I want to go in life. I flee and I refuse to listen to my inner voice, although I know that I find answers to all my questions when I listen to it. I prefer to live in helplessness and as a victim instead of acting responsibly. I deny my power and reject the opportunities to advance, out of fear of the unknown. My body sends me a message and I become **Aware** of it.

I accept↓♥ to breathe normally, I let myself go, I abandon myself. My life transforms itself and I rejoice. I free myself of all my fears. I joyfully breathe in life. I re-connect with a feeling of inner security. I accept↓♥ to advance with determination and I enjoy life!

HYPOACUSIS *See: EARS — DEAFNESS*

HYPOCHONDRIA *See also: AGORAPHOBIA, ANXIETY, DEPRESSION, HALLUCINATIONS*

I am a **hypochondriac** if I am excessively concerned about my health. Thinking that I might be sick can become an obsession for me.

While my attention is focused on this possibility, it prevents me from listening to the criticism and gossip of others concerning me. I feel a deep insecurity or fear about the loss of control that the onset of a disease could represent for me. I don't accept↓♥ to suffer from a disease because I know deep down that I am already suffering in my inner being. This fear can become so great that I may tune out reality and have hallucinations.

I accept↓♥ to resume contact with myself. Using an energy approach or psychotherapy will help me to regain more self-confidence and to manifest my divine capacity for openness to life.

HYPOGEUSIA *See: TONGUE*

HYPOGLYCEMIA *See: BLOOD — HYPOGLYCEMIA*

HYPOPHYSIS / PITUITARY GLAND *See: GLAND [PITUITARY]*

HYPOSALIVATION *See: SALIVA — HYPER- AND HYPOSALIVATION*

HYPOTENSION *See: TENSION [ARTERIAL] — HYPOTENSION*

HYPOTHYROIDIA *See: GLAND THYROID — HYPOTHYROIDIA*

HYSTERIA *See also: FAINTING, NEUROSIS, RAGE, TANTRUM*

I am **hysterical** when I experience a neurosis and express my psychological conflict through my body, whether it is in the form of a temper tantrum, convulsions, loss of consciousness, etc.

When I have an attack of **hysteria**, I don't know what direction to take, I tune out reality, I seek refuge in my imagination and I may tend to express my inner conflict in public. I unconsciously express my repressed tendencies and I want to attract the attention I am not receiving in my everyday life. **Hysteria** appears after a long period of non-assertion and non-expression of my needs. I have belittled myself so much that I have always backed away from others. I have also disconnected from myself to avoid suffering. But when I can't stand any longer to feel rejected, different, misunderstood and unloved, I explode. I resent myself for feeling so helpless and incapable, but my anger and my violence are directed at others. I want the others to listen to me and **love** me. This is especially true if I belong to an ethnic, religious or other minority. When I am in this state, it displays the inner pain or grief that I may be feeling. I need to heal my inner wound in order to recover a better balance, greater harmony and greater inner peace and make these torments stop.

I accept↓♥ to become **Aware** of the fact that **Love♥**, joy, spontaneity and self-expression are gaining more place in my life. What I ask for from others, I must give myself. I am learning to listen to my needs and to fill them myself. If I respect myself, others too will respect me. I ask for guidance in choosing a therapeutic approach that will enable me to reach this state of well-being.

HYSTEROPTOSIS *See: PROLAPSE*

I

ICTERUS / JAUNDICE *See: JAUNDICE*

ILEITIS / CROHN'S DISEASE *See: INTESTINES — CROHN'S DISEASE*

ILLNESS (mental) *See: INSANITY, NEUROSIS, PSYCHOSIS*

IMPATIENCE *See also: BLOOD — HYPOGLYCEMIA, FRIGIDITY, NERVOUSNESS*

Impatience denotes an inner stress, insecurity or tension that shakes me and affects my nervous system. I become more irritable, quicker in what I have to say or do. "Am I impatient with myself, or with others?" Why do I always need to go faster? It is as if I wanted to catch up on time. When I feel a limitation or that someone wants to curtail my freedom, it irritates me, which manifests itself by my abrupt manner and my **impatience**.

I accept↓♥ to take a few moments to relax and find the source of my irritation.

IMPOTENCE *See also: ANGUISH, ANXIETY, FEAR*

As a man, if I am incapable of achieving or maintaining an erection during intercourse with a lover, then I am suffering from **impotence**, also called **erectile dysfunction**.

This certainly causes me to feel dissatisfaction in my sexual relations. Medically, though **impotence** can be **organic**, deriving from a **physical** or **psychological** cause, I must consider that the cause derives from a psychological or metaphysical (beyond the physical) factor, even an unconscious one. **Impotence** is often related to the fear of trustfully giving or abandoning myself to a woman[1], or losing control over myself or with the other person. I am afraid of being vulnerable, so 'intimacy intimidates me'. I may feel anguished at the idea of 'getting my female companion pregnant'. Being a man, I often have many responsibilities and may feel much pressure and stress at work, and society in general requires me to perform and surpass myself. Transposing this demand to my sexuality, I may feel a sexual pressure urging me to surpass myself, which creates great inner tension causing me to lose control. I reach the point of dreading intimate relations. Conversely, a man approaching retirement may see signs of **impotence** appear and then no longer feel good for anything, or useless even. I am feeling in **decline**. I depreciate myself: as I no longer have the opportunity to surpass myself at work, I can no longer perform in bed. The same thing may happen if I lose my job suddenly and

1. Or to a man, if my sexual relations are conducted with a man.

unexpectedly. In one special area, my life has lost all its meaning. As I don't dare discuss it with my partner, I reach the point of experiencing much guilt and confusion until I fear losing the other person. Feeling great anguish during my **Love** relations may provoke a block that makes me experience **impotence**. This anxiety may derive from the fact that during sexual intercourse, I am more in contact with my emotional side. As a man, I am not used to functioning with my emotions. I am more consciously in contact with my injured inner child who may be feeling insecurity, fear, rejection or misunderstanding. Also, if in my previous **Love** relationships I experienced failures that I found humiliating, I may then feel that I am not equal to the situation in my next sexual encounter. My insecurity, my feeling of incapacity and failure, of self-hate, guilt or neglect may also lead me to experience **impotence**. I may experience my wife's departure as an emotional as well as a physical separation. As physical sexual contact is no longer possible, my sexual organs lose their sensitivity. **Impotence** may also have its source in a past event that marked me: I may have been physically or psychologically abused in my early childhood; I may remain resentful about a previous affective relationship, feeling I was the victim of a betrayal. **Impotence** is also a way to wield power over someone by holding back sexually from an abusive or over-demanding partner. I may feel that my territory (my possessions, my immediate environment with which I identify) is in danger. I may feel a loss of interest in women in general, which could carry over into a physical form, should the lack of interest endure. Lastly, if I identify my partner with my mother, and my mother occupies too much space in my life, being subservient to her and afraid of not pleasing her, feeling **impotent** to make her happy and please her, this may transform itself into sexual **impotence**. As my wife is an exact copy of my mother, I unwittingly commit psychological incest, inevitably leading me to **impotence** on several levels. My Oedipus[2] complex was probably not properly resolved. I may feel threatened by my spouse, often emotionally but it may also be physically. What will happen if I abandon myself to her? Will I lose my feeling of potency? Will I be 'eaten alive'[3] (in the proper sense as well as figuratively: physically, emotionally or financially)? The fear of failure freezes me. I am filled with emotions and don't know what to do with them. I feel an obligation to have satisfying sexual relations, and the burden is heavy to bear. I feel I must please the other person at all costs. I may still feel resentment from past experiences with previous partners. My body is making me reassess my values about sexuality and **Love** in general. Being a man may evoke the image of my father, but I realize I am different from him and can live my own life instead of vicariously living his.

I accept↓♥ to define my place, to make contact with my emotions and let go of my control so that the energy can freely circulate throughout my body instead of staying in my head, to bring physical and mental relaxation. The

2. The **Oedipus complex**: in the child's early development, generally between the ages of 3 and 6, it is characterized by a strong affective attachment to the parent of the opposite sex: the son to his mother, the daughter to her father.

3. **To be eaten alive**: An expression meaning that I am being abused.

impotence I am experiencing may help me to become **Aware** of my true worth as a person and not as a 'sexual animal'. It enables me to see that I can be creative in other areas of my life. I am led to reassess my deeper values and priorities. Once I have become **Aware** that I can find true **Love** in different ways and that I deserve it, the **impotence** will go away and I will have made contact with my inner **potency**.

INCIDENT *See: ACCIDENT*

INCONTINENCE (fecal, urinary) *See also: BLADDER DISORDERS*

Whether **incontinence** is **fecal** — an incapacity to hold in one's stools —or **urinary** — involuntary losses of urine — both situations involve control. Life may be teaching me to be more flexible and let go of people and situations. Loss of control, whether fecal or urinary, forces me to become **Aware** of this. I must leave aside my rigid thoughts that are only a shell that I draw over myself to protect myself from my sensitivity when I can't control the situation. As **incontinence** results from the fact that a muscle can't act effectively any longer, there is therefore a mental deficiency or weakness. I may experience a huge disappointment leading to despair. I give up, I back down and I no longer control my emotions. Instead of being responsible and taking action, I am wallowing in guilt, letting go and being passive. I no longer feel that I have power over myself or over events. In the case of **fecal incontinence**, I can ask myself what person or situation is 'giving me a pain'. I may be in strong reaction against authority and the fact of having to put up with it leads me to experience this situation of **incontinence**. For me, authority may be life itself leading me to make changes I don't want to make. I can go and see who, in my childhood, represented authority for me and against whom I may have been reacting. If I am an adult experiencing this situation, I ask myself if I have difficulty in deciding my life and the directions I want to take. Feeling limp or feeling that I have too many responsibilities, I unconsciously wish to become a baby again, let everything go and no longer take anything on my shoulders because I need someone to take care of Me! In the case of **urinary incontinence**, this uncontrollable and unconscious release of negative emotions that urine represents can be a way to get more attention. The underlying cause of this may be a feeling of rejection, of having no merit, of insecurity or fear of the future. I feel that I lack affection. I may then also fear being 'crushed', which adds to my feeling of helplessness. A situation makes me anxious and I feel defenseless. Feeling limited or being punished intensifies my ailment. I will build myself an imaginary world where the bad figures prevail. I feel vulnerable, and resist **Love** and tenderness because they don't exist in my Universe. Or I believe I don't deserve it. I fear authority in all its forms. I fear losing what is mine or being separated from someone I **love**. It is as though I were marking out my territory. Urine represents negative emotions that are normally released when they are no longer necessary or wanted. This release, often nocturnal, implies a conflict at a deeper level, of which I am not even **Aware**. Incapable of 'controlling' the leak of urine or stools, I am incapable of controlling what happens in my life, especially my emotions, and that scares me. It is important for me that these inner fears and insecurities express themselves and that I ***hear*** them. I may also too easily let go of things or persons dear to me, without having the courage or the strength to go and get what I want. Expecting much from life, I am disappointed and 'let myself go', in my body as well as my mind. Do I feel that time, or chance, is slipping through my fingers?

Great fear or nervousness can also cause **incontinence**, especially in **children**. They are very sensitive to what their parents feel, so parental concern or anxiety is sensed by children of all ages. As a child, being unable to express my feelings in words, I may use 'yellow ink' to convey indirectly that something is going on inside of me, and this gives me a certain feeling that I exist. I do receive attention, though accompanied by blaming, screaming or discord. As a child, **enuresis** often appears at the birth of another child. This indicates that I find it difficult to position myself in the family, I no longer know what my territory is or to which one I belong. If my father ***trained*** me not enough or too much, I feel lost and unattached and lose urine in my sleep, mainly at night. I then feel guilty and hide in my corner, but what I really want is for Mom to take care of me.

I accept↓♥ that it is impossible to control everything that goes on in my life. I learn to trust and I learn to like novelty and the unexpected. If I am **a parent with a child suffering from bedwetting**, I must reassure him and remove any feeling of guilt. I lead him to find his own inner strength and authority. I look at my own life and I see what anguish I am personally experiencing and that my child can sense. I realize that fear solves nothing, and that there is a solution to this situation that is making me anxious. I trust the fact that I am guided at each instant. **Enuresis** can be made to disappear from my life by taking charge of myself and my life. I alone can have authority over my inner world. I allow my feelings to roam because they are the source of my inner power. It is only by recognizing and accepting↓♥ them as part of who I am that I can create my life as I want it to be.

INCONTINENCE (in children) *See: BED-WETTING*

INDEX *See: FINGERS — INDEX*

INDIGESTION *See also NAUSEA, POISONING [FOOD], SALMONELLOSIS, STOMACHACHE*

The stomach is the place where my physical body assimilates food. If I have **indigestion**, my body rejects this food, and I am affected by nausea that reveals my ailment, vomiting, abdominal pains or bloating related to the negative air around me. The same occurs with the reality, the thoughts, the feelings and the emotions I experience, which will also cause **indigestion** if I have difficulty in dealing with them. There is an 'overflow' somewhere in my life. There is a disorder, a disharmony within me. What is the situation or the person that I am having difficulty in digesting, catching or assimilating in my life? What is going on in my life that I can't stand any longer because it is too much all at once and it has become intolerable? What is the newness that I refuse to integrate in my life? I may even reach the point of revolting against this situation or this person that I severely criticize. It may also be something unpleasant that I saw or heard and that doesn't 'go down well'. I must take a position in a situation and so far, I have been incapable of doing so. I don't tolerate people being inconsistent in their actions and their words. I don't know how to manage this situation; the words I want to express remain stuck inside of me. Anxiety, insecurity and aggressiveness 'turn my stomach upside down' and as I can't digest normally, I will physically eject food as I reject the new ideas or situations I experience. I feel physically or emotionally threatened. Everything makes me anxious because I am not in contact with my inner power. As I don't digest what is going on inside of me, I will find it difficult to digest what is going on outside of me.

I accept↓♥ to go and see all the treasures that are inside of me. I look at myself head-on and I see that all the emotions that inhabit me make me a unique and extraordinary being. By being **Aware** of who I am, I can change what I want in my life. I learn to put **Love** in all these situations, because there are some things I must become **Aware** of. **Love** is the ingredient that will help me to digest and pass through the situations in my life, in harmony with my being. I can thus take the decisions that will lead me to achieve my greatest goals.

INDUCED ABORTION (IA) *See: CHILDBIRTH — ABORTION*

INFARCTION *(cerebral) See: BRAIN — CEREBROVASCULAR ACCIDENT [C.V.A.]*

INFARCTION *(in general)*

An **infarction** is generally the death of part of an organ's tissues, also called **necrosis**, caused by the obstruction of the artery bringing blood to this region. Though regions such as the intestine, the spleen and the bones may be affected, the most exposed regions are the brain, the lungs and the myocardium, the **heart♥**'s envelope.

As blood circulation is suddenly stopped by a clot or a deposit of lipids (a sort of fat) in an artery, this means that joy is no longer circulating in this region, even resulting in the death of tissues. According to the region affected, I can ask myself what has led my body to tell me: "That's enough, I can't take it any longer, a part of me is dying". I have lost something vital in my life, with which I identified. I may also feel that I am tireless, and my body is reminding me that I have pushed it far beyond my capacities.

I accept↓♥ to check what needs I may have neglected and how I could get things back into order in my life to enable me to wholly experience events filled with joy and satisfaction.

INFARCTION (myocardial) *See: HEART♥ — INFARCTION [MYOCARDIAL]*

INFECTIONS (in general) *See also: APPENDIX III, FEVER, IMMUNE SYSTEM, INFLAMMATION, PAIN*

Infection is defined by the localized or generalized development of pathogenic[4] germs in the organism, whether they are bacteria, viruses, fungi or parasites. This state occurs when the immune system is unable to combat this invading germ.

This germ can be related in my life to a situation or a person with whom I am experiencing an inner conflict about which I have spoken to no one. As it has not been resolved, it will appear suddenly in the form of an **infection**. An **acute infection** follows a violent but short-lived emotion. A **chronic infection** refers to a very long-standing emotion. I had to make compromises to remain in balance, but now I must make a choice, because this indecisiveness and inaction are taking up all my energy and I must draw from my reserves. I willingly curtailed my own freedom to accommodate others, but I can't do it any longer. The fact of experiencing irritation or disruption weakens my immune system, which can't prevent an invasion from taking place. I must ask myself the question: "What is irritating or affecting me so deeply? What is this conflicted tension I am feeling at work or in my family and that is disturbing me so? What is **infecting** my life to the point that I can no longer protect myself adequately? Am I afraid or vulnerable because of a situation or a person that is poisoning my life?" An **infection** indicates that there has been an accumulation of sad feelings and worries over a long period of time. The **infection** appears when I 'can't take it any longer'. There is a conflict between two aspects of my personality. This is reflected in my life where there are definitely one or several situations that must also change and evolve so that I may recover inner peace. A **viral infection** (by a virus) shows me that someone else has taken control over my life. This **infection** forces me to get some rest and to reassess my life. Why am I not living according to my own beliefs and deep values, but blindly following others? A **fungal infection** (caused by a fungus) reveals how far my own anger and my feeling of helplessness are acting as parasites inside of me and eating me up from inside. I refuse to see my full potential, and I let myself be affected by others. I must accept↓♥ the changes taking place in my life and let go of the great anger I want to experience. This anger is all the more meaningful if the infection is accompanied by pain or fever. It is important to go and see which part of my body is affected. If it is an infection of my sexual organs for example, I am experiencing a conflicted situation that irritates me and makes me feel very angry about my sexuality or how I perceive it. The **infection** will persist as long as I haven't resolved the situation, and I may delay in finding a solution because I am afraid of the consequences and the changes it will bring about in my life. An **infection** often occurs following a weakening of my immune system, which means that it is my **Love** for myself that is involved. I must ask myself what attitudes and thoughts I must change or what actions I must take to bring more **Love** into my life. As I know that happy people

---

4. **Pathogenic:** Capable of causing a disease.

have a strong immune system, I do my best for **Love** to grow in me so that **Love** will become my shield and my protection.

I accept↓♥ to clean up my life, 'disinfect' it and let go of the attitudes and behavior that are not beneficial for me.

INFECTIONS (urinary) *See: URINE — URINARY INFECTIONS*

INFECTIONS (vaginal) *See: VAGINA — VAGINITIS*

INFECTIONS (viral) *See: INFECTIONS (IN GENERAL)*

INFECTIOUS MONONUCLEOSIS (IMN) *See: BLOOD — MONONUCLEOSIS*

INFIRMITIES (congenital)

An **infirmity** is a weakness, an absence, an alteration or the loss of a function.

A person dealing with a **congenital infirmity** has great challenges to meet in life. It is important to go and see what part of the body is affected. It will give a clue to the special challenge I have given myself. This **infirmity** may also result from unresolved conflicted situations that my parents were experiencing when I was a fetus or even before, by my grandparents or great-grandparents, and that I am re-living in order to integrate them and learn the life lesson that is attached to it. I am in a personal and family situation where the life structures are very strict, often due to the social pressure to which I feel compelled to adhere. I fear the look and the criticism of others.

I accept↓♥ to have the right to be different and that the important thing is to follow the way of my **heart♥**.

INFLAMMATION *See also: APPENDIX III*

Inflammation is a local defensive reaction of the organism to a pathogenic[5] agent, and is characterized by redness, heat, pain and tumefaction (swelling).

It is the bodily expression of an inner **inflammation**. I am **inflamed** and **enraged** by something or someone: most often it is the 'fire' of the liver or the gallbladder that is in excess, which expresses itself through my body. I must ask myself what aspect of my life is making me 'red and boiling with anger', and will ultimately make me feel guilt, if it is not already the cause of the **inflammation**. It is important to look at what part of the body is affected to get additional information on the cause of the **inflammation**. I feel stuck and limited. My life is rigid and too structured. The **inflammation** gives me an indication that I am living a situation in my life that I don't want to let go. I am resisting change. I am struggling angrily. What I previously needed to support me and help me advance may no longer be required. The contradiction I am living **inflames** me. It irritates me and I become exasperated! It is

5. **Pathogenic:** Capable of causing a disease.

important for me to also check if I had a sexual difficulty in the past, repressed and unresolved, or a feeling of loss that I didn't accept↓♥ and that makes me feel very irritated. It will then be possible for me to be **Aware** of this situation, and have a new and positive understanding of it. I question myself about my beliefs and wonder if I am experiencing an acute inner conflict in which I am against the other people around me.

I accept↓♥ to be different and to express my opinions even if they may differ from those of others. I assert who I am and maintain my uniqueness. I am learning to trust myself and to live more spontaneously.

INFLUENZA / FLU *See also: BRAIN — ENCEPHALITIS, FEVER, HEADACHES, MUSCLE, RESPIRATION DISORDERS*

This condition results from the presence of a virus causing fever, SNEEZING, shivering, headaches, muscular pains, sneezing, breathing difficulties, etc. The **flu**, which affects my body more violently than a cold, can force me to stay in bed for a certain period of time.

As the **flu** is an infectious disease, it is related to anger and is a sign that all bets are off! I can ask myself to whom, or what, I may have taken a dislike. The particular symptoms that appear indicate more specifically what I am currently experiencing: fever is related to anger, sneezing is related to criticism or wanting to get rid of someone or a situation, etc. It is often a conflicted family situation: something was said or a situation was experienced that I 'can't swallow' because certain rules or limits were violated. A quarrel therefore ensued where I felt that my vital space was being violated, or where I risked losing something or someone that belonged to me and that I was clinging to. The influence of certain persons in my entourage can lead me to doubt my judgment or my capacity to accomplish certain tasks. If it involves members of my family, it is still more difficult for me, because all my life I have tried to build my own personality by detaching myself from my family. Because I always seek their approval (mainly that of my parents), I may become confused about who I really am and about the choices I must make. I feel that my inner defenses have disappeared. I am disturbed by an individual who personifies a certain authority over me. Many cases of the **flu** are attributable to beliefs or fears rooted in society, as for example: "I felt so cold today, I'll surely catch the **flu**!" I must ask myself why I have the **flu**. Do I need a rest or some time to pause? Do I force myself to stay in bed in order to not have to face my responsibilities at work or in the family? I have scant trust in myself and I let myself be influenced, or even invaded, by others; the **flu** virus does the same thing, infiltrating my body because my immune system has been 'weakened' by my 'weak' self-esteem. I am in a situation where I am resisting, as I have great efforts to make in my everyday life and I feel like giving up. The **flu** can also appear following a situation where I felt a great disappointment or frustration that leads me to no longer sense what goes on around me (congested nose) or a person ("I can't stand the smell of her.") and also causes more difficult breathing. On the other hand, the fever frees my body of toxins not otherwise released.

I accept↓♥ to express my emotions and let my tears flow to decongest my whole body and let harmony prevail.

INJURY *See: ACCIDENT, CUT*

INSANITY *See also: PSYCHOSIS*

Insanity, also called **madness** or **psychosis**, occurs when I can't take it any longer and **I reject the world in which I live**. I feel abused and persecuted on all sides, mainly by my own family. For me, life is just suffering. I shut myself into my own Universe where I feel quite well. Nothing can affect me. It is my way of cutting myself off permanently from my family and the outside world. It is escape and evasion. This is found especially in **megalomania**, which is associated with an exaggerated sense of my own worth or of the cause in which I am involved. The cause of this lack of realism is lack of self-esteem. I feel small and I project my ideals onto an illusion.

I accept↓♥ to free myself from this **insanity** by receiving **Love** and understanding. If I believe that 'insanity is overcoming me', I must take myself in charge and accept↓♥ that there is a reason for everything that happens to me and that this enables me to become more responsible, freer, more in control of my life. I can thus deal more easily with the new situations that I encounter.

INSOMNIA

The **incapacity for sleeping** corresponds to a deep fear of abandoning myself and letting go. I feel insecure and I want to exercise control over everything that goes on in my life. When I sleep, however, my 'mental faculties' sleep also, for my senses are more alert and open to the unknown. That is why, by keeping my mind busy with all sorts of ideas and situations, even fictional ones that I invent, I prevent sleep from overtaking me. My life is tinged with anguish and guilt, even sometimes with a little paranoia. I have the impression that a person in my entourage is ***malevolent*** toward me, so I feel I must be constantly ***vigilant***. I sense a danger during the night, which prevents me from finding ***sleep***. I often feel that I am not all right. This may result from a feeling that my ego or my survival was previously threatened in some way, which is understandable if I experienced any deep traumas, especially between ages 3 and 5. Chances are that I feel extreme nervousness and that I find it difficult to take a position and make decisions. When I go to bed, there is only me with myself: I no longer have any children, a spouse or work colleagues. I am 'cut off' from the outside world and I hear only what is inside if me. If I am experiencing **insomnia**, if I deny my inner sounds and what is going on inside of me, and which I am preventing myself from expressing outwardly, then my mental activity and my conversation with myself can't stop, and I thereby make sleep escape me. By asking myself too many questions and incessantly questioning myself about: "And if I'd done this, or said that? What will happen if…?" I thus manifest my lack of trust in myself and in others. I live in torment instead of living in the confidence I deserve, trusting that the best will happen to me. It is also as though I were dying each time I fall asleep, which awakens fears about the unknown in the night. Insomnia can be strongly related to conscious or unconscious guilt. For one reason or another, I may feel that I "don't deserve to rest". It may be because I feel guilty of not succeeding in life, of not doing everything I should for my children, etc. I may also have programmed myself to think that "sleeping is a waste of time": "I have so many things to do". The thymus gland is closely related to ***sleep*** and, thereby, to the energy of the **heart♥**. **Insomnia** can thus also be related to my capacity for loving myself and for trusting in **Love** and thereby in life itself.

I accept↓♥ to relax, to breathe easier, release control and find 'peace of mind' in order to allow ***sleep*** to take place in my life. I learn to trust myself and I know that "the Earth will continue to spin" even if I allow myself some moments of rest. I let go, knowing that I am fully guided and that my inner voice knows what is good for me.

INTESTINAL AILMENTS *See also: CANCER OF THE COLON / OF THE INTESTINE, INTESTINES / COLITIS / CONSTIPATION / DIARRHEA, INDIGESTION*

The **intestine** is the center for absorbing and integrating food (it keeps what is good for the body and expels the rest); this food is present in physical form (foods) as well as emotional (emotions, feelings) or mental (thoughts). Anything that causes me sadness, fear, confusion, revolt, shame or any other clashing thoughts or feelings can find release and create **intestinal problems**. As this is where digestion takes place, if I am thwarted and feel myself the victim of a 'low trick', a 'dirty trick' or I have the impression that someone has played a 'mean trick' on me, I will have an ailment in the **intestines** because I simply won't digest it! I will be especially affected if the 'dirty player' is a member of my family. **Pains in the intestine** often appear following a separation, involving my spouse, but it may also be a business associate, a child, a teacher, etc. As I can't digest this situation, it will manifest itself by a problem in my **intestines**. I could '**die of hunger**', and I would still persist in refusing to accept↓♥ what happened. If it is my **small intestine** that is affected, I may tend to judge the situations I encounter with very sharp opinions involving my notions of 'right' and 'wrong'. I have 'hardened' myself through the severity I experienced when I was younger. I also tend to feel that I have missed many things in my life. I have difficulty in defining and ***assimilating*** my true needs. The **intestines** (especially the **large intestine**) are also related to **my ability to let go**, feeling secure enough inside to be spontaneous. **My intestines symbolize the fact of allowing events to circulate in my life**. I may have a very strong need to **hold in** and **control** what happens to me. I cling to certain things, persons or situations, often even to the point of feeling jealous and possessive, and my **intestines** are congested by everything I hold in and is no longer useful, which can cause **constipation** or **tuberculosis**, for instance. I let myself be 'eaten up' by criticism and affected by gossip and malicious rumors. I resist change because gaining more autonomy scares me. I make myself endure grief and pain because I find it difficult to turn over a new leaf with respect to a person or a situation. **Bad intestinal absorption** indicates that I don't know what is good for me. I prefer to submissively obey a leader or a religion rather than live on the basis of my own beliefs and values. When I resign because I don't know what meaning to give to my life, an **intestinal perforation** may appear.

I accept↓♥ to be autonomous and tell myself that I have all the necessary resources inside of me to create what I want. The only person over whom I can wield control is myself!

INTESTINE (cancer of the) *See: CANCER OF THE INTESTINE*

INTESTINES — COLIC *See also: GAS*

Colic is one or several contractions resulting from a **great inner tension**, from a situation that makes me vulnerable and annoys me so much that intestinal congestion appears, with pains in the stomach, the glandular canals and the urinary system.

I am impatient and irritated about a situation or a person. It annoys me and 'gives me a **colic**'. I don't have control, and it bothers me. I doubt my capacities, I lack self-confidence, I am afraid of not being up to it, and I don't know how to solve a problem. A typical example featuring **infant colics** involves me, as a mother, when I am afraid of not taking care of my baby properly, or not doing enough. The baby senses my inner anxiety and becomes anxious itself (a child suffering from **colic** must be surrounded with calm, patience and **Love**).

I accept↓♥ that in life, everything happens for the best. And so I **let go**, I do my best with **Love**. What I saw as problems and insecurities become simply experiences that help me pursue my development and grow. Exercises of respiration, relaxation and meditation can help me regain contact with my inner being, realize all the forces that are in me and make my **impatience** disappear in the presence of a person or a situation that **annoys** me.

INTESTINES — COLITIS (mucosity of the colon) *See also: INFLAMMATION, INTESTINES — COLON*

Colitis (-itis = anger) is a sometimes ulcerous inflammation of the colon, the **large intestine**.

The role of the colon can be compared to the way I behave and deal with my own Universe. When I am incapable of being myself in the presence of authority and in my personal relations (spouse, parents, teachers, boss, etc.), I control my gestures and actions because I fear the reaction of the person whose approval and **Love** I want. I get to the point of living passively and believing in fate. I feel powerless with respect to a person or a group to whose authority or power I feel subjected. I am the assistant, and not the Number One, the head. I suffer situations that are indigestible for me. It is as though I were being struck repeatedly. I feel oppressed and rejected. I tend to have obsessive-compulsive behavior. I cling to the past and instead of moving forward in life, I am 'on hold'. **Colitis** often manifests itself in children who fear the reactions of their very severe and demanding parents. I feel in want of my mother's **Love**. I have **such a need for affection, Love and appreciation** that I want to **please at all costs** (even to the point of stifling my personality and my basic needs). I am not myself, and I don't dare to express my emotions; I repress them. I am very demanding for myself, and the fact of always pushing my capacities to the maximum brings me great stress. I often choke back things that I find indigestible. This **affective dependence** leads me to feel anger that eats me up inside, along with frustration and humiliation. If I experience these feelings intensely, an **ulcer** will appear. My emotional reactions warned me that I should change my attitude, but I didn't understand. Now, it is a physical signal. How should I act? **Hemorrhagic colitis** (commonly named the **hamburger disease** in some countries) indicates that the conflict especially involves one or several members of my family or a group that I consider as my family.

I accept↓♥ that happiness comes from what I feel inside. **I am learning to love myself** and be myself, and **I take my place**. I let go of my preconceived ideas and prejudices. I am acquiring independence and autonomy and I realize that I am more and more happy because I am now acting in accordance with my own nature.

INTESTINES — COLON (ailments of the) *See also: CANCER OF THE COLON*

The **colon** (or **large intestine**) is located between the small intestine and the rectum. This is where the digestion of food ends and the residue is prepared to be evacuated.

When it is affected, I must ask myself: "What am I holding in so much?" I have been in a situation for several years and must now detach myself from that situation, in part or totally, to make place for new conditions or situations. This may involve my personal life or my work. I fear deprivation, solitude and pain. I must turn a new leaf on a dirty or degrading situation that was painful and vexing and that I still can't explain for myself. I may have felt my reputation sullied and it annoys me. The **irritable colon** indicates that I am feeling great nervousness that may be blown out of proportion if I am faced with the unknown. I don't know how to set limits and I may feel that my intimacy is being scorned. I then become controlling to give myself a feeling of security. If there are **abnormal amounts of mucosity**, I must ask myself what I am accumulating this way (including emotions) that fills an inner void but also prevents me from staying the course on my life goals. **Oxyuriasis** (an infestation of the **colon** by a pinworm or seatworm), which affects young children especially, throws **Light** on my feeling of being abused. I am confused in my relations and my ideas because of my attachment to the past and to people. I absolutely want to please a relative. This leads me to confusion and I scatter my energy, feeling far and remote from the other. There is a situation or a person from whom I must cut my ties.

I accept↓♥ to let the past evacuate itself, I abandon my old thoughts in order to allow my inner wisdom to emerge. I become increasingly **Aware** of my inner riches by letting go of a history gone by and integrating new experiences. By allowing the movement of life to circulate in me, I know that whatever happens, I will be able to face the situation and emerge from it, grown in stature and richer.

INTESTINES — CONSTIPATION *See also: CANCER OF THE COLON*

Constipation takes place inside the **intestine** when the muscular movements that carry out elimination are slowed down, which causes a congestion of waste materials.

These waste materials are but the physical manifestation of my dark thoughts, my concerns, my anger and the jealousy that are cluttering me up. **Constipation** is often associated with a diet poor in fibers. This indicates a great will to **control** the events of my life, resulting from inner uncertainty and insecurity. I am **a very troubled person who needs the approval of others**. I may have an obsession with details, needing to check everything several times to reassure myself that 'everything is under control'. This leads me to question myself about my identity among the people who surround me and about my place in society. My insecurity even makes me tend to be petty and egotistical. Situations that promote **constipation** may occur when I face a difficult financial situation, when I have conflicted relations or when I set out on a trip, because that is when I am most likely to feel worried and 'un-anchored'. Often, I experience a duality between "I want to leave" but at the same time "I don't want to leave". The unknown scares me. I **cling to my old ideas** and my personal belongings. It may be a person I want to hold on to. What I already know affords me a degree of control and gives me an **illusion of security**. I hold onto the past, of which I feel I am a ***lamentable*** slave. I don't feel up to it, I am powerless to change certain situations and it "makes me **sh_**". I am so afraid of being judged that I repress my spontaneity, I prevent myself from moving forward. I thus repress my 'problems' and my past emotions, for fear of seeing them re-surface and having to face them. I live under pressure. I feel stuck in a situation and it makes me tense. I tend to accumulate reserves of fear over my material deprivation. As the fact of holding back my stools demonstrated a certain control or power when I was a **child**, I may still want to do the same thing later on as an adult, even unconsciously, as a sign of defiance against authority in general. When have I allowed myself to take my place and be myself? When was the last time I felt free and full of spirit? What's holding me back? Why this reticence in loving, in holding back from giving, or giving of myself, in friendly as well as emotional relationships? Why all this guilt?

I accept↓♥ that I absolutely must **let go** of everything that no longer suits me, and ***release my grip***. I accept↓♥ here and now to free myself of the past, to move forward and lead a more exciting life. I feel much more relaxed because I trust in life.

INTESTINES — CROHN'S DISEASE / ILEITIS *See also: APPENDICITIS, INTESTINES — DIARRHEA*

Ileitis is defined as an inflammation of the ileon, the last part of the small **intestine**, and is characterized by intense pains. In the case of bacterial or viral diseases, it can resemble an appendicitis attack. Infections related to AIDS and tuberculosis can cause an inflammation of the ileon, but the acute chronic cases involve **Crohn's**[6] **disease**.

It can be a form of self-punishment following a feeling of intense guilt. There are 'dark thoughts' of anger and despair. I want to prevent my children from becoming autonomous and I do everything I can for that. It involves my self-esteem: I feel 'not up to snuff', 'not OK', a 'good-for-nothing'. I depreciate myself so much that I come to think that nobody loves me and that people want me to feel inferior. I reach the point of 'stooping low'[7]. These feelings will add themselves to a situation where I feel deprived, materially or affectively. I feel that the object of this deprivation was stolen from me in a despicable, disgusting manner. To this may be added the fear of dying. Revolt will then brew inside of me. Throughout my whole body I sense a feeling of hate that weighs heavily and that I may refuse to see. A lie may be its cause. This only increases my fear of being rejected by others. As I find it difficult to integrate myself in a group, I stay silently in my corner with my worries. I feel like a king (queen) in my castle: I cling to my **crown** and hide behind it. I feel threatened by the whole world and I hide behind a mask, a title or a false image. I want to please others to give myself some power and hide my helplessness. I am always on a war footing. I can't accept↓♥ how nasty my family was with me and it makes me want to heave. As I have the impression that I am nothing, this disease may help me to receive the attention I need and that I don't feel I am getting. My self-esteem is low and I am energetically too open, in my stomach, to receiving anything, including what is negative in my entourage and can affect me. I reject myself so much that, in terms of energy, it is as if my stomach has become a trash can and I am allowing the people in my entourage to dump their negative energy into me. I let myself be dumped into because I don't take my place enough and I reject situations, which makes me experience diarrheas. I am deeply in search of my personal or spiritual identity, and the seriousness of the disease tells me how far it involves an aspect of my life that is fundamental and essential.

I accept↓♥ to find out how I can increase my self-esteem and enable myself to truly find my identity and my rightful place in my family or in society. It will help me find more calm and harmony in my life. The fact of truly finding my rightful place will provide me with a natural protection from my environment, and I thus discover the security of my 'I AM'. Life is beautiful and I too have the right to live!

---

6. **Crohn** (Burrill Bernard): A digestive tract surgeon at Mount Sinai Hospital in New York (1884–1983). The disease was precisely described in the United States in 1932.

7. **Stooping low**: To obey, to submit to, someone else.

INTESTINES — DIARRHEA

Diarrhea is an acute or chronic emission of overly frequent stools. **Diarrhea** manifests itself by such a rapid displacement of food from the stomach to the **intestine** that it doesn't have the time to be completely assimilated. **Diarrhea** can be brief or chronic (when the period of **diarrhea** exceeds 3 weeks).

This state is often caused by fear or the desire to avoid or flee a situation or a reality that is wholly unpleasant or new for me. A flow of new ideas arrives and I don't have time to integrate them properly. I wish that some things would go faster in my life, which makes me feel very impatient. I feel trapped by something new to me, and it turns my inner sensitivity upside down! I may feel stuck in my obligations to the Law. I **rẽject** myself, I rail against myself and I am desperate! I was targeted with a dirty trick that I just can't digest and I prefer to evacuate it as fast as I can. I felt myself 'hit in the gut' and petrified. On top of everything, I currently have a very lousy image of myself. I feel guilty. I am overwhelmed by these events. In my intimate relations, I find it difficult to accept↓♥ the **Love**, the tenderness and the kindness of others. I am experiencing a dependence that makes me powerless to act. I really need something different, to change for something new. It is not the food, but rather my thoughts, **that no longer suit me**. I want to eliminate something dangerous or dirty. As I can't 'evacuate' this with words, my body expresses itself in its own way! If I constantly express ideas or feelings of rejection (the fear of ***feeling*** rejected or the desire to reject others) or a situation where I feel stuck, then chances are high that I will have **diarrhea**. I may feel so overwhelmed by events that I want to end it as quickly as possible. At the same time, I release the unpleasant emotions linked to it. I may feel helpless and I prefer to escape rather than have to 'face the music'. I find it difficult to say no, to respect myself; the **intestine** refuses to digest and immediately evacuates what I wanted to leave outside of myself. I seek my identity, which I want to bring in line with my parents' expectations. If I don't listen to life and its signals (as some persons live), spontaneous **diarrhea** may also manifest itself. I also feel these emotions in the case of **cholera**: as I am **not Aware** of my creative power, I place my security in something outside of myself (a god, a government, etc.). I feel helpless and desperate because I have no resources. I believe I am condemned to live in misery.

I accept↓♥ to take the time to see, to feel and to listen to my **heart♥** to see what is going on in my life. I thus integrate and assimilate the situations of my existence and my past. When I truly slow down, I realize to what extent I was passing right through (just like the food) and was not taking the time to see the goodness and the beauties of life. My body is warning me that I must trust in life and that I am constantly supported. I accept↓♥ my inner creative strengths. I accept↓♥ to deserve happiness, to have my own living space, with respect for myself and for others. This way, wherever I live in the world, I can create a better world where it is good to live.

NOTE: Some travelers visiting developing countries catch **traveler's diarrhea** or ***turista***. Discovering immense poverty and misery opens the **heart♥** and unconsciously upsets the mind as well as the physical organism. It is often an unconscious reaction that shows me to what extent I can be attached to a certain form of comfort or to a certain pace or lifestyle.

INTESTINES — DIVERTICULITIS

Diverticulitis (-itis = anger) is an inflammation of the small cavities (**diverticules**) in the walls of the colon (the large **intestine**).

This ailment is related to **anger** held back in my everyday life. I am currently experiencing a situation in which I feel a prisoner and to which I can see no end; this causes tension, pressure, pain and sorrow. I feel trapped. My **intestine** becomes fragile, like my emotions. I am constantly on the alert and expecting the worst. I am secretive in what I share with others. I won't allow anyone to penetrate into the nooks and crannies of my personal life. The first step toward a solution is acceptance↓♥. How can I resolve something if I refuse to accept↓♥ its existence?

I therefore accept↓♥ the situation as a reality and I remain open to the divine channel that brings me the **Love** necessary to integrate this experience. I let go of my old resentments. By my acceptance↓♥ and my openness, various solutions become available to me because I am no longer blinded by anger.

INTESTINES — DYSENTERY *See also: INTESTINES / COLIC / DIARRHEA*

Dysentery is an infectious and contagious disease with an ulcerous inflammation of the large **intestine**.

Dysentery indicates how focused I am on the future and disconnected from my present (and from myself), and that I reject my past. I hold firm to my positions and I stand up against people who have different opinions. **Amebic dysentery**, the most commonly familiar form, which is due to an intestinal parasite, shows me that I have someone who is clinging to me. That person is a real 'parasite'. Unless I am the one who is clinging to others… I have always done my best, but I have often stood in the sidelines. I would like it very much if someone would take over from me, for there are things that I can no longer stand or that I ***feel*** I no longer have the physical or psychological capacity to pursue. **Bacillary dysentery** (which is derived from the word 'stick'), due to an intestinal bacterium, is an indication that I am incapable of defending myself. I allow others to take advantage of me. I am going nowhere, I am 'dried out', financially and affectively. I develop a hard, dry attitude to protect myself.

I accept↓♥ to be in contact with my present emotions and to be true about the things I want to change in my life. I ask for help if I need it, I take my responsibilities for myself and I regain mastery over my life!

INTESTINES — GASTROENTERITIS *See also: STOMACH / DISORDERS / GASTRITIS, INTESTINES — DIARRHEA, NAUSEA*

Gastroenteritis is an acute inflammation of the **gastric (stomach) and intestinal (intestine) mucous membranes**, characterized by vomiting and diarrhea of infectious origin. It is possible to determine an 'external cause' and relate it to the ingestion of contaminated water or food.

However, I must also go and see the 'inner cause' that made me experience this event. Here, the irritant is far more important than in a case of gastritis, for it affects not only the food's point of entry, but also the starting point of the integration process, which shows that I am so irritated and frustrated by what is happening to me that I can't absorb anything at all. I therefore want to reject a situation or a person — if not life itself — and I am 'red with anger', which makes me experience diarrhea and vomiting. I find it difficult to accept↓♥ events and the fact of dying one day. I may hold on to certain mental patterns that have now become obsolete. A person or a situation that is indigestible for me turns against me by inflaming me emotionally. I am haunted by certain thoughts that are eating me up inside. I feel constant uncertainty. Despair overcomes me and my sensitivity is extremely upset. I am afraid of myself and of what inhabits me. I perceive myself as bad, and I am afraid of having many enemies. I feel very uncertain and I prefer to melt into the crowd rather than stand up even if I make a few waves around me. I don't dare to live my life as I want to. Maybe it is authority that I have difficulty in digesting, for I tend to live according to established laws with no possibility for me to depart from them, following my old beliefs.

I accept↓♥ to open myself to a new reality and new ideas and learn once again to trust in others and in life, by being able to manifest my disappointment instead of letting it brew inside and create all sorts of pain for myself. I stop expecting approval from my entourage.

INTESTINES — RECTUM *See also: ANUS*

The **rectum** is the terminal segment of the large **intestine** after the sigmoid[8] colon and ends at the anal orifice.

If someone or something in my life thwarts me and I find that questionable or 'dirty', I will want to expel this thing or this person from my thoughts and my life. If I can't do so, pains or bleeding will appear in my **rectum**. If I experience this situation very acutely, as an ***impardonable*** dirty trick that I just can't let pass, there may appear disorders in the **rectum,** or even a **cancer of the rectum**. It may be the departure of a loved one that I don't accept↓♥ for I need to be in contact, communicate and share with that person. I am clinging with all my strength to a person or a situation. I find it difficult to forgive what happened, which is preventing me from letting go and moving on to something else because I felt humiliated. Still, I may feel disgust and repulsion. Why then hold on at all costs? The situation experienced very often involves one or several family members. In such situations, it is usually the **upper sigmoid rectum** that is affected. Either I may want to let go of something or someone from my life but I feel incapable of doing so, or it may be something

8. **Sigmoid colon**: A segment of the colon, in the form of a handle, descending the left side of the pelvic cavity and continuing into the **rectum**.

or someone external that is compelling me to make 'it' a part of my life, and this makes me feel very irritated. I am learning to remain open and try to understand the reasons for the situation that upsets me. I see that even if I feel that someone acted badly, this person probably had good reasons for acting as she did and her motives were sound. When the **lower rectum** is affected, it is a situation where I wonder what my rightful place is, where I am going in life and what my real power is. My sexual orientation may be questioned. There is a great questioning about who I am, my identity or the direction I should take, because when I was younger, people had been very directive with me. I may feel very alone and abandoned. There is no recognition in my family, I am seeking my place. I feel I have 'fallen between two stools'. Not having my place in my family, I feel apart from others and I am afraid of being abandoned. Am I living my life, or someone else's? The stakes are very high, and I can get so tense that all my muscles are stiffened. It is important to note that this state of being can often refer to an event or a state from my childhood: the elimination role is primordial for a child and represents my ease or unease before any authority, notably my parents, and a fear of losing control. The ailments experienced during **defecation**[9] reflect the way in which I hold back or release my inner discomforts and the hidden sides of my personality.

I accept↓♥ to acknowledge my qualities and I know that whatever decisions are made, the results will always be for the best. I must show **forgiveness** or **clemency** either to myself or to someone else. It is a little as if I was giving **absolution** to free myself of everything negative that I held in for so many years, and from which I now want to free myself. I can thus recover my inner peace and be the ***ruler*** of my own life.

INTESTINE (small) DISORDERS *See also: INTESTINES — COLITIS*

The **small intestine** is the part of the **intestine** that follows the stomach and precedes the large **intestine**. This is where the absorption of food takes place.

This corresponds to the integration and **assimilation** of the information that reaches my **conscience**, and what I decide to do with it. I analyze what is good for me and what I must reject. If I am disturbed or anguished, if I feel compelled to set aside my values or my priorities to please others, my **small intestine** will react. I am constantly faced with choices and decisions. If I am afraid of lacking something, if I allow others to decide in my place instead of trusting my inner voice, my **small intestine** will no longer be able to work effectively. By my closed mind, my criticism and my refusal to let go of my past, I refuse to integrate new ideas and new experiences in my life. I may feel separated from my family or my spouse; it is as if a structure has disintegrated. When the annoyances become intolerable and I can't digest them, **cancer** appears. I want too much to understand, to analyze what is going on and the reasons for things, and it eats me up inside. The fact of not feeling ***accepted***↓♥, especially by my family, saddens me deeply. Certain ***hidden*** or undiscussed issues or questions that could have been resolved are 'rotting' inside of me.

---

9. **Defecation**: The expulsion of fecal matter.

I accept↓♥ to confidently open myself to new experiences. I allow this energy of movement to re-enter my life. I can thus advance lightheartedly and listen to my inner voice that knows exactly what is beneficial for me. I thank the Source for everything I receive and I taste the present moment.

INTESTINE (small) — ULCERATIVE COLITIS (UC) *See also: INTESTINES — COLITIS*

Hemorrhagic rectocolitis (**HRC**) is an inflammatory disease of the digestive tube that exclusively affects the rectum and the colon (or large **intestine**). It usually manifests itself by an alternation of diarrhea and constipation. The stools contain blood. It is a chronic affection, where surges of inflammation of variable seriousness alternate with often prolonged phases of remission. Inflammation is the organism's reaction to an aggression, whatever the aggressor may be. The inflammatory reaction corresponds to the influx of the organism's defense cells, called immune cells (the white globules, some of which secrete antibodies), whose role is to eliminate the aggressor.

Who or what is attacking me? I have the impression that I am poisoning myself from inside with the tensions to which I am submitting myself. There is something about my family that I don't digest and I can't get rid of it. They are clinging to me and I can't stand it any longer!

I accept↓♥ to take my place and stake my position with the others, especially the members of my family. I assert my needs and I feel free in my choices.

INTESTINES — TENIA

The **tenia** or **tapeworm** is a parasitic worm that is found in the **intestine** and that can be a few inches to several yards long. The parasitic disease that is due to the infestation of this worm is **teniasis**.

Also called the **tapeworm**, the **tenia** develops in persons who have the impression that ideas or ways of thinking contrary to their own are being imposed on them. I feel far and somewhat remote from my mother and I want to please her by being always clean and honest. However, I feel sad and misunderstood, abused and dirty. I may have the impression that '**parasites**' are prowling around me. As I find it difficult to assert myself and say no, I let my energy be 'eaten away'. The concerns and sorrows that I have difficulty in letting go will also foster the appearance of **tenia**. This bitter taste makes my digestion difficult, my lungs allow some corrupted energy to pass through and the parasitic worms install themselves, producing irritation and nervousness. Could I also be a parasite for certain persons, believing that I absolutely need them to be able to succeed in life or to protect myself? I am living on illusions and deceit. I easily criticize. I am like a worm, 'spineless': I must rely on others. I deny who I am, it is as though a stranger were living in me. I have become remote from my being and I feel a great emptiness.

To heal myself inside, I accept↓♥ to take care of my ideas, I make place for pleasure and joy. I take my rightful place in life. I reclaim my power. I run my life as I desire. I live in truth and I return to the true values.

INTOLERANCE to GLUTEN

Gluten is the protein of wheat flour that, in the production of bread, constitutes the elastic mass that imprisons the bubbles of carbon dioxide and, when coagulated by heat, sets the texture of the soft inside of the bread loaf.

If I am **intolerant to gluten**, I must ask myself if I am feeling stuck, with others constantly 'in my bubble', my vital space, especially my friends. I can't breathe any longer for being so tightly surrounded, with everyone 'stuck to my skin'. I am experiencing a duality because I like people, mainly because they support me, sustain me and protect me. I sometimes feel that those who surround me want to fashion my life and even manage it. I feel I am a prisoner of myself, and therefore of the others, by this very fact. I feel like letting everything go and pushing them all away from me. What am I trying to hide from myself? I am very sensitive and I easily allow myself to be invaded. I admit that I have reached my limits. However, I must learn to take my place and give myself space.

I accept↓♥ to examine what my true needs are and to assert them with all the persons around me. I can assert my individuality and take my place while respecting others. I choose to live moments of solitude to renew contact with my inner world. Consciously, I know that is where I will find all the answers. My feeling of freedom grows every time I listen to my inner voice that knows what I need, and I give myself the means to satisfy them myself.

INTOXICATION *See: POISONING [FOOD]*

IRREGULAR WALK *See: CLAUDICATION / LIMPING*

ITCHING (anal) *See: ANUS — ANAL ITCHING*

ITCHING (vaginal) *See also: VAGINA (IN GENERAL)*

Vaginal itching is related to sexuality and to the female principle. If it itches, it is because something is annoying me with respect to my sexual relations; my partner is making me impatient. As I do in the case of ordinary **itching**, I ask myself what is irritating me, bothering me and annoying me.

When **itching** appears, I accept↓♥ to find the cause and learn to communicate and hold an open-**hearted♥** conversation to express what I feel.

ITCHING / PRURITUS *See: SKIN — ITCHING*

-ITIS (disease names ending in) *See: APPENDIX III*

J

JAUNDICE / ICTERUS *See also: BLOOD / DISORDERS / BLOOD CIRCULATION, LIVER DISORDERS*

Icterus, commonly called **jaundice**, is an excess of bilirubin caused by a massive destruction of red globules in the blood, due to a congenital anomaly in their membrane or to an aggression. It can also result from the destruction of liver cells or an incapacity for eliminating bile (retentional syndrome). The result is a yellow coloration of the skin and the whites of the eyes.

As it is related to the cleaning of the blood system, I therefore have difficulty in 'cleaning' my emotions. I feel very intense bitter emotions of envy, disappointment and frustration, to the point where I "become **jaundiced** about such and such a situation" and I "turn yellow". I experience a lot of resentment. I become so sharp and excessive in my ideas and opinions that I cling to them, creating an imbalance inside of me. I am in conflict with the power exercised in my place by authority in society, which I prefer to flee rather than join it. I want to move away from a situation that is intolerable for me. I refuse to change. I feel guilt and shame. I feel a prisoner, in an emotional, social or physical yoke. I question myself about the road to follow and I question myself about who I am and the directions I should take. My negative spirit becomes narrow-minded and I have difficulty in taking an overall view of a given situation or of my life in general. I have lost courage, and I feel so much a prisoner of my unexpressed and unchannelled emotions that I need to be alone in order to 'refuel'. The '**jaundice of the newborn'** is also related to frustrations, disappointment or resentment. I want to escape, but it is impossible for me: I am tied to a situation or simply to my mother. As a child, I may have taken upon myself my parents' thoughts, as for example if my parents wanted a boy but had a girl, I may feel responsible for my parents' disappointment and I have the impression that I am lacking protection.

I accept↓♥ to open myself to the people around me, for I have much to learn from them.

JAW AILMENTS *See also: MUSCLES — TETANUS / LOCKJAW*

The **jaws** are bones essential for **eating**, to begin the process of digesting and assimilating what I eat, whether it is food or the reality around me.

They enable me to swallow realities, inasmuch as I am able to swallow them, physically as well as emotionally. They represent my capacity and my strength in choosing to open myself to something or someone. My **jaws** therefore make possible safe exchanges with others. They open the way to truth and self-assertion. All the inner power that I manifest is symbolized by my

jaws. The **upper** one refers to my relation to my father. The **lower** one refers to my relation to my mother. Because they must meet as opposites to be effective, the **jaws** symbolize my capacity for facing the struggles or oppositions that I encounter or those that inhabit me. **Jaw problems** can appear when I **clench my teeth** because there's some repression and I hold in all the energy related to anger, obstinacy, stubbornness, and maybe even an unconscious desire to get revenge on someone or something. Or maybe I want to avoid crying out my inner pain. Things are not going as I want them to, and rage overcomes me. I incessantly 'chew over' the same problems without finding any solutions. I hold on to my immature emotions and behaviors. Then **jaw tics** may appear, which show me that I am 'talking in silence'. What do I absolutely want to keep for myself? What are the emotions that I am imprisoning? I see events with a certain narrowness of mind. I am not in contact with my inner power and I try to cling to an authority external to myself. Where has my sense of responsibility gone? My feeling of powerlessness produces a feeling of inferiority and jealousy. When they are **painful**, it is because I am using a forced smile to hide my desire to attack or bite someone. A **fracture of the jaw** follows from my tendency to precipitate things and decisions. I feel rushed by life and others, but I am the one who wants to go too fast. I can be withering in my comments to others. However, I feel muzzled and powerless to really express my true inner feelings of sorrow and pain. If I have a difficulty with the **joints of my jaws** (called the **TMJ**, **temporomandibular joint**) (they appear to be unaligned), I must ask myself if there is a gap, a difference between what I think and what I dare to say openly. I am experiencing an inner duality between telling or hiding the truth and my deeper feelings. There is a distortion between my emotions and my thoughts; I am torn between what I would like to do (wishes) and what I must do (duty). The dreams I used to have about my future life are totally different from the reality, and great disappointments and questionings follow from this. I am losing hope of reaching my ideal as an individual or as a couple in society. When I **grind my teeth**, I am feeling insecurity. I am anxious and I repress my emotions a lot. This is especially true among children toward their parents. My **jaws** may also become **decalcified** and **softened**. They show me how I too can be 'soft' in certain situations, especially when I have the impression that people laughed at me and paid no attention to what I was saying. There follows a very great depreciation for me. I may also feel dominated and incapable of expressing myself because of my timidity or my fears. I may also have been forbidden to speak, which I interpreted as: "I must have nothing very interesting to say". When my **jaws block**, I am incapable of expressing myself or of controlling what goes on around me, and I repress my emotions. My **jaw** may be paralyzed by fear or sorrow after a situation where I felt powerless to speak or act in order to prevent a situation from happening. A **blocked jaw** may have locked at the very moment when I tried with all my strength to ***interdict*** and prevent a word from being spoken or an event from happening. I felt paralyzed for not being able to say something. I feel ***muzzled***. When there is a **cancer of the jaw**, this incapacity is felt intensely, especially in my family where my words carry no weight. If my **jaws are too narrow**, the development of my personality suffered from bullying. My obligation to be the best puts me under great pressure. My intellect is constantly stimulated, contrary to my emotional side, which is in deficit. I must relax and allow the energy to circulate freely.

I accept↓♥ to express myself freely. I am fully guided in what I have to say and I reclaim my rightful place. I live in honesty, in my **heart♥** and in truth.

JEALOUSY

The dictionary defines **jealousy** as "a feeling of vexation mixed with envy", related to the fact that someone else obtains or possesses something I would have wanted to obtain or possess.

It results from inner insecurity, poor self-esteem and poor self-confidence that make me doubt my capacity for creating things in my life or fear losing what I have (notably my spouse). I come to develop aggressiveness and frustration. My distrust of others is exaggerated, my mental discussions are badly managed and my beliefs are often mistaken. I am very sensitive to the criticism and gossip that result from the **jealousy** of others toward me. I become **Aware** that my fears lead me to exert control over a person or a situation. In fact, it is my anxieties that are exercising control over my life.

I accept↓♥ to trust in life, I get rid of my old beliefs and I take appropriate means to heal these inner wounds by individual or group psychotherapy or by an energy-based approach that will help me to connect better with my own inner power. I realize that this **jealousy** is imprisoning me and poisoning the lives of others. I will then feel freer, more confident and more able to carry this freedom and this confidence over to others in order to experience more harmony with myself and with the people around me.

JODHPUR THIGHS *See: CELLULITIS*

JOINTS (temporomandibular) *See: JAW AILMENTS, MOUTH DISEASE*

JOINTS (in general) *See also: ARTHRITIS — ARTHROSIS*

A **joint**, or articulation, is a part of the body where two or several bones are joined in a way that permits movements adjusted[1] to the anatomy of the human body (synonyms: joint, junction, juncture).

The **joint** represents **facility**, **mobility**, **adaptability** and **flexibility**, lending grace and fluidity to movement. All these simple qualities are possible with a **joint** in perfect condition. However, it also has its limits. As bone represents the 'densest' form of energy, the most fundamental in my existence, **articular** problems are involved in all the physiological components of the human body (tissues, blood, etc.). Thus, an **articular disorder** indicates a **resistance**, a

---

1. The closely meshed seams joining the bones of the cranium are generally considered to be motionless **joints**.

holding back, a certain stiffness in my thoughts, in my actions or in the expression of my often repressed emotions. An **inflammation** appears if I am afraid of moving forward: I become incapable of moving, I have difficulty in changing direction, I play the game of being emotionally detached, I don't act spontaneously, I hesitate or refuse to abandon myself to life and give my trust. Hence the anger that often results from my refusal to communicate my frustrations and disappointments. When I move painfully or with difficulty, my body is saying that I don't want to understand (or accept↓♥ to understand) something that is limiting me in expressing my Self. I feel stuck, ***locked up*** in a facet of my life. I have difficulty in being articulate, in seeing my ideas clearly and being able to express them. I feel like a 'kid'[2] with very few options. **Joint pains** (**arthralgia**) show that some emotions and shocks were endured for a long time and are now intolerable because there are too many of them. These **pains** indicate a withdrawal into myself, a lack of flexibility (with myself or with others) or a lack of adjustment. **Stiffness in the joints** tells me how I can also be 'stiff' (rigid) and intolerant in my way of thinking, and that it would be to my benefit to lay down my blinders in order to see life more positively. I may be living too much in terms of external structures and authority instead of listening to my inner voice, which should be my supreme authority. I have the impression I am carrying the whole world on my shoulders. If my **joints crack**, I resent myself for having done or said certain things, even if nobody else has reproached me for anything. If my body experiences **degeneration in a joint**, I withdraw into my head, my rational mind, and thus cut myself off totally from this existence that I refuse. By looking at the affected body part in order to understand my rigidity, I can activate the process of **accepting↓♥ that I have something to understand**. For example, painful **wrists**, **elbows**, **shoulders** or **hands** indicate that I must stop a certain action or job. I want to curl up within myself (**elbows**) because I am tired of doing what I am doing or of being what I am; I no longer want to be responsible for it (**shoulders**). The **hips**, **knees** and **feet** (lower limbs) indicate that I no longer want to pursue life with the difficulties it involves. I must remember that focusing attention on a single spot (i.e. unconsciously applying energy or emotion to a single **joint**) can make this energy crystallize and immobilize the **joint**. In this case, the process of **acceptance↓♥** from the **heart♥** is essential to integrate my **Awareness** of this disease and thereby free myself of it. A **joint** is a place where two bones meet. An ailment or a disease involving it denotes my inflexibility with myself or with another person or a situation. By looking at what body part is affected, I can find the facet of my life with which I would profitably be more flexible. Is it the **joints** of my **fingers**, my **wrists**, my **ankles**, etc.? The accumulated emotions and shocks suddenly become intolerable and indicate a withdrawal into myself. The painful and obsessive thoughts focus and crystallize at a specific point in my body.

---

2. **A kid**: Like someone who is 'less than nothing'.

By accepting↓♥ to listen to myself, I can thus reclaim my true power and acknowledge all the good that is in me. I can advance, develop and make the needed changes in my life in a fluid and harmonious manner.

JOINTS / ARTICULATIONS *See: ARTICULATIONS*

JOINTS — STRAIN / SPRAIN

Sprains are due to a lesion in the ligaments of one of my **joints**.

The **joints** represent **flexibility** and my capacity to adjust to the different situations of my life. The **wrist** and the **ankle** are expressions of energy just before it manifests itself physically. A **sprain** signals me that I am applying the brakes and that I don't want to do what is asked of me. I **resist** or I feel **insecure** about the direction I am taking (**ankle**) or in what I am doing (**wrist**) at this time or what I could do in a new situation. I am ready for anything to not give in, but when the pressure is too high, it is my **ligaments** that bear the brunt and can even reach the point of tearing. I feel guilty and want to punish myself because I am resisting. I am experiencing a mental tension that I can no longer tolerate. I feel like resigning. Depending on my degree of resistance, stubbornness, anger, guilt or mental tension, I will have a **benign strain**, also called a **twist**, where the ligaments are simply distended, or a **serious sprain**, where the ligaments are **ruptured or torn**. In the latter cases, I am experiencing a rupture or a tear with a person or a situation. Someone is trying to 'tear something away' from me, which I refuse to let go. I become **Aware** of what I was doing and feeling when it happened. I can ask myself: Am I on the point of doing something that it would be preferable for me to give up? Is my way of dealing with a situation causing me real tension or anxiety? Am I seated on an unstable and mentally disturbing basis? Am I refusing to admit my mistakes involving a person or a situation? Am I relying on proper grounds or on my fears? Have I **sprained** justice? Has there been a **sprain** involving my integrity?

I accept↓♥ to take the time to reorient myself or make the necessary changes so that I can feel well and move forward freely. I accept↓♥ the presence of this **sprain** to lead me to make changes. If my acceptance↓♥ is given, my healing will be quick and complete. But if I depreciate myself and feel useless and 'good for nothing', because at this time I can't walk or can barely walk, then the healing will take much longer. That is why it is in my best interest to see this situation (the **sprain** and what it involves) in a positive and constructive fashion.

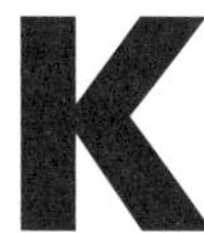

KAPOSI'S SARCOMA *See also: AIDS*

Kaposi[1]**'s sarcoma** (or **Kaposi's disease**) is a malignant proliferation of conjunctive tissue. It is a rare affection with a slow clinical development. There also exists a rapidly developing form in persons who have AIDS.

As conjunctive tissue acts as a support for other body tissues (nutrition, defense), I look at the facet of my life in which I feel left to my own devices. I abandoned myself during an event that marked a turning episode in my life. I need support, moral as well as physical. I feel persecuted, fragile and unprotected. I am tired of my role as the 'family provider', whether for my children or other family members for whom I am responsible. Revolt grips me when I face my helplessness.

I accept↓♥ my limits and I seek the help I need. I know that I can choose myself, I do so consciously and I take the time to please myself and get some rest. I thus have more energy to carry out the tasks that my inner voice guides me to do. I recover my freedom and my joy in living.

KERATITIS *See: EYES — KERATITIS*

KERION *See: HAIR — TINEA*

KIDNEYS — ANURIA *See also: KIDNEYS [RENAL PROBLEMS]*

Anuria occurs when the **kidneys** stop producing urine or when an obstacle prevents the flow of urine between the kidneys and the bladder.

If I suffer from **anuria**, I may be feeling 'naked' and unprotected from life; my risk of being afraid is increasing more than usual (**kidneys** = seat of fear) and I tend to cling to my old beliefs. Furthermore, urine represents old emotions to be eliminated from the body. If I hang on to my old possessions, my beliefs, my fears, my doubts or my quirks (very powerful on the metaphysical level), I manifest **anuria**, namely the suppression of urinary secretion (commonly described as: the kidneys are blocked). Anxiety can be so high that it is as if I had to 'hold in' for fear of letting go my emotions of sorrow, often represented by the liquid to be allowed to circulate. The intensity of the stoppage (a complete stoppage means death) will give me a good indication

1. **Kaposi** (Moriz): An Austro-Hungarian dermatologist and histologist (Kaposvar 1837 – Vienna 1902). In 1870, he described pigmentary xerodermia. Several affections came to bear his name: vacciniform pustulosis, hemorrhagic sarcomatosis and a variety of chronic lupus with hypodermic nodules. He published a book on dermatology in Vienna in 1879. That same year, he directed the dermatology clinic of the Allgemeines Krankehaus, making Vienna the world center for dermatology.

about the old patterns I must discard in order to open myself to new thoughts. I withdraw into myself and my **heart♥** is full of sorrow. I am dependent on others and I still believe they make me happy. I can go as far as cutting myself off from my emotions. I prevent them from manifesting themselves in order to not feel them. This involved great stress for my physical body. Emotionally I am like a desert. My life has become dull, with no adventure or excitement. I feel cut off from my curiosity.

I accept↓♥ to let my emotions flow in me whatever they are, because they are part of my divine essence. Then I clean up and get rid of all emotions, relations or possessions that are not beneficial for me and replace them with something new and positive. I trust in life, which provides me with everything I need. I heed my intuition that dictates to me the road to follow.

KIDNEYS — NEPHRITIS *See also: ANGER, FEAR, INFLAMMATION*

The term **nephritis** used to apply generally to all the diseases of the **kidneys**. However, this term is also used to designate an inflammation of the **kidneys** (which is now better known by the term **nephropathy**).

It embodies fright and great anxiety about life and death. It involves frustrations, feelings of failure or disappointments that were not channeled but deeply repressed in me. I overreact or become overexcited about something that thwarts me, over which I feel powerless, not knowing what life lesson I should draw from it. I treat myself roughly because I resent myself for not being able to assert myself and say no when I feel like it. I intoxicate myself with things that I choke back. Well-hidden secrets make the **kidneys** work much harder.

I accept↓♥ to trust life. I express myself and have greater self-confidence. I live in peace.

KIDNEYS — RENAL CALCULI *See: RENAL CALCULI*

KIDNEYS (renal problems) *See also: CALCULI / STONES (IN GENERAL), FEAR, RENAL CALCULI*

The **kidneys** maintain an equilibrium (a balance) in the body's inner environment by filtering toxic substances from the blood and compensating the 'inputs' to the inner environment by 'outputs' (secretions of urine).

They help me face life. They take part in controlling arterial pressure. The **kidneys** stimulate the production of red globules. In the figurative sense, as the **kidneys** rid the body of its waste, it is as though they were cleaning out my body by evacuating the negative ideas that inhabit me, expelling everything that ***pollutes*** me, and thus helps to purify it. The **kidneys** filter the emotions and enable me to live in joy when the cleaning is done constantly and naturally, letting go of old angers and old sorrows. If I have a good relation with my inner world, my **kidneys** function well. The **kidneys** represent stability, discernment and balance. A bad functioning of my **kidneys** denotes retention of my old emotional patterns or a holding back of certain negative emotions that only need to be released. My relation with my partner is often conflicted and I feel vulnerable, desperately seeking a certain balance. Sexuality can be a way for me to flee my problems. I expect others to make me happy. I feel ***liquefied***, as if all my strength has been removed. My old contained emotions most often manifest themselves by **stones in the kidneys**, also called **renal calculi**. I am always doing 'calculations' (**renal**!) to know what belongs to me or what I risk losing. I am afraid someone will 'break my **back**'[2]. I want to impose my limits and my boundaries so I won't 'lose' an inch! It often happens that it is all my unexpressed sadness that solidifies over time because I haven't let go of an anguishing situation that makes me insecure (emotionally and financially), a letting go that would have afforded me a new understanding of it; it was anger then that manifested itself, took over this sadness and froze it instead of expressing it and letting it flow like the water of a stream. I may feel like a boat that has ***run aground*** and can no longer move forward. I have the impression that I am falling in ***ruins***. I am filled with remorse; I would like so much to go back in the past to change things. The **kidneys** are also known as the 'seat of fear'. When they weaken or are damaged, there may be a fear that I don't want to express or that I may not even want to admit to myself. My discernment is thus affected. I have the impression that I am ***concerned*** by situations that in fact have nothing to do with me. I therefore tend to go to extremes, either becoming very authoritarian with a pronounced tendency to criticize or, on the contrary, becoming submissive and indecisive, feeling powerless and going from disappointment to disappointment. Life for me is 'unfair'. I have difficulty in making decisions. I may have difficulty in judging what is good for me and what isn't and that I should eliminate from my life. I find it difficult to live with myself and others. I can't always tell the difference between truth and illusion, which leads me to experience disappointments and frustrations. If my **kidneys** stop filtering the blood, it is as if my body wanted to keep this fluid as long as possible in order to not lose it or for fear of lacking some. I must therefore ask myself what situation could have generated a fear associated with a liquid (for example, if I am already afraid of drowning, the liquid here would be water). It may also be the fact of having come close to gulping down a toxic liquid. It may be a situation involving money, as people often refer to '**liquid assets**'; or I experienced, or saw someone experience, a situation where they had to '**liquidate their debts**', and I passed judgment, so my **kidneys** will be affected. The **kidneys' collecting tubes** are affected if I feel that I have to struggle for my existence. I feel dispossessed and dejected following a landmark event in my life. I feel ***afflicted*** with all the troubles of the world. **Kidney problems** often appear following an accident or a traumatic situation where I was afraid of dying. When fear sets off an existential conflict, **cancer** appears. I feel that I am left with nothing, with emptiness. I feel that I have lost everything and that my whole world is crashing down. I feel shattered, for I am faced with having nothing left. I am no longer happy in my family, and my deep vitality has flown away. I am afraid of not being able to face life, so I cut

2. **Having one's back broken**: Having one's career broken.

myself off from my own feelings. The **kidneys** also symbolize collaboration (as there are two and they must work in close collaboration). I must ask myself how my relationship with my partner is at this time. Do I hold him (her) responsible for all my troubles? Do I tend to 'dump my waste' on others and poison their lives with my 'problems'? Or on the contrary, do I cling to my past, which ***exhausts*** me and puts me off-balance? I easily criticize, and I am a defeatist because I feel that my life is filled with failures. If such is the case, my **kidneys** will have difficulty in functioning and I may even suffer from a **renal failure**. I will then have no choice but to 'collaborate' with a machine, the hemodialysis generator, that will help me in purifying my blood. I must think over my whole system of relations with my entourage.

I accept↓♥ to take charge of myself and learn to discover my true needs. I take responsibility for my life and stop blaming others. I am able to live with my choices. My discernment is sure and accurate. I collaborate 100% with life and my back is solid. I let my emotions flow like the ***river,*** knowing that they are fully part of my being.

KILLIAN'S POLYP *See: NOSE — KILLIAN'S POLYP*

KISSING DISEASE *See: BLOOD — MONONUCLEOSIS [INFECTIOUS]*

KLEPTOMANIA *See also: DEPENDENCE, NEUROSIS*

If I tend to compulsively commit thefts for no utilitarian reason, I am suffering from **kleptomania**.

I am feeling a tension that comes from an inner emptiness combined with a feeling of guilt. Then, for me the end justifies the means, and it is as though I were challenging myself to be able to appropriate for myself something that is forbidden. It gives me some relief, even if remorse can come to me later on. It is possible that unconsciously, I may in fact be hoping to be 'caught red-handed', because for me it is a way to attract attention. The fact of committing a forbidden act can be a way for me to demonstrate my revolt against authority and taunt it. This authority that I didn't accept↓♥ when I was young was either my father's or my mother's or that of the person who was in charge of my education. My thoughts are so disordered that they manifest themselves by a lack of control over my gestures. I use my charisma to extract or appropriate things that don't belong to me instead of using it, for instance, to convey a positive and hopeful message through my words.

I accept↓♥ to engage in therapy so that I can identify this inner emptiness or this revolt against authority, and be able to put **Love** back into the situation. I will thus experience greater inner peace and others, too, will be better off for it.

KNEE(S) (in general) *See also: LEGS*

The **knees** are the joints on which I **kneel**, abandoning myself to the normal hierarchy or to what is above me and also to the movement and direction that are taking place. When I walk, the **knees** lead the whole body into the movement. The **knees** therefore manifest my degree of flexibility and serve to absorb the shocks when the pressure is too high. They also represent my degree of perseverance, but also my indecision. They will be affected if I depreciate myself for my physique or my sports performances. If I have difficulty in bending my **knees**, I thereby show a degree of rigidity. It may come from my ego, which is very strong and full of pride. I am afraid of losing my freedom. A **knee** that bends easily is a sign of humility and flexibility. It indicates that I easily listen to my inner voice. The **knees** are necessary to maintain my social position and status. Good **knees** indicate that I am open to my entourage and to change.

KNEE AILMENTS

Damage to the bones or to the soft tissues is related to a deep inner conflict and involves, at a deeper level, the abandonment of my ego and my pride. An ailment in my **knees** tells me about my difficulty in making a choice between my own individuality (ME) and that of a group (US). It may be I in relation to my couple, my family, a circle of friends, a religious, social or political organization, or both parts of myself (female and male). When the **menisci** are affected, I experience an inner duality that makes me nervous and tense. I often find myself caught 'in crossfire'. I cling so tightly to something or someone or to what others may think of me that it prevents me from moving forward. The **dislocation of a knee** shows me how off-balance I feel with a person or a situation, and my **knee** can no longer bear the weight of my body. **Knees that give out** show me how easily swayed I am, and how little confidence and conviction I have. Whatever discomfort I experience in my **knees**, I ask myself before whom or what I feel I must ***abdicate***? It may be before an authority external to me. It may also be simply before life, for I have the impression that my burden is too heavy. I am collapsing under the weight of my responsibilities, and my **knees** want to ***bend*** in spite of myself. I must ***stand by*** my words and gestures, but that sometimes requires some effort. I may experience a failure with one of my biggest dreams or great ambitions, and this realization makes me bend my **knees** in abdication. If my **knees crack**, I may have the impression that I am cracking[3] or that I am afraid I might crack under the weight of my responsibilities, the pressure, the efforts, etc. As I am very much a perfectionist, I see this somewhat as a failure, or at least I am disappointed in myself or my performance. In the case of **hygroma**[4], which especially affects nuns or people for whom religion holds a great place, I must ask myself what conflict I am experiencing about my spirituality and the implications that follow from it in my life. The pain I feel each time I **kneel** (to pray for example) reminds me of my inner conflict and the need to decide for myself what I want in my life and make the appropriate changes. It may even reach the point of a spiritual rift. The emotions I repress are only asking to be expressed. I must take a stand

---

3. **To have the impression of cracking**: To have the impression of failing.

4. **Hygroma**: An inflammation of the serous bursa (also called BURSITIS).

about a facet of my work (whether at home or at the office) that I don't like, and this bothers me, while also seeing its positive sides. **I am afraid of betraying someone if I choose myself or if I take care of myself**. If I want to eliminate the **ailments** that affect my **knees**, I must accept↓♥ to open myself to the world around me and accept↓♥ to have to change my way of being in certain respects. I become **Aware** of the anger I have carried and repressed for years. I must learn to go with the flow and let go of my old ways of thinking.

I accept↓♥ to ***kneel*** before someone or a situation, or maybe simply before life in general, in order to be able to receive help and open myself to a new reality that I previously couldn't see because I was imprisoned in my own world. And I have all the potential I need to accept↓♥ new responsibilities. If I feel frustration and guilt because I realize I always want to be right and my desire for greater social power is insatiable, I stop and question myself about my true values, in order to return to essentials and enable myself to come back to my **heart♥** instead of allowing my rational side to decide everything. I thus give myself permission to make creativity live in me, and I give power back to my intuition that knows what is good for me. From now on, I am protected by my inner authority. I now have the capacity for bouncing back in any situation!

LABIA (vaginal) *See: PUDENDUM / VULVA*

LABYRINTHITIS *See: BRAIN — BALANCE [LOSS OF]*

LARYNGITIS *See: THROAT — LARYNGITIS*

LARYNX *See: THROAT — LARYNX*

LARYNX (cancer of the) *See: CANCER OF THE LARYNX*

LASSITUDE *See also: BLOOD — HYPOGLYCEMIA, FATIGUE (IN GENERAL), TENSION [ARTERIAL] — HYPOTENSION*

I feel **lassitude** when my body is tired and I feel like giving up. Boredom and discouragement overcome my brain. I am weary and I no longer feel like being 'where I am right now'.

«What has brought on this **lassitude**?» I am dissatisfied with my affective relations with my spouse or my friends. I am weary from adjusting to others all the time. I am experiencing a duality between putting my needs first or those of others. Often, my blood becomes impoverished because the joy of living is no longer present.

I accept↓♥ to rekindle my taste for life by doing things I like, pleasing myself and listening to soft music. It will help me lighten my mood. I resume contact with the **Soul** that I am, which will guide me to recover my joy in living.

LAZINESS

Laziness is a tendency to avoid all activity and refuse any effort.

It is related to weariness about my life in general, a slackening, for I don't feel like making any efforts or forcing myself to do anything. By avoiding being engaged in action, at the same time I avoid being criticized and having to put myself in question. I stay in my bubble and in a state of monotony.

I accept↓♥ to take action. I start acting and doing things to give myself energy, spirit and joy in living. I thus discover my talents that had so far remained hidden, and this gives me a great feeling of personal achievement!

LEANNESS / THINNESS *See also: ANOREXIA, WEIGHT [EXCESS]*

Under-eating can lead to **thinness** and excessive food consumption can transform itself into **obesity**. In both cases, the small intestine ***assimilates*** food poorly.

Nervousness, anxiety, the consumption of medications, great fears or very great joys are factors that can make one individual become fat while another becomes thin. If I am a **thin** person, I am often very emotional, with a very great sensitivity, and I don't always know how to express my feelings, because having already been hurt, I want to protect myself so as to no longer have to suffer from the ***sarcasm*** of others. I live in constant ***dejection***. I tend to reject myself and to ***pursue*** certain things or persons. I easily disdain what surrounds me. I thus maintain a certain distance from others. I am embittered by life. I may feel that I must ***get out*** and ***abandon*** someone or something in order to survive, hence a feeling of ***cowardice***. I may also have the impression that I am the one who was ***left*** and ***abandoned***. In **anorexia**, there is often a link with the mother or the image of the mother. This same sensitivity is found in an **overweight** person, whose more imposing physique creates at once a protection and a barrier. People who are **anorexic** refuse to live and prefer to die rather than accept↓♥ **Love**. **Obesity** is linked to one's self-image and sometimes to the image of the father. In either case, I must find the cause in order to 'assimilate' life in a healthy and balanced manner.

By welcoming and **accepting**↓♥ myself as I am, I can relate or reconnect myself with others in a **conscious** manner, which will warm my **heart**♥.

LEFT SIDE *See: FEMALE PRINCIPLE*

LEFT-HANDED

Left-handed persons are generally so named because they use their **left** hands and arms more than their right hands and arms for activities such as writing, playing music, doing sports, etc.

In the old days, our education stressed the importance of being right-handed, and people would say that being right-handed was 'being OK' and **left-handed** meant 'being not OK'. The French word ***gauche*** means '**left**', but it also means socially **awkward** or **clumsy**, which is its meaning in English. We are now passing from the age of Pisces into the Age of Aquarius, i.e.[1] we are moving from our rational sides to our more intuitive and creative sides. It is known that preventing a child from being **left-handed**, if that is its natural tendency, can lead the child to develop tics, awkwardness, affective disorders, difficulty in speaking or reading, and a feeling of guilt or inferiority. If I experienced such feelings because I was forced to be right-handed, I should restore peace with myself by giving myself understanding and acceptance↓♥ in what I endured. As the **left** side embodies the affective, intuitive and sensitive side, in short the 'female' side of my being, then if I am **left-handed**, whether I am a man or a woman, my creative side is very developed and I have a special aptitude for learning music, singing, in short, any form of art. It is innate in me. The personality of a **left-handed** person may also be more introverted and

---

1. **i.e.:** That is / In other words (*id est* in Latin).

reserved, whereas the right-handed person tends to be more extraverted and outgoing with others.

I only need to accept↓♥ my creative potential and make good use of my great sensitivity for everything to fully emerge. In any case, I accept↓♥ myself as I am, **Aware** that I have special strengths that make me a unique person.

LEG(S) (in general) *See also: SYSTEM [LOCOMOTOR]*

The **legs** symbolize my movements and my autonomy. My **legs** move me forward or backward and give me my own direction, stability, solidity and a firm base. **They therefore represent my power and my capacity for moving forward in life**, while leaving the past behind me. My **legs** enable me to go, or not go, to meet people, to get closer to them or farther from them. My **legs** are also related to the mother (Mother Earth). The **left leg** represents the emotional side and the fact of not being able to go someplace even if I want to. The **right leg** represents the rational side and the fact of not wanting to go someplace even if I must. My **legs** express my relation with the act of moving forward. They also reflect the orientation I take in my life (work, family, sexual orientation, etc.) and the directions to take to get there. They also represent the field of my **relations** with my entourage. An **ailment** in my **legs** may indicate that I am too rooted in my everyday routine, my comfort zone. Weak **legs** indicate that little energy is circulating in them, which denotes a lack of self-assurance in me, an inability to remain standing and be strong before a certain situation or a certain person. I then tend to depend on others. I seek support and motivation in others instead of finding them within me. The size of my **legs** also gives me information: if I have **small legs**, I find it more difficult to connect with the physical, material world, and would rather delegate the related responsibilities than have to bear them. On the contrary, if I have **stout legs**, they are bearing too much weight: the responsibilities I have decided to take on (mainly the material ones) and not only mine, but sometimes those of others, which I have accepted↓♥ out of 'obligation'.

LEG AILMENTS

When I am having difficulty with my **legs**, I must stop and ask myself the question: *"What is the current or upcoming situation that is making me afraid of the future?"* I resist change, I feel paralyzed and limited, and I may be so scared that I feel like taking to my heels; but is that really the solution? With whom am I having **relational** difficulties that are a source of tension and conflict? Difficulties with my **legs** can reveal my feeling of not being ***supported*** by others, and maybe especially by my mother. I am ***collapsing*** under my responsibilities. I will therefore find it difficult to stand on my **legs**. There are some displacements that seem very difficult to carry out: for example, if I wonder whether I should move far away from my father or if I wish to move closer to such and such a person. I don't want to budge. I am afraid that my so well-structured living environment will undergo too many changes. I have high aspirations, but I think I don't have what it takes to reach them. I am at a dead end. I feel that I am a burden for others. When I am doubtful or afraid of the road I am taking, I may even **break a leg**. I move ahead and develop every day, at every moment, and the **problems in my legs** only show obstacles that I must now remove in order to pursue my way toward greater happiness and greater harmony.

Whatever new situation comes up, I accept↓♥ to learn how to channel my inner security; I can trust myself and overcome my resistance to change.

LEGS — LOWER PART (calves)

The **lower part of my legs** is at the level of the **calves**, which are undergirded by the tibia and fibula bones.

The **calves** enable me to move forward, so there is movement. They also represent a protection against my past while I move forward in life. If I have **pain** or **cramps** in my **calves**, I am forced to slow my pace. Am I trying to stop certain events that await me and make me afraid? Do I feel that events are accelerating and everything is going too fast? Am I having difficulty in adjusting my position in relation to a person, a situation or a belief? In any case, I tend to 'retrench' myself in my old thought patterns, and I may feel tugged and tensed by external pressures. When the **muscle of the calf** is affected, I ask myself if I am focusing my attention too much on one problem in particular. I am 'spinning in place'. I am stubborn and don't listen much to what my inner voice has to tell me. I am very bitter about a situation (involving an inheritance, for instance) and joy has deserted my life. My happiness is conditional on others instead of coming from inside of me. I refuse good things happening to me. If the **tibia** is affected, how immobilized am I? The **tibias** are like pillars holding up my body. Do they uphold it happily, or is it just a colossal burden? The **tibias** represent my torments, my difficulty in being mobile. I tend to follow others and do little to improve my life. I feel I have made do with little in life, and that depresses me. I ask myself questions about being a parent. I may also feel attacked, and I would like to give someone a good kick! I stay motionless, with goals that are more materialistic than human and spiritual. I have little self-confidence and I have difficulty in being myself. I don't know what road to take. I feel threatened and I would want to attack. I want to detach myself from my mother and get out of my dependency, for I find it hard to bear. If the **fibula** is affected, I am in a situation where I am caught in the middle. I feel torn by a choice. I want to be independent but something is preventing me from doing it. My body tells me that I can trust the future and that life takes care of me.

I accept↓♥ this strength within me, and I fully trust others for I have full trust in my unlimited potential. I choose the life I want to live, a new way far more easy and enriching. I accept↓♥ to look and move in all directions. I focus my attention only on beautiful things. I am my own pillar and life upholds me always!

LEGS — UPPER PART (thighs) *See also: THIGHS (IN GENERAL)*

The **upper part of my legs**, forming the **thighs**, is undergirded by the **femur** bone. It reflects my tendency to hold on to things, most often related to my past. My **thighs** represent especially my male side, which contains all my energies and inner strengths. If my power is being questioned and I have to yield in certain situations, I must reassess my limits, which I find difficult to accept↓♥. Depending on what I allow to happen, or prevent from happening, in my life, my **thighs** will react. If I am constantly reliving the past or feeling guilty about certain events, this will have the effect of accumulating in my **thighs**, which become larger. I may also have kept resentment or bitterness, for I felt betrayed. It is as if my past was holding me back and preventing me from going forward. Being anxious and poorly confident, I am afraid of moving forward, for I am no longer supported. Often, my past prevents me from being intimate with myself and others. I cut myself off from my sensitivity and my deep essence. My injuries and traumas make me 'drag my feet'. I don't fully experience my sensuality and my sexual desires, which is a source of anger and frustration. The fact of having children of my own may reactivate all those injuries of the past, and my **thighs** will be affected. **Large legs** can also be a sign that I am accumulating too much (materially and emotionally as well as intellectually), that I am keeping things 'just in case!' out of insecurity, for fear of lacking something or someone. As squirrels do, I hoard reserves in often unfounded anticipation of a possible shortage. It is good for me to sort things out so I can keep only what is beneficial for me. I have an ailment in my **thighs** when I inwardly hoard too much of the energies and talents that I should use more extensively instead. My creativity is stifled, my seminal power, physical as well as emotional, is neutralized by my passivity and my exaggerated obedience to authority (which can be that of my parents). I may feel powerless, and I wonder just how far I have accepted↓♥ that my parents or my teachers define my life instead of taking charge of my destiny myself. When there is a **fracture of the femur**, my basic structure is affected. I am in ***opposition*** (physically or verbally) against something or someone I must ***confront***. I feel I am stagnating or maybe even losing ground. My ***adversary*** is stronger than me and I must ***bend***. I will come to wish that someone will take me in charge because whatever I want to do or wherever I want to go, I hit a wall. People are unconcerned about me or my needs. That's why I am always being asked to do more, while I receive so little in return.

Now I accept↓♥ to fully live my life. I reclaim the space I had left to others. I release all these long-contained energies. I unleash my creativity. I feel all the liberating power of freeing my inner forces as I wish. I can feel safe only if I rely on my strengths and not on others. The more I take action, the more alive I feel!

LEGS — VARICOSE VEINS *See: BLOOD — VARICOSE VEINS*

LEPROSY *See also: CHRONIC ILLNESS, NERVES, SKIN / (IN GENERAL) / DISEASES*

Leprosy, also called **Hansen's**[2] **disease**, is an infectious disease. "I have **leprosy**, I feel that I don't have everything I need to come to terms with my life and my responsibilities." "Why have I caught this infection? Do I have chronic **leprosy** due to Hansen's bacillus, which affects the skin, the mucous membranes and the nerves?" It is mostly frequent in tropical countries. It has a contagious 'family' character and its incubation period is long (3 to 5 years). If I am affected, I feel dirty and impure and don't feel up to the mark. I suffer from isolation and I even disgust myself. I destroy myself. "Was it present in my family? Was there any communication there?" Has the suffering caused by this lack of communication affected me to the point of wanting to destroy myself? My sensitivity was affected and I felt 'skinned alive'. In any case, do I deserve to live? I tend to ask myself this question often, and I will let myself drift[3], feeling incapable of changing anything in my life. I live like a victim instead of being the creator of my life. I feel condemned, criticized by a god, society or my entourage. I thus feel powerless to change anything at all. I carry the entire responsibility for all the ailments of the world on my shoulders. I resolve the accumulated baggage from my family's past and I find MY place in society.

I accept↓♥ from now on to nourish myself on thoughts of **Love** and harmony in order to grow a new skin that will better reflect the divine being that I am. I reclaim the power that I left to others very long ago, and I take responsibility for my life. I acknowledge my creative energies. I accept↓♥ my body as part of my divine being. I accept↓♥ that I deserve the best!

LEUKEMIA *See: BLOOD — LEUKEMIA*

LEUKOPENIA *See: BLOOD — LEUKOPENIA*

LEUKORRHEA *See also: CANDIDA, INFECTIONS, SALPINGITIS, SKIN — ITCHING*

Leukorrhea is also called vaginal discharge.

It is a vaginal infection that shows either a refusal to have sexual relations or guilt or aggressiveness toward my partner, or the fact of not having any. It often results from my impression that I am powerless before my spouse, and as I feel I have no power over him, this disease becomes a sort of tool for manipulation that will make me feel I control the situation and therefore my spouse himself, because it is I who decides if I can have sexual relations or not. I have such a need for **Love**, but I expect it from outside instead of giving it to myself. As I am not in contact with my needs and desires, I play the victim. I place them after the needs of others. I am submissive and I may even let myself

2. **Hansen** (Gerhard Henrick Armauer): Norwegian physician and botanist (1841–1912). In 1869, he discovered the bacillus of leprosy in a nodule. He publicly reported his discovery to Christiana's Medical Society only in 1874. He was then named Inspector General of leprosy for Norway.

3. **Let oneself drift**: The expression refers here to the fact of 'becoming resigned', not to 'becoming detached'.

be exploited, if I am not the one exploiting my spouse. My creative energies are completely ignored. The fact that I am a woman does not mean that I must submit to others. I can no longer stand always 'adjusting' to others and making concessions, notably in my couple.

I accept↓♥ to take my place, acknowledge my true worth and convince myself that I am the only person who can exercise control over myself and my life.

LICE *See: CRAB LICE*

LIGAMENTS *See: JOINTS — STRAIN / SPRAIN*

LIMPING *See: CLAUDICATION*

LIPS

In the **lips**, I can perceive an **open or closed mind**, what I want, or don't want, to say. I can perceive tension, worries, sorrows or fears by the cracking or dryness of the **lips**. They can be plump if I have joy, pleasure and **Love** in my **heart♥**, or rather thin when I am more reserved or even rigid with my desires and the pleasures of life. In a woman, the **lips** of the **vagina** show the repercussions of the same disorders, except that any ailments or diseases linked to them will more likely involve the expression of her sexuality and her femininity.

The lower lip represents my male, rational side, and the upper lip represents my female, receptive, emotional side. The state and the form of my **lips** indicate if I open up easily to others, if my anxieties are gnawing at me without my being **Aware** of it. Do I tend to 'purse my **lips**', questioning and judging the opinions of others? Or do I tend instead to 'bite my **lips**' because I don't trust enough in my own judgment, my own good sense? I may experience an inner conflict involving my sensuality and the place I allow it in my life. Am I abusing a certain power? If I have difficulty in pleasing myself, my **lips** will be affected. If I receive an unwanted kiss, if I must 'blow into the balloon[4]', if I feel betrayed by someone close to me (the Judas kiss), my **lips** will be affected. In this case, I have the impression that someone in authority is abusing their power.

I accept↓♥ to express my feelings, the negative when I am dissatisfied (or else my **lips** may swell) as well as the positive, such as compliments, my affection, my appreciation. For it is with my **lips** that I can give a kiss and show my affection to the people I **love**. I feel safe, and I dare to say and show who I really am.

4. **Blow into the balloon**: An expression that means to take a breath analyzer test.

LIPS (dry, chapped, cracked)

I have **dry lips** when I feel great fatigue, when I have a 'muted' fever, when I feel alone, when I am worried or when I regret having said certain words. My joy in living goes away and I feel little pleasure in my sharing with others. I no longer can share my emotions with others or with the person I share my life with.

This loss of joy will be all the greater if my **lips** also go as far as to **bleed**. If my **lips crack**, I ask myself what 'division' I have allowed to open up within me. It may be a gulf that exists between my real world and my imaginary one. I want to stay in my ivory tower for fear of being injured. **Cracked lips** may be found in a child whose parents are separated and who needs gentleness. I make up a fantasy world of illusion that helps me escape my negative emotions, my 'ghosts' who control my life. I make concessions and water down my demands, but I have had enough of all that.

I accept↓♥ to be in contact with reality and the people around me. I allow myself to communicate more intensely with others and to 'embrace life' with more **Love**. Instead of living in the past or the future, I learn to taste the present moment. By making gentle contact with who I am and with others, I will no longer need to live in unreality. By unifying what was previously divided, my **lips** live again and recover their perfect state.

LITHIASIS (biliary) *See: BILIARY CALCULI*

LITHIASIS (urinary) *See: RENAL CALCULI*

LIVER DISORDERS *See also: BILIARY CALCULI, JAUNDICE*

The **liver** is the largest gland in the organism, appended to the digestive tube and playing a role in several important biological functions, including the secretion of bile and the purification and detoxification of the blood. The **liver** represents my **faith** and my **confidence** in my possibilities.

Liver disorders originate from my own attitude. My accumulated frustrations, my hates, my jealousy, my contained aggressiveness are so many triggering factors for **liver problems**. These fears disguise one or several fears that can't be expressed otherwise. I tend to easily **criticize** and **judge** myself or others. I complain constantly. I resist someone or something. I feel much dissatisfaction. I have difficulty in accepting↓♥ others as they are. My joy in living is often nonexistent because I envy others, which disturbs me and makes me sad. I tend to be depressive. But how ready am I to make efforts, materially as well as in my spiritual development? Do I feel ***able*** to make the necessary changes, or do I feel that I lack the courage? I still haven't understood that **what I reproach the other with is but the reflection of myself**. It is only my mirror. I complain all the time and ask others to change. Where is my good faith? Where is my own effort? I am also lacking in joy of living and simplicity.

I may develop a **cancer of the liver** if all the emotions that are harmful for me have been 'gnawing' at me for some time. It may often happen that this cancer results from a conflict involving the family or money, especially when I am afraid of lacking something. It often happens that the emotion accumulating inside the **liver** is anger. I don't feel respected and recognized, which generates great frustration. I question myself about the meaning I want to give to my life. Do I still have the '**faith**' to fulfill myself and be happy? Is my life ***devoid*** of meaning? What is good for me, and what should I eliminate from my life? What are my limits and my possibilities? Am I destroying myself or nourishing the joy and the life that inhabit me? Where does my feeling of powerlessness come from? Why do I cling to others or to situations instead of trusting, and believing in, myself? I don't want to give up my people. All this holding back of emotions generates anxiety in me and pollutes me. In the case of **cancer of the liver**, there is a strong feeling of discouragement, despondency, even despair. I fear so much losing something or someone that I hold on to them as much as I can. I don't have **faith** in myself. I am afraid of ***deprivation,*** and the ***absence*** of the people I **love** bears heavily on me and seems like an ***eternity***. This fear leads me to overly ***accumulate*** in order to avoid any ***deficiency***. I build up ***reserves***; I want to ***devour*** everything for fear of being needy. I have an omnipresent and almost obsessive desire that I can't satiate, which leads me to overeat, which in turn disturbs my **liver**. I worry about everything and I find life unfair. **Cancer** indicates that I need to make great changes in my life. I have such a negative image of myself that others remind me of it by treating me as I treat myself. This can take the form of persons who constantly show me no respect.

It is ***now*** time for me to become **Aware** that I must accept↓♥ myself as I am and learn to **love** myself more. Being able to **love** and understand myself opens the way to understanding and loving others. I find a new joy in living. I stop criticizing others and accept↓♥ to take a new direction in my life where joy and the positive are my role in life. I acknowledge my desires, learn to respect myself, and these new positive energies will make the illness I am experiencing go away.

LIVER ABSCESS

An **abscess** in the **liver** is an accumulation of pus in the liver.

As the **liver** is related to criticism, a **liver abscess** indicates a great dissatisfaction in my life, which may result from the fact that events are not going as I wish, that I worry too much over certain situations, or that the joy and **Love** that nourish my life are not enough. I have an overflow of emotions. I have a dark view of life and I am delighted with my inactivity. I persist in keeping something or someone, if not my old thoughts. I give too much space to my negative thoughts and I don't live in the present and in my physical body.

It is a message that life is sending me so that I will accept↓♥ to develop my flexibility and my openness and to lead me to seek the **Love** and understanding that I need in order to discover more of this **Love** that is in me. I accept↓♥ to take action, to live my passions and achieve my dreams. I thus allow life to live more in me. I have **faith** in myself and in my full creative potential.

LIVER CALCULI *See: BILIARY CALCULI*

LIVER — CIRRHOSIS of the LIVER

Cirrhosis is an inflammatory disease of the **liver** caused, especially, by an abusive consumption of alcohol. It is characterized by lesions disseminated in the **liver**. The cells are destroyed and replaced with fibrous tissue. In **cirrhosis**, the **liver** can either increase (**hypertrophy**) or diminish (**atrophy**) in volume.

Cirrhosis is found in a person who feels pushed by life, events or certain situations that force them to advance. As I feel pushed against my will, I resist and cling to my opinions. I feel resentment and aggressiveness. This disease is a reflection of my anger and my resentment against life and what is happening to me. I am filled with latent inner aggressiveness and I constantly feel guilty because I am convinced that my life is a failure. I spend my time blaming myself and criticizing others. I harden myself so much that I can no longer see the **Light** at the end of the tunnel. I have lost my spontaneity and I refrain myself because I don't dare do things that I like, in the name of morality, the rules to be followed or simply the routine I have developed over the years and that imprisons me in my comfort zone. I am very insecure and anxious. What's the use of living? Why fight for my place? I am only one digit among so many others. Certain events of my past have left a deep trace and my wound is so great that that I don't feel like opening myself up to **Love** for fear of suffering again. I repress myself so much that I tend to escape through alcohol. Life could be '**so rosy**', yet I see it so black. My **faith** in myself has vanished, and I let myself passively drift. I am trying to destroy myself, rejecting my life or what I have become.

In order to help myself take up with life again, I accept↓♥ to live the present moment and see the good things happening to me now. I open my **heart♥** and focus my attention on each gesture, each action here and now, and I learn to not be my most severe judge. By being more tolerant with myself, I will also be so with others, which will bring far more harmony and happiness into my life. I examine my true intentions, I remain open to **Love** and I forgive myself in what I am. I assert who I am and reclaim my freedom to be what I want to be. I am taking action. I let go of this heavy and harmful past. I have **faith** in myself and accept↓♥ to start over a new life full of freedom, spontaneity and **Love**.

LIVER CONGESTION *See: CONGESTION*

LIVER — HEPATITIS *See also: ALCOHOLISM, INFECTION, INFLAMMATION, JAUNDICE*

Hepatitis is an inflammation of the **liver** caused by a virus, by bacteria, alcohol, medications, a transfusion of infected blood or, in drug addicts, polluted hypodermic needles, and it affects the whole body. The symptoms are weakness, jaundice, a loss of appetite, nausea, fever and abdominal discomfort.

The **liver** is the 'giver of life', cleansing the blood of its poisons and excesses, and maintaining my emotional state (the blood) in proper balance. The **liver** is the place where I can accumulate poisonous emotions and excessive hate. It is the **seat of anger**. Words or diseases ending in '-itis', such as **hepatitis**, indicate irritation and anger. **Hepatitis** can be linked to my personal relations or to a difficult situation. I am desperate and I am questioning the image I project. When I fret for trifles, it makes me feel great anger, resentment, rage and even hate, which can lead to violence against myself or against others. All these emotions often have their source in my feeling of failure involving one side of my life, or in my revolt against the injustice that prevails in the world. I resist opening my mind and seeing things or events differently. I have difficulty in telling right from wrong. Do I truly respect myself in what I am and what I am experiencing? Do I have the impression of losing myself, so submerged am I by everything that surrounds me, and I reach the point of losing contact with my divine self and no longer knowing what direction to take? I may feel myself caught between two worlds. I feel cut off from the unity, from the father above and the mother below. I may feel resentment against some members of my family who are ***interfering*** in my life. **Viral hepatitis A** has its source in a resentment I may feel toward food as such, or a problem involving food and that I consider as vital for me. An example that comes to mind is an ex-husband who refuses to pay alimony. The notion of escape is very present in my life and prevents me from living in truth and respect. **Viral hepatitis B** highlights a resentment felt about something or someone that was imposed on me. I may have ***put off*** until later an event that was important for me, and I experienced a great disappointment and maybe also a feeling of rejection. It is as if I had been 'injected' into a situation that I refused. For example, I may have been forced to take part in a dance competition. I was ***ejected*** from a comfortable situation and then found myself in another situation that didn't suit me at all. I felt trapped and powerless to react. I am anxious and certain events of my past have marked me so much that I tend to define my current life in terms of those experiences that I find negative, rather than trust and accept↓♥ that things can go well for me. I am 'poisoned' by my own difficulty in letting go of the past, by my attachment to material things and to my social image. It may take the form of my need for having several sexual partners. I thus avoid investing myself completely, fearing commitment and thus avoiding being hurt or being 'stung'. **Viral hepatitis C** appears following a great resentment about something unknown or secret, such as: "Who are my parents? Where was I born?" I may feel strong resistance against new situations in my life that lead me to make changes. I may want to cling to my prejudices and preconceived ideas.

I make use of the time of rest that I must set aside to take stock of my life. I free myself of the prejudices and angers I had kept inside of me. I accept↓♥ to adopt new attitudes that will enable me to achieve my full potential. I eliminate everything that is harmful for me and I accept↓♥ that joy be part of my life because I deserve it!

LOCOMOTION *See: SYSTEM [LOCOMOTOR]*

LORDOSIS *See: SPINAL [DEVIATION OF] — LORDOSIS*

LOSS of APPETITE *See: APPETITE [LOSS OF]*

LOW PRESSURE *See: TENSION ARTERIAL — HYPOTENSION [TOO LOW]*

LOWER BACK *See: BACK DISORDERS — LOWER BACK*

LSD (consumption of) *See: DRUGS*

LUMBAGO *See: BACK DISORDERS — LOWER BACK*

LUMBALGIA *See: BACK DISORDERS — LOWER BACK*

LUNG(S) (in general) *See also: BRONCHI*

It is by the action of my two **lungs** that life circulates in me. They are therefore the air filters for my whole body. I inhale life and I return it to the Universe. Properly functioning **lungs** enable me to aerate each of my cells. It is with my **lungs** that I become **Aware** that 'I' exist. They represent my capacity to topple all the walls that I built up myself or that society set in place, as well as my capacity to adjust. They can therefore recognize a distress in living, and this can enable me to air these negative feelings that I must purify with the **Love** that I inhale.

LUNG DISEASES *See also: ASTHMA, BRONCHI — BRONCHITIS, SCLEROSIS*

Lung conditions such as **pneumonia**, **bronchitis**, **asthma**, **fibrosis**, etc., are the sign that I have a very deep fear of choking or dying. I am living at odds with life and my deep aspirations. It is as if my purpose in life was obstructed. I am afraid of facing life. I feel so anxious that I confine myself to living within a very restricted territory that also seems uncertain. I may feel that I have lost my territory[5] or am in the process of losing it, which makes me feel trapped. If I lose it, it is like dying: I am no longer anything! I therefore have a certain difficulty in finding my place and managing my relations with the world

5. **My territory**: My spouse, my family, my friends, my work, my house, my ideas, etc.

around me. I feel I am losing myself. As the **lungs** serve for my breathing, a bad functioning of the **lungs** will cause a difficulty in transferring oxygen from the air to the blood, a vital function for my survival. This bad functioning only highlights death, which scares me and with which I should deal on more familiar terms. I tend to smother my ***tears***. Sadness weakens my **lungs**. If I have a pain or a **difficulty in breathing**, I must ask myself if I am feeling smothered or oppressed in my life. Do I feel I am lacking air or feel ***asphyxiated***, especially in my relations with the members of my family? Do I feel limited or feel that I don't deserve to be happy? I feel like 'screaming my distress at the top of my **lungs**'. I don't like conflicts and dualities, and I tend to be too conciliatory just to avoid disputes. I feel sad and depressed and I must learn to acknowledge my personal worth and to do things that please me. My **lungs** will be affected, especially my breathing, if I previously felt abandoned as a child. If I am an orphan, my trust in life and in adults in general may be shaken, and my **lungs** will manifest this inner injury. I may have difficulty in facing changes in my life and experiencing separations, especially if the separation from my mother at birth (which physically takes the form of the first breath) was experienced traumatically. My **lungs**, which should play an important role in the process of becoming autonomous (breathing on my own), may interpret this situation as a sort of death to some extent. Am I able to live independently, without always needing someone to do things on my behalf? I may harbor ***macabre*** ideas that can give rise to a **tumor**. Although society espouses the idea that cigarettes are what cause **lung diseases**, it is rather the anxiety over death, experienced after consuming tobacco, that causes the disease. In the case of **pulmonary embolism**[6], there is a shattering of joy and of the accumulated sadness that I maintain. I am revolting against my feeling of helplessness. It is as though someone were preventing me (obstructing) the passage to carry out a project or get to a specific place, and depression follows. I no longer feel at home. My emotions and ideas are obstructed.

I accept↓♥ the fact of being constantly protected and guided. Instead of taking pleasure in maintaining old memories that make me melancholy and may further amplify my feeling of being alone and isolated, it would be better for me to look at everything I have and all the abundance that is present in my life. I have the right to have a territory, my own personal place that belongs to nobody else, as they in turn have their own territories. This is how harmony can exist and I can fully flourish. I reclaim the power that is mine and breathe life 'with full **lungs**'!

LUNGS (cancer of the) *See: CANCER OF THE LUNGS*

LUNGS — CONGESTION *See: CONGESTION*

---

6. A brutal obstruction of one of the branches of the pulmonary artery.

LUNGS — EMPHYSEMA (pulmonary)

Pulmonary emphysema is especially characterized by a respiratory difficulty on exertion.

When I am still a fetus and my **lungs** are still forming, this marks my commitment to being here, my agreement to say yes to life, all of which takes place through my breathing. If I fear life or if I want someone else to take care of my own life, my **lungs** may encounter certain difficulties. By breathing shallowly, I protect myself from having to deal with reality. I feel anxious and I am afraid because I feel threatened. As my **lungs** dilate and contract, they demonstrate my capacity for widening, sharing and entering life, or for contracting and isolating myself and withdrawing from life. To be affected by **pulmonary emphysema** means that I have difficulty in breathing and that I feel oppressed by the effort. By breathing, I draw life into me. Why do I have difficulty in taking in life? In what aspect of my life do I feel unworthy? Is it my way of ***fleeing*** life? Life no longer attracts me and I have no interest in it. I have some great fears and one of them is to assert myself and claim my place. Why has life lost all its meaning for me? I feel stuck and stifled. I haven't learned to be myself and to take my rightful place; I live according to others. I am feeling a deep absence of communication. Words are '**strangled**' in me, hence a feeling of powerlessness. My frustrations and my dissatisfaction are stifling me. I have the impression that I don't deserve to live. I am bearing a very heavy burden.

I accept↓♥ to become **Aware** that everyone has their place and that I must take mine. I **accept↓♥ to love myself more**, assert myself and express my needs, in a word, to be ME. The oppression I felt is replaced by air and life entering my **lungs**. I see once again the possibilities that life offers me. I rediscover a taste for happiness.

LUNGS — LEGIONNAIRE'S DISEASE

Legionnaire's disease is an infectious disease, the first epidemic of which was observed in July 1976 among a group of war veterans gathered for a convention in a Philadelphia hotel. It is due to a small Gram bacillus, then unknown and now named *Legionella pneumophila*. **Legionnaire's disease**, or **legionellosis**, is a disease resembling pneumonia. After an incubation period of 2 to 20 days, it starts up brutally, develops rapidly and can lead to death (lethal in 16% of cases).

Being in contact with other combatants (like me) made me recall painful memories and sadness over human suffering. I felt powerless before death. Memories were suddenly awakened and my fears and inner conflicts about work rose back to the surface. A feeling of anger and injustice imprisons me, prevents me from breathing and fully taking part in life in general. The situation is heavy to bear and I feel guilty of not having done more. I feel like running away but I am forced to stay. I bear the shame of taking part in wars with which I disagree.

I accept↓♥ to make peace with myself and free myself from those memories. I work through my bereavements and stop gnawing at myself inside. I ask for help and give myself the right to breathe and participate fully in life. I realize that life is precious, I taste the present moment and I give thanks.

LUNGS — PNEUMONIA and PLEURISY

Pneumonia is an infection of the **lung** provoked by a bacterium or a virus, whereas **pleurisy** is an acute or chronic inflammation of the pleura, the membrane enveloping the **lungs** (the word **pleuritis** was previously used to name localized dry **pleurisies**).

As the **lungs** are the organs of respiration that produce the transformation of 'my' air for my whole body, I am experiencing an inner conflict that is gravely weakening me. I must therefore identify the emotion or the feeling that is irritating and limiting the functioning of my relation with the air of my inner life, because these blockages are preventing me from living fully. These feelings deeply anchored within my being, and represented by the inflammation, may be telling me that I am deeply 'offended' and 'irritated'. This irritation is an integral part of me, it is like a reflex, and it brings me many negative feelings. I must ask myself what is the situation or the person that makes me feel so much hate and is often present in my work environment. My ability to breathe becomes very affected by my emotions, my fear of being alone or overwhelmed, by my revolt against life. I feel I am 'mixed up' in my personal relations. I may feel stifled by all my responsibilities, and I don't know how to get out of it. I am overcome by discouragement and despair and I even ask myself what the meaning of my life is and if it is truly worth the effort to live it. I feel that anyone can invade my space and take something from me. I feel that I am not living fully. I ask myself questions about my personal progress and I am seeking a new meaning for my life, wanting it to be richer interpersonally and wondering what the place of spirituality is (not necessarily religion) in my everyday life. I feel vulnerable and I am not clear yet about how to achieve my ambitions. I project a 'strong man' image but deep down, I feel helpless. I am tired of living, and despair is overtaking me. I want to live my own life and not the one plotted by my parents. I am anguished because I find it very difficult to make contact with my entourage. My job no longer satisfies me and doesn't fit my aspirations. The **pleurisy**, which is often characterized by fluid between two leaves, speaks to me of the ***tears*** that I was unwilling or unable to express in a situation where I experienced despair in mourning someone who was dear to me. I want to show my ***outer shell*** to **protect** myself and show that I am strong, but deep down inside, I feel like a ***defenseless*** child. I am in contact with the pain that follows a tragedy and often remains unexplained. This tragedy usually involves a member of my family. I may also be facing a deteriorating situation that is coming to an end, whether it is a couple or a business, etc., and I want to look after the persons involved.

I accept↓♥ that I need to take some time for myself and 'clean up' my life. I keep only those responsibilities that are properly mine and I return to their rightful bearers those that I took on my shoulders but were not truly mine. I give myself the right to ask for help. Life will thus be easier and more beautiful.

LUPUS / SYSTEMIC LUPUS ERYTHEMATOSIS (SLE) *See: SKIN — LUPUS*

LUXATION / (joint), DISLOCATION *See also: ACCIDENT, ANGER, BONES, PAIN*

A **luxation** or **dislocation** involves the displacement of the two bone extremities of a joint. It may be a shoulder, an elbow, a finger, a knee, a vertebra or a hip. A **luxation** or **dislocation** often follows a blow, a shock or a forced movement.

Depending on the location where the **luxation** has taken place, I must ask myself what fear or what emotional shock has given me the impression of being trapped as though I were being 'put into a box'. I want to escape and get out of an obligation, but I feel forced and trapped by this situation. It is as if I was wearing a straitjacket and trying with all my might to get out of it. My body acted conversely by absorbing the emotional repercussion. Do I feel that I no longer have my place in this world? Am I destabilized in my emotions by a person or an event? About who or what am I being so uncompromising? If the **luxation** affects my **shoulder**, I ask myself to whom I want to get closer. If it is the **jaw** (dislocation of the temporomandibular joint), I feel trapped in a situation where I can't advance or retreat. I am torn between reason and passion.

I accept↓♥ to become **Aware** of my inner freedom and I allow inner **Light** to shine on all situations that seem to limit me, in order to ***dissolve*** and dissipate my fears and develop more harmony with life.

LYMPH (lymphatic disorders) *See also: CANCER OF THE GANGLIA [OF THE LYMPHATIC SYSTEM]*

The **lymph** contains white globules, proteins and lipids (forms of fat). It fights infections and rejects anything that is bad for the body.

An **infection of the lymphatic vessels** (**lymphangitis**) shows me how much I have controlled my emotions and my environment, but I can't take it any longer! I am discouraged! I feel like a large elephant stuck in a small house: I want to get out of it, I want to be free! **Lymphatic edema** manifests my feeling of insecurity. I project an image as being above it all, but this makes me very fragile, because I am basing my life on a masquerade instead of experiencing it from my **heart♥**. Then, I am confused and I no longer know what road I should take, which makes me vulnerable.

Lymphatic disorders tell me to pay attention to my thoughts, to manage my emotions properly and to accept↓♥ joy circulating freely inside of me, like the sap in a tree. I must return to the essentials and focus my attention on the true values of life rather than on the material things or the things that I feel I am lacking.

LYMPHOMA *See: HODGKIN'S DISEASE*

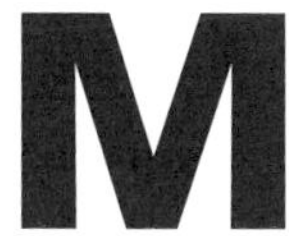

MAGIC MUSHROOMS (consumption of) *See: DRUGS*

MALAISE / AILMENT

A **malaise** or an **ailment** is not an illness but rather a discomfort that I feel and that can vary in intensity.

It is an 'un-ease' or an 'un-wellness' that I feel, and I am in conflict with myself or with a situation in my life. The way to decode an **ailment** is the same as for a disease. The clinical symptoms are less clear however, and can range from 'feeling out of sorts' to fainting. As with an illness, a **malaise** originates from a conflict or a conscious or unconscious trauma. The **ailment** may be temporary, but it may indicate an inner conflict that should be resolved before the message is conveyed more powerfully in the form of a full-blown disease.

MALARIA / PALUDISM *See also: BLOOD DISORDERS, COMA, FEVER*

Malaria manifests itself by high fevers.

It fits with criticism and repression against a person or a situation, for I had to separate from something or someone that I liked. Communication is totally cut off for me, however much I need it. Resentment has taken control of me, and my mind is taking pleasure in 'ruminating' these feelings that are harmful for me. I can't make any true choices about my emotions and my relations. I see myself as powerless. I have lost hope in a situation and no longer have any faith in myself or in life. It is as though I were incapable of converting my ideas and aspirations into actions. My male, active, go-getting side is 'hibernating'. Everything I see looks negative and dark. I am letting death come. To get free of this fever, I must go inside to release the tension, and resolve this situation.

I accept↓♥ to change my point of view about life. I must acknowledge all my possibilities. I indulge myself in little pleasures. I let go of all my resentments in order to recover inner peace.

MALE PRINCIPLE *See also: FEMALE PRINCIPLE*

The **male principle** is represented by the right side of the body and the left hemisphere of the brain. It is also called the Yang side in Chinese medicine, or the rational side in the West.

It represents my relation with the **male principle**, my own as well as in relation to the men in my life: father, companion, etc. The dominant qualities are courage, power and logic; it is related to knowledge, speech and reasoning.

It is the rational, autonomous, materialistic side of a human being. It is represented by the sun. It also represents the intellectual aspect, the active side of my person that takes the ideas and intuitions of my female side and implements them. It manages the 'why' of things. It chooses the directions. **Each human being, man as well as woman, possesses a male side (YANG) and a female side (YIN).** Ailments on the right side show me a conflict with my notion of virility and rivalry if I am a man and, for a woman, they show a duality involving my occupational life and the stereotypes I want to escape from. As I have developed my **male side** by analyzing and wanting to 'become like my father' (learned behavior), chances are high that we both display very similar traits with respect to the qualities and characteristics listed above.

I accept↓♥ that it is when I can balance my **male side** and my female side that I can achieve true fulfillment.

MALFORMATION (in general) — in the HEART♥

A **malformation** is an anomaly that has existed in a part of the body since birth and is due to a developmental disorder during the fetus' intra-uterine life. Contrary to the deformations acquired after birth, **malformations** are always and by definition congenital, namely already present at birth. They may be hereditary or were acquired following a conflict, a trauma or a shock during the individual's uterine life.

What affliction was in me during my formation? A **malformation** indicates a need to be especially **Aware** (often about a fear) related to the body part concerned (go and read the text concerning this body part). As I am in resonance with my parents, they too may have the same conflict. For example, a **congenital malformation of the heart♥** indicates that I am taking life very lightly. The **heart♥**, which represents **Love**, is a pump that draws in and passes on. I put aside my emotions and my spiritual depth. Life for me isn't worth much, and **Love** is but a very vague concept that doesn't apply to me. The lack of **Love** is directed mainly against oneself, against others or against life in general. I am here to learn to forgive and open myself up to this form of energy that is **Love**. Right from the start, I closed myself off from this fluid circulation inside of me.

I accept↓♥ to resolve the circumstances of my birth and to adjust to what I must overcome in order to feel this energy and this **Love**. I learn to forgive and take care of my **heart♥**. I accept myself as I am and I adjust by doing my best, without criticizing myself, and I become **Aware** that I am a part of the great whole. The more **Love** I feel for what I am, the more able I am to pass it on to the people around me. I accept↓♥ to fully embrace life. To taste each instant and explore each facet of life, physical as well as emotional. I accept↓♥ to experience **Love** in all its forms, to understand with my **heart♥** the true value of earthly life.

MANIA *See also: ANGUISH, ANXIETY*

Manias are habits that hide anguish and anxiety. This agitated state brings on an over-excitation in movements and an inflamed mood. It is a way to seek peace and calm. It can be a form of escape because I force myself to always develop in the same context, thus preventing myself from exploring new avenues, in order to always feel safe and in control of the situation. I am afraid of using my go-getting, independent, innovative side. I lock myself into habits that keep me in the confines of the familiar, in a certain comfort zone.

I accept↓♥ to determine the source of this anxiety in order to find more inner calm and more harmony. I will thus see life with more peace and serenity. My actions and attitudes will be more in agreement with my inner wisdom.

MANIC-DEPRESSIVE PSYCHOSIS *See: PSYCHOSIS*

MARFAN'S SYNDROME

Marfan's[1] **syndrome** is a disease, described as hereditary and genetic, that impairs the fibers of the conjunctive tissues and is responsible for skeletal, ocular and cardiac anomalies; the disease is found in very tall persons with abnormally supple joints, who present cardiac anomalies, mainly in the aorta, which frequently require an operation. **Marfan's syndrome** is most often associated with cardiac (inter-auricular communication problems), pulmonary or skeletal malformations.

Are there any family secrets that were hidden from me, or that I hide myself? There is a link that was not established with the past. The way of the **heart♥** was blocked by a lack of communication, by shyness or shame. What is the reason preventing me from communicating with my parents or my heirs?

MARIJUANA CONSUMPTION *See: DRUGS*

MASOCHISM *See: SADOMASOCHISM*

MASS / LUMP / SWELLING *See: HUMP /LUMP*

MASTICATION *See: MOUTH (IN GENERAL)*

MASTITIS *See: BREASTS — MASTITIS*

MASTOIDITIS *See also: EARS — OTITIS, FEVER, INFLAMMATION*

Mastoiditis is an inflammation that occurs at the base of the temporal bone, the mastoid, just behind the ears.

1. **Marfan** (Anthonin Bernard Jean): French pediatrician (1858–1942). He described 'dolichostenomelia' in 1896, better known by the name of **Marfan's syndrome**. There is also **Marfan's disease**, congenital syphilitic spasmodic paraplegia.

Mastoiditis can occur when I refuse to listen. I am annoyed and frustrated by what I have just heard or would have liked to hear about someone or something that bothers me. I feel sad and, if I am a child, I may not understand what is being said, which provokes insecurity. My fear, or my impression of having been tricked, makes me not want to hear whatever is being said. I prefer to ***extract*** myself from certain conversations to protect myself, but I find myself limited thereby.

I accept↓♥ that "I am at peace; harmony and joy circulate in me". Thank you!

MASTOSIS *See: BREAST DISORDERS*

MEASLES *See: CHILDHOOD DISEASES*

MEDICINE

Medicine is the science and art of preventing and curing diseases[2]. Thus, although a preventive and predictive **medicine** does exist, **medicine** deals mainly with diseases, traumas, infirmities and the means to cure them.

When a physician can put a diagnosis on an illness I have, it is then easier to choose the sort of treatment that can apply. The previous century enabled **medicine** to make gigantic bounds, with important discoveries in chemistry and biology and with the help of the new technologies. In many cases, **medicine** has proved quite effective where it was possible to determine a diagnosis. However, when my ailment or disease can't be clearly identified, it can happen that **medicine** is powerless to help me. I may then search for the causes of this ailment or disease with the help of ideology, psychokinesiology, energy readings or other forms of investigation by calling on responsible persons with a recognized professional ethic.

MELANCHOLY *See also: ANGUISH, DEPRESSION, GRIEF, PSYCHOSIS, SUICIDE*

Melancholy is a state of deep sadness.

I find myself at fault, I am feeling seriously depressed and I can hardly stand this mental pain. My moving about, even physical, is affected by it. I am faced with a dissatisfaction, an annoyance or a sorrow that bring a lack of joy. This sadness leads me to feel 'mixed up in my emotions', which become increasingly gloomy. I feel I am going in circles. I have a sickness of the **Soul**. I want to be recognized at my full worth but I go rather unnoticed.

I accept↓♥ to affirm that "joy inhabits my whole being". I set realistic goals that will help me find more energy in myself, dissipate the sadness and make room for more joy and satisfaction. I make peace with myself, and my **Soul** is light and 'ready for takeoff'.

MELANOMA *See: SKIN — MELANOMA [MALIGNANT]*

---

2. Definition derived from the *Merriam-Webster Dictionary*.

MEMORY (failing) *See also: ALZHEIMER'S DISEASE, AMNESIA*

Memory is the faculty to store ideas and emotions and bring back to **Awareness** whatever I want to recall.

After an emotional shock, I may conceal certain fears or sorrows from my **memory**. I avoid, for example, recalling a painful separation, an unbearable tragedy, anything that is painful to remember. It is the subconscious that is preventing the conscious from recalling, from ***holding on*** to information. It is a way for me, however unconsciously, to escape from a form of reality that I would find difficult to experience. My brain decides to keep only the 'winning solutions', those with no pain attached to them, or that won't reconnect me to unpleasant situations where I feel that I failed. I need to feel backed and supported by others. I feel that I am not up to it, and I let go of things important to me for fear of not succeeding. Flight is easier than anguish and sorrow.

I accept↓♥ to take full responsibility for my life, **Aware** that each situation is here to help me know myself better and feel more completely free.

MÉNIÈRE'S DISEASE — LABYRINTHITIS *See also: TINNITUS, VERTIGO AND DIZZINESS*

Ménière's disease[3] is marked by true rotary vertigo, with the sensation of being in an amusement park ride because of an impairment of a labyrinth (usually an increase in the pressure of fluids in the labyrinth) associated with tinnitus and lowered hearing. Its symptoms resemble those of **labyrinthitis**, which is an inflammation of the labyrinth, a cavity of the inner ear. It is often associated with great physical and mental fatigue or with over-work. I have too much information and details in my head, so there is chaos and 'overheating'.

I am not in contact with the physical world and there are blanks in my thoughts. I feel like in a labyrinth, I refuse to hear the messages of my inner voice. I also tend to reject the advice of others. I prefer to escape, sometimes very suddenly, into my own world. I wander and go in circles and don't know where to go. I have lost my road map. Am I starting to negate myself? I can't take it any longer! I want to plug my ears. For too long I have had to endure, remaining silent and repressing my needs and desires, but now I have reached my limits. I can no longer hide and stay motionless. I observe the situations of intolerance or imbalance in the different spheres of my life. What change would be important for me to make in order to recover my balance without making me dizzy? Why do I listen to others but don't want to share my suffering and my sorrows with them?

I accept↓♥ to give myself some physical and intellectual rest. I choose to take a pause and allow the movement of life to circulate in me by making the necessary choices. I thus find balance in all the senses of the word.

---

3. **Ménière** (Proper Paul): French physician and otologist (1799–1862). In 1861 he published the article in which he described his famous syndrome: "Report on inner ear lesions giving rise to symptoms of apoplectiform cerebral congestion".

MENINGITIS *See: BRAIN — MENINGITIS*

MENISCI *See: KNEE AILMENTS*

MENISCUS

The **menisci** are formed of fibers and cartilage, one on the inside and the other on the outside of the knee. They ensure the proper adjustment of the bones with joint surfaces that don't fit: it is therefore a sheath, a support.

When there is a **tear**, it is because I am resisting in the way I adjust myself; I am rigid and I don't want to yield (to situations, to others, etc.) to authority. **Premature wearing down** can also occur. The **knee** is related to the movements of life. When my **menisci** give out, it is because I prefer to break off rather than adjust. An **ailment** in a **meniscus** shows me that I depend on others in certain situations, being poorly self-confident. I comply with the requirements of others. I am abrupt and tense, and the least unexpected tension affects my menisci. I am used to being the conciliator, arranging things so that harmony will prevail or that disputes will be resolved *amicably*. If I think I have failed in this role as a go-between, my menisci will react. I let go of my rigidity and try to understand why I am so stubborn.

I accept↓♥ to adjust and change the way I am in certain aspects of my life. I am increasingly flexible instead of wanting to force events or persons. By becoming **Aware** of my potential, I increasingly trust life, which gives me everything I need. I can achieve all my aspirations by listening to the only authority that exists: my inner voice.

MENOPAUSE DISORDERS

In the autumn of life, a woman's body changes, and I must accept↓♥ it. It is a highly emotional period that especially involves my feelings about being still loveable and desirable, but mostly about being loved and desired. I take stock of my life, and I may have regrets for not having done this or that, or I have the impression that I haven't fully taken advantage of life. I feel that I must resign myself to receiving less **Love**, notably through sexuality. It is as though my body were ***falling silent***, being no longer able to experience passion. In the first half of my life, often called the 'active period', I am engaged in action, I 'do' things, I procreate, I build. It is my rational, active, organizing side, also known as my male, or 'Yang', side, that predominates. But now, I feel diminished, and I may want to pursue all my domestic chores and my social tasks, instead of making way for all my femininity, my gentleness and my creativity that are my female, Yin, side. I would like to launch myself into life on my own authority and give myself first place, but it scares me because I am going into the unknown. I am under pressure, and I want to react by resisting or acting indifferent in order to protect myself. The **hot flashes** that I experience during **menopause** manifest an inner conflict, and my female side is being stifled by the symptoms that my male side elicits ('men-oppose'). This inner duality can illuminate the opposition I experience with certain men whose behavior I can't tolerate. This heat that surfaces is full of emotions that could appear during my menses. Now, I must find another way to express those emotions. It may be through oral communication or my physical and sexual desires that are always quite present. These **hot flashes** remind me that my needs for human warmth through sexuality are a priority and that I must take care of them. Unconsciously, the fact of undressing because I am too hot reminds me of the situations where I would undress to attract the man I loved. The **sweating** that results from these hot flashes releases all my emotions that no longer have any reason for being. The only effective way to make them disappear is to once again become the useful, experienced and wise woman, for my **stubbornness** in not following the flow of life may transform itself into a headache or a migraine. Even if I am no longer a child-bearer, I must find my spiritual direction. I need to find the **Woman** in me. It is a little like in retirement: I now have the time for working entirely free, making other plans and taking up other challenges. I discover new meanings in the words 'Freedom' and 'Individuality' that enable me to be ***reborn*** to a new life. My attention is now focused on me and my spouse instead of focused solely on the children (in many cases) and the family. I discover a new reason for living. It is a little like a new beginning: I can do things that I like and that I have chosen. It will enable my blood to flow normally and allow my **heart♥** to fill with self-**Love**. These hot feelings of frustration, insecurity and anger can be replaced with cooler feelings of freedom, gentleness and trust in the future. The fear of aging can become more present and real. I can even unconsciously make menstruations reappear to help me return into the past and cling to a physical youth that has long disappeared. It is therefore important for me that I accept↓♥ to kiss goodbye to my youth so I can fully live the present moment. I become **Aware** that instead of being the end of something, this stage is in fact a **PAUSE** that enables me to assess my life, take stock and resolve the situations I have always tried to escape from. I may rediscover and fully experience my sexuality, which could eliminate my symptoms of **frigidity** and **vaginal dryness**.

I accept↓♥ the transformations in my body, as well as the spiritual ones in my inner life and in my social and family life. I live in simplicity. I savor each moment and I have the power to change my life with all the experiences I have had so far, through which I have gained extraordinary wisdom and treasure. I become **Aware** that **menopause** is a birth to who I truly am. I no longer have to live for others, but I can live for myself. The more I advance in age, the more wisdom teaches me joy, calm and pure unconditional **Love**, and it is only by developing these states of being that I can truly remain young all my life. It is the youth of the **heart♥** and not of the body.

MENORRHAGIA *See: MENSTRUATION — MENORRHAGIA*

MENSES / MENSTRUATION / PERIOD DISORDERS *See: MENSTRUATION DISORDERS*

MENSTRUATION DISORDERS

Menstruation is the discharge, through the vagina, of blood originating from the uterine mucous membrane. It occurs periodically in non-pregnant women from puberty until menopause.

Menstrual pains (**dysmenorrhea**) may be related to **guilt** and **anger**. These feelings may have their source in an experience where I was sexually abused, especially before puberty. If I refuse my condition as a woman, if I am indignant over the submission of women in society or the rules with which I must comply, if I resent men, my father or the person who was the main male figure when I was a child, my **menstruations** will be very painful. I am very perfectionist and I expect the same behavior from others. On the other hand, if I also feel that my parents are disappointed over having given birth to a daughter, I may do my best to look like a boy in order to be loved by my parents. My affective life is unstable and I am afraid for my future. I may **unconsciously delay my menstruations or make them stop**. I refuse my femininity and maybe my sexuality too, believing it to be dirty or sinful. Every ***month***, even unconsciously, I may be disappointed at not being pregnant, for it is generally the loss of blood (related to a loss of joy) that indicates whether I am pregnant or not. There results a vague feeling of solitude, not feeling 'accompanied' by a baby 'on the way'. This disappointment at not being pregnant originates in the innate memory of the species, which intends me to be made for procreation and to ensure its survival. Thus, the losses of blood, metaphysically related to a loss of joy, indicate to some degree my sorrow, even unconscious, of not having been pregnant, linked to my genetic programming for the preservation of the species. In the past, **menses** were a positive sign that a woman was not pregnant, especially in non-marital situations. If my losses exceed my 'normal range', namely if they diminish or even **halt the menstruations**, or on the contrary if they **increase** them, I must then check to see if I am experiencing any of the stages mentioned above that I may go through in my life and that could explain this change. My difficulties with **menstruations** often originate from the resistance I feel about my sexual power or my potential for maternity and creativity. I feel helpless, not ***predisposed*** to stand by my needs, and I repress my emotions. The shame I feel makes me live as a victim. I have difficulty in letting go and '**fixing** problems'. The sadder I feel, the more abundant are my menses.

The more I accept↓♥ that it is simply my body's response to programming, the more harmoniously this period will unfold. As a woman, I must accept↓♥ to live in harmony with this body that works in cycles. I allow the flow of my emotions and creative energy to run free. I focus my attention on the positive, and thus create a new life.

MENSTRUATION — AMENORRHEA

Amenorrhea is the absence or the suppression of menses, also called **menstruations**, in women.

Amenorrhea, which occurs at an age when I have my menses, can be related to a rejection of my femininity, to a shock or to the inconveniences of being a woman; to guilt, possibly induced by words or actions of my sexual partner; or to feelings experienced during certain **menstruations**. I am feeling a certain fear, discomfort or guilt. I may fear losing my child for the benefit of the family. To put that right, I program myself mentally to make my menses stop, by refusing life, by deciding to stop procreating. I may be refusing to experience what my mother experienced with my father, and I refuse to unwittingly serve as a '**progenitor**' (as a mere 'tool of reproduction') in my current relationship, for I recall the pain I felt when I used to see my mother so sad in her **Love** relationship. I refuse to go through that experience. I am in conflict with my creativity and my desire to please. I have this deep need to be admired, which I fight with all my strength.

As a woman, I have to **heartily♥** accept↓♥ my partner and trust him, especially if he **loves** me and is open with me. I accept↓♥ life expressing itself through my femininity.

MENSTRUATION — MENORRHAGIA *See also: FIBROMAS*

Menorrhagia is an abnormal increase in the abundance and duration of the menses, which can derive in some cases from the presence of a uterine fibroma.

There is a difficulty with blood coagulation, a blood loss that I can't control, a feeling that something eludes me. **Menorrhagias** are related to the non-acceptance↓♥ of having children or to great losses of joy because I can't bear a child, whether because of my infertility or because I use a means of contraception to avoid becoming pregnant. I am losing my place as a woman. I am seeking my identity. There are two sides of me that want to meet and become reconciled: the inner angel and the demon. What do I truly want? How can I fill this need for tenderness and pleasure? What is the situation in my couple that I can no longer stand and that I need to change?

Whatever my situation, I accept↓♥ to make peace with who I am and the point I have reached with the children.

MENSTRUATION — PREMENSTRUAL SYNDROME (PMS) *See also: PAIN*

The **premenstrual syndrome** appears during the period preceding **menstruations**. It takes the form of nervousness, pains in the back, the head and the stomach and mood swings. The hormonal imbalance causes physical changes that mimic a state of pregnancy (water retention causing weight gain, swelling of breasts, etc.).

It is the process of rejection and guilt that is beginning to surface. For a woman, the menstrual period is a reminder that she is living in a world dominated by men. I must prove that I am a strong and radiant woman and at the same time, I would like so much to not have to work and prove my worth! I may be tired of being submissive, when I would rather be able to dominate and control, as many men can. It thus indicates how the **premenstrual syndrome** brings about situations that make me ask myself questions about how I perceive myself as a woman in my relation to my femininity, especially if I want to succeed in a professional career. I may be troubled and confused and I allow myself to be influenced by the stereotypes imposed by society. I find society's rules very '**painful**'. What role do I want to play? Can I allow myself to lead an active life and also allow myself moments of relaxation and pleasure?

I accept↓♥ myself, I **love** myself as I am and I allow room for development.

MESCALINE (consumption of) *See: DRUGS*

METABOLISM (slow) *See: WEIGHT [EXCESS]*

METEORISM *See: GAS*

MIDDLE FINGER / THIRD FINGER *See: FINGERS — MIDDLE FINGER / THIRD FINGER*

MIDDLE OF THE BACK *See: BACK DISORDERS — MIDDLE BACK*

MIGRAINES *See: HEAD — MIGRAINES*

MILK CRUST *See: SKIN — ECZEMA*

MILK-ALKALI SYNDROME *See also: ACIDOSIS, APATHY*

The **milk-alkali syndrome** or **Burnett's**[4] **syndrome** provokes renal failure by an excessive intake of **milk**, calcium or **alkali**. It remains reversible for a long time if I stop this excessive consumption.

I try to fill an inner void left by my unfulfilled felt need for maternal **Love**. My state of fatigue and apathy reminds me how important this need was for me. This doesn't mean that I had a mother who didn't **love** me, but that I may have had an even greater need. Reacting to this lack, I may have had an attitude of domination toward my mother or women in general. It may also be that I try to make up for whatever was bitter in my life by anything that most resembles what was gentle in my childhood and reminds me of my mother's **Love**.

I accept↓♥ right now to take care of myself, as my mother would do it. I accept↓♥ the soothing delights of life, knowing that I am an exceptional person who deserves the best.

---

4. **Burnett** (Sir Frank MacFarlane) (1899 -1985): An Australian professor *emeritus*, an immunologist and virologist, he received the Nobel Prize in 1960 (physiology or medicine) for "the discovery of acquired immunological tolerance".

MISCARRIAGE / SPONTANEOUS ABORTION *See: CHILDBIRTH / ABORTION / DELIVERY*

MONGOLISM / TRISOMY 21 / DOWN'S[5] SYNDROME

Mongolism is a congenital disease in which the newborn child presents morphological anomalies (the appearance of the face is often enough to diagnose it, along with the single palmar fold), and it will affect the child's intellectual development with the presence of debility; cardiac anomalies may also be associated with it.

If I am **mongoloid**, I feel anguished in this artificial world and I find it difficult to accept↓♥ some of its bothersome or threatening features. There are so many responsibilities involved in the fact of growing up that I prefer to remain in a child's world, a world where simplicity, spontaneity and carefree joy prevail. I am not required to become involved or to measure up to the norms of society. Even before birth, I sense that I am, or my parents are, different from the others; I want to be separated from the world and to stay as close as possible to my mother who knows how to protect me. My aggressiveness only mirrors my frustrations at being unable to reach all my goals. If one of my children is affected by **Trisomy 21**, I ask myself how far this child has come to teach me the true human values and to do everything with **Love** and gratitude.

I accept↓♥ to engage each experience with openness and trust in others, and in life. I allow trust to grow with each new encounter, in each of my contacts with persons, animals or objects. I thus feel increasingly alive as I become ever more a part of this world. I learn to set my priorities and my values in their proper places and I let go of the judgments of others. I thus feel better and I glow with joy.

MONONUCLEOSIS *See: BLOOD — INFECTIOUS MONONUCLEOSIS*

MOTION SICKNESS *See: TRAVEL SICKNESS*

MOUNTAIN / ALTITUDE SICKNESS *See also: APPETITE [LOSS OF], BLOATING, EARS / BUZZING / TINNITUS, HEADACHES, NAUSEA, VERTIGO*

When I go to high **altitudes**, there may occur a number of related disorders originating from the fact that oxygen is rarer there and my body has difficulty in breathing in more of it: a degree of openness or adjustment is lacking. When I climb that high, I change levels of **Consciousness**, which can provoke a shock for me. The disorders I experience are but the reflection of my anxieties and my **conscious** or unconscious inner injuries. It is certain that the more my

5. **Down** (John Langdon): A British physician (1828–1896) who published in 1866 an article titled "Observations on an Ethnic Classification of Idiots", in which he classified idiots according to physical and ethnic characteristics, and gave a detailed clinical description of the disease he named "Mongoloid Idiocy".

physical body is in top shape, the easier it will be for me to withstand, even physically, these changes of inner **Consciousness**.

I accept↓♥ to remain calm and confident in myself and in life; to open myself to new horizons and further develop the feeling of freedom inside of me.

MOUTH (in general) *See also: GUMS*

The **mouth** represents openness to life and makes it possible to make contact with the mother by suckling her breast. It is a sensitive and selective sensory organ. It is the entrance for food, air and water. It is thanks to it that I can speak (lips, tongue, vocal cords), communicate and express my emotions and my thoughts. It is a sort of bridge between my inner being and the world around me (reality). It symbolizes my intimacy and my vital space. My **mouth** is the manifestation of my personality, my appetites, my desires, my expectations, my character traits and the pleasure of being alive. It enables me to open up to everything that is **new**: sensations, ideas and impressions. It is thus a two-way passage, and the difficulties I experience basically have a twofold dimension, inner and outer. It is interesting to note that the **way I chew** food reflects my way of being and behaving. If I 'gobble' food without chewing it, I am rather impulsive and details hold little meaning for me. On the contrary, if I masticate endlessly, I am a perfectionist and I linger too much on trifling details. I may thus have the impression that I have control over the situations of my life. This way, I no longer taste life: I break it down into a thousand pieces, constantly dwelling on the past. If I bite off large mouthfuls, I am 'working at double speed' and taking lots of responsibilities on my shoulders. I will often be running several projects at the same time. Absorbing food in very small mouthfuls indicates self-restraint for fear of rushing or taking on new tasks that I find very difficult for me.

I accept↓♥ to eat slowly while tasting the food, so that I can better taste life and its delights.

MOUTH DISEASE *See also: CANCER OF THE MOUTH, CHANCRE (IN GENERAL), HERPES (IN GENERAL), THRUSH*

My **mouth** is the door to my digestive system and the respiratory tract where I accept↓♥ to take in everything that is necessary for my physical (water, food, air), emotional and sensory (excitations, desires, tastes, appetites, needs, etc.), existence. Thus, **mouth ailments** indicate that I show a certain narrowness of mind, that I have rigid ideas and opinions and that I find it difficult to take in and **swallow** what is **new** (thoughts, ideas, feelings, emotions). There is a situation that I can't 'swallow': it is often words I heard that bothered or hurt me, or words that I would have liked to hear but remained unspoken.

The inequality and disharmony in the relationship between my parents trouble me. I therefore want to reply or respond, but I don't do so because I feel uncomfortable in the situation or because the opportunity simply doesn't present itself. I therefore remain 'stuck' with what I have to say. The gestures or words of others that hurt me and about which I would have wanted to hear explanations, which never came, can provoke ailments in my **mouth**. There is a confrontation between me (what I say) and my entourage (how the others receive it). Do I dare tell things as I experience them, at the risk of losing the **Love** of others, or am I capable of respecting myself in what I am and dare to show it to the rest of the world? I may feel misunderstood because I don't know how to ***communicate***. My body is sending me the message that I may be conveying unhealthy ideas with my **mouth**, and that I should change my attitude about myself and others. The typical example is the **oral chancre or ulcer** (herpes) that usually manifests itself following the stress or trauma resulting from an intense nervous period or a sickness. It shows me the sad and irritable manner in which I take everyday reality. I am feeling irritated either about something that was done or said to me, or about something that I should have said. Someone or something left me an after-taste in my **mouth** that still affects me. I am ***astonished*** and I don't know quite how to react. **I may be feeling stuck**: I may be feeling **caught** in the situation (**blocked**), or I have been ruminating for some time over an unpleasant situation, or I really need to recover my complete freedom by saying what I have to say even if it risks displeasing me. Meanwhile, I feel invaded from all sides. I may also be hungry for **Love**, affection, knowledge, spirituality, freedom, etc.

If I feel that what I need is unreachable or unrealistic, my famished **mouth** will react to the sense of lack that I feel. If the **corners of my mouth are chapped**, I am going through an inner struggle: is it to be protected and made safe by others, or to take my place and have to listen to my own authority, my inner voice? I may feel frustrated, tense and aggressive because I don't dare assert my disagreements. If my **mouth is dry**, I tend to be anxious and prefer to flee reality. I can live disconnected from my body and my emotions. Having a **dry mouth** allows me to avoid swallowing things I find unpleasant. Many things in my life disgust me; I am cut off from pleasure. A **mouth with a coated tongue** is a sign that everyday life is stifling my joy in living and my taste for starting up new projects. An **affection in the temporomandibular joint** (cracking, for example) **highlights** my fear of contradicting others, especially persons in authority. I avoid confrontations and prefer to repress my tears. If I **chew the inside of my cheek**, I am trying to get rid of something I am ashamed of.

I accept↓♥ that instead of living in a ***stupor*** or in fear of being hurt, in any situation I will trust in my inner strength and my capacity for finding workable solutions. From now on, I take my place while remaining open to what is beginning for me, to what is **new**, provided that it is in harmony. I bite ***hungrily*** into life. I accept↓♥ my tenderness and my gentleness and I express myself confidently.

MOUTH — APTHA

Aptha is a superficial lesion on the oral mucous surface, characterized by a small white protuberance, often surrounded by a red edge, and can also appear on the genital mucous membranes. It is associated with a fever that does not break out.

It appears because I easily react (sensitivity) to my surroundings, to 'vibrations', to the ambience of a situation. I **suffer with my mouth silently closed**. It is also a sign that I am **having difficulty in taking root** and am not succeeding in expressing myself, in saying what I want or even reacting, because I don't believe I have the power to do it. I don't feel **apt** to accomplish great things. My insecurity leads me to be 'mute' about what I am experiencing, knowing that saying things could bring major changes in my life or could also turn against me. I have something in my **mouth** that is burning me but I must keep it there, I have no way to eject it. I may have sensed a base deed and was unable to respond. It is as though I had no other choice but to digest it! It may have been experienced through my sexuality. When I was young, I may have felt uncomfortable at one point about a situation where I was unable to react or to assert myself. If I encounter a similar situation again today, recalling that first experience even unconsciously, **aphta** will appear. My words are futile and incomplete because I am too nervous. I remain silent, without even thinking about revolting! Yet, I can't go on, I am 'at the end of my tether'. My sensitivity is very intense and I wear masks, I play a role for fear of coming into contact with my deepest feelings. I am anxious and everything irritates me. I may feel guilt, which brings me low self-esteem. I would like so much to accomplish things, but I resist so much! I become **Aware** that I usually refuse any new ideas, even when they could bring positive changes in my life. If I sense an injustice, disgust or a hidden dissatisfaction (in my **mouth**) and I feel like blowing off steam, I can do so while remaining open and in tune with myself. I must choose my words, however: I might risk using words that are nasty, false and aimed at destroying. I am responsible for expressing myself non-violently; otherwise, it could turn against me. However, as these white protuberances are very painful, as soon as I open my **mouth** to express myself, I feel them and it hurts me.

If I want to avoid seeing them return more seriously, I accept↓♥ to express myself openly and calmly right now. I replace guilt with confidence in my capacity for adjustment, my understanding and my intuition that I listen to more and more. I thus make peace with my emotions and with the way of expressing myself that suits me best.

MOUTH — BREATH (bad) / HALITOSIS *See also: GUMS — GINGIVITIS, THROAT [SORE], NOSE AILMENTS*

Bad breath, also called **halitosis**, is the direct consequence of my difficulty in dealing from the inside and from the outside with the situations that I experience. This difficulty may originate from the fact that I stand on my positions about certain ideas that I don't express and that rot in place. The difficulty may also arise from the fact that I can't get back the upper hand in a period of major change in my life and that my old ideas have stagnated too long relative to the speed of the changes I am going through. I check just how far I am able to 'take on' the situations of my life. Do I feel I have to act against my convictions? It is important for me to communicate with the persons involved to tell them about my emotions and my thoughts in order to get rid of my **bad breath**. It is often related to thoughts of malicious gossip, disgust, hate or vengeance that I have against myself, another person or life itself, and of which I am ashamed. I **resist** very hard, and the poison I produce shows itself outwardly by a nauseating stink that persists until I let go of my negative emotions and my taste for revenge. The air that I breathe in and that nourishes my cells is charged with all my thoughts, positive as well as negative. What thoughts eating away at me inside are infecting my **breath**? These thoughts may often be unconscious. Something is rotting, either inside of me or due to a situation involving another person. When a person is constantly enduring this situation, I should tell them about it to make them become **Aware** of it and remedy this problem that may have persisted for some time. Knowing this, the person will have the opportunity to experience forgiveness: either forgiving themselves for entertaining unhealthy thoughts, or forgiving another person for having resented them so much.

It is good for me to remember that once **Love** and honesty have become the basic ingredients of my thoughts, my breath will become fresh again. I accept↓♥ to free myself of the unhealthy thoughts of the past. Now, I breathe the freshness of my new positive thoughts of **Love**, for myself and for others.

MOUTH — PALATE

The **palate** is the bony roof of the oral cavity. It plays a role in phonation and swallowing.

It will be affected if I thought I had received or acquired something (a new job for example) with certainty, but which was then taken away from me, and I have difficulty in 'swallowing' this situation. I will therefore feel very frustrated and disappointed because I believed that this thing was already mine, but it was taken away from me. I may have had the impression that I had my place in a family or an organization, but someone else took it from me and I no longer have it. It is as though my **palate** was not large enough for me to be able to keep everything I have caught or conquered. I don't have access to what pleases me (thing or person). I feel like I am being punished for a bad action on my part. I feel a great injustice. A situation affects me, for I am in conflict with laws or authority.

I must accept↓♥ to ask myself why this situation occurred. Was I expecting too much? Must I try to regain what I thought I had lost, or may it be better like this? I must answer those questions for harmony to return and my **palate** to heal.

MOUTH — THRUSH *See: THRUSH*

MUCOSITY of the COLON *See: INTESTINES — COLITIS*

MUMPS *See also: CHILDHOOD DISEASES (IN GENERAL), GLANDS [SALIVARY], INFECTIONS (IN GENERAL),*

The **mumps** are a contagious viral infection that most often manifests itself by inflammation in certain glands, notably the salivary glands. Children are most frequently affected.

There is something or someone in my life that makes me feel irritable and frustrated. I am feeling disparaged and criticized and I sometimes feel like having my turn at spitting in people's faces. Unless it is someone else who would like to do the same to me or my ideas! I have difficulty in catching or swallowing the things that I like very much because I can be prevented from doing them, or forbidden to do them. The **mumps** generally affect children more than adults, as they have much difficulty in expressing their anger and frustration. I am constantly struggling with myself. I judge myself severely, perceiving myself as fragile or abnormal. I deny my instincts and my awakening sexual energy. This limits my range of influence.

Instead of scorning myself, someone else or a situation, I accept↓♥ to look at what I can learn from it. I allow my inner energy and natural desires to flow and I can thus gain closer contact with my creativity and inner joy.

MUSCLES (in general)

The **muscles** are controlled by mental force; it is the life, the power and the strength of our bones. It is the reflection of what we are, what we believe and think of becoming in life. The **muscles** represent the effort to be expended and the work that must be carried out in order to move ahead. The **muscles**, which correspond to my mental energy, are necessary for moving and taking action. They symbolize development and vitality. **Ailments** in my **muscles** show me that I feel powerless about a situation, as though I were in a **straightjacket**. I feel diminished in my physical, intellectual or emotional strength. This causes a diminishing of my performance or my capacities. All my experiences and my related feelings are also impregnated in my **muscles**. My inner state (tense, nervous or relaxed, for example) corresponds exactly to the state of my **muscles**. They react strongly to any overstress I experience. As my whole body is made up of **muscles**, it will take on the form of my thoughts and the attitudes that I convey. If I easily let myself go to depression, negativism or fear, I will adopt an equivalent posture. On the contrary, if I have joy in living and spirit and I am positive, my **muscles** will be firm and flexible. If I accept↓♥ to transform myself and live in the present instead of clinging to the past, my **muscles** will be healthy. My **muscles** envelop my bones; so they also represent all my deep feelings that are part of my emotional life. If I am not in contact with them and favor instead the material and artificial side of life, my **muscles** will suffer from it. Then I tend to be on guard and I am permanently nervous. **Convulsions**[6] may result from this. I want to rationalize things too much and

6. **Convulsions**: Sudden and involuntary contractions of **muscles.**

it is as though I were 'overheating' and the excess is externalized by these **convulsions**. The **stretching of a muscle** tells me that I am experiencing enormous tension and I feel forced to please others. I know I should do things differently and follow another road, but I persist in not changing, for fear of the reactions of the others. If I reach the point of suffering a **pull** or a **tear** in certain **muscles**, the pressure is still more extreme, and I persist in going in one direction while my inner voice tells me to go in another. I am stubborn and I hold on to something that is no longer beneficial for me. **Muscular pains** remind me that I 'set the bar very high' for myself. I am shaken by certain events and my suffering is such that I must make major changes in my life. My outer pain expresses my inner pain. I want to surrender. I am ***demotivated*** and ***discouraged*** because I am living in regrets and remorse. My dreams are ***vanishing***. When there are **muscular diseases**, I must refer to the body parts affected in order to determine the cause that is expressed. I go and see to what mental situations, to what patterns or behaviors this part of the body is related.

I accept↓♥ that my body resumes contact with my whole world of emotions and that I become my own authority. My **muscles** recover their health when I trust my inner wisdom and when I take the time I need to read the events. This removes the emotional tension I experience as well as the one in my **muscles**. I live from my **heart♥**. I change my way of living. By being more open to life and more flexible, my **muscles** too will be so.

MUSCLES — CONVULSION *See also: BRAIN — EPILEPSY*

A **convulsion** is a sudden and involuntary contraction of **muscles**.

I am struggling with an inner duality that leads me to act irrationally. During a **convulsion** attack, I no longer control my body and my emotions. Beyond the fears, there are spasms, agitation and suffering, and my whole body reacts. I don't know what direction to take and my body is trembling as I no longer control anything, I feel in a void.

I accept↓♥ to stop and take the time to see what, in my life, is causing all this stress and agitation. I take the time to stop and focus my attention on the dualities of my existence. I take the time to taste life, I choose my priorities and I make decisions accordingly so I can honor them. I recover peace and joy in living.

MUSCLES — DYSTROPHY (muscular)

Muscular dystrophy is a disease where the **muscles** weaken and degenerate, sometimes rapidly. The most frequent and severe form is called **Duchenne's**[7] **myopathy**.

It is related to **such a great desire to control situations and people** that I lose all control. I feel that for me, all is already lost and my body is so fatigued

7. **Duchenne de Boulogne** (Guillaume Benjamin): A French physician (1806–1875). A pioneer of neurology, he described a form of myopathy and studied the effects of localized electrical stimulation for diagnosis and therapy.

by this stress that it gives up and progressively destroys itself. I am not good enough, or I don't believe myself **capable of being up to the mark**. My life is dull and no longer interests me. I am really afraid of not succeeding my life and I no longer make any efforts. As a result, my **muscles**, which represent action, become sick and it is now my own fear that is taking control and I allow myself to be controlled by society. I feel that we are mere puppets and that misery is part of my life. Just see how the others treat me! By not enjoying life, by not keeping this vital space I need so much, by restricting my possibilities, I am sinking in quicksand. I can no longer advance and I can't count on anyone. I can't manage my own vital strength to reach my goals. I distort my memories of the past to suffer less. **Muscular dystrophy** is a severe disease, often defined as incurable, but its state can later be stabilized and resorbed if I put in the necessary efforts.

I accept↓♥ to let go, to **remain open and face my own fears here and now**! When I have faced my fears and identified them, I no longer need to manage everything. I accept↓♥ to go ahead and free myself from the need to control, which in fact is but the projection of my fears.

MUSCLES — FIBROMATOSIS

Fibromatosis originates from fibrous tumors (fibromas) or from an increase of fibers in a tissue (fibrosis) that produces stiffness in my **muscles** and my fibrous tissues, which in turn provokes intense pain.

The soft tissues concern my way of thinking. The pains I feel are warning me that I am experiencing much stress and tension, hence my intense mental fatigue. They make me realize that **I am lacking in flexibility**, that **I am rigid and anxious**, especially in my thoughts and my attitudes. Because of my own inner conflicts, I prevent energy from circulating freely in my muscles. I become **Aware** of these tensions: where do they come from? Is it a mental fatigue related to what I do, to my way of being and expressing myself? Do I not dare suggest certain projects that might raise controversy, not counting all the time and energy involved? I should cover all bases, and that bothers me. The body part affected helps me find the cause. I may have to change directions.

I accept↓♥ to be open, and I will feel the knots of tension disappear. I am here to develop. The fact of becoming stiff is causing me all these pains. I live the present instant and I learn to trust.

MUSCLES — MYASTHENIA

Myasthenia is a chronic neurological affection characterized by fatigability in the form of muscular sagging. There is a blocking in the transmission of the nerve impulse to the **muscles**.

Even if I rarely experience such a disease, when it does occur it is because I am experiencing discouragement and lack of motivation and I am 'tired of living'. I feel I will never be able to do what I want or I will never be able to achieve my dreams. I am exhausted: I was under tension for a long time and now, I flinched!

I accept↓♥ to become **Aware** of what is discouraging me to the point of letting myself waste away. Once I have found out why, I can more easily change the situation. If I don't find the exact cause of my conflict, I can still seek sources of motivation that will eventually lead me to find the solution to my conflict.

MUSCLES — MYOPATHY

The general term of **myopathy** concerns all congenital illnesses resulting from an alteration of muscular fibers.

Muscles, from a metaphysical standpoint, are closely related to my mind, to the way I think. I constantly depreciate myself and I have no motivation. I want to prevent a situation from developing or I want to stop all movement in someone or something that is currently part of my life; that's why my **muscles**, which enable me to perform movements and **move about**, will deteriorate. Someone may also want to prevent me from performing a movement or force me to stop. I am anxious because my own incapacity for doing certain things and my lack of strength revolt me. My fear of ***failing*** at my task anguishes me. I work hard to build solid bases in my life and I must be even more tenacious and perseverant. It is by looking at the affected body part and what it prevents me from doing that I will have a good indication of the nature of the thoughts that I must change.

I accept↓♥ to admit it always occurs to widen my field of **Consciousness**, to enable me to experience more **Love**, freedom and wisdom. I give myself permission to fully live my life based on my own values and inner strength.

MUSCLES — MYOSITIS

Myositis is an inflammation of the **muscles** that produces muscular weakness and rigidity, **muscles** being related to effort.

It originates from the stress about the efforts I must produce in view of some physical, intellectual or emotional work, which I don't necessarily feel like doing because it demands lots of energy, but with which I feel 'stuck'. As I feel bound to do it and don't really feel like making an effort, I feel very little motivation. I need calm, solitude and introspection, but that hardly fits with my rather rapid pace of life. It provokes reactions in others who don't understand me. They find me mysterious and enigmatic. It is as though there were a storm around me and I must protect myself against any threats.

I accept↓♥ to take my time, I ask for help or I give myself more time to carry out my tasks in order to allow my **muscles** to rest and restore my energy. I detach myself from the doubts and questionings of the people around me, and I am the Way that suits me and brings me inner peace.

MUSCLES — TETANUS / LOCKJAW *See also: MUSCLES — TRISMUS*

Tetanus is an infectious disease due to the infection of a wound or even to a sting by a bacterium. A person affected by **tetanus** first sees the jaw **muscles** contract very painfully[8]. Respiratory and cardiac **muscles** are affected later.

This shows a great inner irritation provoked by thoughts that are harmful for my well-being. I cling to my old ideas. I live partly in ***darkness***, which is becoming unbearable. Instead of expressing them, I swallow and stifle them inside of me. I think too much and stay in place. I fall back on outer structures and authorities instead of taking my place. At the same time, I refuse life and I refuse to live according to my deeper impulses and passions. I am in a family situation where either I feel I am a burden for the family, or something external to me is a huge burden to me. I question myself about my role as a family provider. I want to stand up to my mother or to my children. I am sure that what I am doing is for the well-being of all, but others may perceive it as selfishness.

I accept↓♥ to allow **Love** to purify me and I make place for harmonization. I take myself in hand. I live from my **heart♥** and I advance with the certainty that everything that happens is for the best.

MUSCLES — TRISMUS *See also: MUSCLES — TETANUS*

Trismus is characterized by the involuntary tightening of the jaws, due to the contraction of the **muscles**. It is often the first sign that I am affected by tetanus.

This situation may occur when I feel aggressive. By refusing to express my feelings, I have a sense of staying in control. I refuse to open up for fear of being judged, rejected or misunderstood. I bite my tongue, regretting certain words spoken or heard. By closing up, I am also closing the door to **Love**. I am filled with sadness. I take care of others rather than take care of myself. I want to look strong to feel worthy, but deep down, I feel small and weak.

I accept↓♥ to trust, to clearly express my desires and make place for **Love**. I dissolve any thoughts of revenge and replace them with forgiveness.

MUSCULAR CRAMPS (in general)

A **cramp** of **muscular** origin indicates that I am **holding in** something that I don't want to let go. It is a great **inner tension** expressing itself by a blockage of **muscular** energy. The muscle itself represents energy, life and strength. I 'block' life by not letting go of these old thoughts that transform themselves in the body as it evolves. I still have some old preconceived principles and I convey them in my everyday actions. I am 'under tension', asking myself a thousand questions. My attention is focused on certain worries that take up

8. This is called spasmodic rigidity.

so much of my energy that I become disconnected from my physical body. It is important to check what body part is affected by the **cramps**.

I accept↓♥ right now to let myself go with my **heart♥**, to open myself more to new possibilities likely to make me advance. I can't change the past but I can change how I interpret events. I am increasingly **Aware** of the beauty present. Meditation and an energy-rebalancing technique will help in releasing these superfluous tensions and better harmonize my energy-based bodies.

MYASTHENIA *See: MUSCLES — MYASTHENIA*

MYCOSIS (between toes) / ATHLETE'S FOOT *See: FEET — MYCOSIS*

MYCOSIS (of scalp, hair, nails) *See: HAIR — TINEA*

MYOCARDITIS *See: HEART♥ — MYOCARDITIS*

MYOMA (uterine) *See: FIBROMAS AND OVARIAN CYSTS*

MYOPATHY *See: MUSCLES — MYOPATHY*

MYOPIA *See: EYES — MYOPIA*

MYOSITIS *See: MUSCLES — MYOSITIS*

N

NAIL(S) (in general)

The **nails** represent the hard tissue and my deepest spiritual energy, my inner strength. I can use them to create my life. I take my time and I don't rush things; this way, I avoid rushing the current of life. This inner strength sustains me. This protection represented by my **nails** is constantly with me. They show me my capacity for being flexible. The **nails** show up on my body at the most 'extended' locations. They may be affected when my activity, my dexterity or my direction tend to change and I have difficulty in facing these changes. They also denote a difficulty in positioning myself in relation to situations or persons. The details of my everyday life can become the focal point of my whole attention. The **nails** thus represent my feeling of **protection** from everything that goes on around me. An **ailment** in my **nails**, an **inflammation** for example, indicates that I am hanging on and that I am having difficulty in letting go. I feel vulnerable. Where is my real power? My **nails** may grow **extremely thick** for I want to protect myself, as a turtle does with its thick shell. I want to arm myself against external dangers and I live in a prison. I want to unsheathe my claws to defend myself. If I am a **woman**, I won't dare defend myself, whereas if I am a **man**, I may hesitate to attack or assert myself. Whoever I am, is it really against others that I must protect myself, or from my own feelings of aggressiveness and self-destruction? I want to close off access to my person for everyone around me in order to protect my vulnerability. If I take excessive care of my **nails**, I must ask myself what image I want to project for others in order to hide a part of me that I find ugly. **Dots** or **white spots** on the **nails** indicate that I have experienced a distressing event. I stifle my frustration for I am afraid of being in action, so I remain passive. I feel the need to defend myself, like a hunted animal. **Damaged nails** are an expression of my feeling of being walled in and feeling almost as though I were buried. **Nails that split up** are a sign of my tendency to want to cling to two places or two persons at once. I am following a road and rules that are harmful for me, but I persist in pushing on. I feel torn inside. I have the choice of using my **nails** either negatively (to attack, to defend myself and to injure, as animals do) or positively, by using them for my dexterity and my creativity. Whatever energy I use, I can discover its state by defining the state of my **nails**.

I accept↓♥ to make peace with this inner strength. I let my resistances go and I stop clinging to others. I can develop this inner solidity only by relying on myself.

NAIL-BITING

If I **bite my nails**, it indicates a very great inner nervousness and the existence of a situation that is eating away at my energy. It may also be a deep-seated insecurity over not being capable of being or doing what is expected of me. If it involves a **child**, it may indicate the presence of resentment or frustration toward a parent, a situation that may also occur after I have become an adult. As a child, I may feel that my family is preventing me from asserting myself and is stifling my creativity. I may feel incapable of taking myself in hand and being self-reliant and I want others to take care of me. I may also be **chafing at the bit** and repressing my aggressiveness; by **watering down my claims**, I can provide an intimation of an imminent overflow of unexpressed emotions. It may be a part of me to which I have taken an aversion. I suppress my need to express my needs, in words as well as sexually, because I am afraid of discovering my true essence. I have difficulty in asserting my autonomy, often with my parents. I no longer want to give or receive any blows. I have the impression I am 'digging my grave'[1].

I accept↓♥ to express all my emotions and seek my security and self-confidence in myself. And so I thrive!

NAILS (ingrown)

It is a **nail**, the lateral edges of which sink into the adjacent soft tissues. It usually affects the big toe.

An **ingrown nail** indicates guilt or nervousness about a new situation. I feel like seeking revenge or opposing someone (often my mother) but I am incapable of doing so. It may also represent a conflict between my mental and spiritual desires. If it is a **fingernail**, it concerns a situation in my everyday life and, more frequently, if it is a **toenail**, it concerns a situation or a decision about the future. In the case of the **big toe**, an **ingrown nail** may embody my concern about some pressure that I believe I must face in the future and about which I already feel guilty, as I fear I won't be able to experience that future harmoniously and successfully. I feel resentful and my guilt leads me to feel I don't have the right to move forward and achieve things. I may also feel regrets over certain decisions I have made. I punish myself with the suffering that an **ingrown nail** causes me. It is important to see which finger or which toe is affected, in order to find more information about the facet of my life to which I must adjust while removing my guilt. The **nail** tends to curl back on itself as I do in my life. I withdraw into my shell and I want to clasp everything close to me. I do want to succeed with my life but I feel incapable of achieving my dreams. Then I tend to be aggressive and frustrated. I believe I must 'do' things to show my worth.

I accept↓♥ to look at all my inner richness, to acknowledge all the strength that inhabits me, and be myself. I no longer need these '**claws**' that continue

1. **Digging one's grave**: To take many useless risks.

to grow all over and that I believed I needed in order to defend and assert myself. Instead of wanting to cling, I should instead go toward others. I move ahead, relying on my inner strength.

NAILS (soft and brittle)

My **nails** represent my vitality, the state of my vital energy. **Brittle nails** express an imbalance in my energy level and in how I use it. **Soft nails** express the lassitude I feel, the indifference that inhabits me. My life is as dull as my **nails.** It is my job to spice it up and to make sure to use my energy well. I become **Aware** that I am living my life halfheartedly, allowing others to decide for me. I am living in shadow, refusing the strengths inside of me. I feel powerless and fragile, like my **nails**. I have difficulty in facing all the emotions inside of me.

I accept↓♥ to take myself in hand! I discover all the strength that is in me. That I am tall and strong and that I can accomplish great things. It depends only on me to be sure of my capacities and to move forward.

NAILS — YELLOW NAIL SYNDROME / XANTHONYCHIA

The **yellow nail syndrome** appears when my **fingernails** or my **toenails** take on a greenish yellow color and become thick and curved. Medically, this takes place when the circulation in my lymphatic system is inadequate, which derives in turn from a chronic respiratory disorder. Because my **nails** are a protection for my fingers and toes, my body is showing me that I must increase my protections because I am feeling fragile and am not facing the events of life (lungs = life) in the small details that occur for me today or tomorrow. I find my life dull.

I accept↓♥ to seek within me what could infuse more passion into my life. I increase my inner vital energy so it will manifest itself to the ends of my fingers.

NARCOLEPSY *See also: COMA, FAINTING, INSOMNIA, SOMNOLENCE*

Narcolepsy is an irresistible tendency to fall asleep[2]. I fall asleep suddenly, for a few seconds to more than an hour. If it is accompanied by diminished muscle tone, also called **catalepsy**, then it is a case of **Gélineau's**[3] **syndrome**.

Sleep becomes a way out from fears and resistances. I say no to development and I refuse to accept↓♥ what is going on in my life. I will therefore **flee** because I no longer feel like seeing or sensing certain persons or situations. Not knowing how to resolve this, and being incapable of asserting myself, I will withdraw into my **sleep**, which is the easiest solution to avoid a danger. I then tend to act as a victim, feeling helpless or thinking that I don't have the necessary tools to face what is scaring me. I refuse to live in reality, which is

---

2. **Narcolepsy** is quite similar to **hypersomnia** (Hyper= in excess and Somnia = sleep). The only difference is that in the latter case, I **choose** to sleep more often and longer.
3. **Gélineau** (Jean-Baptiste Édouard): A French neurologist physician (1828–1906). In 1880, he described the syndrome that bears his name by introducing the term "**Narcolepsy**".

so constraining. I must re-evaluate my life, and I refuse to let go of certain persons or situations.

I accept↓♥ to take myself in hand and forge ahead, even if I must ask a friend or a relative for help, so that I can take action and create my life as I want it to be. I resume contact with my senses, my emotions, my life, with the world around me and with nature. I release my fears and accept↓♥ to live each instant fully **Aware** that everything that happens to me is an experience for my development. I stop fleeing and I appreciate being here and now.

NASTINESS / MEANNESS / MALICE *See also: RIGHT [I AM]*

Nastiness is a morbid desire expressing hate for the purpose of hurting, either with words or through action.

I thus want to prove to myself that I am 'OK' and that 'I am right'. It may originate from great injuries, which leads me to turn my bad temper and my frustration against others. As I resent life or other persons for my suffering, I want to get revenge, believing I will derive some satisfaction from it. It is my way of expressing my aggressiveness externally in order to seek more inner peace. I need change and freedom of action, but at the same time it scares me, and I close myself off. I am therefore experiencing a great inner duality. When I can identify such behavior in myself, I can ask for help in order to feel better with myself. For even if I express my irritability by **nastiness**, I realize that it only relieves my suffering temporarily.

I accept↓♥ that my suffering belongs to me and that instead of seeking vengeance, I will listen to my emotions and their primary source. This is how I can learn the life lessons that I need in order to grow. I can thus develop attitudes of openness and kindness with the people around me and enjoy greater inner peace.

NAUPATHY *See: SEA SICKNESS*

NAUSEA and VOMITING *See also: PREGNANCY DISORDERS*

Nausea is defined as a nervous spasm preceding vomiting. It is an urge to vomit along with a general uneasiness.

I experience a feeling of sadness and I feel pain about a reality that is upsetting my life and that I want to be able to avoid. **Nausea** is a sign that I am feeling **disgust** or that I feel an aversion to something, a person, an idea, a situation, or maybe even an emotion, for I don't feel safe. I am feeling revolt, anger, fear, frustration, or bewilderment over it, and it 'stays on my **stomach**'. I must become **Aware** that I have absorbed something of my reality or my being that creates a desire to express it immediately. And if this is not done through spoken words, it will manifest itself through fits of **nausea**. When it is just too much and resentment is too great, the effect of **vomiting** is triggered, because I tend to manifest physically my rejection of this situation that I find unfair. This rejection may target something external, but it may also involve a part of me that I want to make disappear. When I **vomit**, I am refusing something or someone. I thus avoid advancing and developing. I look at what or whom I am resisting so. It may be one of my parents whom I would like to 'get out of my life' because what we ***used to have*** in common seems to have disappeared. Am I afraid of not being up to dealing with what is in store for me? Why do I refuse what is new? Do I feel forced by others to say or do things? I may feel sick to my stomach when I see how helpless I am to take action or to take control of my life. I may no longer want to have anything to do with this superficial life. If I **vomit bile**, a situation is now intolerable and I have had enough of watering down my needs. Early **pregnancy** is often accompanied by **nausea** and in this condition. I must accept↓♥ the changes that the newborn child's arrival will bring into my life. Am I refusing this child, or is it some part of me (my powerlessness, my insecurities, etc.) that I want to deny? Do I have enough strength to take care of this child? By being the owner of my life, I can pass on the same values to my baby. I ask for peace and I accept↓♥ to digest the emotions and the conflicts that this event produces in my everyday life.

I learn to accept↓♥ each facet of my person. It is the only way to build my life in my own image and to let go of the past. I trust life and the future. I always have my **freedom** of choice. When I do what I like, I no longer have to resist. I welcome all the beautiful things that life wants to give me.

NAVEL / BELLY BUTTON / UMBILICUS *See: UMBILICUS*

NECK (in general)

The **neck** is the part of the body that supports the head. This body-spirit link is also the bridge that enables life to manifest itself and is its living expression, the one that allows the most fundamental movement. It embodies **flexibility**, **suppleness** and **anticipated direction**. It is multidirectional and broadens my external vision of the world. I can see everything around me and with the flexibility of my **neck**. I can view a situation from all angles (front, rear). My point of view becomes more objective. A healthy **neck** enables me to make better decisions. Everything that gives life passes through the **neck**: air, water, food, and blood and nerve circulations. It connects the head and the body and allows free self-expression, the spoken word (voice) and **Love**. The **neck** thus separates the abstract from the concrete, the material from the spiritual. It is important to keep my **neck** healthy, for it enables me to see my surroundings with an open mind, leaving aside any form of stubbornness and narrowness of mind (stiff **neck**). Otherwise, if I force myself to look in one sole direction, trying to stubbornly maintain my view of things at all costs, my **neck** will react and I may not arrive safely at my destination. Standing up to someone and ***defying*** my entourage puts useless pressure on my **neck**. I don't have to '***stick out my neck***' in situations where I am not involved. I am **Aware** that I tend to stand up to others. As my throat is located in my **neck**, if I have any difficulty in swallowing my emotions, if I 'choke them back', this can create a tension in my **neck** where the energy center for communication is located. As the **neck** represents conception, it also represents my feeling of belonging, my right to be on this earth, and it thus gives me a feeling of security and fullness.

NECK (stiff) *See also: SPINE (IN GENERAL) — NECK*

The **nape** of the **neck** is the region of my body through which all energies (waves) must pass to spread throughout my whole body. The **nape** of the **neck** is at the top of my spine. The spine is my body's structural support.

The **nape** of my **neck** is thus the pivot of my head. It enables me to consider all the facets of a situation. If it is supple, I can be completely open to the world that surrounds me and face its requirements. It corresponds to my self-confidence. If I am afraid of suffering a mishap, the **nape** of my **neck** will be affected. If I suffer or see an injustice, the **nape** of my **neck** will react likewise. I may find myself at a moment in my life when I 'don't know which way to turn'. There are many surprises and unexpected incidents (often in the family), and I tend to act the martyr. A **stiff neck** is a clear sign of a refusal or a congestion of energy. The head can no longer turn in different directions. I may feel I am lacking support and I tend to be stubborn and rigid in my way of thinking and to have my way. This leads me to be passive, trying to avoid moving forward and taking action. I must give free rein to these various thoughts that block my head and that only want to be carried out by my physical body. I feel I don't have all the qualities needed for achieving my desires and my ideas, which risk remaining at the stage of 'projects' or impracticable dreams. If the **nape** of my **neck**, as a pivot, rests on values and principles external to me, it will be rather weak. The **nape** of my **neck** enables my head to survey different life options or landscapes that lie before me. I must look lovingly at these different landscapes, without criticizing them, quite freely, as a river allows its water to flow through it in a perpetual to-and-fro rhythm, with no constraints or restrictions.

I accept↓♥ the different sensations that come to me and I let them flow freely. I also accept↓♥ all the riches that I have inside of me; I no longer have to worry about what others think of me, for I am now fully **conscious** of the extensive potential that inhabits me.

NECK — TORTICOLLIS / STIFF NECK *See also: BACK DISORDERS — UPPER BACK, NECK [STIFF]*

When I have a **torticollis**, there is a contraction of the **neck** muscles that causes a more or less pronounced pain and limits the **neck**'s rotation movements.

A **torticollis** shows that I am feeling insecure. **I resist viewing from all angles the situations I experience**. My **neck** muscles contract, my **neck** stiffens and I can no longer turn my head. My inflexibility prevents me from enjoying the help that people offer me and that would enable me to get some things that seem difficult for me moving in the right direction. I prefer to hold my head straight and associate my pain with a 'sudden chill'. It is in my best interest to become **Aware** that this 'chill' affected my **heart♥** instead, thus provoking a blocking of energy. I may also be trying to **flee** an uncomfortable situation that requires me to assert myself and stake a position. I may also feel powerless to live with it. I want to move forward, but I also want to back off, because I see an obstacle ahead that scares me. I am experiencing a great inner annoyance. I rely more on others than on myself, which leads me to have a rigid and stubborn attitude. It is also important to stop and notice the direction in which I refuse to look or the thing that I obstinately persist in seeing, saying or doing and that 'suits me quite well'. Am I turning away from my personal goals and values? I am afraid of seeing the truth head-on and taking my responsibilities. I find myself in a situation where I have a choice to make, but it seems impossible. The moral torture tied to it is indefinable. Is it possible for there to be a person, a thing or a situation that I would want to look at, and at the same time not want to look at because of my timidity, my shame or my moral sense that is very strong? If stiffness prevents my head from turning from **left to tight**, I may ask myself to whom or to what I am refusing to say no. If on the contrary I have **difficulty in nodding yes** with my head, maybe it is because I reject new ideas right off.

My body tells me to accept↓♥ to see and enjoy this instant and recognize all the new things that are part of my life. I accept↓♥ to learn a new way of seeing things or new ideas; my life improves and my **torticollis** vanishes.

NEEDS (in general) *See: DEPENDENCE*

NEPHRITIS *See: KIDNEYS — NEPHRITIS*

NEPHRITIS (chronic) *See: BRIGHT'S DISEASE*

NEPHROPATHY *See: KIDNEYS — NEPHRITIS*

NERVE (optic) *See: NERVES — NEVRITIS*

NERVE (sciatic) *See also: PAIN, BACK DISORDERS — LOWER BACK, LEGS / (IN GENERAL) / AILMENTS*

The **sciatic nerve** starts in the lumbar part (lower back) of the spine; it goes through the buttock, the thigh and the leg and extends down to the foot.

The pain I feel paralyzes me. The pain may act more intensely in one leg than in the other. I may be financially worried at that time because I am going through an important transition in my life that makes me experience great insecurity. If my **right leg** is involved, it may be because I am afraid of lacking funds and being unable to face my responsibilities in what lies ahead for me. I may also feel I am 'losing support', especially if this follows a betrayal. I feel compelled to go in one direction even if I don't feel like it. If the pain is located in my **left leg**, my lack of money may intensify my feeling of being unable to give everything to fill the material needs of the people I **love**. So there are some things that I want to do, but cannot. I fear that their **Love** for me will be affected by this. I delude myself, believing that I am very spiritually motivated and detached from worldly goods (a sort of hypocrisy). However, **the fear of being short of money** pursues me and makes me very **anxious**. I work very hard, carry great responsibilities and despite all my efforts, I still have some financial problems. My body stiffens: I feel **stuck**. It is as though I were gripped by the throat, helpless in a situation, with the impression that somebody else has power over this situation and not I. I feel confined in my freedom and my creativity. I constantly call myself into question. What am I not doing? Do I have the necessary knowledge and talent for facing a new situation? My **insecurity** leads me to **revolt** and to resent life. I come to develop a feeling of inferiority. I may refuse to 'give in' to a person or a situation. Insidiously, aggressiveness sets in and my communications with others suffer from it. Anger boils up inside of me. I feel like ***stopping*** everything! I had better **calm my nerves**, because right now, I have the impression that my **nerves are all in knots**. I become **Aware** of my inner **confusion** and pain (internal as well as external) about the directions of my life in the here and now. This pain often results from my stubbornness in wanting to hold on to my old ideas instead of opening myself up to change and new perspectives. I am concerned with the welfare and happiness of the people around me, but to the detriment of my own happiness. This situation is frequent in pregnant women, who experience inner confusion and pain concerning the direction their lives are now taking: and so doubts, fears and worries may surface. Do I feel supported enough in the new responsibilities I will now be taking on? How can I decide who or what I should want to get closer to, or on the contrary get away from, as either option could bring many changes into my life? I become **Aware** that I have imprisoned myself in a vise to avoid being happy and developing my full potential. I avoid living from my essential being, from my authentic self. I push aside my whole intuitive, impulsive and creative side. I prevent myself from moving faster because of my fears. I seek security outside of me and in material, artificial things. I don't need to judge myself, but to accept↓♥ myself as I am.

I accept↓♥ that **the source of my true security is in me** and not in my possessions. I let go and I trust in the Universe, for it holds abundance for all and at all levels: physical, mental and spiritual. By trusting the Universe, I am trusting life. I choose to accept↓♥ flexibility, I discover true wealth: the one I have inside of me. The true worth of a human being is measured by his, or her, magnanimity. I accept↓♥ my limits, I become **Aware** of my fears and integrate them. I decide to advance in life and I let myself be safely guided for my greater good.

NERVES (in general)

The **nerves** are organs that receive and send information throughout the body, originating from feelings, thoughts and the senses. Conscious activities are controlled by the peripheral **nerves** that have their source in the spine, which is the 'home base' of the nervous system. Unconscious activities, such as **heart♥**beat or respiration, are controlled by the autonomic nervous system.

Through meditation or deep relaxation, I can achieve conscious control over this system. I may be affected in several ways because the nervous system covers several functional activities. The **nerves** are like my body's electrical system. If my circuits are overloaded because there is too much tension, this affects my organism's functioning. This tension may derive from the fact that I have concerns about the future, and also from my fear that some of the projects I want to carry out may not be completed. This **tension in my nerves** reveals my inner state: I feel in **detention** (prison) with respect to a person, a situation or simply myself. If the **sensory nerves** are affected (those leading from the sense organs), I want to desensitize myself from something or someone. If it is my **motor nerves** (reaching into the muscles), I am having difficulty in performing certain movements. The **nerves** are therefore at the basis of **communication** and if they don't function adequately, I can ask myself in what sphere of my life I had better communicate and receive what others have to say. If my **nerves are in knots** or my **nerves are on edge**, it reminds me of my great sensitivity and, though I may have felt hurt in the past, I accept↓♥ to learn to trust others and life.

NERVES — NEURALGIA *See also: PAIN*

Neuralgia can be defined as a faulty contact on the course of an electrical wire. Electrical wires represent all our **nerves**. It is an acute pain in a **nerve**, caused by an excessively high tension along its course.

If the **nerve** is cut off, it is because the free communication or circulation of energy in me is interrupted. There is a separation, a spacing apart. A 'chill' has set in between me and another person. A degree of animosity, along with aggressiveness and resentment, prevents me from coming into contact with that person. My thoughts are irritating and burning. I feel that "my **nerves** are going to crack". The location of the pain points to the sort of emotion involved. A feeling of guilt and the desire to always remain within society's set norms will often be the source of a spell of **neuralgia**. I fear authority. If **neuralgia** is located in an **arm** or a **hand**, this indicates that a pressure (such as an engagement) or another emotion (such as helplessness) is preventing me from taking a harmonious decision or direction in my life. If the **neuralgia** is in a **leg**, a **calf** or a **foot**, the emotion is blocking a further step in a new direction, and therefore the free circulation of energies in my life. **Facial neuralgia** shows me that my face is 'frozen hard', and I hide my emotions to protect myself. I may also constantly have something right in front of my face that reminds me of a painful event in my life. **Dental neuralgia** shows me that giving in to others leads me to revolt. I become indifferent in order to avoid having to make decisions.

I accept↓♥ to become **Aware** of my inner emotions that prevent a natural flow. In what situation do I feel stuck? What behavior or habit am I trying to get rid of? By becoming **Aware** (from the body part affected) of the aspect of my life that is affected by anxiety or insecurity, I can remediate it more easily and find the solutions and all the **Love** that the situation asks of me. I let go of this prison that I built myself so that I can fly with my own wings. I allow each of my inner emotions to flow so that I can accept↓♥ them, integrate them and change them positively. I thus remain in perpetual contact with my divine essence and I can then accomplish great things!

NERVES — NEVRITIS

Nevritis is the inflammation of one or several **nerves**.

The part of my body that is affected by the **nerves** involved indicates what aspect of my life I must become **Aware** of. Even if the **nevritis** may appear to have its source in an infection, alcoholism, in certain illnesses or in the secondary effects of certain medications, it is desirable for me to find out what is making me experience anger in my communications with myself. I also refuse others in what they are and do. I feel under attack and want to defend myself. I detest the ***unexpected***, which is why I try to ***anticipate*** everything, giving myself a false sense of control. I prefer to live ***anonymously***. This way, others don't see me and I avoid criticism.

I accept↓♥ to resume this inner communication by giving myself the understanding I need. I thus find more peace in my life and in my body. I live in truth, transparency and with an open **heart♥**.

NERVOUSNESS

Nervousness is a sign indicating that I lack trust in myself, in my entourage and in the future. Wanting to do things too fast or talking very fast betrays my **nervousness**. I am afraid of "not getting there". I want to assert myself, charge ahead and get there first, but as I never felt supported or encouraged when I was younger, it pursues me today, and any situation that brings up something new or unfamiliar triggers this **nervousness**. When I am **nervous**, I lose this connection with my inner self. I become irritable and unstable.

I accept↓♥ to trust life and know that I don't need to control everything perfectly for life to be beautiful and loving. I become **Aware** that my **nervousness** hides instability, the fear of an event I dread or a fear of losing someone or something dear to me. I must thus get free of this, while trusting my inner self and relaxing regularly.

NEURALGIA *See: NERVES — NEURALGIA*

NEURASTHENIA *See also: BURNOUT, DEPRESSION, FATIGUE (IN GENERAL)*

Neurasthenia, or **nervous exhaustion**, is a state of extreme physical and psychological fatigability. Its symptoms take the form of a difficulty in making decisions and confusion. Though I present no organic disorder, I may experience difficulty in digesting, physical pains, extreme emotionality and great weakness. **Neurasthenia** resembles **depression** on several points. I will tend to withdraw into solitude and mope about.

I don't want to make an effort, for I tell myself that it won't change anything. It is my negative attitude that produces this illness. I feel myself in a deadlock. I want to excel and stand out, but I seem to ruin my chances of advancement every time, and I get discouraged.

I accept↓♥ that instead of focusing my attention on "everything that is not going right in my life", I should instead give ***Thanks*** for what I do have. I must take myself in charge, set up projects and accept↓♥ the fact that I have all the potential, the perseverance and the courage I need to reach all the goals I set for myself. Joy and happiness can then take far more space in my life.

NEURITIS *See: NERVES — NEURITIS*

NEUROPATHY *See: SYSTEM [NERVOUS]*

NEUROSIS *See also: ANGUISH, HYSTERIA, OBSESSION*

A **neurosis** is a nervous affection characterized by psychological conflicts, which determine behavioral disorders but alters only very slightly the personality of the person affected.

Like depression and psychosis, a **neurosis** is caused by uncontrolled emotions or by the quest for an identity to replace the one I refuse. Even if I remain in contact with reality and go on living in society, I may have a feeling of anxiety, my judgment may be altered and my sexual life may suffer from it in the form of impotence or frigidity. I feel alone, with nobody to support me. I feel empty, disconnected from my emotions. I refuse to feel pleasure. I prevent myself from truly living and at the same time, death scares me. I may develop dependencies, for I need an escape valve to release everything I am resisting. The inner struggle is constant and exhausting. If I repress a part of me, I must balance it with behavior that may be obsessive. I am annoyed because many people, including some in authority, disagree with my way of doing and thinking.

I accept↓♥ to take back my rightful place and to need people to give me attention in order to feel worthy. I also need to find a meaning in life, which will enable me to free myself from the tensions I experience. I will be free, as I will focus my attention on my goal, my source of happiness and satisfaction. I must thus accept↓♥ my deep nature, which is to **love** others and **love** myself without having to understand life from A to Z to accept↓♥ myself as I am.

NEVUS / MOLE *See: SKIN — MELANOMA [MALIGNANT]*

NODULES

A **nodule** is a well-delimited, almost spherical and palpable cutaneous or mucous lesion that can lodge at various depths in the skin (dermis, epidermis or hypodermis). It is commonly found on the vocal cords or in the ear.

This **nodule** helps me to become **Aware** that I feel disappointed and resentful about a project I was unable to complete because I met a major obstacle that forced me away from my goal or did not allow me to reach it. This may be work-related as well as emotional. My communication (vocal cords) may be involved; I wanted to say certain things but didn't dare say them, or I feel that I spoke too much and "put my foot in my mouth". It may also be something I heard (a **nodule** in an ear) that bothered me to the point of "stopping the construction in its tracks". The important thing is to decide that everything happens in good time. I check to see if the rigidity I show in my life can be the cause of my inner malaise. If I go too hard on myself, one day I will feel like revolting. I sometimes feel that the expectations of others toward me are practically unrealistic and I must be someone else to survive in this world. A **nodule** usually appears at a place on my body where I don't want to be touched, for the fact of being touched by someone (even someone I **love** or trust, a physician for instance) reminds me of my first shock, a painful event. My feeling of insecurity may have been intensified then. I may have met with a refusal, which was very hard to take. I don't receive the recognition I crave, and I doubt my creative powers.

I accept↓♥ what slowed down my rush in order to overcome it. The main thing is to reach the goal I have set, whatever pitfalls and delays appear along my way. I will be all the more proud and happy with myself. I let my facade drop and I learn to be myself. I decide the projects that are close to my **heart♥** and important for me and not only for others. By reclaiming my place, I will be able to express my needs and I will have all the energy and strength I need to achieve all my goals.

NOSE (in general) *See also: BODY ODOR*

The **nose** refers to human instinct, especially involving survival. As it enables me to smell, it also helps me to sense what is going on inside and outside of me. If I have a **sharply sensitive nose**, it becomes my helm. It detects what I have to do in my life; it is thus constantly seeking. My **nose** shows me how I take my life in hand, if I am in control of my life and destiny. The **nose** is the organ through which air (life) reaches my lungs. Air is very important. We breathe through our two **nostrils**, but can also breathe through the mouth. A breathing difficulty can inform me about the difficulties I have in my life. If I refuse to live or have difficulty in dealing with my entourage because what I smell or feel doesn't suit me, my capacity to breathe through the **nose** will be impaired. It is as though I tried to expel a conflicted situation through my **nose**. Do I feel I am being 'led by the **nose**'? If the **left nostril** is causing me a problem, I must seek the message on the emotional or affective side, for that is where my emotions enter, whereas the **right nostril** informs me of a rational difficulty, for that is where understanding and analysis enter. A danger to be sensed will block my **left nostril**, and a danger to be deciphered will affect the **right nostril**. As with animals, the **nose** senses danger and predators; smell enables me to detect prey or, on the contrary, my own scent will cause me to be detected by others. Smell, sensing, danger and survival are thus related to **nose** ailments. I can sniff out a bad deal or a danger, sense that a plot is afoot or that something is being hidden from me. Anxiety therefore results from this situation involving an intruder. In any case, I may even have to hark back to the moment of my birth to discover the source of my **nose** ailment. If I had to undergo a **nose** operation to allow me to breathe better, it was like saying yes to my intuition, to my sensing, to life.

I accept↓♥ to take an open and self-confident attitude. I can thus heal any **nose** ailment.

NOSE AILMENTS

The **nose** is the organ of smell. It is the sense that enables me to live and be in contact with the atmosphere, the outside world. Smell is one of the most powerful senses I have and it is related to my first energy center (chakra) located at the level of the coccyx. The **nose** is the double opening on life! The right and left nostrils are the channels of the interior and the exterior. If my body sets up a barrier in my breathing channel, it is to indicate to me that I am isolating myself from someone around me or from a situation that affects or bothers me or that I don't accept↓♥. I want to cut myself off from something that can affect my secret and intimate side, involving my thoughts or my physical or emotional self. "I find it stinks!" Or it may be a person whom I don't consider 'in good odor'. This person I can't stand may simply be me (or certain features of my personality that I reject)! I may thus come to lose my **olfactory faculty**. This leads to melancholy and sadness, for I am thus cut off from scents that I like. I want my intimacy to be respected. However, I must ask myself whether I don't "stick my own **nose** into other people's affairs", whether I myself am '**nosing** everywhere'. It may be a person or a situation that I criticize, that I judge as 'stinking' and about which I may feel resentment and even disgust. I 'smell' a situation coming, there is an event being plotted that I am afraid to confront. I am experiencing a situation where something or someone will emerge, and this makes me feel uneasy inside. I have difficulty in feeling the closeness of a person. My inner peace is troubled by an intrusive presence that I want to move away from me. It may be at the sexual level, where I find it difficult to spot a 'predator' or a 'prey', as the case may be. It may also be a scent that I don't like, maybe because it reminds me of an event that I would rather forget, and that I describe as foul. My sense of smell is closely related to my holographic (three-dimensional) memory of events. My sense of smell makes it very easy for me to recall pleasant, as well as unpleasant, events. When I can no longer smell, I want to cut off information before it reaches my brain, to no longer be in contact with a situation that can awaken anger in me. Therefore, any painful memory involving a specific scent may cause an ailment in my **nose**. It may be a nauseating odor, but can also be the pleasant scent of a person from whom I had to separate and that still affects me today. When my **nose is blocked**, I can no longer taste food. I must therefore ask myself whether I still feel like living or what, in my life, is leaving me with a 'bitter taste'. With my **nose blocked**, I may wish unconsciously to not recall certain events I experienced, in order to avoid re-living the painful emotions of my past. I may want to resist someone or a situation. I force too much, instead of listening to what my inner voice tells me to do. I have the impression that I am being 'led by the **nose**'. As my **nose** is directly related to my intuitive and emotional side, I must ask myself whether I have become closed to my intuitions and perceptions. It is as though I drew a veil over my emotions and feelings. I allow my biases to lock me into a limited framework instead of remaining open to new possibilities. By «blocking» my respiration, I «block» my understanding, which may very well suit me. If I felt hurt, I may cut myself off from one part of myself and I may then tend to see more value in the external and superficial side of things. I may become arrogant, stubborn and tend to mock others, simply because I have cut myself off from my wisdom, from my intuitive side. I smother my aggressiveness and my frustration. I want to change my life completely, but I don't express my deepest feelings. Thus, a **dry nose** indicates that I can't openly express my **Love**. If I **fracture my nose**, am I afraid that a separation may occur, either my parents or other members of the family? If I **break my nose**, there is someone I want to expel from my life. I may also want too much to outdo my father and show him that I have succeeded. My lack of understanding for him can lead me to regret having him as a father. My fear of failing is great. I didn't see an aggressor approach me, and I was thus unable to defend myself. A **deviation of the nasal septum** indicates that my life is badly partitioned and that I tend to get everything muddled up (especially my work and my affective life).

I accept↓♥ this state of restriction in my breathing to free others from their decisions, which it is not for me to judge or criticize. I therefore stop judging people and situations, their choices and their decisions, as I free myself of my own choices and decisions. This allows life to flow freely in me and allows **Love** to grow. I fully accept↓♥ who I am and all the experiences I have been through. With my new understanding of events that were difficult for me, I accept↓♥ that they form a part of my history, and I can start breathing freely again.

NOSE BLEEDING

As the **nose** is the organ channeling air to my lungs, and blood is the transporter of air and oxygen throughout my organism, **nose bleeding** (**epistaxis**) shows me that I am allowing joy and the **Love** of life to escape out of my body, outside of my being. **I therefore have a loss of joy about something that I feel**. This certainly indicates a great disappointment in my life. I feel I have been emptied of all my blood and all my joy in living. I have a feeling that tells me that that I am not recognized, accepted↓♥ or loved at my true worth. I play the victim and tend to distance myself from others. I feel locked in and rushed by the things to be done. The fact that blood is dripping like this from my **nose** attracts the attention of others. If I am a **child**, I find it difficult to take my place in front of the person who represents authority for me. I always seek that person's approval.

I accept↓♥ to learn to acknowledge and **love** myself, and therefore to understand that I owe my happiness only to what I think of myself. An age-old belief tells me that a bad emotion or situation is now going out of my life.

NOSE CONGESTION *See: CONGESTION*

NOSE — KILLIAN'S POLYP *See also: TUMORS*

Killian's polyp[4] is a benign tumor that develops in a sinus or in the corresponding nasal cavity and has the effect of obstructing the affected side more or less completely.

As with tumors in general, I had an emotional shock over what I felt. The pain makes me withdraw and leads me to feel anew some situations that could affect me. I locate the **polyp**, this ball of flesh, and I can find out what may have disturbed me, on the left side, with the affective and emotional element, or on the right side, with the rational or responsibility-related element.

If I must have the **polyp** removed, I thank my body for the information it gave me and I accept↓♥ in my **heart♥** the coming into **Awareness** I had to achieve.

NOSE RUNNING DOWN THE THROAT

Any liquid in my body represents an aspect of my emotions. If **my nose is running down my throat** instead of the liquid flowing out of my body, this indicates that I 'swallow back' my emotions or my tears. I tend to huddle up in myself and to 'weep on my sad fate'. I am attached to something or someone. There is an overflow of tears that want to run, but I have difficulty in letting them go: I want to show that I am very strong and in control, but the reality is quite different. My sensitivity is always present and if I repress it, sooner or later it must express itself. I have such a need to be taken care of! What I show others is all the opposite of what I experience inside of me, and I thus cut myself off from the world around me.

It is important for me to take charge of myself and to do things for myself, in order to renew my taste for living and accomplish my mission. I must be true with my entourage. I fully accept↓♥ my emotions. I start taking care of myself again if I want others to give me their human warmth.

NOSE — SINUSITIS

When I am affected by **sinusitis**, I experience a blocked **nose** involving the facial **sinuses**.

This infection of the **sinuses** is related to helplessness in front of a person or a situation: **I can't stand her** or **I am doing a slow burn**. I imagine the sensation of having strong mustard in my **nose**, choking me and burning. I

---

4. **Killian** (Gustav): A German otorhinolaryngologist (1860–1921). He practiced in Berlin and then in the United States, where he invented bronchoscopy in 1897 and esophagoscopy in 1898.

can also sense a danger or a threat that raises fear in me. Whether the danger is real or imaginary, the result will be the same. "It smells vile to me". The truth is hidden or twisted, and that makes me uncomfortable. Am I in a situation where I feel there is no way out, that I am boxed in? Do I desire to have a child but have the impression that it is impossible, or do I already have a child but would want to be closer to it, ***united*** with it? I may have the impression that "something doesn't smell right", that "something fishy is going on" or that people are doing things ***behind my back***. I resist what nourishes me, for I refuse to let air enter into my ***nose***. My creativity will also be very low and I will tend to work more rationally. I am feeling very irritated because I feel limited, with no room to maneuver. I feel forced, compressed, "squeezed like a lemon" in my vital space (**maxillary sinuses**) as well as in time (**frontal sinuses**). I find myself in a situation where a hierarchy prevails: as I feel subjugated and receive less information than if I were among the decision-makers, I feel I am sensing and testing the wind without really grasping all the elements of each situation. As I don't understand everything, I can sense some things, but I get no confirmation of what I feel, which bothers me a lot. Instead of listening to my inner voice, I allow my old thought patterns to dictate my behavior. I then repress my emotions of anxiety and my fear of not being loved. I feel caught in a stranglehold. My powerlessness leads me to hide myself in illusion and revolt. I feel I have ruined my life. **Sinusitis** 'explodes' when I can't stand it any longer and I am ready to explode emotionally. I can no longer live in the safety of the rigidly organized life I have created for myself. I can no longer stand living by depending on others whom I use as 'life preservers'. I need new ***reference points*** and to assert my authority. The message I must understand is that I must feel **Love** around me and inspire it deep inside of me.

I accept↓♥ to talk about myself. I no longer need to constantly seek compromises. I trust my inner voice to know what is good for me. I let gentleness take place in my life. I trust myself and at last, I can see the **Light**!

NOSE – SNEEZING *See: SNEEZING*

NOSE – SNORING *See: SNORING*

NOSTALGIA *See also: MELANCHOLY*

Nostalgia is melancholy caused by regret.

When I am **nostalgic**, it usually means that I look through a confused cloud of emotions, outside of the present time, with the feeling that I am missing something. It is a form of daydreaming. This 'dream' must not become a regular escape from the present moment. I cling to the 'good old memories of the past' to help me 'weather the storm'. By clinging to the past, I can no longer see anything beautiful that may be in store for me. My optimism and my spontaneity go away. I can't enjoy the 'here and now', and I allow countless opportunities for meeting new persons or trying new experiences to slip by.

Nostalgia can easily transform itself into negativism, and my friends may then move away from me. This **nostalgia** may not harm me, provided that I experience it only occasionally and without exaggeration.

I accept↓♥ to fully savor the present moment so that each second that passes can be enjoyed as a unique experience from which much can be learned.

NUMBNESS — TORPOR / TORPIDITY

Numbness is characterized by a limb that is insensible, heavy, tingling and that often cannot move.

Physical **numbness** is the reflection of my mental **numbness**. I suffer, I am injured. I am in such pain that I have decided to no longer feel, to no longer let the energy flow. **I dull my feelings**. I withdraw because a part of me is injured and I no longer want to feel it. I therefore make myself less sensitive. I become inactive about what goes on around me and inside of me. I am afraid of being harmed. It is a partial 'death' intended to avoid suffering. These injuries have often been present since childhood, have become aggravated over the years, and I carry them as a burden. I have not learned to **love** myself and I have closed myself off from **Love**, instead of sharing this **Love** and my compassion. It is a form or escape. It may represent for me an inner coldness, a desire to hold back **Love**, a lack of dynamism. As I feel I have no power over myself, I tend to want to control others and hold them back. It often happens that over the years, the dreams and ambitions of my youth disappear, or rather that I choose to '**dull**' them, having lost any hope of ever achieving them. I place myself in a situation of lethargy. Nevertheless, they are still present, and if I am in a period of raising questions, these dreams may come back to haunt me because they were never achieved, and even unconsciously, I don't want to come into contact with them again in order to avoid re-living the pain of having had to give them up. The **numbness** only wants to remind me that these dreams are still alive, and that it is still time to achieve them to give a new meaning to my life. The body part affected and the side affected (left or right) enable me to identify the location of my injury.

I now accept↓♥ to rediscover my spontaneity about life, that I must **awaken** in me more **Love**, dynamism and enthusiasm about the aspect of my life that is involved. I will thus increase my quality of life in this world, which is my right. I accept↓♥, here and now, to learn to **love** myself more and truly open myself to **Love**, instead of **holding back** this **Love** and my compassion. I raise the barrier that I had installed for so long. The more I learn to **love** myself, the more I realize that there is a return: I receive **Love** and friendship. This serenity I had sought for so long on the outside is now bursting out of me, and I communicate it to others.

NYSTAGMUS *See: EYES — NYSTAGMUS*

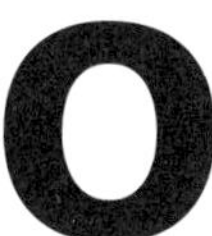

OBESITY *See: WEIGHT [EXCESS]*

OBSESSION

Obsession is an illness of the mind. When I am **obsessed** by something or someone, all my attention and energy is focused on that subject. These ideas are repetitive and threatening, but I remain **Aware** of their irrational nature. Nothing else matters.

If I have an **obsessive personality**, chances are high that I am a person full of doubt, who has great difficulty in making decisions, and that I experience a **Love**-hate ambiguity about myself and others. The **obsessions** can take on very different forms: it may be a phobia about something or someone, it may be mental ruminations about "what might happen if…", the madness of doubt, or a compulsion to commit certain acts that may be innocuous, but may also be criminal or even suicidal, but are then practically never acted upon. Most of the time, I have an anxious fear of 'something that could happen' through negligence or a personal misdeed and that must be avoided. My priority is to maintain my **obsession**, albeit unconsciously. My thought system is paralyzed. I am nourished by the object of my **obsession**. I thus fill an inner void and a great insecurity. For me to experience an **obsession**, I must be feeling a sort of inner tension and concern; at that point, it might be time for me to find a focus of interest in my life that could provide me with more calm and inner peace. I can thus better enjoy whatever life brings me. If I am an **obsessed** person, I judge and criticize myself very severely. I panic at the idea of what may happen in the future, but my fear is often unfounded. This anguish prevents me from fully living my life and developing. I force myself to remain in my comfort zone and I hesitate to undertake projects and have dreams, for I have decided in advance that something negative will occur that will prevent them from materializing. I know that I have reached a stage in my life when I must let go of things or persons that no longer suit me. I must let go of what is negative for me, but I hang on to them for fear of the unknown.

Today I decide to take charge of my life. I look objectively at all the good things that have happened to me and I accept↓♥ that life only wants what is best for me. I deserve it and I trust myself. By freeing myself of what has no place in my life, I get ever closer to my divine essence. I thus reconnect with my inner power and security. I no longer need to be **obsessed**; I need only trust my inner voice that always guides me toward what is good for me.

ODOR (body) and SWEATING *See also: NOSE*

In general, all the fluids contained in the human body represent my emotions. In this case, an **unpleasant body odor** is the sign that harmful emotions are overflowing and that I must express them instead of holding everything inside of me. It may be irritability, dissatisfaction, hate, frustration, resentment or disgust about a person or a situation. I am very sensitive about the gossip and criticism directed against me. It may also be the sign of a loosening or an intense emotion related to the body part where sweating occurs. If I have little self-confidence and I also fear criticism and rejection, my **body odor** risks being unpleasant. As this situation makes people retreat from me, I can ask myself what reason I may have to want to keep them at a distance. Persons with a **pleasant body odor** generally have good thoughts and are in harmony with their entourage. I may be a person who received a life with a high spiritual mission and I may die 'in good **odor**'. People may then actually smell a flower-like scent emanating from the corpse. Similarly, if I am reading spiritual texts, or if I am in a state of meditation or contemplation, or if I feel in a very happy state, I may then give off a scent such as that of a carnation, a rose, sandalwood or various other aromas. Other persons may or may not smell the scent I give off. Though it is rare, I may be a person who is able to sense illnesses and even feelings in another person. Some old country doctors used to say that they had to 'smell the humors'. Thus, each illness had a special **odor**, just as illnesses have a special color in the magnetic field called the *aura*. If there is **abundant sweating**, it is the sign that I am feeling much inner nervousness and insecurity or having great anxieties. I allow everything that I repress and that remains imprisoned inside of me to come out through the pores of my skin. It is often anger and shame. I am unsure of the road to take in my life. I am on the defensive, as I am afraid of being hurt or trapped if I express my emotions, especially in public. However, I am becoming **Aware** that I am actually the one I want to protect myself against: I repress my emotions so much that they want to re-surface, and that is what I want to avoid. I distrust others, when I am the one I actually distrust. With the water coming out of my skin, I want to 'wash' a situation where I felt separated from others and experienced a feeling of smearing and injustice. I break out in **cold sweat** when I am paralyzed by fear and experience great difficulty in my relations with my entourage.

I accept↓♥ to assert myself and express my positive and negative feelings in order to free myself and make place for something new, and allow thoughts of **Love** to nourish me. Around me, I have only people who wish me well. I eliminate my only enemy, myself, by loving myself more and becoming **Aware** of all the possibilities in me.

OLFACTION *See: NOSE*

OPIUM (consumption of) *See: DRUGS*

OPPRESSION

When I feel **oppressed**, I sense a weight on my chest, at the level of my lungs. I may also feel I am smothering.

It may be my emotions overwhelming me, my concerns weighing heavily or my revolt rumbling. I may feel overwhelmed by the authority and the 'power' by which I feel abused. Faced with a person or a situation, I may feel the **pressure** from a deep inner insecurity that urges me to resolve the situation as quickly as possible. I fear criticism and I lock myself into a certain way of doing things in order to go unnoticed and not make waves.

I accept↓♥ to reclaim the power that is rightfully mine. I become **Aware** of the freedom I have. I release my negative feelings to make place for calm and **Love**.

OPPRESSION (pulmonary)

This state shows the presence of an imbalance between my inner pressure and the external pressure. **It is a very strong feeling that is blocking the free circulation of life in me**. I must therefore become **Aware** of it and ask myself if this strong pressure is coming from inside of me and what, in this probably very basic feeling, is preventing me from breathing regularly and deeply. Something is burning me; it is as though my lungs were overheating. This sensation is amplified by my uncertainties and my insecurities.

I accept↓♥ to let go, to not force myself to be this way or that, or to do so many things. To help me dissipate this pressure, I inhale the **Light** that clarifies and the **Love** that purifies these emotions, which will thus be balanced.

ORAL / BUCCAL HERPES *See: HERPES (IN GENERAL)*

ORCHITIS *See: TESTICLES (IN GENERAL)*

ORGANS (genital) *See: GENITAL ORGANS (IN GENERAL)*

-OSIS (disease names ending in -osis) *See: APPENDIX IV*

OTITIS *See: EARS — OTITIS*

OUTGROWTHS / EXCRESCENCES *See: Polyps*

OVARIES (in general) *See also: FEMALE DISORDERS*

The **ovaries** represent my desire to give birth to children and also my creativity, my ability to create, my femininity, the fact that I am a woman and that I am fulfilled or satisfied as a woman.

OVARIES (disorders of the)

Ovarian problems indicate a deep conflict involving the fact of being a woman, the expression of my femininity, or the fact of being a mother. I may have neglected the creative side that I have in me. It is as though I were cutting myself off from a part of myself, for the **ovaries** are the starting point in the creation of life and they are located in the pelvis, which is the region where I can give birth to a child, but also to new aspects of myself, where I can rediscover myself. I may therefore have an inner conflict involving the creation and discovery of my own path. Rather than be myself, I prefer to play a role that protects me from dangers. As I have locked in all my potential, I have also locked in my creativity. I feel tied up by the others, but I am the one putting on my own handcuffs. I feel under the spell of ***fatality***. I may want to compensate by overproducing ova. An **ovarian cyst**, which is an abnormal collection of fluid in an **ovary**, shows that emotions have accumulated, and I am constantly brooding over the same thoughts or troubles. Am I experiencing an internal conflict over becoming a mother? What is the reason that makes me hold back from having a child? Have I recently witnessed an event that may remind me of a traumatic sexual experience? If I do not feel worthy of having children, I may **stop producing ova**. A **cancer of the ovaries** can develop following an event where I experienced the *LOSS* of a person dear to me. I feel that my life or the life of someone I **love** was ***ruined*** or is ***in distress***. The corresponding disease of a **cancer of the ovaries** for a man is a **cancer of the testicles**. It happens quite often that it is one of my children who died in an accident or following an illness or an abortion. It may be a person with whom I have no blood ties but whom I **love** as much as though it were my own child. The **feeling of loss** may be about an abstract entity as, for instance: *"Since he's had this new job, my husband is no longer at home, he comes back late, we hardly speak any longer, his job is always on his mind. I have lost my husband! If it goes on like this, his job will have done our marriage in"*. Therefore, "I have lost" the man I knew before and with whom I was happy, which is no longer the case today. It may be the loss of a project that was close to my **heart♥** and that was aborted. Besides, if I were the initiator of this project, I would refer to it as being 'my baby'. My feeling of guilt over the event in question is often a marked and triggering factor of the illness. I am now having difficulty with commitment, because I felt torn apart by a person of the opposite sex. A **cancer of the ovaries** follows a painful situation that hurts me in my image as a mother and produces helplessness and a sense of failure. Even the foundation of my life with respect to creativity is called into question. As with a tumor, many things do not please me, but I refuse to make the appropriate changes.

Whatever the situation, it is important that I ***immediately*** accept↓♥ all the feelings inside of me, and express them so that my inner injury can heal and I can turn to the future with a more positive outlook and many projects to carry out.

OVER-OXYGENATION *See: HYPERVENTILATION*

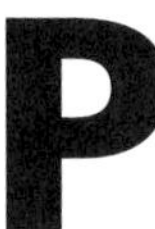

PAIN

Pain is one of the means that the body uses to draw my attention and tell me that I must stop and become **Aware** that there are changes I must make in my life and in my way of perceiving and judging myself. Whatever the **pain**, it is related to an emotional or mental imbalance, to a **deep feeling of guilt or sorrow**. It is a form of inner anguish, and because I feel guilty of having done something, of having spoken or even of having 'unhealthy' or 'negative' thoughts, I ***punish*** myself by unconsciously manifesting **pain** of varying intensity. The question I must ask myself: "Am I really guilty? And guilty of what?" The **pain** currently experienced only serves to mask the true cause: the feeling of guilt. My thoughts are very powerful, and I must remain open in order to properly identify these instances of guilt. My task is not to avoid them, but to confront them, for these are fears that I will need to integrate sooner or later. A **pain** also indicates that something is unaccomplished or flawed. It is a **subtle lure**: I believe I have understood, but there remains a further step for me to take before I can be actually in Truth and therefore in well-being and non-**pain**. I may indulge in this discomfort instead of simply facing my emotions. Instead of wanting to numb the **pain** with all sorts of medications, I can immerse myself in my **pain** and discover what it wants to teach me. I thus confront the fear that is imprisoned in this **pain**. If I become **Aware** of it, I can then free myself of it. I need to trust, and let go of, a person or a situation in order to release the inner tension. Physical **pain** often follows an experienced separation that intensifies my sensitivity. I experience it brutally. If I strike someone, this **painful** contact, though it is more emotional than physical, leaves an imprint, and the **pain** may appear in the person who struck the blow as well as in the one who received it. **Pain** in the **bones** indicates that the situation is affecting me at the deepest level, whereas in the muscles, it is more a **pain** of a mental nature. A **pain** connects me instantly to my mental suffering and forces me to stop and feel what is going on in my body. In a sense it is positive, for it allows me to 'connect' with myself as a **Soul** and to become **conscious**. When a **pain** is '**chronic**', it simply means that, since the onset of the **pain**, I have not yet confronted the true cause of this **pain**. The longer I delay becoming **Aware** of it, the more regularly the **pain** will return until it becomes 'chronic'.

It is important that I accept↓♥ to identify the origin of my **pain** and to remain open in order to resolve the 'real' cause of my **pain**. The place where the **pain** is located gives me some indications about its real cause.

PAIN (cardiac) *See: HEART♥ — CARDIAC PROBLEMS*

PALATE *See: MOUTH — PALATE*

PALPITATIONS *See: HEART♥ — CARDIAC ARRHYTHMIA*

PALSY (cerebral) *See: BRAIN — CEREBRAL PALSY*

PALUDISM *See: MALARIA*

PANCREAS *See also: BLOOD / DIABETES / HYPOGLYCEMIA*

The **pancreas** is located at about 4 inches above the navel[1]. The **pancreas** synthesizes enzymes that help in digesting food. This is where the insulin level is maintained, to aid in stabilizing the sugar level in the blood. If it is out of balance, **diabetes** or **hypoglycemia** will appear (see these diseases for more details).

It symbolizes freedom, power, self-mastery, my definition of my 'self'. When I experience a lot of emotions, I may have difficulty in digesting. When this state endures and I live in sadness, I may develop **hypoglycemia** (related to a lack of joy). The seat of the Ego, of my emotional energy and my feelings, this energy center is constantly in motion. It picks up the vibrations of others (positive or negative) that influence my mood. It is the center of emotions and desires. The **pancreas** represents my capacity for expressing and integrating **Love** inside of me and my capacity for dealing with the opposite feelings (anger, for example) without creating pain. A difficulty in my **pancreas** indicates that there is disorder and confusion in my emotions, which is why I am having difficulty in digesting. I wish to keep control and power over others, I become agitated inside and I suffer a loss of self-esteem. I wage an inner battle with obstacles, I am afraid of new challenges and I exhaust myself struggling, which brings on a lowering of energy. I like my freedom. A bad functioning of the **pancreas** often follows traumatic events such as the loss of a loved one, a shock that I took but that destabilized me. It represents the primary instincts that I repressed. It is often a situation involving another member of the family and where the issue is to acquire more power or money (in the case of an inheritance, for instance). I may be the one at the center of the conflict (I receive rebukes, they want to 'expel' me) or it may be someone else (and I am the person who is grumbling). This situation, where I bear an emotional burden, can lead me to produce calculi. The **pancreas** is related to obsessions and ruminating. I keep repeating and brooding on the same thoughts without finding any solutions. I find a situation in my life ***abject*** and unfair. If I experience a situation that is very hard to swallow and **I find it *ignoble*, *odious*** or ***sordid***, I may go as far as to develop a **cancer of the pancreas**. In this case, I am ***revolted*** and I resist with all my strength to remain on my positions. For instance, I may have lost my name or I may have searched in vain for my roots.

1. The **pancreas** is related to the energy center (chakra) of the **solar plexus** that is located at the base of my sternum, a few inches above-my navel.

It is related to my joy in living: I am feeling disillusioned, and I am so afraid of failure that I prefer to do nothing. By having no goals and no expectations, I avoid being disappointed. Do I allow new situations to easily take place in my life, or do I resist change? What are the changes or the adjustments I must make that would enable me to better assimilate the emotions that inhabit me? How do I accept↓♥ to embrace all the gifts of life? Is it easy for me to feel pleasure with all my senses, or do I refuse happiness instead because I feel ***unworthy***, even of the ***name*** I bear? I tend to be ***disdainful***. I am indignant about certain situations. I may even be ***humiliated*** and have difficulty defending myself. Do I tend to want to follow two masters or two teachings at once? I must become **Aware** of my needs and take action in order to get what I want. This will help me to become **Aware** that my fear of neediness is groundless, because from now on, I am living in abundance in all respects. I must find a balance between what I give and what I receive, between my work and my leisure time. I don't need artificial stimulants to 'nourish' myself (drugs, food, sexuality, etc.), I need only learn to **love** myself as I am. I need to allow myself to enjoy small pleasures. I must examine my perceptions and opinions about sugar and about the sweet things in life in general. Is sugar harmful and poisonous in my view? Do I refuse to have a good time or enjoy gifts because I feel I don't deserve them, or people might think I am a materialistic person? My acrimonious relation with sugar and its affective representations (**Love**, gentleness, tenderness) results in affecting my **pancreas**.

I become **Aware** that when my **pancreas** is in harmony, I feel a sensation of balance, peace and well-being. I feel in my right place and comfortable in my life. I accept↓♥ that everything in life is an experience. I adjust to situations, I let go of my emotions and I stop controlling everything, situations as well as persons.

PANCREAS — PANCREATITIS *See also: APPENDIX III*

I am feeling much rage against life because it no longer offers me any sweetness. I want to reject it. I feel an enormous anger, feeling imprisoned because of a person or a situation. I am at a dead end, and I prefer to remain in place with all my emotions that make me feel powerless because I don't know how to deal with them. I prefer to give up rather than make an extra effort. I am full of insecurity. I let myself go. I no longer have any tone, physically as well as in my thoughts and my emotions. Instead of waiting for sweet things to come to me, it is up to me to get some for myself, knowing that I deserve them. I choose to live. I dispel my dark thoughts.

Instead of fleeing my emotions, I embrace them and look at what they want to teach me. I see all the sadness concealed behind the anger. I drop everything that no longer suits me in my life and I build new frameworks for living (in my personal, family and professional lives). I thus create a new life full of happiness and joy.

PANIC ATTACK *See: FEAR*

PARALYSIS (in general)

Paralysis is an impossibility to act, a stoppage in the functioning of the activity of one or several muscles. It can affect an organ, a system of organs or the whole body.

This illness is related to escape: am I trying to avoid or resist a situation, a person or my responsibilities? **It is often fear that paralyzes me**. What I am experiencing may appear so intolerable and unbearable that I want to 'cut myself off' and make myself numb, as I feel that there are no feasible solutions because I am incapable of fully bearing my responsibilities. I may also feel, or have previously experienced, a deep trauma that is asking me to 'stop living' because this is too much. Life sometimes asks me to take some time off to reassess my priorities; and if I turn a deaf ear, paralysis may take over and force me to stop. It is also possible that an intense hate or a lack of self-confidence may lead me to no longer act. This way, I can't make any mistakes. I want at all costs to achieve an unfeasible desire: and my body stops, to give me a sign that it is preferable for me to accept↓♥ this fact. I may also be very rigid in my way of thinking, and if everything doesn't go as expected, my reaction is to withdraw and escape. It is important for me to become **Aware** of the pressure that haunts me, about what is happening or is going to happen, in order to control it and enable the **paralyzed** part to 'start living again'. I may feel '**paralyzed**' in a situation where I can't move or that offers me no latitude over the choices or the actions to undertake. The fact of lacking initiative or not finding a solution in a situation **paralyzes** me. Where should I go? It may be preferable to stay in place. The affected body part gives me some additional indications about the source of my ailment and my fear. If my right leg is **paralyzed** for example, it may be my fear of what is in store for me in my future job, in my family responsibilities or my responsibilities as a citizen. If I can't escape a situation or can't find a solution, my **legs** will **paralyze**. If I can't repel, or hold on to, a situation or a person, my **arms** will be affected. If I no longer feel like talking or drinking but don't know how to go about it, my **mouth** will **paralyze**. When I experience **paralysis**, I feel that my whole world is ***collapsing***. It is as though someone were giving me a ***slap in the face***, which often produces a **facial paralysis**. The latter expresses my visceral fear of showing my feelings, of which I am ashamed. I am **paralyzed** at the prospect of being seen in my true **Light**. **Infantile paralysis** highlights the fact that the baby feels like a prisoner. **Quadriplegia** or **tetraplegia**[2] highlights my deep feeling that whatever I may do, I can't be up to snuff and can't satisfy everyone's expectations. Though I 'split myself 4 ways[3]' and 'bleed myself white[4]', nothing works. I become **Aware** that I am **paralyzing** myself with my own negative attitude toward who I am. I feel like a victim, '**paralyzed**'. The fact that I am in poor contact with my **heart♥** and my emotions prevents me from advancing

2. A paralysis affecting all four limbs simultaneously.

3. To take great pains to do something right.

4. To give everything I can, to deprive myself for someone else.

and developing. I stay in my shell, clinging to the past. Anxiety **paralyzes** me. I want to anesthetize my inner pain.

I accept↓♥ to see the nature of the situation in my life that is '**paralyzed**' and that I need to change or improve so as to increase my inner well-being. I let go of the past, which I want to 'freeze', and turn to the future, knowing that the best is yet to come. I take charge of myself: I do things for myself. Instead of wanting to control others and the outer elements of my life, I take control of my own life. I learn to accept↓♥ the **Love** of others. I bite into life!

PARALYSIS (infantile) *See: POLIOMYELITIS*

PARANOIA *See: PSYCHOSIS — PARANOIA*

PARKINSON'S DISEASE *See: BRAIN — PARKINSON'S DISEASE*

PAROTID GLAND *See: GLANDS [SALIVARY]*

PATELLA

The **patella** is a bone, triangular in form, which makes possible movements of flexion-extension with the knee joint. If my **patella** is **painful** or **deformed**, I may experience anger, disappointment and irritation about my dreams that seem out of reach or impracticable. I 'bend my knees', I feel beaten. There is a situation that seems to be stagnating, blocked in the present moment, and I am waiting for it to improve, but I doubt very much that this will happen. I may refuse to give in to authority, being unwilling to get down on my knees. I feel dominated by my family. I feel myself sliding down a hole and I don't know how to get back out of it. My autonomy is limited.

I accept↓♥ that the moment has come to take some time for myself, to stand up and take initiatives in order to achieve my dearest dreams. It is by believing in them that they can take form for me.

PECTORIS (angina) *See: ANGINA PECTORIS*

PEDICULOSIS *See: CRAB LICE*

PELVIS *See also: HIP DISORDERS*

The **pelvis** is the bony part that simultaneously joins and separates the lower and upper parts of the human skeleton. It is the **origin of all of the body's movements** of displacement, locomotion and action.

It corresponds to the fact of my feeling secure while **dashing into life**. The **pelvis** represents **power** in all its forms. It is the receptacle containing the energies of power that sustain the ego. A difficulty in this area shows me that I may be afraid of advancing in life. I may cling too much to the past. As this is where a child is carried during pregnancy, it is possible that my ailment in the **pelvis** may be related to an aspect of my own gestation where I felt frustrated by my parents, especially my mother. I may have taken on many responsibilities, and I am re-creating this state in my current life by wanting to be 'everybody's mother'. An ailment in the **pelvis** may also be related to the fact that, for some reason, I cannot welcome a person. It may be a newborn child, but it may also be someone I would like to accommodate in my home, but that is impossible. A danger is therefore threatening my family's safety and my sense of independence. The **pelvis** is associated with the center of sexual energy and with pleasure in all its forms. I cut myself off from the pleasant sensations of life when I feel I don't deserve them. I may also have felt betrayed, or thought that a dirty trick was played on me: I will then be on the defensive. If I have a **wide or very wide pelvis** (with large buttocks), I unconsciously believe that life or the situations in my life **limit** my power. I therefore try to get it back. I try to compensate physically by reflexively blocking all the energies at this location (fear, insecurity, anger, helplessness). There may follow a discomfort or a conflict involving my sexuality. It is important for me that the energies flow more harmoniously in my body and that I sincerely believe I have done everything I could.

Even if I can get more power, I can become **Aware** and accept↓♥ in my **heart♥** that **there is no power** to be taken other than mental power. If I want to free all these energies and achieve a better energy balance, I begin to **love** myself as I am and show joy, trust and faith in everything I do. I empty this container of power and I allow life to circulate. On the other hand, if I have a few difficulties with my **pelvis**, it is possible that I may be underestimating the importance of my basic needs such as lodging, food and sexuality. I must reconsider the importance I should give to the different aspects of my life so that it can rest on a solid and healthy base.

PENIS AILMENTS

The **penis** is the male organ intended for copulation. It represents my male side, my power, the procreating male and also affective security. When a disease is located in the **penis** or the **testicles**, it indicates a deep conflict in the expression of my masculinity. Did this conflict begin with my mother? I make the connection with the maternal **Love** that I received and that was not what I had expected. Did I have to surpass myself to be loved? Did I adjust to what I believed was expected of me as a man? Am I happy with being the man I am? I have become a little fatalistic in my affective relations. I feel I can no longer control anything and I withdraw into myself.

I accept↓♥ to discard the mask of the strong man and I question myself about my relation with the two aspects that are in me: the male and the female. I accept↓♥ this vulnerability that is in me and I make contact with my inner wise person. I give myself unconditional **Love** and accept↓♥ myself as I am. I use my creativity in its entirety, in its male as well as in its female aspect, and I beam with the joy of being in possession of all my resources.

PERICARDITIS *See: HEART♥ — PERICARDITIS*

PERIOD DISORDERS *See: MENSTRUATION DISORDERS*

PERITONITIS *See also: APPENDICITIS*

Peritonitis is the chronic, most often acute, inflammation of the peritoneum. It usually provokes a pain that is felt like a dagger thrust in the abdomen, and is often accompanied by vomiting.

This abdominal pain tells me that there is an affective disorder, a crying need to resolve my fears of being abandoned. I haven't heeded the advance signals sent by my body. **Peritonitis** shows me that these pains match the intensity of my unresolved emotions. They are so intense and strong in me that they explode of their own accord. My suffering bursts out into the open. It is a form of self-destruction, a way of saying: take care of me. Why am I so hard on myself? I am irritated and aggressive 'because of the others'. I feel attacked, as though I were, or would be, given a 'kick in the stomach'. I feel the need to protect myself, to grow a shell. I may also have an illness that is gnawing at me from inside.

Instead of seeing myself as a victim, I accept↓♥ to be a container for **Love**, responsible for my own joys and sorrows. I examine the situation that concerns me with a new eye and I let go, whatever the circumstance or the person involved. I stop criticizing others because they don't meet what I expect of them. I use the intelligence of the **heart♥** to speak calmly with the person in order to understand and resolve this situation. Whatever the other's receptivity, I choose to allow **Love** to flow unconditionally, in me and around me. I accept↓♥ to take charge of my happiness, whatever the circumstance. I am the only one responsible for my life. When I let go of my own accord, my body relaxes, I manage my emotions far better, and everything thus becomes fluid and harmonious.

PERSPIRATION / SWEATING / SUDATION *See: ODOR [BODY]*

PHARYNGITIS *See: THROAT — PHARYNGITIS*

PHLEBITIS *See: BLOOD — PHLEBITIS*

PHOBIA *See also: ANGUISH, CLAUSTROPHOBIA, RAGE*

A **phobia** is an unjustified fear, characterized by anxiety about an object, a situation, an act or an idea.

If I have a **phobia**, I **may** have received a very strict and repressive education and I may have repressed certain aspects of my sexuality when I was a child. A **phobia** usually implies a fear of death. In fact, the object of my **phobia** is dangerous for my survival, otherwise it would not exist. When this **phobia** appeared in my life, I experienced huge anger about a situation where I felt helpless. This affected my vital need for security, which was completely ignored. Often I can recall a special situation where I felt great fear about the **object of my phobia**. However, it is also important to consider it in the proper sense as well as in the figurative sense in order to discover the emotional charge (often great anger) that is linked to it. If I have the **phobia of spiders** for example, I ask myself what the outstanding feature of **spiders** is: it is their capacity for spinning a web to capture their prey. I may personally be afraid of being caught in a trap by a work colleague or a member of my family, etc. As some **spiders** are ***venomous***, I may also not tolerate people who ***poison*** my life and prevent me from being Number One. If I have the **phobia of dirtiness** or of **microbes**, I detest everything I consider '**filthy**', whether it is in my sexuality, my physical body or anything I consider immoral. I tolerate "no blemish on my record" and I therefore demand perfection for myself and for others. If I have the **phobia of serpents**, I loathe the animal itself as well as people who behave like **serpents**, namely who take all possible circuitous ways to reach their goals and are totally unpredictable. The **serpent** is associated with sexuality.

I accept↓♥ to confront this anxiety, even if it may require me to consult a therapist to guide and accompany me in my endeavor. I become **Aware** of the real or imaginary object of my fear. I trace back to the origin or the cause of this fear. I allow my feelings of anger and powerlessness to express themselves in order to reconnect myself with my divine power of creation. My anguish thus dissipates and I resume control over my life.

PINEAL *See: GLAND [PINEAL]*

PITUITARY *See: GLAND [PITUITARY]*

PLEURISY *See: LUNGS — PNEUMONIA AND PLEURISY*

PLEURITIS *See: LUNGS — PNEUMONIA AND PLEURISY*

PMS (premenstrual syndrome) *See: MENSTRUATION — PREMENSTRUAL SYNDROME*

PNEUMONIA *See: LUNGS — PNEUMONIA AND PLEURISY*

PNEUMONITIS *See: CONGESTION*

POISONING (food)

Poisoning or **intoxication** occurs when a toxic substance enters my body; a set of physical disorders follows.

When a **poisoning** occurs I must look at **who, or what, is poisoning my existence**. It is not so much the **food** that is concerned as the reflection of my own thoughts. Besides, among the persons who partook of the same **food**, not all have suffered from **poisoning**. I become **Aware** of the situation or the person who bothers me so much. I try to find toward whom or what I am being drawn and what **poisoned thoughts** I entertain toward this person or this situation. What is **poisoning** my existence? What am I to understand about this situation? Why am I so fatalistic? A **poisoning** throws **Light** on my highly developed artificial, false side: I am merely playing a role. My values are those of others, so I avoid creating any waves. Authority or social rules may be **poisoning** my existence. I feel in prison in one area of my life. I ask myself how far I can go in what I express, for I am **Aware** of the weight of words and of what that involves.

I accept↓♥ to reduce the '**poisonous** situation' to its simplest expression and summarize it in a word: sadness, frustration, jealousy, etc. As everything that I don't accept↓♥ comes back into my life, and increasingly strongly so, until I have accepted↓♥ it, I had best **open up here and now** and accept↓♥ this situation with my **heart♥**. I then realize that this person or situation is there to help me surpass myself and move forward. I allow all the **poisons** to come out of me: all my attitudes, my actions and my emotions that no longer suit me. I regain control over my life in simplicity and truth.

POLIOMYELITIS

Poliomyelitis is a contagious disease produced by a virus that settles on nerve centers, mainly the spinal cord, causing paralysis that may be lethal once it reaches the respiratory muscles. **Acute anterior poliomyelitis**, which is an impairment of the anterior horn of the spinal cord, is commonly called **poliomyelitis**. As it is mostly found in children, it is also called **infantile paralysis**.

If I am affected by this disease, the virus paralyzing me is **jealousy** and **helplessness**. I envy what someone else or others are capable of accomplishing. I'd like to slow them down, but I am the one I am slowing down and paralyzing. I don't like to have to account for myself, to have to obey authority, or to have no alternatives. I allow others to get the better of me. My vulnerability makes me feel constantly in danger. I want to accomplish so many things, but I feel paralyzed. I believe I don't have any power over my life. I am always on guard. I want so much to prove my worth. Despair is very present and intense.

I accept↓♥ to not envy others: I am an extraordinary person with huge capacities. I have as many qualities and strengths as others and must accept↓♥ them. Rather than **flee** and focus my attention on others, I regain full power here and now over my life and accept↓♥ that abundance is an integral part of my life.

POLYOREXIA *See: BULIMIA*

POLYPS

A **polyp** is a benign tumor growing on a mucous membrane in the mouth, the nose, the intestines or the uterus.

The resulting outgrowth is a physical sign showing me that there is a person or a situation in my life that bothers me and that I feel like avoiding and fleeing, but this is not possible. On the contrary, I feel caught and stuck and **can't extricate myself from it** for fear of being abandoned or displeasing others. I deny my inner power, and that makes me feel overly supervised and regimented. I have emotions that solidify in me. They are like 'knots of sorrow' that I must untie.

If it is in my **nose**, I ask myself what odor is announcing a danger and affecting me. I want to protect myself and I need the support of others. If it is in the **intestines**, I feel that others want to prevent me from reaching my goals. I have come to follow others instead of driving forward and being a leader: I thus risk less being disappointed.

I accept↓♥ that something or someone is bothering me, and I ask myself what I can learn from all that. How could I feel freer? By facing my responsibilities, the **polyp**, or **polyps**, will disappear.

PORT-WINE MARK / STRAWBERRY MARK *See: SKIN — PORT-WINE MARK / STRAWBERRY MARK*

PREGNANCY DISORDERS *See also: BLOOD — DIABETES, CHILDBIRTH, NAUSEA*

Though pregnancy is usually joyous and enriching; it can also be terrifying, with its hidden worries, its doubts, fears and concerns, especially when it is the first time. These hidden feelings will find a way to break out if, as a future mother, I am incapable of expressing them verbally. I may sometimes feel that the challenges to be met are so great as compared to what I am capable of taking on that I may unconsciously reject the child. I think I must leave my youth behind me, therefore along with my freedom. I see all the responsibilities I will have to take on. Here are a few examples of **ailments** I may experience during my pregnancy: **heartburn** indicates a difficulty in swallowing the reality of what is happening; **constipation** shows my fear of letting go, that I try to hold on to things as they are now, while knowing that the coming of a child will bring major changes into my life; a **painful sciatic nerve** manifests my fear of moving forward in the new direction where life is pointing me; **gestational diabetes** is the result of the sadness I feel during this period. I may also feel dissatisfied or afraid of experiencing rejection as I see my body changing this way, and I want the fact of 'being oversized' to stop. **Nausea** indicates how the transformations of my body are making me feel disgust. I reject my self-image that is transforming itself. I am anxious about the delivery and my ability to be a mother.

I learn to trust and I accept↓♥ to have all the necessary tools in order to live through this marvelous experience in joy and harmony. I accept↓♥ to commit myself to this child soon to be born. I also accept↓♥ the changes that will take place in me and will make me a new person.

PREGNANCY — ECLAMPSIA *See also: BRAIN — EPILEPSY, TENSION ARTERIAL — HYPERTENSION [TOO HIGH]*

In late **pregnancy**, **eclampsia** may appear, which is a serious affection typified by secondary convulsions associated with a severe surge of arterial hypertension and cerebral edema. Usually occurring during a woman's first **pregnancy**, it is like an **epilepsy attack**, with loss of consciousness, stiff limbs and convulsions.

It is a little like being struck by ***lightning***. **Eclampsia** will hit me if I am a woman who, through insecurity or guilt, will reject **pregnancy** or anything that may represent the coming of the child. I may also feel resentment toward my spouse, for I hold him guilty and responsible for the **pregnancy**. In other cases, it may be I as a mother who, having difficulty in accepting↓♥ my child's imminent coming into the world, will reject myself, as I feel incapable of taking on my new responsibilities. I feel in prison and I want to free myself from it. I fear death: mine and that of my child. I feel powerless, and I prefer to hide behind someone else instead of going up front and forging ahead. The dilemma here however is that I can't trust anyone else to deliver this child into the world: I, and only I, can do it. I must face all these emotions rushing about inside, and I don't know very well how to react. I am sensitive to gossip and criticism. If I need much attention, will this child come and take away from me what I receive from others? Will it become the center of attraction, while I become like a ghost? I feel very vulnerable and I do want this child, but I also want to have my own space.

I learn to consider the coming of my child with a positive attitude, knowing that I have all the resources necessary for helping her in her development. I take the time to visualize how the pregnancy and the childbirth will go; and that, I am certain, is how it will take place. This is how I can create my life and give my child a solid base. I am strong enough and I am receiving all the help I need.

PREGNANCY (ectopic)

An **ectopic pregnancy** develops outside of the uterine cavity.

In this case, it may be that, as a mother, I am feeling anxious about the delivery and I am holding back from giving birth. I desire this **pregnancy**, but I fear it at the same time. I may feel that the nest I am offering my child is too small or that we'll find ourselves in an untypical situation. I may fear that my spouse is cheating on me or has done so in the past. Or am I the one thinking about cheating on someone?

I accept↓♥ to let the normal process of life take its course and allow energy to flow freely inside of me so that the elements of life can take their proper place according to the divine plan.

PREGNANCY (false) / PSEUDOCYESIS

I may experience in my physical body the same states as a pregnant woman even if I am not actually pregnant, and this is then called a **false pregnancy**.

A **false pregnancy** shows uncertainty and insecurity over my responsibilities as opposed to my desires. I may desire to have a child, but do I feel up to it, do I feel capable of taking on and fulfilling all the child's needs and desires? Maybe not. If the **false pregnancy** occurs while I am a bachelor, I must also go and see if I am experiencing difficulties concerning my sexuality. I may feel like having a child, but I don't feel like having an affective relationship with another person. I may also be afraid of all the responsibilities involved in having a spouse even if I do want one. I tend to tell myself fibs and play confidence games on myself. My body reacts to my imagination. I like to play a role and pass myself for someone I am not. I allow myself to be invaded by others. Though **false pregnancies** appear mainly in women, this phenomenon will sometimes occur in a man. I can ask myself how that can happen. It is important for me to remember, whether I am a man or a woman, that I possess both sides within me, the YIN side (woman) and the YANG side (man). Even if I am a man, I may develop my maternal instinct and certain fears associated with it, and thus develop the symptoms of a **false pregnancy** out of empathy or energy symbiosis. I then identify what insecurities my inner child is currently experiencing. I may thus reassure it and give it the **Love** and attention it needs for everything to return to normal.

I accept↓♥ to be born to myself. I allow the emergence of my desires and my inner depths that only want to come out of the dark. I thus increasingly take my rightful place in the Universe.

PREGNANCY (gemellary) *See: CHILDBIRTH — ABORTION*

PREGNANCY[5] (prolonged)

When a **pregnancy prolongs itself** beyond the usual period, as a mother I may unconsciously desire to continue carrying this child for as long as possible, enjoying this state where I feel my child is safe and where the bond between mother and child is so strong. I want to keep my child sheltered from the 'stormy squalls' of everyday life. I may be afraid of these new responsibilities that await me with this new child who is going to be born. Will I be up to the situation? Will it change something in my couple? Will I be a good mother? My concerns over this birth may cause me to delay the coming of the child. It is also possible that my child is feeling so comfortable in this secure environment that it feels like staying in there as long as possible. I can then enter into contact with the child's divine aspect and comfort it, assuring it that I will do my very best to take care of it, that I will continue to **love** it and that I am eager to hold it in my arms. I must detach myself from my child and

5. **Pregnancy** lasts about 9 months or 273 days after the date of fertilization.

convince myself that it has all the necessary tools to face the challenges it will encounter. All it needs is my **Love** and my affection.

PREMATURE CHILDBIRTH *See: CHILDBIRTH [PREMATURE]*

PRESBYOPIA / FARSIGHTEDNESS *See: EYES — HYPERMETROPIA AND PRESBYOPIA*

PRESSURE (arterial / blood) *See: TENSION [ARTERIAL]*

PROBLEMS (cardiac) *See: HEART♥ — CARDIAC PROBLEMS*

PROBLEMS (palpitation) *See: HEART ♥ — CARDIAC ARRHYTHMIA*

PROCTITIS *See: ANUS — ANAL PAINS*

PROLAPSE OF THE UTERUS *See also: PROSTATE [PROLAPSE OF THE]*

A **prolapse** indicates a pathological downward displacement of an organ, with a slackening of the elements that maintained it in place. It is frequent in the prostate, the uterus, the vagina, the rectum, the urethra or the bladder.

I then experience great **carelessness**, **neglect** and **lack of control**. The muscles collapse because my level of energy is so low that it can't maintain the elasticity of the organ any longer. I am tired and I feel a huge **inner despair** that is linked more especially to the facet of my life represented by the affected organ. For example, the **prolapse of the uterus** (**hysteroptosis**) expresses all the weight I bear as a mother, when the children's problems never seem to resolve themselves and I am tired of having all those worries to manage. I **love** my children but I am tired and I can't take it any longer. I am thirsty for freedom, to be released from those constraints. I have great ambitions that I can't reach. The **prolapse of the bladder** (**cystocele**) shows me the heaviness of my unexpressed emotions. My self-confidence is so low I grovel before others, and so does my **bladder**. I am deeply saddened for I think I have neglected my duty. I prefer to drop out and break off contact, physically or emotionally.

I accept↓♥ to find the means to take charge of my life and be active. I can seek out what I really like, whether it is an art, a sport or a hobby, in order to recover my vitality and my joy in being alive.

PROSTATE (in general)

The **prostate** is a gland of the male genital system that is located under the bladder and secretes a fluid that constitutes one of the elements of sperm.

It thus represents the male principle and power. A healthy **prostate** shows that I clearly know where I am going and listen to my inner voice. I feel my emotions and I can expel the overflow. I can be myself, master of my life.

I accept↓♥ that authority is inside of me and guides me in the choices I must make instead of letting myself be carried away by artificial values.

PROSTATE DISEASES

The **prostate** is related to my feeling of social power and sexual capacity. As **prostate disorders** are more prevalent among older men, I must ask myself: do I feel satisfied and comfortable in my sexuality? Am I experiencing frustration, impotence or maybe even confusion about my sexuality and also about my search for a possibly younger partner? Should I best give it all up? I may now be feeling useless, ineffective and incapable of being a 'real man'. I may also feel that I am not up to my children's needs, or simply a poor father. Am I still ***desirable***? I live in the intense fear of not being within the sexual ***norms*** that society has established, especially if I or one of my children are homosexual: unconsciously, I know that the species is in danger due to non-procreation. Am I comfortable with my sexual desires or the size of my genital organs? I must learn to rid myself of guilt and stop putting pressure on myself about the 'performance' that society wants me to achieve. I must become **Aware** of my worth, not only for my sexual 'exploits', but by looking at all the good human qualities that I possess. I may have the impression that I am badly '***mated***' with my spouse, that we form a mismatched couple, especially in the sexual area. We form an ***amalgam***, an odd mixture. Do I repress my emotions and my creative impulses? Do I refuse any ***erotic*** acts in my life? I may experience a platonic **Love** that is not expressed in my physical body. If I don't know my needs and my desires, it is as though I were disconnected from my own person. I feel forced to **prostrate** myself in front of someone or even before the God in whom I believe. That is humiliating! I stop pressuring myself over things to be done or things I no longer have to do: am I feeling vulnerable over money because I am going into retirement? Do I feel useless, being now much less in the midst of action than when I was on the active labor market? If I have a **difficulty in the prostate**, I must ask myself if I am experiencing difficulty and guilt in front of my grandchildren or my own children who, though they have become adults, are still for me 'little' and 'fragile'. I fear they are in moral or physical danger, especially in any situation related to sexuality and that appears in my view as dirty or outside of the customary norms established by society. I still want to be their ***protector***. I feel that I am being prevented from getting close to them. If I have no children or grandchildren, the difficulty may be experienced with a nephew or a neighborhood child whom I consider as being 'part of the family'. I tend to want to ***adjust*** myself to the expectations of others. I also want others to conform to my values or to those of society. I have the impression that I have ***enormous anomalies***, and I don't know quite what to do to be within the norms. I often feel that I am ***strange***, different from others. I don't like my image as a father. An **adenoma** occurs if I have a great sorrow about one of my children or if I feel that I am losing my 'power', at work or in society. I still have to learn to trust, and the fact that I am afraid of something 'serious' or 'bad' happening to the people I **love** only attracts the object of my fear even more. I trust in the fact that we're all guided and protected inside, including those about whom I worry. I will thus avoid developing a **cancer of the prostate**. The latter appears after I have first experienced several failures in my affective relationships. Deep inside of me I feel I have lost this male dimension necessary for seducing and attracting a female companion. I am frustrated and bitter, but these feelings are usually turned back against me. My life no longer has any meaning (often upon having retired). I have lost confidence in my resources and in my image as a father and as a man. I have cut myself off from my creativity and my right to happiness and enjoyment.

I accept↓♥ to learn to enjoy life. Not only sexually, but also with all my senses. I can be in contact with my creativity and achieve great things. I also accept↓♥ to truly feel all the emotions inside of me and learn how to fully embrace them. They are part of me. I thus regain full power over my life.

PROSTATE (prolapse of the) *See also: PROLAPSE [OF UTERUS]*

When the **prostate** descends, it puts great pressure on the bladder. It indicates that I have difficulty in releasing the feelings of uselessness that I have built up inside, with urine representing the release of my negative emotions. I feel confused and find it difficult to express my desires.

I accept↓♥ to increasingly acknowledge my worth and I know that my contribution to society is inestimable.

PROSTATE — PROSTATITIS *See also: APPENDIX III, INFECTION, INFLAMMATION*

Prostatitis is the inflammation of the **prostate**. I may feel disappointment or frustration, either with what my partner expects from my sexual exploits, or with myself, for I resent myself for not being more 'virile' and more highly 'performing'. I find myself old, 'worthless', 'finished'. I can't 'possess' my partner. My values or MY worth are based upon material and superficial things. I thus cut myself off from my emotions because I fear them.

It is therefore important for me to accept↓♥ that my sexuality may have changed and evolved over time, but may still be as exciting and whole as ever.

PRURIT *See: SKIN — ITCHING*

PSORIASIS *See: SKIN — PSORIASIS*

PSYCHOSIS (in general)

Psychosis is a major mental disorder that gravely impairs one's psychic existence in one's relations with oneself and the outside world, and includes an alteration of one's conscience of self, others and the outside world, affect, intelligence, judgment and personality, which will take the form of a marked disorder of outward behavior, with the subject living as though a stranger in this world. **Paranoia** and **schizophrenia** are **psychoses**.

If I suffer from this illness, I want to flee who I am and escape from this body that I don't accept↓♥. I feel so uncomfortable that I feel I no longer have an identity, having let myself be invaded by the people around me. I have poor self-esteem and I try by every means to get people to **love** me and to receive attention. I no longer dare to be myself. By renouncing myself, my relations with others and my life in general, I become obsessed and fixated on something or someone who moves me away from my inner pain. A **psychosis** may also result from an event where I experienced an emotional shock so great that I wanted to cut myself off from reality, with my mind unable to understand "why this could happen to me". And I hid events and emotions in my subconscious, but they are still there, and sooner or later I will have to face them in order to integrate them and learn the life lesson that is attached to them. It is by freeing from their mental prison these events that unconsciously control me and make me act impulsively, that I can regain full control over my life and live in peace with myself. A **manic-depressive psychosis** is an alternation between bouts of excitation (mania) and depressive episodes that take the form of melancholy. I am afraid of ruining my life and having no future. It often manifests itself after I have lost something or someone that was dear to me. I quickly go to extremes because I feel disconnected from my inner power and I am therefore incapable of taking charge of my life. An **infantile psychosis** can result from a disturbed relationship between a child and its parents. As a child, I may experience rejection related to my mother's unconscious revolt or because I have been subjected to sexual revelations too premature for me to integrate them, for instance. As a child, I lock myself up in a state of indifference, inertia and stagnation with respect to my mental development, or I retreat into a separate world that becomes no longer communicable and that I use as a means of protection. It is as though I were unable to find my place and take charge of myself. I withdraw into a 'protective separation', having experienced a deep rejection or an 'affective drought', with the impression that I can't be what my parents want me to be, controlled as they are by their own fears, desires and fantasies concerning me, their child.

I accept↓♥ to open myself gently to my inner world. I acknowledge the power I have over my life. The pains experienced in the past are part of each person's development process and I must accept↓♥ it: it is the only way to leave pain behind me and build my life on new positive bases. My sensitivity becomes a tool of transformation, for I thus gain access to different levels of consciousness. I can trust life because I am fully protected and guided.

PSYCHOSIS — PARANOIA

Paranoia is defined as a **psychosis** characterized by delusions of grandeur, distrust, touchiness, psychic rigidity and aggressiveness, and induces ***delusions*** of persecution. **Paranoid** behavior can be considered as a syndrome that originates from a feeling of inferiority, which carries the meaning of a protest, a compensation, a revenge or a punishment. However, if I am **paranoid**, I continue to keep my intellectual capacities.

I have obsessions, fixed ideas (monomanias), on which my attention focuses. I notice each little detail, however trifling, that can take on insane proportions. I feel constantly stalked and spied upon, which leads to a ***delusional*** state. If I am affected by **paranoia**, I feel I am the victim of everything that happens to me and I am constantly on alert. I feel that I am being ***watched*** and constantly followed. My view of the outside world is ***distorted*** (I think about what others think of me). My despair and my distress lead me to ***cry out in desperation***. I feel ***pushed to the wall***, not knowing in which direction I can run away. I always anticipate the worst and I hide behind a ***shell***. Having not received all the success and admiration I had expected, my resulting emotional injuries make me flee, and cut myself off from, a reality that I have difficulty in dealing with. I am inconsolable about a situation that I experienced. It may be a situation where I had to face death, my own or someone else's. I still feel it up close to me, as though it were watching me. I feel myself living between two worlds, and I no longer know what is real or imaginary. I no longer ***trust*** anyone. I look for 'exit doors' to avoid facing reality. There is one side of my person that I find difficult to accept↓♥. It embodies all my anxieties, my feeling of helplessness and my repressed anger. I flee my own emotions. "I am nothing". I had to learn from very early on how to live in a dangerous, disapproving environment. I may even have been 'thrown out' of my home, my school or my circle of friends. Being no longer able to look myself in the face, I flee the truth in an unreal world. I will tend to be ***jealous*** of others.

I accept↓♥ that my obsessional negative thoughts are bad for me and that I should instead increasingly take on my responsibilities in life, for I am able to create it as I want it to be. I create my life with positive thoughts. I am sincere and true with myself and with my entourage. I welcome all the emotions inside of me.

PSYCHOSIS — SCHIZOPHRENIA

Schizophrenia is a way for me to hide my true identity from myself and from others. If I am a **schizophrenic**, I often grew up in a very rigid family context in which I lost my true identity. No longer knowing who I am, I then decide to become someone else. It is a denial, a total refusal[6] of my '**I AM**'. What I am experiencing is so intense that my **schizophrenic** state becomes an emergency solution for an unbearable stress; **I feel there is no solution to my situation, so my only chance for survival is to flee**. As a person suffering from **schizophrenia**, I often have a very strong intellect and I need to understand what is happening to me, beyond simply accepting↓♥ it. I usually live in a climate of threat; and feeling threatened, I distort reality, otherwise I panic and fear grips me. I feel the need to protect myself from the world around me. My vision of it is very different from the reality. I feel that the only way to get control is to live in solitude. I build myself a world in which I control each part of my personality as I wish. I am never entirely myself when I am with others. I hold a ***fabulous*** fictional power over myself until those parts of me that I wanted to forget come to the surface again. This hidden personality demands

6. There are varying degrees of intensity of the illness.

to express itself and make itself heard. That is why I have the impression of hearing voices or being possessed, because reality is unbearable, and I withdraw into some form of ***delirium***. I must stop ***denying*** reality. I am not possessed by entities, it is only the part of me that I always stifled and is demanding to come out of its hiding place. The fact of being 'divided' becomes unbearable. Attracting people to me, while trying to push them away at the same time, is very tiring. Having great psychic gifts, I develop them to excess. We all experience **schizophrenia** to some greater or lesser degree. In fact, when I registered an inner injury during my childhood (especially from 0 to 12 years) in the form of rejection, submissiveness, anger, misunderstanding, abandonment, etc., I will tend to distort reality later on in my life as an adult, when an event reactivates this injury. It is as though I developed mechanisms, sometimes unconsciously, to avoid re-living the pain or the memory of this previously experienced pain. Among these defense mechanisms, there is the act of automatically changing the subject whenever a mention comes up of a situation where I felt hurt; I may show incoherent behavior when a subject is brought up, such as looking for the salt in the refrigerator, which will be dismissed as a 'distraction', etc. I should try to rediscover the marvelous being that I am and accept↓♥ responsibility for my life.

I accept↓♥ to be able to live securely and that the key to my liberation lies in me accepting↓♥ every part of my being, for together they form a whole. Though there are some things I like less, I know I can change them. But to do so, I must drop my masks and look at myself straight on. I thus no longer need to react excessively, for my whole being now has a voice and can express itself. I trust myself and I know that there is only good inside of me. I let go of the notion of 'evil', which I allowed to infiltrate my life and no longer fits my new reality.

PSYCHOSOMATIC ILLNESS *See: DISEASE [PSYCHOSOMATIC]*

PUBES

Pubic hair partly hides the genital organs and the pubis. If it is **thick**, it denotes a fear about my sexuality, something I want to hide. On the contrary, **sparse** or **absent hair** denotes a vulnerability about my sexual life or in my relations with my spouse.

I accept↓♥ to flourish in my sexuality by expressing my fears and trusting myself more and more.

PUBIS / BONE (pubic) *See also: ACCIDENT, BONES — FRACTURE, TENDONS*

The **pubis** is a segment of bone that forms the anterior part of the iliac bone, the wide and flat bone that forms the pelvis. It serves to naturally protect the genital organs.

As several abdominal and thigh muscles are attached here, a **tendonitis** can sometimes occur, which represents a disappointment related to my sexuality, between what I want and what I actually experience. A **fracture** here involves a greater fear or guilt in the actions I do, or don't, carry out regarding my sexuality. A **condition affecting my pubis** reveals my fear of being injured in my intimacy. This often occurs when I have recently met a person and chances are high that a deeper relationship may develop. I may feel abused. This may reawaken a stress I experienced during puberty. I question myself about my capacity for being a good, performing sexual partner. I also ask myself questions about having a child and how much I see this still unborn child as a burden. I may have the impression that my 'performance' is far from perfect.

I accept↓♥ to learn to recognize my true sexual needs in order to enable me to better flourish in what I am. I become **Aware** of my limits and I accept↓♥ to open up to others, knowing that I am constantly protected.

PUDENDAL FISSURE *See: PUDENDUM / VULVA*

PUDENDUM / VULVA

The **pudendum** (or **vulva**) includes all of a woman's external genital organs. Just as the lips on a person's face are considered as the doors of the mouth, so also the **vaginal labia** represent those of the genital system.

A feeling of emptiness, exhaustion or lassitude can provoke an inflammation (**vulvitis**) or other disorders in the **vulva**. I feel vulnerable and helpless, I reject all physical contact, I feel joyless inside. I close the door on pleasure. The origins of **ailments of the vulva** are normally of a psychological nature. Anxieties and fears often inflame a **vulva** after having had to make many decisions. I am tired of having to decide, and it is a way of showing my powerlessness and my feeling of being diminished by events. I find it difficult to be present with my **heart♥** when the time comes to be intimate with my partner and I no longer feel like being close to him: the injuries of the past are still present and I prefer to keep some control over my body and my emotions.

I accept↓♥ to feel appreciated and I accept↓♥ responsibility for my choices.

PULSE ANOMALIES *See: HEART♥ — CARDIAC ARRHYTHMIA*

PUS *See: ABSCESS — EMPYEMA*

PYORRHEA ALVEOLARIS *See: GUM DISORDERS*

PYREXIA *See: FEVER*

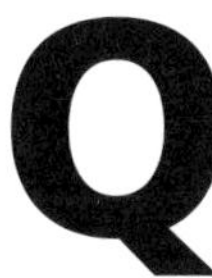

QUADRIPLEGIA *See: PARALYSIS (IN GENERAL)*

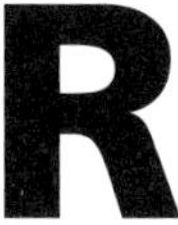

RAGE

Rage is an epidemic disease that affects certain mammals (foxes, cats, dogs, etc.), which transmit it to humans, generally by a bite. A morbid fear of water, or **hydrophobia**, is one of the first signs of **rage**, together with a fear of air movements, **aerophobia**.

If I have **rage**, chances are high that I am 'full of **rage**', anger or bitterness, directed against myself or a person or a situation. I feel powerless and compelled to do something that I find repugnant. I want to project a perfect image of myself, for I have no confidence in my own capacities. I prefer to depend on others even though I resent authority. I felt injured by a person who had authority over me, and now I want to get my revenge. An inner storm is **raging** and the bases or foundations of my life are weak and in danger.

I accept↓♥ that I can settle my differences and disagreements by other means than force and violence. I learn to calmly communicate my needs, my opinions and my feelings while respecting myself and respecting the other. I welcome my emotions, whatever they may be.

RAYNAUD'S DISEASE *See also: BLOOD — BLOOD CIRCULATION*

Raynaud's disease[1] is characterized by a brutal and painful constriction of circulation in the small arteries of the hands and feet, but mostly and almost exclusively in the fingers, creating pale and numb extremities that can turn blue or purple. The fingers whiten at first and take on color when the painful circulation resumes; the repetition and duration of the fits can induce gangrene in the fingers. The blood thus circulates poorly in the extremities.

The emotions that should circulate in the blood are stagnant. When one or several of my fingers are affected, I can go and look for the meanings of the fingers in question, which will throw more **Light** on the area of my life that is involved. The affected limbs feel abandoned and experience a sensation of loss. I must then ask myself these questions: "Am I experiencing rejection in my life? Am I afraid of expressing myself and taking my place? Have I terminated a **Love** relationship to which I am still clinging? Do I feel abandoned by someone or by life (it may be death that claimed the person, and this freezes my blood, refusing to mourn my loss)? Why do I feel the need to move away from people? Is it to not feel forced to do things? Why are physical and emotional contacts so difficult for me? What am I trying to protect myself against?" Maybe I feel too vulnerable or not important or enterprising enough

1. **Raynaud** (Maurice): A French physician (1834–1881) who first described the manifestations of this disease in 1862.

for people to be interested in me in any case! I am experiencing great indecisiveness, which prevents me from moving forward. I am afraid of going back home because a danger awaits me. I need to make peace with my mother or the person who plays her role in my life.

I accept↓♥ that to some degree, I have cut myself off from the Universe around me, and I need to find my place and become a part of this Universe in which I play an important role. If I go to meet it, my extremities will once again be nourished with **Love** and understanding. I am sure all my actions and decisions are the best for me and my development. I accept↓♥ to stride forward and put my ideas and dreams into action, even those that seem the craziest. This is how I build a new reality and create new opportunities. My life is thus rich and stimulating.

RECEDING GUMS *See: TEETH — TOOTH AILMENTS*

RECTUM *See: INTESTINES — RECTUM*

REDNESS *See: SKIN DISEASES*

REGRETS

If I feed on **regrets**, I nourish my body with sadness, sorrow and discontent over what I should have done, said or thought, or not. I am facing an exasperating reality. I feel that I have lost something or someone for good.

My **regrets** gnaw at me from inside and lower my level of energy. They create a fertile soil for illness.

I accept↓♥ to have a positive attitude, knowing that I always act to the best of my knowledge. I learn from my past, which enables me to improve myself, to take on experience and become wiser.

REMOVAL / ABLATION *See: AMPUTATION*

RENAL CALCULI (stones) OR URINARY LITHIASIS *See also: KIDNEYS*

Renal calculi, also called **kidney stones**, are related to the kidneys, the seat of fear. It is the formation of **stones** or crystals from abundant quantities of **salt**, calcium, oxalates and **uric acid**.

Uric acid represents old emotions to be evacuated. A **calculus** can form in the various parts of the urinary system. It is a mass of solidified energy created from aggressive thoughts, fears, emotions and feelings about someone or a situation. As the kidneys are filters of emotions from the body's waste, the abundance of uric acid salts indicates the great quantity of solidified aggressive feelings, for they have been held in for a long time. "I have experienced frustrations and aggressive feelings in my relations for so long that my attention is focused solely on that". My affective life is a failure and I tell myself that happiness is only for others. A balanced person has a 'solid back', but different character traits can cause **calculi**: I am very authoritarian, often extremely so, **hard on myself and on others**, I make my decisions and choices reactively, I cling seriously to the past, and I lack willpower and self-confidence. I am drastic in my opinions and choices. **Renal calculi** often involve an inner conflict between my resolve and my decisions that bring an excess of authoritarianism: knowing that I am weak and fearful, I 'mobilize' all my available strength in the same place in order to carry out certain tasks, and once the period of stress has passed, this concentration hardens to form **calculi**. I repressed all my spontaneity, which has hardened in order to live according to others. Everything is **calculated** and planned in advance to avoid surprises and gain a feeling of control over my life. There is therefore a 'Me' who has one of my personalities that lives in society, and there is the other 'Me' who lives hidden in a closet and is made up of all the emotions I repress. My creative energies accumulate and my aggressiveness does so as well. All the unsaid thoughts that are clamoring to be released and express themselves are transformed into **renal calculi**. I feel that I am being watched and that I must be on alert at all times. I tend to live in isolation, feeling guilty or unable to communicate. I forbid myself to do many things. I allow others to invade me or to invade my life, and I can't demarcate what belongs to me.

I accept↓♥ to recover some inner peace if I want to stop having **calculi**. I should brood less on certain conflicted situations and certain problems for, in so doing, I prevent myself from moving forward. I must resolve them definitely and view the future calmly and flexibly. It is a matter of **Awareness** and attitude. I live spontaneously, like a child, and my life is filled with happiness and surprises.

RESENTMENT

If I feel **resentment** toward a person or a situation, I am experiencing a deep indignation and I feel like getting revenge. I will even cultivate these negative feelings, perceiving myself as the person who was bullied or injured and is a victim. My life should be better, I should have reached the upper ranks of society, "but somebody prevented me from doing so!" I hold others responsible for my own life. Why waste one's energy in hating someone?

It is in my best interest to accept↓♥ events with my **heart♥** and turn toward the future instead or incessantly ruminating over the past: if not, my **heart♥** will harden and my body will react with an ailment or a disease.

RESPIRATION (in general)

Respiration is a function that governs the exchanges of gases between me as a living being and the external environment. It is therefore an entranceway for life so that it can penetrate inside of me. If I can breathe deeply, it represents my ability to give life and strength to my emotions. Superficial **respiration** indicates a fear or a resistance with respect to life, especially in moments of distress or panic, and shows that I tend to repress my emotions. I live my life as I breathe, which can be done superficially, devoid of meaning, or following the rhythm of the seasons. The rhythm between 'taking in' (breathing in) and 'giving out' (breathing out) is done harmoniously; the communication pathways between me and the external world are open and free.

RESPIRATION DISORDERS *See also: ASTHMA, LUNG DISEASES, SUDDEN INFANT DEATH SYNDROME, THROAT DISORDERS*

My **respiratory difficulties** denote a conflict between the place I occupy in life and the one I would like to occupy. It may also be a conflict between my material and spiritual desires or a conflict between my desire to live and that of 'letting everything go'. I may feel smothered by the things I force myself to do or by the persons I feel compelled to meet, which can cause a '**shortness of breath**'. Are my limits well set out or on the contrary, do I allow others and life itself to dictate who I must be? Furthermore, if my **respiratory difficulties** are cyclical, I must ask myself what event or what person is their triggering element; what is 'cutting off my breath', or can I possibly want people to 'allow me to breathe'? I may become so exasperated that my **respiratory problems** will become, often unconsciously, a way for me to manipulate my entourage to get what I desire. I may feel limited. I will also find it difficult to breathe if I hesitate to give and share things or feelings. I am afraid to take, absorb or fuse within me any new things or even life itself, with all the joys it can bring. I despair of ever laughing someday. My **difficulty in breathing out** denotes my withdrawal into myself, as I don't occupy my rightful place. I no longer have any deep aspirations and in a sense, I am awaiting death, my 'last breath'. This is typical if I experience **sleep apnea**. In this case, I sense that there is 'something in the air that doesn't smell good'. I sense a danger without being able to identify it, and I want to be able to feel safe, as when I was in my mother's womb.

I accept↓♥ to let go of my resistances, to go with the flow and abandon myself by trusting life. I am then better able to find my proper place in the Universe. I let go of what is no longer good for me. I accept↓♥ that I have changed and developed and that, despite my life having changed in several respects and some of my dreams having vanished, it is now time for me to look confidently to the future, to take my rightful place and assert who I am today. I say Thanks to everything I have experienced so far, knowing that Life is taking care of me.

RESPIRATION — ASPHYXIA *See also: ASTHMA, RESPIRATION DISORDERS*

Asphyxia is a respiratory disorder manifested by a shut-down of **respiration** or an obstruction (conscious or not) of the ducts that bring oxygen to the lungs and permit **respiration**.

This very spontaneous state is related to a distrust toward life and its unfolding and to certain deep fears manifested during childhood. This state can result from the insecurity of remaining stuck or 'fixed', as if I felt 'fixed' (**as 'fix'-ia**) in a situation where I am smothering and incapable of moving. It is even possible that **asphyxia** may be related to a 'mental fixation' on sexuality, for in the state of **asphyxia**, it is often the throat that manifests the block; and it is related to self-expression, creativity and sexuality. I am feeling ***despondent*** and I don't know very well how to get out of my lethargy. Because I am afraid of the future, I may want to remain in the past, at the time of my childhood or adolescence, according to the period that was happiest for me.

I accept↓♥ that I am now ready to see something else, to move, to no longer have any **fixation** and to trust life! I must take my responsibilities and stop **fixing** my attention on my childhood frustrations. They are present, and I do what is needed to integrate them.

RESPIRATION — CHOKING / SUFFOCATION

Suffocating indicates that I am feeling stuck and lacking air and space. The **throat** corresponds to the center of energy related to truth, self-expression, creativity, and indirectly to sexuality. I may feel 'seized by the throat'; an idea "went down the wrong way"; I feel very criticized. I have repressed my emotions so much that there is an overflow. Nevertheless, I still try to repress them. These emotions however are very present in my life and I unconsciously feed them until they **choke** me. It is possible that some situations are so difficult to swallow that they too **choke** me. I '**choke**' on certain situations of my past that still make me suffer and are still fresh in my memory. I find it difficult to be integrated in society, in my work or in my family. Why am I so afraid of being myself and expressing myself? Is it for fear of being rejected because I believe I can't be loved for myself?

I must absolutely let go and accept↓♥ to allow everything buried in me to rise back up in me. The solution is to learn to communicate and express my needs. What a relief I already feel! And I realize that others can't guess my thoughts and that our respective needs can always be satisfied in mutual respect and harmony.

RESPIRATION — TRACHEITIS

Tracheitis is an inflammation of the inner mucous membrane of the **trachea**, which conducts air to the larynx, the bronchi and the bronchioles. It is generally associated with a spell of laryngitis, bronchitis or rhino pharyngitis.

My affected upper airways show that I feel suffocated. As air is life, I feel great sadness and often anger. I feel misunderstood by my entourage, which gradually leads me into a depressive state. I feel I am **short of air** and living as an obligation, not free to decide my life for myself. It is as if both hands were tied behind my back. I am caught in a reason/passion duality. I **choke** on trying to control others. I need space, maybe even to be away from some persons to feel better, as I feel very irritated. My body tells me to breathe freely and make place for **Love**.

I accept↓♥ autonomy and freedom for myself and others and regain my ***dignity***.

RETENTION (water) *See also: EDEMA, SWELLING*

Water retention is often caused by a bad functioning of the kidneys.

My body 'makes reserves', which illuminates the fact that I may be able to store things or emotions because I hate losing something or someone. I keep my crying inside. I show great self-restraint and I 'take care' to not bother my entourage. I avoid 'giving in to temptation', but this produces frustration and instability. My insecurity may be the unconscious reason for this 'stocking up'. I also tend to criticize myself or criticize others. This derives either from my difficulty in asserting myself or, on the contrary, from my ego that is a little too big and makes me take my own place and those of others. I thus disguise my anxieties. My relation to authority is also very chaotic, as I often feel myself the victim of an injustice.

I accept↓♥ to take responsibility for my life and to learn respect and humility better. I learn to take the place that is mine by divine right, in the confident knowledge that everything is available, so long as I ask for it.

RETINITIS PIGMENTOSA *See: EYES — RETINITIS PIGMENTOSA*

RETINOPATHY (primary pigmentary) *See: EYES — RETINITIS PIGMENTOSA*

RETREATING into ONESELF

Retreating into myself can be a marvelous way to stop, take some time for myself and discover my needs. It can also be called introspection. However, if this period is prolonged and, instead of being a moment for growth and self-knowledge, it becomes an occasion for closing out the world, mulling over negative ideas, indulging in self-pity and playing the victim, I then risk experiencing a deep psychological and physical malaise.

I accept↓♥ to remain open to the Universe while respecting my own needs in order to live in joy and harmony.

RHEUMATISM *See also: ARTHRITIS — RHEUMATOID ARTHRITIS, INFLAMMATION, JOINTS*

Rheumatism is defined as an acutely painful and generally chronic affection that impairs the proper functioning of the locomotor system. I have stiffness in my joints, which makes my movements more difficult.

This manifests my rigidity, my inflexibility and my stubbornness toward certain persons or situations. I am afraid of being injured, so I will project an image of myself as being 'on top of it all' and 'all is well', even if deep down, this is not the case. In my own world, I will consider myself as the victim of the injustices that befall me. I constantly mull over 'my little troubles', which leads to **criticism** against myself or against others. I am a martyr. I give myself no chances; I am demanding, and I find that life has a sour taste. I must ask myself if I am tormented about a situation where I experience some ambiguity: "Will I do it or not?", "Will I punch him or not?" I am experiencing a conflict of separation inside of me; for example, I want to be close to my child but I can't do so. If I strike my child and then regret it later on, chances are high that the hand that did the gesture will be affected by **rheumatism**. My self-esteem is therefore at its lowest point, for I constantly depreciate myself. I worry about others, especially when it concerns my children. I rely on them because they are often my reason for living and my reason for moving forward. If they are injured, if they stumble or experience failures, I fear they may not be able to get back up, and I ask myself: "What more or what else should I have done for them? I should have been able to help them." My guilt and responsibility are great, and so is my depreciation. I must do a hundred times more and be a hundred times better to go out and earn my self-esteem, my worth and the **Love** of others, which I feel I am not receiving in any case. I live in an imaginary world and I am not satisfied with my life. I am frustrated and disappointed because I feel powerless to change things in my life. I would like to be the first and manifest more independence and courage, but I feel incapable of doing so. I feel that I don't deserve to be happy and that I must in any case endure the ordeals of life. Do I have the impression that someone tried to manipulate me or betrayed me? **Acute articular rhumatism** (or **Bouillaud's disease**[2]) highlights the fact that I am afraid of losing the **Love** of someone dear to me because he is about to go away.

I accept↓♥ my great need for **Love**. I learn to take care of myself and stand by my emotions, for they are all positive and they enable me to know myself better. I get in the driver's seat of my life and, instead of the victim I was, I become the creator of my life. I know that all is possible. It is enough to only be patient and accept↓♥ to advance at my own pace and avoid putting pressure on myself while making changes necessary for my well-being.

RHINITIS *See: COLD [HEAD]*

RHINOPHARYNGITIS *See: THROAT — PHARYNGITIS*

RIBS

The **ribs** are a part of the **rib** cage. They protect the **heart♥** and the lungs (vital organs) against damage and external injuries and aggressions.

A **fractured** or **split rib** therefore indicates that protection is diminished and that I am vulnerable to external pressures against **Love**, my autonomy and my need for space. I have exceeded my limits or have allowed others to overwhelm me. I feel stuck between myself (my spiritual and emotional **sides**)

---

2. **Bouillaud** (Jean-Baptiste): French physician (1796–1881). He was the first to demonstrate the link between polyarthritis and endocarditis in his book, published in 1840, *Clinical Treatise of Articular Rheumatism and the Law of Coincidences of Heart Inflammations with this Disease*. **Bouillaud** recommended, in cases of heart♥ affections of acute articular rheumatism, a curious treatment based on blood-letting and leeches.

and the physical world in which I live. I feel fragile and open to all forms of attacks. I may feel that I have no control over my life, I am short of resources and exposed to danger. **Contusions** occur in moments of great fatigue and weakness, mainly when I feel injured by life: it is a physical trace of an inner injury. I want to cry out my pain and my sorrow. Often, when I **fracture** or **split** a **rib**, I experience a special situation involving a member of my family. It is often a situation where I compare myself to someone else: I don't feel up to the mark, '**rib** to **rib**'. I under-estimate myself or I have the impression that others are demeaning me. "Do people really like and esteem me? The location of the affected **rib** will give me an indication of the person concerned. If it is the **lower ribs**, there is probably a conflict with a child or a grandchild. A **middle rib** (lateral) represents instead a conflicted situation involving a brother or sister or a cousin (collaterals) and the **upper ribs** represent a parent or a grandparent. If the affected **rib** is in front of the body (**anterior part**) or the sternum is affected, there is something in my future that is creating a great tension or worry for me, such as actions to be taken for example, or the impediments that the authorities could use to oppose the implementation of some of my projects. If it is located **on my flanks** or in the **central part**, the situation is occurring in the present moment. If it is in the **rear** or **posterior part**, there are feelings from my past that still greatly affect me. I identify the situations that are creating so much pressure. I ask myself what person or situation has exerted such a pressure on me that one or several of my **ribs** were **broken** or **split** because it was too much. I should have distanced and detached myself from this source of pressure because I could no longer stand it. I must ask myself if it is the others, or I, imposing this on me. I am seeking my place in society and I am facing a duality between the image I must project and what I really am. Do I remain in the superficial, or do I decide to live according to my deeper values? Am I always trying to win a good popularity rating with others? I doubt myself and I tend to revolt. I am rather rigid instead of heeding my inner voice and living spontaneously.

I accept↓♥ to look at the event simply and to express frankly what I feel while listening to others. I know now that communication is a tool that enables me to respect myself while respecting others. I stop comparing myself with others and I accept↓♥ to be myself. I am the only person who can have power over me!

RICKETS / RACHITISM

Rickets is a disease of growth affecting the skeleton and caused by insufficient bone mineralization (a metabolism disorder of phosphorus and calcium) due to a deficiency in vitamin D.

If I am affected by this disease, the physical malnutrition I am experiencing highlights the one I am sustaining on a personal and affective level. I have the impression that what I produce with my creativity or my sexuality has no vitality. I am experiencing a void or a lack of tenderness and **Love**. I may feel that I am alone in the world and nobody understands me. I therefore do not have the support I need and I feel vulnerable. As a result, I live for others. I feel inferior to others and it is easy to play the martyr. This disease affects me mostly as a child and highlights the fact that my mother can experience the same emotions as I do.

I must remember that I am constantly protected and that Universal **Love** is present all over. I must accept↓♥ this **Love** and let it nourish me so I can get rid of the disease, which by then will no longer have any reason to persist, for I will have understood that I must first give myself **Love** before I can give it to others. True wealth is within us.

RIGHT (I am)

If I manifest a permanent attitude of "**I am right"**, I must ask myself: "Why am I closed to the opinions of others? What do I want to protect myself from?" I must become **Aware** of the fact that the people around me can remain calm with me, keep their distance, take care to not offend me, and even go as far as to think that **I AM SICK**. The age of reason is said to arrive around age 7: "Can it be that a part of me has remained a child in my reasoning?"

I accept↓♥ that, by listening to others, giving myself a chance to change my mind and accepting↓♥ that others too can have worthy opinions, I increase my degree of **Love**, openness and freedom in mutual respect and sharing.

RIGHT SIDE *See: MALE PRINCIPLE*

RINGS UNDER THE EYES *See: EYES — RINGS [UNDER THE EYES]*

ROSACEA *See: SKIN — ACNE ROSACEA*

ROUNDED SHOULDERS

Rounded shoulders commonly give rise to names such as the '**Hunchback**'. In addition to what applies to **shoulder** pain, **rounded shoulders** symbolize the fact that I am backing down before life and its burden. I can no longer stand bearing all that weight and I believe it is hopeless. In addition to bearing all my many problems, I have the impression that I must also unfairly carry the burdens of the people around me. "Their fates are in my hands!" I still carry much guilt from my past. If my **shoulders** are also **tense**, there is a constant state of tension inside of me. I am thus constantly on the lookout, ready to deal with any unforeseen situation, and thus taking on the responsibility for the happiness of others. I expect something to fall on my head. I accept↓♥ that it is high time for me to take care of myself and let others take care of their own happiness. This form of pronounced **deviation of my spine** can also serve to remind me of an **obligation** of **humility**. Whatever the previous reasons for my condition, I must learn to develop humility, for this energy block originates from great past angers that still affect me today and are accompanied by much irritation about certain persons or situations.

As I am 100% responsible for what happens to me, I accept↓♥ my choice, consciously or not. It is no doubt the greatest challenge of my life. I am attuned to my inner voice and it guides me in what I must do to be happier. A massage or an energy treatment can help me to center myself in the present and to make contact with my higher self to acknowledge my own needs.

RUBELLA / GERMAN MEASLES *See: CHILDHOOD DISEASES*

RHYTHM (cardiac) DISORDER *See: HEART♥ — CARDIAC ARRHYTHMIA*

S

SACRUM *See: BACK DISORDERS — LOWER BACK*

SADISM *See: SADOMASOCHISM*

SADNESS *See also: BLOOD / CHOLESTEROL / DIABETES / HYPOGLYCEMIA, GRIEF, MELANCHOLY*

Sadness is defined as "a natural or accidental state of sorrow or melancholy".

It is important to remember that "everything that is not expressed is imprinted". An unexpressed **sadness** may lead me to a lung disorder. A deep **sadness** can lead me to become **diabetic**. It is my entire body that refuses the joy of living. I only focus my attention on the dullness of everyday life. I feel that nothing smiles at me, I feel the bleakness permeating me, my **heart♥** tearing itself apart; this immense void seems to want to increase inside of me to make room for this knot of pain. I am disconnected from my creative power. I am submitting to life instead of taking action.

I accept↓♥ to let this **sadness** break out, I need some 'spiciness' in my life, some heat that will make all the tears in me start to boil up and leave my body, as steam rises to the sky. I can thus fill this void of gentleness and tenderness. As the dark thoughts dissipate, I recover my dynamism and my joy in living.

SADOMASOCHISM

Sadomasochism involves a relationship where one of the partners expresses their **domination** (**sadism**) and the other expresses their **submission** (**masochism**).

If I am a **masochist**, I derive my sexual pleasure from physical or psychological suffering that I undergo voluntarily, which gives me the sense of having some power or hold over the other. Deep down, I feel really empty, incapable of creating my life and having satisfying relations with others, at all levels. I have this same feeling of powerlessness if I am a **sadistic** person, but it expresses itself differently. I developed a hard side to protect myself from others. From early on, I had to defend myself from certain persons who exercised power over me. I had to repress my emotions and my pain. While growing up, I wanted to punish others for my past. By engaging in **sadomasochism**, I sometimes find a sort of balance in my relations. However, if I feel the need to engage in this form of relation, I certainly want to free myself from a suffering or some inner stress and even, in some cases, from a suicidal impulse, either by exercising control or submitting to it. I thus free myself from certain anxieties. A part of me is still in its period of adolescence: I rebel and I want to show others that I am under control. There is also a pleasurable side to the pain. Is that truly what I want in my life? These programs risk appearing again in my life at the most unexpected moments. Thus, under high stress conditions, I may identify control or submission as the solution. I must beware of the fact that **I become whatever I focus my attention on**. This behavior, which may appear negative, can risk amplifying these negative attitudes in me.

I accept↓♥ to develop, in my subconscious, the following program: I feel free when I am controlling and I feel better afterward; or in the other case, I feel free when I am 'willingly' submissive and I feel better afterward. I accept↓♥ my desire to free myself from my fears and limitations, and that I should develop humility more than submission, and be guided rather than controlling. I can thus seek satisfaction for my greater personal well-being.

SALIVA (in general) *See also: GLANDS [SALIVARY], MUMPS*

Saliva has the power to eliminate the development of microbes. By its moisturizing power, it can also facilitate the production of sounds in the throat and makes swallowing food easier. It promotes the first stage of digestion by transforming starches. Too much, or not enough, **saliva** makes it ineffective and useless. If I suffer from depression, I often tend to eat quickly and swallow my food whole, which provokes a shortage of **saliva** and a sensation of choking. I always feel that '**my mouth is watering**' or that '**my tongue is hanging out**' for something or someone without my desires ever being appeased.

I accept↓♥ to trust myself in my decisions, to decide that I will allow joy to enter and replace my regrets, and to move ahead confidently. By taking action to get what I want, I give back to my **saliva** all its power.

SALIVA — HYPER- and HYPOSALIVATION *See also: MOUTH DISEASE*

Hyposalivation is a lack of **saliva**. **Saliva** is the watery, somewhat viscous fluid that moistens the mouth and the food we eat. The salivary glands secrete the **saliva** that helps digestion. I can breathe through my mouth instead of through my nose. This results in drying the mouth and the upper airways.

As the mouth represents my opening on life, I can ask myself in what respects my desires or my appetites are currently 'dried out' and why they are not appearing in my life as I would like them to. I may find that life's events are not nourishing me enough and that I am losing interest in my life. If it is **hypersalivation**, I ask myself if my mouth is often 'watering': I have plenty of fantasies, desires and projects, but they are late in taking form. I need affection. I want to say and do all sorts of things, but I feel limited in my actions. I am looking out because I doubt myself. My great need for **Love**, even unconscious, can express itself outwardly by **hypersalivation** during the night. In any case, I feel under tension and I am dissatisfied about my relation with every living being and with life itself. I need different experiences to be 'satiated'.

I accept↓♥ to become **Aware** of the gifts of life and freedom that I have. Life gives me everything I need to properly integrate the situations I experience. I leave aside the opinions of others and live spontaneously. I savor the present moment. I enjoy life; I slake my thirst and taste each instant of happiness. I make peace with all these inner desires and I am taking action to make them realities.

SALMONELLOSIS / TYPHOID *See also: INDIGESTION, INFECTIONS (IN GENERAL), INTESTINE — DIARRHEA, NAUSEA, POISONING [FOOD]*

Salmonellosis is an infection that starts in digestion, with a contamination originating in fouled water or food. Its most severe forms are **typhoid** and the **paratyphoids**. The symptoms are varied: vomiting, diarrhea and infectious and toxic syndromes.

I can ask myself what is causing me to experience so much irritability. Though I could easily believe I am not responsible for this happening to me, since it was the food that was infected (an external cause), I must remember that chance doesn't exist, and that the external elements are only here to help me trigger the ailment I am currently experiencing in my life over a situation "that I can't digest and that makes me angry". I am living on the defensive and I am extremely tense. I feel in prison, powerless to take action on the spot. A situation, often involving my family, sickens me and, as I can't express myself, the illness serves to expel what no longer suits me. I am full of irritations. I seek out my true origins, I want to return to my origins or my beliefs, but I am prevented from doing so. I am revolted against this 'foul name' that I bear because I have the impression that it prevents me from doing certain things. I must be up to the task and stay within the limits of what is 'acceptable'. I allow myself to be devoured by society and its rules. I must express what I feel, the emotions that are increasingly invading me and infecting me, for I no longer see any solution. I am carrying a lot on my shoulders! My life is a whirl of emotions.

I accept↓♥ to put harmony back into this situation that I have been able to identify; my health will thus be improved. I will be richer with an experience that helps me develop more wisdom. By acknowledging my worth and accepting↓♥ myself as I am, I feel safe and I radiate peace and well-being.

SALPINGITIS *See also: CHRONIC ILLNESS, FEMALE DISORDERS, INFECTIONS (IN GENERAL)*

Salpingitis is an acute or chronic infection of the **uterine** (**Fallopian**) **tubes**.

The **tubes** symbolize the encounter with my spouse and the communication it can generate. This disease is often related to impotence involving a sexual partner. Do I sense or fear that my sexual partner is cheating on me? Do I suspect that someone close to me, such as my spouse, my father or one of my brothers, or a friend, has tricked or betrayed me by their attitudes or actions, making anger rise in me? Whatever the situation, it very often involves some aspect of sexuality that I found **despicable** or **degrading**. As the tubes are the meeting place of the seeds of the woman and the man, I have a relational difficulty with certain encounters in my everyday life. I feel that the bases of my couple are very weak. Can we have children some day? Or keep our family united?

I accept↓♥ to put some **Love** in the situation to be able to see the truth in the experience that life brings me. I will thus find myself happier, with more joy in living and serenity.

SARCOIDOSIS

Sarcoidosis, also called **Besnier-Boeck-Schaumann's**[1] **disease**, a rare illness, mainly attacks the skin and the lymph ganglions.

I am going through a period of changes, I find it difficult to adjust and I get discouraged because I feel that the 'housecleaning' isn't getting done fast enough. I ask myself how far I can go in my self-assertion and how far I should struggle for my beliefs. This makes me depreciate myself and I alternate between periods of submission and aggressiveness in the actions I take. I would like to "eat my cake and have it, too".

I accept↓♥ to make place for something new; and to do so, I must dare to let go of what is no longer beneficial for me. This may include both material things and my way of thinking, which is sometimes closed and criticizing. I learn to make choices based on where I am, here and now. I fully stand by my choices and I know that I am the maker of my own happiness.

SARCOMA (Ewing's) *See: BONES (CANCER OF THE) —EWING'S SARCOMA*

SARS (severe acute respiratory syndrome) *See also: LUNGS — PNEUMONIA, RESPIRATION*

The **severe acute respiratory syndrome (SARS)** is a serious lung infection characterized by the sudden onset of a fever exceeding 100°F and respiratory symptoms: coughing, breathlessness and difficulty in breathing.

I am afraid, breathing poorly, choking and running a fever. My temperature rises when I feel trapped somewhere, in my couple, at work or elsewhere. I know I must reconsider my vital space because the situation in which I am is choking me. I am afraid to settle or to commit myself. I feel invaded by all sorts of people who poison my existence. It is becoming urgent for me to be more **Aware** of certain things and free myself from these fears so that I can fully take charge of my existence. I ask myself questions about my fears regarding commitment.

I accept↓♥ to consider the situations where I can find 'my' place, or that the time has come for me to disengage myself, to let go, to break off or to change something in my behavior. I learn to choose myself based on my needs and I recover my state of harmony by breathing with full lungs.

---

1. **Besnier** (Ernest Henri): A French dermatologist (1831–1909). **Boeck** (Caesar Peter Moller): A Swedish dermatologist (1845–1917). **Schaumann** (Jörgen Nilsen): A Swedish dermatologist (1879–1953).

SCABIES *See: SKIN — SCABIES*

SCALP *See: DANDRUFF, HAIR — TINEA, SKIN — ITCHING*

SCAPULA / SHOULDER BLADE

The **scapula** (or **shoulder blade**) is a flat, wide, thin bone that is part of the skeleton. With the clavicle, the **scapula** joins the arm to the trunk.

Pain in this location can indicate a revolt against authority, for I feel stuck or crushed by it. **Difficulties** (**fractures** or other) in the **scapula** may originate from an opposition between what I am, represented by the trunk, and what I want to express, embodied by my arms, which are the extensions of my **heart♥**'s energy. **Tensions** (or **knots**) in the **left scapula** indicate that I am in disagreement with my spouse or my children, and **tensions** in the **right scapula** indicate that something is thwarting me at work. An **ailment in the scapula** indicates that I tend to let myself be 'trampled on' or 'walked on'. I need a ***shield*** to protect myself. There is a situation in my life where I feel totally inferior to others, less good, less competent. I live passively, which diminishes my energy level.

I accept↓♥ to consider what I am overall, in order to show harmony in my life, in the actions I take. I take some time to calmly meditate and do some introspection into who I truly am. I learn to be comfortable with solitude, for it allows me to regain contact with my divine essence. I will more easily express my needs later on.

SCAR *See: SKIN — SCARS*

SCARLET FEVER / SCARLATINA *See: CHILDHOOD DISEASES (IN GENERAL)*

SCHIZOPHRENIA *See: PSYCHOSIS — SCHIZOPHRENIA*

SCIATIC *nerve See: NERVE [SCIATIC]*

SCLERODERMIA *See: SKIN — SCLERODERMIA*

SCLEROSIS *See also: INFLAMMATION, SYSTEM [IMMUNE]*

Sclerosis is a hypertrophy that hardens the conjunctive tissue that is necessary and present in the whole body.

It is important to become **Aware** that if I am affected by this disease, it is me that I am attacking, which may induce the **sclerosis** to extend to most of my organs. This hypertrophy provokes a sort of burning energy that brings out long-repressed rage. The tissues harden, which suggests the hardening of my thoughts and attitudes, thus creating an energy imbalance. I also harden my positions toward life and the people around me. I am inflexible and find it very difficult to adjust to new situations. I prefer to ***cling*** to my old ways or thinking. I no longer have the same flexibility, mainly about what goes on in my family. I may feel invaded by others. My whole body or any of its parts may be affected by **sclerosis**. It is therefore important for me to become **Aware** of what I am experiencing inside. My closing myself to **Love** may indicate that I feel unworthy of this **Love**, that I feel guilty and am ashamed of living.

I accept↓♥ to open myself to **Love**, I acknowledge my divine worth, I am everything, I am capable of everything. I reconnect myself with my curiosity and with what makes me passionate.

SCLEROSIS (lateral amyotrophic) *See: CHARCOT'S DISEASE*

SCLEROSIS (multiple)

Multiple sclerosis is defined as a demyelination[2] of the myelin sheath surrounding the body's nerve fibers including the brain and the spinal cord, by an apparently auto-immune inflammatory process. The entire body is affected and the attacks (bouts) may occur at different moments of the person's life.

It is as though my body were ***trapped***, placed in a cage and increasingly limited in its sequences of movements. If I have **multiple sclerosis**, I am generally affected by great suffering that makes me see life in discouraging terms. Something or someone is paralyzing me and I feel stuck. I am no longer ***dashing*** into life. Life is short on sweetness and honey. A deep revolt animates my whole being. I feel compelled to do everything myself; being a perfectionist and intransigent, I refuse to make mistakes and I barely accept↓♥ help. I find it difficult to accept↓♥ constraints, especially those that come from my family. I have an ironclad willpower. I become **Aware** that for this to be so, I must be very hard on my thoughts and remain distanced from my emotions. Any thought of failure terrifies me. I have difficulty in forgiving myself and forgiving others. I may chide myself for having allowed an opportunity to slip by. I fear being left behind or ditched. **I am very afraid of being 'dropped'**. I may also be afraid of falling, in the proper as well as the figurative sense, and fear that this fall may lead to death. All these fears involving a vertical displacement and leading me to believe that my life is in danger can trigger **multiple sclerosis**. It may be a fall from a ***ladder***, the risk of falling into a chasm, a sudden loss of altitude in a plane, something falling on my head, etc. Symbolically, 'falling in **Love'** or my 'plunging popularity' becomes dangerous for me. A fall can thus be physical, moral or symbolic. I find all these situations ***upsetting*** and ***distressing*** and I am ***staggered***. I am afraid of falling from a great height or having 'death fall on me'. I may also feel ***degraded*** by someone else or I am afraid of losing my grades or a privileged position at work, for instance. I feel I no longer have a future. Very often, I may judge myself or judge others very severely, which leaves me with **a great feeling of depreciation, of being belittled as a person.** When I feel ***diminished***, I have the impression that life is crushing

---

2. **Demyelination**: A diminishing of myelin, the protective substance made up of lipids (a form of fat) and proteins that encases certain nerve fibres.

me and I tend to ***crawl*** instead of standing straight. I may even stop and ***come to a halt***, no longer having the strength to advance, to ***move*** myself. It is thus in my legs that the disease shows its first signs and that I may have the impression of being crushed. Being less and less capable of ***walking*** and moving about may give me the feeling that I am no longer safe this way. The fact of no longer being able to move forward may prevent me from facing a situation that I want to avoid at all costs. For instance, if I don't have the physical capacity to rescue a company in difficulty, it allows me to avoid once again facing a failure in which I would depreciate myself. Whatever my age, I am not allowed to undertake projects, grow, or give my opinion. I take on my shoulders the burden of achieving the desires of my mother or my father: I become "their arms and their legs". I quickly realize that I am powerless to play this role. I reach the point of not finding myself good enough for them. My defense against all these inner fears will be to **want to control everything**, to want everything to go as I want it to. **Criticism**, often directed against myself, imprisons my life. I believe that suffering is part of my everyday lot and that I don't deserve any rest. My efforts to surpass myself are constant and nevertheless always insufficient. My tired body thus refuses to pursue this 'struggle of the strongest' and wants to make me understand that I may also need others and that I must learn to trust. I resist happiness and acknowledging my worth. I repudiate myself. The fact that I have already been disparaged and ***belittled*** makes me believe that I am not worth much. I am like a tree that bends. I feel wiped out. I destroy myself so much in thought that now, it is the disease that is destroying me. Inflammation implies a **burning** and very emotional rage that can affect my whole existence. I can ask myself: "Do I really want to be free?" This way, I can unconsciously take revenge on someone who ***gravitates*** in my world and hasn't shown me enough **Love**! This form of cage in which my body finds itself possibly protects me from admitting my true feelings! By remaining silent this way, I feel compelled to take certain roads in order to please others instead of moving forward in the direction I want to take. Instead of being in movement and changing, I remain stagnant and inert. As I no longer want to feel anything, my sensory nerves are impaired. My emotional repression can lead me to become incapable of moving forward in my emotions, thus resulting in muscular and mental confusion. When I am affected by **multiple sclerosis**, I become dependent on others. I become like a child who needs someone to take care of its basic needs. I must ***cling*** to others and ***grab onto them*** to not fall, physically as well as emotionally. I must ask myself if my responsibilities as an adult are too heavy to bear. I may prefer to return to a state of dependence instead of always having to make efforts to get or keep what I possess. I was so happy when my mother looked after me. I found her ***admirable***. But I will never again see the gentleness in her eyes. I now have the feeling that my life is endlessly agitated and ***effervescent***. My body tells me to let go, to free myself from my chains. The key is inside of me. I accept↓♥ to trust my inner guide and I recognize in each person the presence of this guide, which leads everyone to act to the best of their knowledge. I then manifest more flexibility and understanding.

I accept↓♥ to give meaning to my life. I take charge of my life again by fully standing up for my feelings. The approval of others is no longer ***necessary***. I welcome the feelings inside of me. They are part of me. I leave behind me the negative comments that may have been voiced about me, from my family as well as my whole entourage. I give myself more gentleness. I follow the flow of life and its sweetness, which enables me to ***develop*** harmoniously. I drop my clown's costume to allow my inner **Light** to shine. My inner ***peace*** grows every day.

SCOLIOSIS *See: SPINE [DEVIATION] — SCOLIOSIS*

SCROTUM *See: TESTICLES*

SCRUPLES

Scruples are found in persons who experience concerns about their consciences; my **Soul is hurting**, I fret a lot. I am full of doubts. I am constantly analyzing myself. This lowers my level of energy and it may have the effect of provoking or accelerating the appearance of the 'twilight of my life' (old age).

I accept↓♥ to choose to live in harmony and to digest new ideas; I regain my liveliness!

SEA SICKNESS *See also: TRAVEL SICKNESS*

Seasickness is the sensation of not having control over a situation, of being tossed about by life's events, a feeling of losing everything. Not having 'both feet planted on the ground', I feel insecurity taking on even greater proportions when I feel uneasy about the future and everything unfamiliar. It shows itself in bouts of nausea. I must ask myself what I can't digest or what I feel like rejecting and haven't accepted↓♥. By fleeing my own emotions and the essence of each thing, I avoid feeling confident and well-anchored in life. I am like a boat that lets itself drift at the mercy of the winds. It is not I who decides which road I will follow, but I let external events take care of it, hence my feeling of insecurity. I feel resentful toward others but basically, I reproach myself for living in impotence. I must ask myself what suffering I feel in relation to my **mother**. Maybe she has left her physical body and I miss her presence. Or our relationship may be tense or conflicted. It also happens quite often that any **travel sickness** (**boat**, **plane**, **auto**, **train**, etc.) is related to my fear (**conscious** or unconscious) of death.

I accept↓♥ to look inside of me to find the answers to my questions. I stop destroying myself with my negative thoughts and the severe way I judge myself.

SELF-MUTILATION *See also: AMPUTATION*

Self-mutilation is a behavior that leads me to inflict injuries or lesions on myself. This attitude may originate from a previously disturbed mental condition, as with psychotics, schizophrenics or mentally deficient children.

However, it may derive from the fact that I feel great guilt in my life, possibly associated with a great irritability turned against myself because I don't feel worthy of being who I am. The hate and anger I feel against myself and the fact of wanting to punish myself and having to suffer are highlighted in my acts of **self-mutilation**. Instead of expressing myself with words, I use **self-mutilation** as a means for expressing my frustrations. I may also use these injuries I inflict on myself to attract attention, which I equate with **Love**. It is as though I wanted to physically manifest my inner suffering in order to free myself from it and bring to **Light** my need to be loved. It may be that even when I was still very young, I took on the role of the victim who deserves to suffer. Life will therefore bring me persons and situations who will make me feel this way. I certainly need outside help in such situations.

I accept↓♥ to ask for outside help and I seek out in my entourage who could help me, directly or indirectly, to recover my self-esteem and the joy in living that I too have the right to take pleasure in. I accept↓♥ to emerge from my silence and express my pain and my suffering in order to free myself from them.

SENESCENCE *See: AGING [AILMENTS OF]*

SENILITY

When I am an elderly person and my physical and psychic faculties are impaired, the condition is called **senility**.

Senility is a disease that can be related to escape. By returning to childhood, I am returning to the security it brings me. I thus choose to let others take care of me and I want them to take me in charge. I already feel helpless in many areas, notably in my difficult communications with others. Instead of living passively as an adult, it is preferable for me to be considered as senile and thus to have a good reason for people taking care of me, with people now treating me as a child. I ask myself: "Was my life worth living? What still remains for me to achieve?"

If I am already impaired by **senility**, I accept↓♥ to become **Aware** that it is not necessary to flee. If I want to reap this attention I want so much, I myself must sow it around me. I benefit from divine protection and I live in peace and security. At each moment of my life, I become **Aware** of the force of the Universe. I can create my life as I want it: I need only take charge of myself and ask for any necessary help in achieving my dreams.

SEPTICEMIA *See: BLOOD — SEPTICEMIA*

SEXUAL DEVIATIONS and PERVERSIONS (in general)

As an individual, I am struggling with a **sexual deviation**, because I wish to reject and repress a large part of my being, and I am constantly waging an inner struggle. I was often injured in my life and I don't realize that I have deviated the accumulated frustration. I feel a prisoner of my pain, of my strict education, of society's rules and of my own limitations, and I want to expand my feeling of freedom and power. My body thereby tells me to accept↓♥ each aspect of me that I associate with a defect.

Each human being possesses a male side and a female side. If I am a man, I accept↓♥ my feminine side, or my masculine side if I am a woman. I become humble and I decide to assert myself without hurting others. I choose to unify my whole being, for each facet of me needs to express itself.

SEXUAL FRUSTRATIONS, ABSENCE of DESIRE *See also: EJACULATION [PREMATURE]*

Often due to a very strict education regarding everything related to sexuality, I sincerely believe that the **sexual** organs are immoral and dirty, and I feel guilt. I may also suffer from a 'performance complex', and the more I try to improve myself, the less I succeed. I may resent the opposite sex, and denying my sexuality or refusing to experience it is my way of getting revenge: I won't give them any pleasure, they don't deserve it! Thus, it is me that I am punishing and cutting off from my vital needs. I may sense a **diminishing or an absence of sexual desire (anaphrodisia)**. My disappointments and lack of interest in life lead me to experience the same thing in my sexuality. It may be a certain level of depression that derives from my negativity toward myself and others.

It is best for me that I accept↓♥ to experience my sexuality in a healthy manner, as it is part of my quality of life. I take the time to do things that please me and give me satisfaction. My zest for life and the good things will thus be **awakened**, along with my taste for intimate and **sexual** relations.

SHINGLES / HERPES ZOSTER *See: SKIN — SHINGLES / HERPES ZOSTER*

SHORT-BOWEL SYNDROME *See: INTESTINAL AILMENTS*

SHOULDERS (in general) *See also: JOINTS*

The **shoulders** represent my capacity to bear a load. My **shoulders carry my joys, my sorrows, my responsibilities and my insecurities**. They refer to the burden of my actions or of those I wish to undertake. As any other person, I am not exempt from carrying a burden. If I make myself responsible for the happiness and well-being of others, I then increase the weight I carry and my **shoulders** will hurt. I feel that I have too much to do and I am never able to get everything done. I may also have the impression that people are imposing things on me or preventing me from acting, either because of different opinions or they simply don't want to assist and support me in my projects. I feel blocked. I often have the impression I am being given '***slaps***' in the face and I can't stand it any longer. I feel powerless and I have the impression that I must 'ground arms'. It is as though people wanted to ***shoot*** me. I see my life hazily and can no longer see all my good qualities. I also have sore **shoulders** when I expedience great affective insecurity (left **shoulder**) or material insecurity (right **shoulder**) or if I feel crushed by the weight of my responsibilities, affective as well as material. I don't feel **supported.** I am locked into a structure and I can't 'break down the door' to get out of it. I am so afraid of tomorrow that I forget to live today. The difficulties I run into and the responsibility of having to create, do and succeed, all this can 'crush' me. I may want to prove to myself that I can nevertheless face up to situations with my **shoulders** squared back and my chest pushed out, but in fact, my back is weak and twisted by fear. I constantly impose perfection on myself, and I even can go so far as to 'flog' myself emotionally if I feel I have slacked off. I may reproach myself for not having been able to keep under my wing a person who is dear to me. I feel much remorse and 'I should of's. I am anxious and I worry too much about the future. If the affected part of my **shoulder** involves the bones (**fracture**, **break**), it will be more related to my basic responsibilities. If the affected part of my **shoulder** concerns the **muscles**, it will be more related to my thoughts and emotions. I also learn to allow the energy of my **heart♥** to circulate to my **shoulders** and into my arms, which will prevent rigidity and pain, for my **shoulders** represent action and also movement, from design to matter. It is through them that my inner desires to express myself, to create and carry out pass, for they originated in my **heart ♥**. The emotional energy must reach into my arms and hands in order to carry out those desires. If I hold back from saying or doing things, if I 'coop myself up'[3] instead of plunging into life, if I wear masks to disguise my fears and apprehensions, my **shoulders** will be tense and more rigid. If it **hurts** especially **when I raise my arms**, I have difficulty in being autonomous and 'flying with my own wings'. My personal identity is called into question not only for myself but also for others, mostly my family, who will sometimes attack me and leave me unbalanced. If my **shoulder bone** is **cracked, fractured or broken**, there is a very deep conflict in my life involving the essence of what I am. I ask too much of myself. I want too much to have control, and the burdens are too heavy to bear. A **tension** or any other ailment I may have in the region of the **shoulders** gives me different indications depending on whether it affects the right or the left **shoulder**. If my **right shoulder** is affected, it is my active male side: I may be experiencing a conflict or a tension over my work or my way of reacting to authority. I depreciate myself about my role or my status, in relation to my family, my couple or society. It is the 'stiff and controlling side' that gets the upper hand, whereas if my **left shoulder** is affected, the tension I feel involves the female, creative and receptive side of my life and my ability to express my feelings. I belittle my image or my own capacity for being a good child for my parents. A **frozen shoulder** means that it is becoming cold and is hindered in its complete use. Do I become cold and indifferent to what I do (just to do it?) or do I really want to do it? There is a deep tension indicating that I really want to do something other than what I am currently doing.

---

3. **I coop myself up**: To confine, especially in a small place. In the figurative sense, it means *to withdraw into oneself.*

I become **Aware** of what is crushing me, I accept↓♥ that I am responsible for ME and I leave to others the task of looking after their own happiness. I immediately stop trying to 'carry the world on my **shoulders'** and I learn to delegate. I also accept↓♥ to learn how to live in the present instant, which enables me to lighten the burden I carry on my **shoulders**. I trust the Universe that provides for my everyday needs.

SINUS (pilonidal) *See also: BACK DISORDERS — LOWER BACK, INFECTIONS (IN GENERAL)*

The **pilonidal sinus** is an infection of my body hair over the muscle near the coccyx, at the base of the spine.

I am feeling frustration, irritation or revolt over a situation where I find my basic needs in danger, as they can't be provided for as I want. This state of deprivation may remind me of a situation from my early childhood, which could even go back to when I was a fetus and where, then too, I had the impression that I was deprived of something or someone who was vital for me at that time. It may be a physical element such as a warm place to stay or comfortable clothes; it may also be of an affective nature, such as the **Love** and tenderness of my parents.

Whatever the situation, it is important for me to accept↓♥ to ask the Universe to help me fill all my basic needs, and for me to trust it completely. I must also accept↓♥ that I experienced a situation of deprivation when I was younger, but which was there to teach me to develop my faith and help me appreciate everything I possessed and possess today and of which I must become **Aware**.

SINUSITIS *See: NOSE — SINUSITIS*

SKELETON *See: BONES*

SKIN (in general)

Skin covers my entire body and delimits what is 'inside' from what is 'outside', namely my individuality. By its surface size, my **skin** is the most salient organ of my body.

It is a protective layer that precisely defines my vital space and faithfully and unconsciously allows my inner state to show through: it is therefore a link in my relation with my entourage (I in my relation to others). My **skin** is the extension of my felt experience, of my inner sensitivity. It is the mirror of my inner life, my calling card. It analyzes all contact information. If I am a gentle person, so will my **skin**. If I am very highly sensitive, my **skin** will also be very **sensitive**. On the contrary, if I am rather hard with myself or with others, my **skin** too will be **hard and thick**. If my **skin** is **irritated**, then someone or something in my life is irritating me. Great insecurity makes my **skin sweaty**, whereas **skin** that **perspires a lot** evacuates the emotions that I hold back and that I need to release. A **disease** that '**touches**' my **skin** indicates that I am experiencing difficulties in communicating with my entourage. I feel a loss in my soundness of health. The state of my **skin** indicates the state of my relations with others. My individuality is called into question, my intimacy and my vulnerability may be threatened. What are my limits? What are my zones of intolerance? My **skin** reacts when I need to touch and be touched, and I experience a deprivation in that respect. That is why I may develop ***eczema*** or ***psoriasis*** at the time of a **separation**, for instance: my **skin** is experiencing stress; it is in a state of need and becomes red with anger, not understanding why it is not receiving affection and tenderness. I am feeling an immense affective **coldness** and having difficulty in ***acclimatizing*** to my new life or my new situation. The quality of my relations with the outside world will thus be represented by the state of my **skin**.

SKIN DISEASES

Skin is like the bark of a tree. It shows us that there are outer or inner problems. It insulates the cells and other elements of my body from my outer environment.

If my **skin** has **anomalies**, chances are high that I am a person who puts great store in the opinions of others and in what they may say about me. As I am unsure of myself and fear being rejected or hurt, I will create a **skin** disease that will become a 'natural barrier' and enable me to maintain a certain distance from my entourage. I want so much to ***join*** a group, my family, my work colleagues, etc., but having poor self-esteem, I create a distance before being rejected. I suffer from the ***absence*** of contact with my mother and I may want to place the blame on my ***father***. As **skin** is a soft tissue that is related to mental energy, it expresses my insecurities, my uncertainties and my deepest concerns. It is important to see what layer of the **skin** is affected, especially in the case of **burns**. An impairment of the **epidermis** refers to a situation where a difficult separation took place; the **dermis** refers, rather, to an event that I perceived as dirty, unclean. Lastly, when the **hypodermis** is affected, therefore closer to the bones, there will be self-depreciation and a diminishing of my self-esteem. The **skin** therefore constantly reflects my inner feelings, hence the expression "being red with anger". My **skin** can change **color** when I am embarrassed or feeling ashamed. It is therefore my physical demarcation line, the mask between my inner and outer sides. If my **skin is dry**, it is because it is lacking in water. Water is the second element (after air) necessary to life. My relations with life are therefore dry and arid. I block myself inside from my relations with my entourage. I may have the impression of 'drying out on the spot'. I hold in my emotions so much (from which I want to cut myself off), rather than allow them to show through my **skin**, that it becomes **dry**, emotionally '**out of gas**'. I must seek joy in my communications with others. **Sweaty skin** expresses a '**skin**-deep emotion'. Flaky **dead skin** (dander, scales) indicates that I let myself follow old mental patterns. If I experience a stressful situation, I tend to fly off in all directions and scatter myself. If **pimples** mark the surface of my **skin**, it is because I am outwardly expressing problems of relations and communications with my entourage, dealing with specific issues. If my **skin** shows signs of **inflammation**, I must then become less irritated with certain situations of inner or outer conflict. If my **skin is oily**, it is because I am holding in too many emotions to myself. In this case, there is an overflow of emotions that expresses itself outwardly despite me. I may want to escape a situation or a person as though someone were trying to catch me, like the little oiled piglet we try to catch and that slips from our fingers. I don't want to be touched. It is therefore a sort of protection. A **hypersecretion of sebum** also indicates my 'adolescent', immature attitude when my emotions are concerned. I am very nervous and don't know what to do. I must allow the energy to circulate so that my negative thoughts can disappear. When my **skin** is affected, it is important that I ask myself if I am experiencing a situation of separation where I fear being separated from someone or something that I "have under my **skin**" and finding myself all alone. It may be a physical separation: for example, my spouse gets a promotion and must move somewhere else. It may also be the fact that I feel separated from a person because of an absence of communication; thus, I may live in the same house as my spouse or my children, but I am feeling a sore emptiness because a great divide separates us and I have the impression that I am living alone. This solitude is often due to the fact that I have withdrawn into my shell, feeling greater insecurity. I then tend to view situations negatively and to mope. I have the impression that I have been **riddled** with blows or that someone wanted to '***screen***'[4] me. It may also result in a loss of sensitivity in the **skin**. **Scratches** or **scrapes** show that I feel torn, '**skinned** alive' inside. I allow myself to be scratched, I don't take my own space enough, and it would be in my interest to set my limits and to make others respect me. By constantly making compromises, I place myself in a position of inferiority and I perceive life as unfair. When my **skin** is under attack, it may react by cutting off its sensitivity to protect itself. For instance, if I have experienced unwanted fondling, my **skin** may want to 'freeze' this region and no longer be able to feel it, in order to avoid remembering this unpleasant situation. Or on the contrary, my **skin** may be **hyper-sensitive**, and the way to protect myself will be to flee, or retreat from, certain situations (to not go in the sun or to have to wear a hat, for example). This is the case, for instance, when I have **freckles**: often, I may feel stained or dirty. This may apply on the moral, affective or physical levels. I may also have the impression that I have tarnished the image of my family for instance, and that by "not making any noise" or by conforming to the expectations of others, I can make up for it. I must take a calm, cool look at the frustrations I harbor so that my **skin** can be cleared and less thick. The more transparent and the truer I become with others, the more transparent my **skin** will be. **Itching** shows me that there are one or several irritating thoughts surfacing on my **skin** and that I must look at them straight on so that they will stop drawing my attention and bothering me. If there are any **changes of color on my skin**, I ask myself to what extent I accept↓♥ my

---

4. **Being screened**: To be carefully inspected.

sensitivity and my intuition. Do I see myself as 'awful'? Shame and guilt prevent me from living spontaneously. I force myself to engage in relationships that are not beneficial for me. My inner being cries out for freedom and the acceptance↓♥ of my whole being. If I have **red flushes**, my integrity is affected, and I would prefer so much to go unnoticed. I am being mocked, and I would like so much to be liked and to be up to the mark.

I accept↓♥ that, instead of buying small jars of so-called 'miracle creams', I will begin by appreciating my qualities and indulging myself with small delights: my **skin** will 'exude' this well-being through its smoothness and its clarity. The more capable I am of freely communicating my emotions, the more supple and radiant my **skin** is. I trust and accept↓♥ the **Love** of others. It is all a matter of attitude. I choose better quality in my relations with the outer world.

SKIN — ACNE *See also: FACE, SKIN / BLACKHEADS / PIMPLES*

Facial acne is related to **individuality** (head = individuality) and also to my inner harmony and to what is happening on the outside. My **face** is the part of me that others see first of myself and that enables me to be accepted↓♥ or rejected. **Acne** can surface when I am emotionally or mentally in conflict with my own reality, especially during adolescence when my personality is not yet fully formed. This conflict is related to self-expression and to my inner nature. **Acne** therefore **is a visible expression of irritation, criticism, resentment, rejection, fear, shame or insecurity, aimed at myself or others, and is a sign of non-acceptance↓♥ of myself. I find myself unattractive or sometimes even disgusting**. All these feelings are in ***effervescence*** inside of me. The inner revolution I am experiencing manifests itself by a revolution of pimples. These expressions are all linked to the assertion of my identity, to **Love** and to my unconditional self-acceptance↓♥. I reach the point where I find my life ***bitter***, constantly concerned about the image I project to others and that they have of me. Instead of experiencing freedom and movement, I retreat into my inner world with all my fears. **Acne** physically manifests itself on the epidermis through infected **skin** lesions. I know that ***fast food*** can promote **acne** and affect the functioning of my liver, the seat of anger. It reminds me that if I eat greedily, I am simply trying to fill an inner void. During adolescence **acne** is often related to inner changes I am living through and occurs at a moment in life when I must choose between the fear of opening up to myself and to others (resistances, choices, decisions) and therefore breaking away from all contact with others (often unconsciously), or to the changes I **must face** in my life, to adjustments related to my inner world and the view I have of my external world. No longer being a child and not yet being an adult, I may feel myself in an uncomfortable position in relation to **my self-image**. It may also be that I am afraid to **lose face** in front of the people around me and am worried about what others think or the judgments they may pass on me. Otherwise put, **acne** manifests itself by an unconscious fear of my sexuality, an attempt to externalize who I really am. I wish to be seen and noticed, but I am not going about it properly. As an adolescent, my behavior is to come into contact with others even if I fervently wish I were doing the opposite. I make myself unattractive to filter out people I do not want in my 'magnetic field' or environment; I set up barriers and only let in those I feel really well with; I want to be left in peace without bothering those I am unconsciously distancing myself from; I turn inwards and want to stay that way; I am not able to **love** myself enough, therefore others are not able to **love** me and I know that something is bothering me and is creating negativity under my **skin**; I compare myself to others and find all kinds of faults in myself (too fat, too big, etc.); I feel limited in my vital space and reject myself; I feel excessively controlled and directed by my parents. I easily rebel against authority and I reject the established rules. I identify with one of my parents to please the other, instead of taking on my own identity. I therefore cut myself off from a part of me. **Acne** can show up on different parts of the body. When it is **on my back**, it represents my past, my habits, my previous fears and anxieties. It is a way to reject myself. Or I may direct my rejection toward those who, I feel, do not provide me with moral support or are inconsiderate toward me. When it shows up at the **top of my back**, it represents repressed anger or annoyance, from which I am trying to find relief. **When it is on my chest**, it represents the future and what is in store for me. **Acne** signifies the **search for my vital space** and the **respect of others** toward it.

By accepting↓♥, at **heart♥**, the changes in myself, I listen to my basic needs (sexual or other) in a healthy and natural way. I will one day discover the person who meets my expectations. I must take my space with my **heart♥** and, if need be, express to others what my space is and how they can fit into my vital space. I accept↓♥ and **love** myself as I am, and stop wishing to please others at all costs. I accept↓♥ to go toward others and I allow them to approach me in complete safety.

SKIN — ACNE ROSACEA *See also: FACE, SKIN / BLACKHEADS / PIMPLES*

Acne rosacea is a **skin** lesion due to a congestion and dilation of small vessels. It is a disorder of the sebaceous glands. The cheeks and nose redden, followed by small pink-rimmed pimples. This form of **acne** is mostly found in women in their fifties. This inflammation in the face is often associated with an unhealthy diet, an excess of alcohol or cigarettes, and may also result from cirrhosis of the liver.

It is my anger manifesting itself, my frustrations over my feeling that nobody listens to me, that my opinion doesn't count, that I am not recognized. I feel cut off from my family and I resist their **Love** and marks of affection. I easily criticize, mainly about my own body, and I must wonder if I give myself the freedom to be myself. Do I express and accept↓♥ my differences? Do I accept↓♥ my femininity, or does it represent a danger for me? I dare to cut myself off from whom? From myself ? Why are my relations with others so complicated? What needs to be improved in my relations with others? Why this need to want to 'grab everything that goes by' (things as well as persons) and give so much importance to appearances and superficiality? I am very emotional and I complicate things for nothing. I am in a transition period and no longer recognize myself, I must adjust to a physical and emotional change. Am I in harmony with this change?

I choose to make peace with myself and I accept↓♥ the cycles of life. I reconnect with my divine essence and accept↓♥ to restore order and make peace with this movement of life. I learn to trust myself more and to truly appreciate who I am. By becoming more autonomous, I achieve my full creative potential.

SKIN — ACRODERMATITIS

Acrodermatitis is a **skin** disease that essentially affects the palms of the hands and the soles of the feet, where four of the 21 minor energy centers (chakras) of the body are located.

I ask myself questions about the sacrifices I impose on myself. Are they truly necessary? Can I offer my time and energy according to my needs and at my own pace? I have a very great sensitivity that can limit my capacity for managing the relations and events of my life. **Acrodermatitis** indicates a need to give more **Love** with my hands, especially to the members of my family, because the energy center located in the palm of each hand is an extension of the energy center of the **heart♥**, which represents **Love**.

I can learn a healing technique using the imposing of hands, which will help me to facilitate the circulation of this **Love** energy that I block for myself. I can also do manual creative activities, such as painting or drawing, to enable this energy to flow more freely through my hands. For the feet, I must envision myself as walking on sacred ground and allowing the energy that inhabits me to flow freely toward the earth, knowing that as I set off this energy circulating, I am also constantly receiving it.

SKIN — ACROKERATOSIS *See also: SKIN — ACRODERMATITIS*

Like acrodermatitis, **acrokeratosis** affects the soles of the feet and the palms of the hands by thickening the **skin**.

I use my mental energy to protect myself from giving with my hands and feeling more in harmony with the earth. I fear change and I don't dare go toward others. I harden myself and I reject any new opportunity that is offered to me. I feel limited and I become impatient and impulsive.

I accept↓♥ to free my mind of my anxieties. I dare to bite into life: I trust and I open myself to give and receive in total safety. My curiosity opens doors for me to new experiences that enable me to get closer to people. I can use the same suggestions made for **acrodermatitis** to get energy circulating again.

SKIN — ALBINISM / ALBINO *See also: SKIN — VITILIGO*

Albinism is the incapacity to produce melanin, which plays a role in **skin** pigmentation (coloration). **Albinism** generally affects the **skin**, the hair and the eyes (when there is a partial absence of melanin, the person has **vitiligo**, and at that point there are non-pigmented spots in certain areas of the body).

"Am I allowing someone to control my life because I think that person is able to do it better than I can or because it is beyond my powers?" I believe I have no right to live. I want to go far away, so heavily does the gaze of others weigh on me. I reject and exclude myself from the world around me. I hold myself responsible for all the faults in the world and unconsciously want to purify myself. I feel like a ghost with no **Soul** or identity of my own.

I now accept↓♥ that I am different and unique, not only physically but because I possess untold qualities that make me a marvelous being. By using my talents in the service of humanity, I am thus more **Aware** of my power.

SKIN — ANTHRAX *See also: SKIN — FURUNCLES*

Anthrax is a **skin** infection joining several furuncles and extending into the subcutaneous conjunctive tissue.

I experience harmful aggressiveness because I feel that my personal freedom has been **unfairly** and **unacceptably** hindered. I want to get the neighborhood 'up in arms' and shout my indignation. I feel caught, pursued, stuck and powerless. An inner struggle is on, reflecting the one taking place outside, often in a situation involving a person or an organization in a position of strength and power. This struggle opposes my head and my **heart♥**. I discard my affective and intuitive side, which should be the prime authority over what I must do in my life.

I accept↓♥ that I must learn how to find my rightful place and have the power to change any situation in my life. I only have to decide so. I learn how to listen to my emotions and my intuition. I rediscover my spontaneity and my inner child's **heart♥**. I accept↓♥ to be myself at all times.

SKIN — BLACKHEADS *See also: FACE*

Blackheads or **comedomes** are small, blackish protusions on the **skin** caused by a hypersecretion of sebum[5].

They are the outer expression of my inner feeling of being 'dirty', 'unclean' and 'not worth much', and indicate that I underrate myself. I am even ashamed of myself, which makes my contacts with others difficult. My feeling of abandonment, solitude and failure weighs heavily. I learn to **love♥** myself as I am and to be proud of myself, and my facial complexion (where **comedomes** are generally found) becomes radiant.

I accept↓♥ to learn how to trust myself more. I am making projects again. All these **dark thoughts** I have about myself and that show up in the form of **blackheads** are replaced by positive thoughts. I focus my attention on my qualities, and others respect me too.

---

5. **Sebum**: A form of fat partly made up of triglycerides, that forms mainly on the epidermis.

SKIN — BLISTERS

A **blister** is an accumulation of water formed between two layers in the **skin**, the dermis and epidermis, following repeated friction in the same place. The water thus accumulated acts as a natural protection for the body.

It thus highlights my lack of protection, notably on the emotional level, or my lack of endurance. A **blister** is a reminder of an **emotional weakness**, and its physical location gives an indication of the level of that weakness. A **blister on the feet** is related to the directions I take in my life and my resulting feeling of insecurity. If it is behind the **heel**, it is related to my mother and my own motherly attributes. I must ask myself if I am really moving forward in my life or just telling myself stories. I am very hard on myself. I make myself suffer, but weep for others. I want to toughen my **skin** as I want to toughen my emotions, to no longer suffer. I resist something or someone. A **blister on the hands** makes me see the irritation and the frustration in what I do or in the way I lead my life. I tend to idealize other persons instead of seeing all the great qualities I possess. By looking at where the **blister** is located, I can ask myself what is **annoying me** in my life, what is causing me friction and provoking sorrow (water) even unconsciously. It may be what I see or feel, and I feel apart from others because my view of life is very different. I want to be a channel and share my knowledge and experiences, but often people turn a deaf ear and are bothered by what I say. A **blister** is there to throw more '**Light**' on what I am living through. I ask myself what emotions are now **skin** deep and about to burst out. There is an inner tension only seeking to express itself outwardly. I tend to restrict myself, which can show up as aggressiveness, often turned against myself.

I accept↓♥ to express my emotions more, by following the flow of life. I discard all my self-imposed limits.

SKIN — BRUISES

Bruises are also called **contusions**. They are red, bluish or black in color, and occur when I bump into a hard object that crushes the **skin**.

This contusion is related to a **repressed expression**, a mental pain or a deep anguish that I don't verbalize. My aggressiveness turns back against me. It can occur at moments of great fatigue when I am unsettled. I am seeking to find what my true power is over life and events. I flee my emotions and I feel that I am nothing, ***melting*** into the crowd. I feel a slave to others, wondering what my rightful place is. I leave to others the authority that I should enact myself by my words and my acts. I flee my true personal worth. My feeling of weakness irritates me to the highest point. I feel **guilty** for some reason, I want to **punish** myself, I take the attitude of a victim, I lack stamina in facing life's events (a predisposition to **contusions**). Life therefore warns me instantly that by striking this object, I am not moving in the right direction (whatever it may be). The object is usually motionless and **I collide with it while moving toward it instead of the opposite way**. I therefore punish myself. Do I look where I am going? Do I move smoothly in life or do I tend to act abruptly? Am I careful enough to continue, or too tired by my bruising and my inner injuries that now appear on my body? Am I calm enough inside? Do I distance myself enough from a situation to accurately grasp its meaning? I am experiencing avoidance and 'I am somewhere else'. I may want so much to do things in order to be loved and appreciated that I focus all my attention on what I am doing and no longer see what is moving toward me. I 'bump my nose' by dint of asking myself questions and feeling that they remain unanswered. I start 'bucking' (becoming stubborn) instead of being persistent. I have '**the blues**'[6] because I need **Love** and affection and I only receive violence and 'low blows' instead. I feel the victim of events that I believe I have to endure. I take pity on my fate. I am good and mad: I have the impression that I have to fight in life, so I mutilate myself, thinking that I am everything I deserve. Maybe I should think over my positions to be able to avoid the obstacles that present themselves on my path.

I accept↓♥ to take control of my life. It is very important for me to choose and stand by the decisions that are in harmony with me and my development. I take better care of myself and I no longer need to hurt myself because I know that I deserve to be happy and taken care of. I regain control of my life. I respect myself and I **accept↓♥** to change my framework for living in order to remain flexible toward life and what it has to give me.

SKIN — CALLUSES *See also: FEET — CALLUSES AND CORNS*

Callosity is a thickening and a hardening of the **skin** resulting from repeated rubbing, therefore from certain **rigid** attitudes and certain thought patterns that I currently have. Several regions of the body may be affected.

The **skin** is related to mental energy; when it accumulates or crystallizes in fearful reaction to some situation, immobility or inertia then ensues, preventing the flow of energy, with no flexibility in my thoughts. I remain open **even if I am afraid**. This fear leads me to close or narrow my objective outlook on life. My biases lock me into my positions. I may reject my role as a peacemaker or my duties to serve others. I protect myself by thickening my **skin**, thus preventing aggressors from entering. I must be **Aware** that by so doing, I also prevent any marks of affection or gentleness from reaching me. The region where **callosity** appears can give me further information: in the **shoulder** for example, I **harden** my ideas and attitudes about the responsibilities in my life. If my **feet** have **calluses**, it shows that I am resisting a change that is coming for me. Instead of being confident, I add a protective layer to 'ward off blows'. As my **feet** give me stability and help me move ahead, when I get **calluses on my feet** (generally on the heels), I feel anxiety because I don't feel supported. I am afraid of losing my **footing** or falling short in my basic needs (security) and I protect my rear (heel) by thickening my **skin**. I unconsciously flee my inner feeling of insecurity. The thickening of the **palms of my hands** also indicates

---

6. **I have the blues:** I am experiencing moroseness, somewhat like depressive feelings.

that I am resisting a change. I protect myself for giving or receiving. I lock up my spontaneity and creativity in rigid structures that limit me.

I accept↓♥ to become gentler with myself. I find the source of my fears, so the energy blocked and accumulated on the **skin** can then begin to spread in harmony with me. My **skin** becomes supple and young again.

SKIN — CHAPPING

Chaps are painful crevices most frequently found on the hands and feet.

I am probably experiencing a pronounced irritation about someone, something or a situation. I feel trapped; I am '**bound hands and feet**' in a relationship and I don't know how to get out of it. As **chapping** is found very often during the winter, being caused by the cold, I may have the impression of having been **burned by fire** by a person or a situation, for intense cold can 'burn' as much as fire. If I have **chapped hands**, it mainly affects my everyday life, whereas on the **feet**, I may apprehend what the future is holding for me. I feel limited in my actions. I want to do plenty of projects, but the conditions are unsuitable for carrying them out. I find my father's, or my mother's, coldness daunting. My contacts with others are painful. I experience a great tension and my **skin,** which also becomes tense, will **chap**. I take the sorrow of others on my shoulders. Feeling vulnerable, I find it difficult to express myself. Why even talk at all? I would like to get rid of this past that weighs heavily on me. To soften my **skin**, I apply balm, and the balm suggested in this case is: "Stop bothering me with a situation about which there is nothing that I can do". My **skin** will thus become soft and smooth again.

I accept↓♥ to become **Aware** of my worth. I speak with my **heart♥**. By taking care of myself, others will too.

SKIN — CHILBLAIN / PERNIO *See also: COLD [EXPOSURE TO THE]*

Chilblain is a localized redness caused by freezing and found in the extremities such as the ears, the nose, the hands and the feet. These purplish red areas are thick, cold and sometimes very painful. **Chilblain** sometimes forms small water blisters on the surface of the **skin**.

Life burns me and I have frozen my reactions. When **chilblain** is on the **hands** and the **heels**, it enables me to move more slowly. I prevent myself from feeling. On the other hand, I cling to those situations and I see nothing else. Physically, I project the image of a go-getter, but feel empty and exhausted inside. I no longer feel like moving ahead, and my taste for living is slowing and coming to a halt. I even wonder why I am living. My strained thoughts are reducing my blood circulation. The cold that caused this **chilblain** comes from a chill between me and another person, often a member of my family: I feel a lack of **Love**; the cold-blooded character of this person freezes my **Soul**. I live in fear, shivers run up my back. I refuse to acknowledge my limits or admit that my vital space was violated. The family disharmony weighs heavily on me.

Rather than see only the negative aspects of my experiences, I accept↓♥ **to let go of the past and open myself up to life**. When I open myself to life, I am able once again to see all the **Love** that surrounds me and to live in harmony with what I am and with my entourage.

SKIN — DERMATITIS

Dermatitis is an inflammation of my **skin**.

An inflammation is a mute anger, a repressed irritation trying to express itself. The anger that consumes me can be as much against me as against the people around me. **Dermatitis** is a way of reacting if someone 'slips' under my **skin**, upsets or bothers me or if a situation causes me any frustration. It highlights a need for physical contact (usually by touch) that demands to be fulfilled or the need to avoid a contact that is imposed on me and that I reject. My vulnerability and my sensitivity are in danger. I am experiencing a discomfort and even a certain duality about the limits in my relationships with others. How far does my freedom go while still feeling secure? As I find it difficult, or if I don't dare, to ask the other person to stop, **my skin 'boils' with anger**, or on the contrary, I may have difficulty in showing my need for human contact, caresses, etc. I feel uncomfortable with my mother: either I feel that she rejects me or that she overprotects me, and it bothers me.

I accept↓♥ that the important thing is to respect my needs and talk about them with the persons concerned, and the **dermatitis** can then resorb itself naturally.

SKIN — DERMITIS (seborrheic)

The **skin** is the body's protective envelope and it also protects my inner organs. **Seborrheic dermitis** is a frequent cutaneous affection characterized by more or less large areas of redness covered by scales that detach themselves from the **skin** (yellowish, fatty squamæ). They predominate in zones where seborrheic secretion is most prevalent (most often on the scalp, the outer nostrils, the forehead, the temples or the sternum). Seborrhea (a hyper-secretion of sebum) predisposes to **seborrheic dermitis**. As sebum lubricates the **skin** and protects it, do I feel a need to protect myself because "the sky might fall on my head"? It shows an excess, a surplus, a surfeit, a secret too heavy to bear, such as: I may have become **Aware** of a fraud that I witnessed or in which I am taking part and I am afraid of being unmasked. I am experiencing a recurring and growing stress in my life that is related to a surplus, an overload from a situation that I can no longer tolerate. Am I taking care of someone to excess, without first seeing to my own needs? It expresses an unresolved inner annoyance; when I have a complex about my physical appearance or there are things I want to hide in my personal life, I reject any closeness to others.

I accept↓♥ to live in truth. By recognizing my own needs and expressing my annoyances and frustrations, I increasingly manifest the transparency of my inner being. Peace can thus settle in permanently.

SKIN — ECZEMA

Eczema is a **skin** ailment capped by red zones, which can appear in adults as well as children. I am a hypersensitive person.

I have not learned to love myself and, as I fear being hurt, I live largely on the basis of what others expect of me. I am afraid of being abandoned. If I have **eczema**, I previously experienced a very intense situation of separation, as for instance during a move to a new home, a change of class at school or a dispute that led to a later separation. It may even go back to the time when I was in my mother's womb. I had great difficulty later on in ***acclimatizing*** to my new living conditions. Sometimes, everything takes place at the level of felt experience, because viewed from outside, there don't appear to have been any great **changes**. I may have felt that my values were ridiculed, and it is as though my deeper being had been rejected. I have the impression that I have no power over my life. I will tend to re-create situations where I feel separated, especially from people I **love**. As **eczema** 'touches' the **skin**, what I miss, even unconsciously, is contact, the touch of the person before the separation, which I have now lost or still have but rarely experience. There is a loss that I still need to come to terms with. It is my **skin** that used to make contact with the other, and as this contact has been ***taken away*** from me, my **skin** expresses its need to be touched in the form of **eczema**. My **skin** tells me: I have been loved, but that was in the past. **Eczema** also shows me that I am feeling ambivalence about touching: I need it, but it also scares me. If the **eczema** is generalized, the separation was sudden, total and appeared earlier than expected. It is as though my **skin** were crying out, sending a **call** for help. If I have **eczema** only on my **hands** for example, I can ask myself if there is a pet I was very close to and that I lost; as I used to take this animal in my hands, the **eczema** is located especially there. I may also experience a situation where I am frustrated because I resent myself for not taking action or not receiving. On the **elbows** or on the **knees**, **eczema** manifests an inner withdrawal that thwarts me. It makes me ***isolate***, withdraw and depreciate myself. Either others forget me, or **I forget myself, but to my own detriment**. I put great store in what people may think of me or how they perceive me. The image I project is very important. I find it difficult to be me. Not knowing where my destiny is leading me creates a lot of worries for me, and anxiety then invades me. I go from despair to revolt or anger. This despair that is 'simmering' is going to 'erupt' in waves. The ***effervescence*** and the impatience that I feel about a situation that I want to resolve express themselves through my **skin** that is boiling inside of me. All these factors ***combined*** lead me to feel **frustration**, **irritation** and much ***sorrow***. My emotions are 'skin deep'. While I am trying to please everyone, I forget to take my own needs into consideration; all that, just to be loved by others. I am thus separated from a part of myself. I act on the basis of the expectations of others instead of doing what pleases me. **I reject who I am**. I don't **love** myself as I am, and therefore the fact that my **skin**, which is visible for everyone, is in bad condition or even 'ugly', will confirm in my physical appearance how I perceive myself inside. The more I reject myself and the more I attract people around me by whom I will feel rejected; my fear of rejection will manifest itself! This makes me 'beat a retreat' and cut myself off from outside reality, though what I truly want, deep inside, is to get closer to people. I may also be emotionally irritated without being **Aware** of it. With the **eczema,** I am going to erect a physical **barrier** between me and the others in order to **protect** myself and avoid feeling threatened or hurt. **In the case of a baby** however, I will develop a **milk crust** (**seborrheic dermitis**) because I need more human warmth and physical contact with the people I **love**, especially my mother. Feeling isolated, I will display **eczema** to get closer to others. I am vulnerable in my sensitivity. I need **Love** and attention. It is important to note that most **eczemas** appear in **infants** between the ages of two and six months. Now, it is precisely at this age that a child becomes **Aware** of its own existence, separate from its mother. The fact that this 'separation' generates insecurity or fear will make **eczema** appear. **As a child**, my need to be touched appears along with the need to have **skin on skin** contact (in the proper sense of the term) with a person who loves me, not a contact with a blanket or clothes preventing this direct **physical contact**. I may feel helpless before "all these large grownups surrounding me". I may feel powerless before them and vulnerable to their reactions. Whether I am an adult or a child, this crust represents what I must let go of to finally become me, this 'me' that was hidden for so long. My personality is imprisoned and I cut myself off from parts of me. I prefer to live superficially, punishing myself while believing I don't deserve any better.

I accept↓♥ to let go of certain attitudes and mental patterns in order to detach myself from my past and focus on the actions to undertake in order to achieve my potential. I must accept↓♥ and **love** myself as I am. **WHAT I DON'T GIVE MYSELF CANNOT BE GIVEN TO ME: SUCH IS THE LAW OF RECIPROCITY.** I therefore identify my true needs and act in accordance with them. I learn to fully live the present instant, knowing that each action I perform today forms my tomorrow. I move forward confidently in life. I thus make a fresh start.

SKIN — ÉPIDERMITIS *See also: APPENDIX III, HERPES, SKIN — SHINGLES / HERPES ZOSTER*

Epidermitis is an inflammatory condition of the **epidermis**, the external part of the **skin**.

A tension certainly exists between what I experience inside and what is going on in my external life. I may feel urged to separate from my past and cut myself off from it. It may be by certain ways of thinking or ideologies, certain behaviors or persons that are no longer in harmony with me. The anger I feel over our differences saddens me, because I don't understand what has happened for us to have moved so far apart from each other.

I accept↓♥ to welcome the changes that occur in my life and I leave behind the old structures and ways of thinking. By studying what my **skin** and my **skin** problems are related to on the metaphysical level, I will be able to understand what I am experiencing in order to remedy it.

SKIN — ERUPTION OF PIMPLES *See also: SKIN — ITCHING*

An **eruption of pimples** is the appearance of small red spots with small outgrowths on the surface of the **skin**.

My **skin** is the first part of me that comes into contact with the world. The redness is related to my emotions and the **itching** is the sign of my annoyance. I am irritated over delays or slowdowns and frustrated by a situation or by someone. This **eruption** can also be related to the shame and guilt that I feel. Did I act too fast? Did I go too far in my words and my actions? Most of the time, there is a state of intense stress about my emotions, and that is what makes the **pimples** appear. As the earth manifests volcanic **eruptions** because an overly high pressure accumulates under the surface of the earth's crust, the **skin** manifests eruptions caused by inner tensions seeking release. If I find myself in a similar situation in the future, my body will remember it and a new **eruption** will appear. I feel thwarted inside, I may feel threatened, I may even reject myself as a person. My insecurity leads me to withdraw, with the hope of possibly not being approached by anyone. Unconsciously, I may even use this as a means to attract attention. I hold back my creativity and my strengths. If I am an adolescent, I may fear or resist external authority. I want to be integrated more quickly as an adult. Whatever my age, my life is organized by others, for I have little faith in my own potential. I need to act, to undertake things and charge ahead, but certain trying experiences of my past, often related to my father, hold me back from taking steps to become more autonomous. The affected region on my body indicates at what level my annoyance is located.

I accept↓♥ to become **Aware** of the cause of the **eruption** and I accept↓♥ to express what I feel. This frees me, and my **skin** becomes clear again. I acknowledge my worth and my inner wisdom.

SKIN — FURUNCLES *See also: INFLAMMATION*

A **furuncle** (commonly called a '**boil**') is defined as an inflammation of the **skin** caused by a bacterium and is characterized by a whitish mass of dead tissue.

I have the impression that something or someone is **poisoning** my existence, and as I repress all my anger and anxieties inside of me, I have "had it up to my neck" and the overflow shows itself in one or several **furuncles**. As **furuncles** affect the **skin**, the anger experienced often results from a situation where I was **separated** from someone or something dear to me and that I no longer want to have any physical contact with (by touch). For example, I may have passed by a moment of glory, where I could have been the '**star** of the show', but I remained in the shadows instead. It may be a promotion or advancement at work that slipped through my fingers. The location where the **furuncle** appears on my body gives me an indication about the aspect of my life that triggers so much anger and about the reason why I am 'boiling' inside because I feel soiled. For example, a **furuncle** on my left shoulder indicates frustration over my family responsibilities and those of my couple. I may have the impression that I have too many responsibilities and that my spouse is not doing enough.

I accept↓♥ to express the anger I feel and to ask for help, if need be, to avoid poisoning myself this way with **furuncles**.

SKIN — FURUNCLES (vaginal)

Any **furuncle** indicates non-verbalized frustration. If it manifests itself in the area of my sexual organs, could I be feeling anger at my spouse (or sexual partner) and the way we experience sexuality (for example, I may be frustrated by the duration, the frequency or the intensity of our sexual relations)? And if I don't have a partner at the time the **furuncles** appear, I may feel angry about the fact that I am not experiencing my sexuality as I want to, for want of a spouse. Whatever my situation is, if I do have a spouse, it is important for me to communicate my needs and frustrations, so that we can both make the necessary adjustments for a more fulfilling sexuality.

If I don't have a partner, I accept↓♥ my current situation as the best that can be for the moment. By taking a positive attitude, I increase my chances of meeting a person with whom I can develop a beautiful relationship and who will be able to satisfy me in all respects.

SKIN — IMPETIGO

Impetigo is a contagious cutaneous infection that most often affects children under the age of 10.

I am going through an emotionally very trying period. Someone is poisoning my existence but I can't express it: so my body speaks up for me. I feel vulnerable and under attack and I wish I could be safe and protected from the outside world. I am experiencing an unfair situation that undermines my balance and I want to push aside or drive away this thing or this person from my life, but I don't know very well how to do so. I detest what I see.

I open my **heart♥** to someone I trust in my entourage and I accept↓♥ to share my secrets. This allows me to free myself from a great sorrow or great suffering. I accept↓♥ that I have my own limits. I make everyone around me respect them, which enables me to find this inner security I need so much.

SKIN — ITCHING *See also: SKIN — ERUPTION OF PIMPLES*

Itching, also called **prurit**, is related to the **skin**, the most extensive sense organ of the human body. **Itching** is an irritation, something that 'gets' under the **skin** and affects me in one particular place or irritates me inside.

I **feel thwarted** by unsatisfied desires, and a degree of **impatience** sets in and makes me scratch, scratch, scratch. This scratching indicates that some situations in my life are not going according to my wishes and that I am separated from the pleasure and enjoyment that I want to find. Things aren't moving forward fast enough for me. I am irritated and dissatisfied with my life and I feel that others are the cause of that. I often look too far away for this happiness that is actually more within my reach. I don't feel that I have control over my life and I resent authority in all its forms. Can it be that I am the one limiting myself by separating myself from my own emotions? Life is urging me to make rapid changes. I feel **insecurity** and **remorse** as a result of all that. What is **itching** me so much that I sometimes tear my **skin** to the point of bleeding (which shows that I need to go and look into the depths of my being to find the answers to my questions)? Is it because I don't have the answer, or because I don't want to see it? Maybe I don't want to end up on the street. What do I have to do to change this state? **I identify the 'cause' of the irritation**. Is it related to my father, my mother or someone I **love**? Is it a situation that I want to change inside? I ask myself questions about my place inside my family. Do I feel I belong to it, or do I feel instead that I am separated from it and that I must go and seek **Love** elsewhere? Have I lost contact with my own emotions? If the irritation is generalized to my whole body, it therefore intensely affects my whole being. If it is in one special location, I find the answer according to the body part affected. In the **scalp** for example, there is a disorder in my thoughts. I trust my mind to find answers to my questions, when I must go and see them in my **heart♥**.

I accept↓♥ these **itchings** for I know that they have a message to convey to me. I no longer need to flee or leave what I am doing for the **itching** to disappear. On the other hand, if it involves allergies, I try to see to what or to whom I am allergic. I will no longer need to feel badly to the point of scratching myself constantly. Deep inside, I know that the openness of the **heart♥** heals many illnesses. I reclaim my rightful place. I allow my creativity to express itself. I accept↓♥ to see what I must change in my life by trusting myself completely.

SKIN — ITCHING around the ANUS *See: ANUS — ANAL ITCHING*

SKIN — KERATOSIS *See also: FEET / CALLUSES AND CORNS / WARTS, SKIN — ACROKERATOSIS*

Keratosis is characterized by a thickening of the superficial layer of the **skin**. On the **skin**, it can appear as rough, reddish surfaces that can form a crust.

As the **skin** is the junction between the outer world and the inner world, I may have such a fear of my environment that I feel the need to protect myself by forming a 'thicker barrier'. The reddish color indicates repressed frustration over what I am going through. I am rebelling against my 'destiny'. I don't 'take the bull by the horns' and grapple with certain difficulties. I may fear that my partner could cheat on me and cuckold me. This would lead me to re-examine my priorities and my structures for living. The bases of my relationships may be more fragile than I think. The place where the **keratosis** forms, whether on the arms, the thighs, the face or the hands, indicates on what aspect of my life I feel the need to protect myself.

I accept↓♥ to send thoughts of **Love** wherever **keratosis** forms on my body, in order to integrate the state of **Awareness** I must achieve. My trust in life will increase in me, and I can recover my **skin**'s natural suppleness.

SKIN — LEUKODERMIA *See also: SKIN / ALBINISM / SCARS / VITILIGO*

Leukodermia, also called **acromia** or **depigmentation**, is a diminishing, loss or absence of normal skin pigmentation, consisting in the appearance of discolored, dull white patches, surrounded by a zone where the skin is more pigmented than normal. It often appears at the location of a scar.

After a major event, my life took on a different color than expected. I felt hurt, betrayed and disrespected in my intimacy. My inner pain follows me and I feel like vanishing so I won't suffer. It may be a tiny white spot, but tied to a deep injury that left its trace. I may feel guilty of having involuntarily rejected a person by my words or gestures. It affects my daily life. The color of some of my relationships has become superficial or non-existent.

I accept↓♥ to take responsibility for my own emotions and let others take theirs. I look at what hinders my joy in living and I make peace with myself. I listen to my **heart♥** and tell others what has hurt me and how I want our relationships to develop.

SKIN — LIPOMA

A **lipoma** is a benign tumor formed by a proliferation of adipous tissues (fat); its usual location is sub-cutaneous and its removal is not necessary. It generally appears between the ages of 30 and 60. Its location gives me some indications on the reason for its appearance.

It often happens that I depreciate and judge myself with respect to certain parts of my physical body, and then **lipomas** may appear at those specific locations, on my stomach for example. Someone may have laughed at me or merely teased me, and it hurt me and I felt offended. As there is an overproduction of fatty cells, I can ask myself against what or whom I wish to protect myself. I feel attacked and unprotected: what are the deeper causes that haunt me? I feel abandoned, unless I am the one creating a distance to be able to go on living in society. By becoming **Aware** of the message of this 'benign' tumor, I can rectify the bothersome situation without doing violence to myself or continuing to attack myself.

I accept↓♥ to remove the injury linked to a previous situation in order to accept↓♥ myself as I am and I let go of my fear of ridicule. I immediately stop overprotecting myself and I accept↓♥ to open myself to change. I discard these moorings I had encoded in my subconscious. I make peace with myself and I open myself up once again to exchanging and sharing with others.

SKIN — LUPUS (chronic erythematosis)

There exist different sorts of **lupus**. However, **lupus** in general is an inflammatory disease that can affect a large number of organs. Its origin is attributed to the auto-immune system. When the **skin** is affected, we speak of **chronic lupus erythematosis**.

I develop **lupus** when I experience a deep discouragement, hate or shame toward myself, which weakens my defense system. My unease is often rooted in a deep emotional guilt that invades me and gnaws at me from inside. I see myself as a bad person and I don't deserve to be happy. I prefer to punish myself rather than assert myself. I give up and surrender for I feel there is no way out, no solution, and I may be frustrated over my powerlessness. I have had such a rough time of it all my life that I can't take it any longer. I am still deeply scarred from it. I feel like a battered **wolf**, drained of power. I want to be left alone. Death is a way out, and I refuse to accept↓♥ **Love** and forgiveness for myself or for others.

I accept↓♥ to learn again how to **love** myself, which is an important, even essential, stage in my healing. I can ask for help from inside of me or ask some competent people to help me in initiating this inner healing process. I reconnect with my inner power and allow my youthful ambitions to manifest themselves! This is how my talents and my full potential can be recognized.

SKIN — MELANOMA (malignant)

Malignant melanoma is also called **nevus** (or **mole**) **cancer**. It is a tumor in the **skin** or a mucous membrane or secondarily in an eye, and originates from cells tasked with pigmenting them (melanocytes). One form of **melanoma** appears spontaneously; the other results, more rarely, from the transformation of a nevus (mole).

A **melanoma** refers to some of the same emotions involved in the case of a simple **nevus** (lentigo), but these are more violent, deeper and more diverse for a **melanoma**. A **melanoma** appears at a place on my body that I can relate to an event where I felt myself being **SOILED**, stained, mutilated, disfigured or ***denigrated***. My bodily security was affected. My **skin** is modified and altered. It is as though my **skin** were recalling a foul physical contact, non-consenting or coerced by society, my family or some other person. The **melanoma** becomes like a shield, a shell to fend off further aggressions. I call into question my bodily and moral ***SECURITY***. I need to be ***cleared*** of something I did or said, or of something that was done to me and that I experienced as a ***stain***. I may also have lived through an event where I felt ***TORN AWAY*** from someone or something dear to me (**skin** diseases are often linked to a separation) of whom I may have lost all ***traces***. I may also be afraid of such a tearing away occurring in the future. For example, family secrets such as the birth of a child out of wedlock may have been suppressed, and the names of the persons involved carefully hushed up. My borders and limits have been breached and I feel vulnerable. My relations with others, especially some members of my family, are 'irritating'.

A **melanoma** often manifests itself following a conflict with a person identified with the male element, either my father or a person who evokes his image. I may be part of a couple but feel divided, torn from my partner. My space has been ***polluted***. I feel '***battered***' and ***filthy***. I may also judge myself very severely and consider myself 'a ***slob***' living in decline; I have no self-esteem and others always pass before me. I feel **belittled**, **DEMEANED** in what I am and what I can accomplish. I allow others to have power over me by listening to their criticism. The situations where I must be close to others, physically and emotionally, are very difficult for me. ***Brushing my skin*** on someone else reawakens my inner injuries. I am in an endless struggle between needing others to the point of becoming dependent, yet wanting so much to be autonomous. I may feel torn away or ***torn apart*** inside of me. I can no longer stand my limitations. I need freedom. I need to ***clear the way***. I feel ***dejected*** because I have the impression I have lost my moral and physical integrity. I tend to be down in the dumps.

To ***stop*** that, I accept↓♥ to return some **Love** into the situation at the root of the **melanoma**. However hard it was when I experienced it, I accept↓♥ to see what gain or wisdom has come of it. I accept↓♥ to ask for ***help***.

SKIN — PIMPLES *See also: HERPES (IN GENERAL), SKIN — ACNE*

Pimples are often related to acne. Whereas acne is usually located on certain parts of the body (face, back, etc.), **pimples** can be found all over the body. They are small reddish bumps that may contain pus, depending on the infection involved. I have **pimples** because I express **impatience**, I want to forestall things, and fast! If the pus shows (**white-headed pimples**), I am **angry** and **boiling inside**. I repress my emotions, which are only asking to express themselves. I am always afraid of making a mistake. I feel thwarted and worried, I may be feeling a small inner sadness and, in the case of **pimples** on the **entire** body, a generalized discouragement. Facial **pimples** are related to individuality. They have the same meaning as facial acne. I reject myself, I filter the persons who cross my 'barriers', I want to be left in peace and not be approached. **Pimples** are the manifestation of thoughts that are toxic for me. I keep everything inside of me, and my **pimples** remind me that this is not beneficial for me. I want to hide, but at the same time, I would like so much to tell people who I am and that I exist.

I accept↓♥ to take the time to say or do things, remembering that I am fully guided. I remember that every human being has the right to express themselves frankly and simply. By expressing my emotions more fully, my body will no longer need to express them in the form of **pimples**.

SKIN — PORT-WINE MARK / STRAWBERRY MARK

These **port-wine marks** or **strawberry marks**[7], also called '**birthmarks**', are very frequent malformations of the small blood vessels, also called capillaries, located in the superficial layer of the **skin**.

7. Medically, these are called **mature angiomas** or **plane angiomas**.

If I had a **port-wine mark** at birth, I can start by examining the part of my body where the mark is located. This usually corresponds to a strong emotion, often of anger or sadness, experienced by my mother when she was pregnant with me, and which affected me too. There is a feeling of shame that goes way back in time and makes me depreciate myself. This shame appears to affect the whole family. It may refer to family contacts that are either nonexistent or constraining and cause much ***confusion***. I am attached to my family. I tend to attack as a way of asserting myself. **Port-wine marks** are often readily apparent, and I would like to ***melt*** into the crowd and not be noticed. As surgery or laser treatments make it possible to cause these **marks** to partially or totally disappear, I will become **Aware** of the relation it has with me, in order to integrate it and to become more fully myself.

I no longer have to stand the shame imprisoned in this redness: I free myself from it and I accept↓♥ to have my own life independent of that of my family.

SKIN — PSORIASIS

Psoriasis consists in an overproduction of cutaneous cells, creating an accumulation of dead cells, a thickening of the **skin**, in thick red plaques or drop-shaped ones, covered by fragments of whitish horned substances. If I have **psoriasis**, I am among the 2% of the world population who have this disease.

I am generally hypersensitive, '**skin deep**', and I have a great need for **Love** and affection that is not filled, possibly reminding me of another difficult period of my life. At that time, I probably experienced a very great feeling of abandonment or separation from someone or something that was dear to me. For **psoriasis** implies that there was a double separation[8], most often from two different persons, or a double separation from a same person. I may have been separated from my two parents when I was a child. It is the **skin** that is 'touched' because for me, being a child, what I need the most is a physical contact with my parents or with any other person whom I **love** and feel close to. The double separation may have been from my mother and one of my brothers or sisters, or from my spouse and a project at work (my 'baby'), or any other combination involving a separation from two persons or two situations that I **love** and greatly value. I may feel separated from myself, from my own identity. Furthermore, I may feel forced to have unwanted contacts with other persons. The fact of being or feeling separated prevents me from having this contact, especially involving touch, and therefore my skin, with these persons I **love**. ***Reunion*** is impossible. Then **psoriasis** will appear. I am now so afraid of being hurt that I want to keep a certain distance between myself and others. I want to avoid losing face. **Psoriasis** is a clever way that my body uses to protect myself against too much physical closeness and protect myself against my vulnerability. It is like an armor that molds and protects my body to the extreme. I am therefore experiencing an inner conflict, an

---

8. **Double separation**: In the case of eczema, it is a simple separation, from one sole person or situation.

ambivalence between my needs and my desire for closeness and my fear of contact that makes me keep my distance. I feel misunderstood by others. I want to control what others give me. I have the impression that I am being 'had', that certain persons abuse their authority, especially if they have lots of money. I must therefore free myself from certain mental patterns and attitudes that have accumulated and now no longer have any reason to exist, being burned out and dead. I have repressed my emotions so much that I live in permanent anxiety. I control my life well enough, up to the point where I must face my own emotions. At that point, panic takes over.

I now accept↓♥ my sensitivity; I learn to do things for myself, not only based on what others expect of me. And although **psoriasis** probably occurred after a painful event or an emotional shock, I accept↓♥ it as part of the natural process of living and growing and in order to become stronger and more solid inside. I come to terms with each of my emotions. I learn to trust myself. I dare to take the risk of opening myself to others so I can receive the gentleness of contact. By being 'in contact' with what goes on inside of me, anguish gives way to trust in myself and in life!

SKIN — SCABIES

Scabies is a cutaneous disease caused by parasites and characterized by itching.

What is itching me to the point of arousing such impatience and annoyance? Is there a situation in my life that I have wanted to change for some time, but without anything happening? Maybe things are not going as I wish, or as fast as I would like. I allow myself to be bothered or infested by a person, a thing or a situation, and it would be best for me to let go and to not want to control everything in my life. What is itching may be the fact that I am having difficulty in tolerating my submissive behavior. Feeling powerless in certain situations of my life, I tend to set my sights on others. I am afraid of asserting myself, and it is as though I were letting something or someone 'dig under my **skin**' without being able to do anything about it. I am afraid of being hurt, and I prefer to stand aside instead of frankly expressing my thoughts and feelings. I retreat within myself a lot, and I am almost shy with others. I look at the location of the scabies on my body in order to discover the source of my ailment. I must allow life to take its course and to tell me that each thing has its moment.

I accept↓♥ that everything is in place and in harmony. By respecting myself and taking the reins of my life in hand, I resume contact with my creative power.

SKIN — SCARS

A **scar** is a permanent or long-lasting fibrous tissue that replaces normal **skin** tissue following a lesion. It is the result of wound healing.

The place where the **scar** is located shows me that the physical injury is related to a psychic injury. The fact of having this **scar** is a constant reminder of this event that has been a source of pain, of rending, of suffering. When there is no more physical pain in this **scar**, there only remains a memory in this portion of life. When I look at this **scar** and the psychic injury resurfaces, I must realize what I have learned from this experience life has faced me with, or what lesson I must draw from this situation. A difficulty in healing throws **Light** on the fact that this psychic pain has left these traces. I have difficulty in accepting↓♥ and forgiving (someone else or myself) for what happened. It still 'infects' my life…

I accept↓♥ to forgive in order to put back more **Love** into the situation and more peace inside of me. This will allow the **scar** to become less swollen and to heal closed, sometimes even to the point of disappearing entirely.

SKIN — SCLERODERMA *See also: SYSTEM [IMMUNE]*

Scleroderma is characterized by a hardening of the **skin** and a loss of its mobility and suppleness.

As a person suffering from this disease, I am often very hard on myself and have often felt hurt. As I experience great insecurity, I believe that I constantly have to protect myself from the people around me. To do so, I harden myself so much that I become a block of ice, and I avoid speaking whenever I can. I am afraid of change and especially of growing old. I may experience a situation where I feel remote and separated from someone or something, and the dragging out of this feeling over time results in **scleroderma** manifesting itself. It is as though this person has torn away a part of me. I feel solitude and emptiness and have the impression of not being alive. I cling to the past and feed my old wounds. Because I hold in too much, the burden becomes heavier day by day. As I am not in contact with my **heart♥** and my emotions, I don't enjoy life. I shrivel up inside, avoiding relations with others and, in some sense, I destroy myself. I feel like a piece of dirt, worthless for not having been able to avoid this separation. Because I fear being judged, I avoid showing my true face.

Healing is found in the opening up to others. Thus, I accept↓♥ to open my **heart♥** to **love**, to feel the warmth and well-being that are all around me, the warmth that goes deep down inside of me and melts this block that was freezing me. I become **Aware** of my worth, and I welcome each part of my being. It is by accepting↓♥ to be fully in relation with myself that I can be in relation with the people around me.

SKIN — SHINGLES / HERPES ZOSTER *See also: CHILDHOOD DISEASES / VARICELLA — CHICKENPOX*

Shingles, also called **Herpes Zoster**, is an infectious disease due to a reactivation of the **Herpes** virus. **Shingles** is identifiable by its eruptions on the **skin**, showing up unilaterally and in strips, along the pathway of a nerve.

As the nerves are our means for internal communications, the pain caused by this eruption means a break of communications in the affected region.

Shingles burns like fire (this fire may be related to anger resulting from criticism or fear). I felt under attack and I am experiencing deep bitterness. A situation or a person has hurt me, provoking **tension**, whereas my body desires **attention**. I may also have the impression of having been dirtied or stained. The pain reminds me of an unwanted contact, a forced submission to some authority. My first reflex is to withdraw and close myself in, believing that I can thus avoid other injuries. I act this way because the situation is making me feel **great inner insecurity**. By acting in this way, I return this aggression, of which I believe I have been the victim, against myself; I am tacitly admitting that my aggressors were right. I feel in constant danger. It is a part of me that I refuse to see. I hold back my creative energy. I want to escape what I take to be my darker side. I accept↓♥ that the purpose of the puffy eruption is to make me become **Aware** that I am feeling an intense emotional reaction or irritation over someone or something that causes me excessive stress and makes my decision-making difficult. Even if I seek harmony in my own relations and in those between others, the only power I have is over my own life. My body tells me to trust the flow of life inside of me.

I accept↓♥ my sensitivity, for it is part of me. I stop being my own enemy and I accept↓♥ to look at myself in the eyes. It is by making contact with each part of my being that I can recover a sense of security. I learn to detach myself from the suffering of others, knowing that they too must become **Aware** of certain issues so as to fulfill themselves.

SKIN — STRETCH MARKS / STRIA

Stretch marks are small streaks (striæ), purplish red at first and then pearly white, with the appearance of scar tissue, crisscrossing the skin that is over-distended. **Pregnancy stretch marks** first come to mind, but it can also involve young girls in their puberty period or persons who are trying to thin after having put on too much weight. There is a tendency to believe that it is mostly women who have **stretch marks**. Such is not the case, as many men, and even children sometimes, have them too. **Stretch marks** are often a matter of "I gain weight and I lose weight." **Stretch marks** are mainly located around the abdomen, but they are also found on the buttocks, the thighs and the arms. I worry about my physical attractiveness. I am lacking in suppleness and elasticity, I don't truly live in the extension of my own deeper nature. I experience great differences of opinion that make me uneasy. I am tense and my skin produces **stretch marks**. I feel hurt or injured because of attachment and vulnerability. I am often the one who wields the rod on myself[9].

I accept↓♥ to give myself all the gentleness I need. I am understanding and flexible with myself and with others.

SKIN — URTICARIA / HIVES / NETTLE-RASH

9. **Rod**: A stick made of wood or metal.

Urticaria, also called **hives** or **nettle rash**, is characterized by the appearance of red patches on different parts of the body. These slightly bulging patches cause intense itching. **Urticaria** is due, as the case may be, to a food intoxication related to the taking of medications or other substances, but this condition may be aggravated by stress and tension.

I may be feeling overwhelmed, I am doing a lot, but what I do is not recognized. I need the attention of others, but I can't stand their criticism. If I am suffering from **urticaria,** I am quite probably a hypersensitive person who is experiencing much rejection. I don't like the being that I am, and my fear of being hurt is so strong that, in order to be loved, I do things based upon what people expect of me. My fear of being rejected becomes real because I reject myself. I often have the impression that people want to get rid of me and out of the way. My **skin,** damaged by these red patches, makes me feel ugly and undesirable. I am like an animal **marked with a branding iron**; I am dependent on my owner. As I live according to others, I refrain from doing things for myself; I don't dare carry out new projects, which further increases my feeling of helplessness. I resent others and hold them responsible for my plight. I feel separated, even torn from someone, and my integrity is affected. However, I want this separation because in this way, I avoid complications.

I accept↓♥ to be the ruler of my life, I become the most important person for me. I move forward and I trust myself. I accept↓♥ to be up ahead and interacting with others. I have all the qualities needed to be a good leader.

SKIN — VITILIGO

Vitiligo is a depigmentation of the **skin**, which is considered to be its most frequent form. Thus, my **skin** becomes ***white*** in patches over certain areas on my body. It can occur on any part of the body, including the face and hands.

It may affect me if I don't feel concerned about the things or by the persons around me. I feel that I no longer have any identity. I have no sense of belonging to my family, my community, my work colleagues or my people. As I have the impression of having been ***stained***, which may represent a feeling of impurity, I want this stain to disappear; and instead of a dark stain, I find myself with a white stain. I have the impression that I have been '**bled white**', that all my resources have been squeezed out, physically as well as emotionally. I may feel like '**disappearing**' or becoming '**transparent**' in order to pass unnoticed. I would want to be ***sterilized***, free of microbes or problems. I may have had one or several sexual experiences where this feeling of staining was prominent. I may also have the impression that I was **separated** from one or several persons dear to me. I find that sad, and their absence weighs heavily on me. I was incapable of stopping or preventing this separation that I experienced brutally. Otherwise however, the consequences would have been catastrophic, for instance death or exclusion. This grates against my strong sense of duty and tradition. My roots, my life structures are disrupted. I have been hindered. I may also have experienced this event as a break, as a tearing away, which is often related to my father or the person who represents him, and more subtly, with the heavenly Father, the God in whom I believe. If I am a man, I want to become a father in the image of someone else, but it is not I. I also have an endless need to elucidate things. I have lost my reference points, my bearings, most often with respect to my father. I feel that I no longer have any protection from him. He is like a stranger to me. I will therefore feel guilty and depreciate myself, feeling soiled and dirty over this situation. If I can allay all suspicion, I can then recover my dignity. The specific part of the body that is affected indicates what aspect of me is concerned. A part of me is completely hidden and ***detached*** from everything, and in the ***dark*** I would therefore want to be '**white as snow**', ***immaculate*** like an innocent and naive child. I mustn't make a mistake or be faulted. I say no to the impulsive and creative part of me. There is a contradiction between what was taught to me and my true personal values. I hide to protect myself. My sensitivity was painfully affected in my childhood and even today, I still feel defenseless. I have built myself a new personality to please others and thus avoid being hurt. Most of the time, my mouth is ***sealed***. Deep down, I feel like killing everyone because nobody understands me. I no longer have a ***clear*** view of the things I have to do because I place too much importance on what others expect of me instead of on what I really want. When I was young, I felt I was a burden for my parents; I believe I was a cause for concern for them, if only over money issues, as my parents had to work much harder to feed the family, especially me.

I accept↓♥ to become **Aware** of the importance of my life. I resume contact with my deeper nature. I am safe when I am myself. I deserve the best, and I allow nobody to hurt me. By respecting myself, others too will do so.

SKIN — WARTS (in general) *See also: TUMORS*

Warts are viral skin infections that cause an excess of cellular production, creating a painless hard mass (a benign tumor).

This mass is an accumulation of barriers I have built up on my path. Barriers of sadness or grudges, related to certain sides of me that I perceive as ugly and detestable, provoking a feeling of guilt. I am ashamed of who I am. I reject my sensitivity and my spontaneity. I therefore feel rejected and misunderstood by others. If it is by my father, the **wart** usually appears **on the hands**, and if it is by my mother, it will often be located **on the feet**. At this level, it may correspond to a situation involving my roots, my country or my family. A **wart** may also appear on one specific limb when I have made a gesture that I regret (the **inside of the hand** for instance). My insecurity makes me retreat into myself. I live in accordance with others. I need to touch and be touched. I am desperately in search of myself. For me, nothing is ***manifest*** or obvious. If, for example, I have **warts** on the **backs on my hands**, I judge myself severely with respect to my own handwriting and that of others or regarding manual work. I have the impression that "my hand is not doing as well as the teacher's" and I depreciate myself because of that. An emotional void is filled by the appearance of **warts**. I feel that I don't deserve anything better than these ugly things, and this is how I punish myself. If I believe that I am ugly, then my body becomes ugly; it is simply a reflection of my inner attitudes toward myself. If I am ashamed of what I do or I wish for something but don't believe that I deserve it, it is possible **warts** will appear. I crave recognition and tend to put "the cart before the horse". These **warts** contain all my repressed creativity and sensibility, which ask only to express themselves. I incessantly ruminate on the same thoughts. I am afraid of solitude and death. It is important that I look at the locations where the **warts** have appeared so I can understand what part of my body or my life is affected. In the **back**, it concerns the past; in the **side of my body**, the present; and the **front of the body**, the future. On my **face**, it involves a situation where my self-esteem is being mocked. As a virus is at the origin of this **wart**, I must ask myself if I am feeling under attack, or invaded by someone or something wielding some sort of power over me. I am disgusted at having been 'had' like that. I feel eaten up inside. **Epidermoid warts** (at the epidermic level) involve an irregular separation over time. At the **dermis** level, it is more often an event where I felt dirty and that is tinged with regret. I will tend to criticize myself.

By accepting↓♥ who I am, a being worthy of **Love**, I will no longer need any **warts** to remind me of this, and they will disappear. I allow my true being to emerge. My creativity expresses itself freely.

SKIN — WARTS (plantar) *See: FEET — WARTS [PLANTAR]*

SKULL / CRANIUM *See: BONES — FRACTURE, BRAIN — CONCUSSION*

SLEEP DISORDERS *See: INSOMNIA*

SLEEPING SICKNESS *See: NARCOLEPSY*

SMELL *See: NOSE*

SMOKING *See: CIGARETTES*

SNEEZING

Sneezing is caused by an excitation or tickling of the inner walls of the nostrils, provoking an abrupt expulsion of air through both the nose and the mouth.

Sneezing means that **something or someone is bothering or irritating me**. I look at what I am doing and who is with me. What is annoying me, the situation or the person? Am I **criticizing** someone or **criticizing** myself? I unconsciously feel the need to extract myself from a certain situation, to free myself or to move away from someone because I am feeling dissatisfaction. What do I want to reject from my life? Who or what do I want to get rid of? What do I need to express or display outwardly? What is the part of me that I am resisting?

I identify the cause and I accept↓♥ to take the place that is rightfully mine and to act in such a way as to restore harmony, either by having a frank exchange of views with the person concerned or by remediating the situation.

SNORING

The noise that I produce while breathing during my sleep, due to an obstacle between my nasal airways and the larynx, is called **snoring**.

If I **snore**, I must ask myself some questions. Am I clinging to my old ideas, attitudes or material possessions? Do I stubbornly insist on staying in a relationship or in a certain situation that is not beneficial for me? Am I tired? Am I stagnating in my old living patterns, which shackle my freedom? If my **sinuses** are **congested**, what is the thing that I find difficult to breathe and that follows me even during the night (my spouse's scent or a perfume, for example)? Or maybe I want to 'catch' my spouse who is sleeping next to me and remove the distance separating us (physically as well as emotionally). I thus try to get closer to her/him. Do I want to tell my spouse during the night everything I was unable to express in words during the day? If I feel my requests are not being heard, I tend to **snore**, and my unconscious continues to express itself all night because I can't express it otherwise. I feel trapped, either in my relationship with my spouse or in some other personal relationship. It is important to see whether the **snoring** is produced during inspiration or expiration. If it is during **inspiration**, it is as if I am calling for help. If it is during **expiration**, I want to move a danger away.

I accept↓♥ to learn how to let go and to make room for something new. I try to make my communications clear and free of any insinuations or any ambiguity. I am open to changes and renewal.

SOMNAMBULISM / SLEEPWALKING / NOCTAMBULISM (somnambulant)

When I am a **sleepwalker**, I ***wander about*** while sleeping, without being **Aware** of it.

When I am a **sleepwalker**, it is because I am experiencing great inner tension, sometimes unconsciously. I may be trying to escape a situation that worries me too much. I 'express' myself this way in order to release this tension. I often experience the fact of being (even unconsciously) 'outside of my body'. When this event occurs, my 'astral body' directs my physical body from this 'out-of-body' position. Which is why, as a **sleepwalker**, I can wander about with my eyes closed and still 'see' the obstacles, for I see them with the vision of my astral body. I think far too much and I experience plenty of dualities. I feel crushed under the '**I have got to'**s. It is as though I were living in a prison from which I want to escape once night has come. I feel I am a burden for my family or for society. The care I need weighs heavily on me. I don't want to be found. I live in my bubble, far from others. I have little self-confidence, and it is difficult for me to move forward in life (advancing in the dark), for I doubt my inner voice.

To diminish this **sleepwalking** in my life, I accept↓♥ to communicate more with my spouse, my parents or a friend about what I am experiencing, or I simply write it down. I can thus find more inner calm and normalize my sleeping hours. I live more spontaneously. I show my creativity, I allow all this repressed energy to express itself, and I know that I can confidently move forward in life.

SOMNOLENCE

Somnolence is related to the liver, which can work in slow motion. I sometimes **doze** after enjoying a good meal.

It is a pleasant way to prolong this moment. I no longer have to think, I let myself drift. However, it is also a sign of slow digestion; I must then ask myself what I am currently finding difficult to digest. It is also natural to see an old man falling asleep during the day, for he is nearing the end of his life. He remains there, fatigued, awaiting death. However if I am a person of adult age and I regularly **doze off** during the day, I am unconsciously refusing to live, I am hiding, I am fleeing in order to no longer have to make choices and decisions and take action. I am limp, inactive and numb. I have retreated into my shell and am doing a lot of introspection.

I accept↓♥ to resume contact with life and become the actor and creator of my life. Otherwise, frustration risks setting in.

SPANISH FLU *See: BRAIN — ENCEPHALITIS*

SPASMOPHILIA *See also: TETANY*

Spasmophilia is a syndrome related to a chronic state of neuromuscular hyperexcitability.

I am easily depressed and I see each event of my life as a tragedy. I feel great insecurity and I have difficulty in managing my emotions and my actions in relation to outside influences. I am constantly thinking about all sorts of problems, whether mine or those of others. I have great difficulty in relaxing, letting go and fully appreciating life. How should I position myself? What is my place in this world? I am disconnected from my needs and full of apprehension. I turn a deaf ear and **Love** of self is absent. I thus also reject the **Love** of others. It is as if my body wanted to express something I have always repressed. I am unhappy and powerless over my incapacity for expressing myself in words or gestures. I am now resolved to release my mind and stop maintaining dramatic asides so I can take part in the movement and make place for something new.

I accept↓♥ to breathe life in to my full capacity, to express my ailments, my sorrows and everything that must come out of me, to make room for calm, peace and gentleness. I accept↓♥ to give myself gratifications, loosen up, have some good time and view situations as experiences. I fully participate in all the beauties of this world and I see life as an exciting adventure, full of joy and happiness.

SPASMS

One or several muscles contract and relax involuntarily and unrhythmically: I then have a **spasm**. **Spasms** form a sort of knot.

I am tensed up; I want to hold on to **Love**, I am afraid of losing this person whom I **love** so much. These **spasms** create a feeling of worry and helplessness in me. This knot of suffering that I can't control comes from many annoyances and irritants that give a bitter taste to my life. My mind lets go during the night, which is one of the reasons for **nocturnal spasms**. It kindles in me certain emotions and some guilt related to my sexuality.

I acknowledge that the knots stifle me and, in order to keep **Love** around me, I accept↓♥ to detach myself.

SPINAL CORD *See also: SCLEROSIS [MULTIPLE]*

The **spinal cord** is the part of the central nervous system that is contained in the vertebral canal inside the spinal column. It starts from the spinal bulb (*medulla oblongata*) and ends at the level of the second lumbar vertebra.

As it carries data from the brain to the body parts concerned, an impairment in this area indicates that I may have some difficulty in putting my thoughts and all my creativity into practice in the physical world. I have such a need to calculate everything and plan everything to perfection, without ever making a mistake, that spontaneity has no place in my life. As my **spinal cord** works this way, my inordinate rigidity will lead to ailments and dysfunctions. I greatly hesitate to move forward: my inner demons are fighting my more sensible side.

I accept↓♥ to listen to myself and to do things intuitively, knowing that I am always doing my best and that mistakes do not exist: everything is an experience to help me grow.

SPINAL DEVIATION (in general)

A **spinal deviation** mainly symbolizes a resistance to fully living my life. I feel that, as a child, I lacked parental support and fundamental structure. I was shaken in my deepest convictions. Since becoming an adult, the way I hold myself in life and my difficulty in allowing life to sustain me and letting go of my old ideas manifest themselves by a **spinal deviation** that curves sideways, forward or backward.

I accept↓♥ to take myself in hand and 'stand up straight' before life, with confidence and determination.

SPINAL DEVIATION — CYPHOSIS

A **cyphosis** is an abnormally rearward-convex **spinal deviation**, usually at the level of the shoulder blades. Besides a bad posture, **child and adolescent cyphosis** is often due to a growth disease called **Scheuermann's disease**[10].

If it affects me, I notice my body is folding up as if I was returning to the fetal position. From whom or what do I want to protect myself? Do I want to get closer to my mother because she does not understand me or because she is repudiating me as her child? I feel too little, not up to the family or to the task I want to accomplish. I want to keep everything for myself for fear of deprivation. I bow low out of timidity or because I do not acknowledge who I am, or I am always on guard, feeling inferior, incapable of claiming my place and living joyfully.

I accept↓♥ to feel safe even in the presence of other persons: I am capable of claiming my place, defining my limits and taking up the challenges that life lays down to me. I 'keep my back straight' and acknowledge myself as a unique and divine being. I thus learn to **love** myself more and to be proud of my achievements. I learn to thank this divine part of myself, which is present deep in my **heart♥**, for this courage that is in me, for I know that I possess all the answers when I remain connected with the **Soul** that I am.

SPINAL DEVIATION — HUMPBACK / HUNCHBACK *See: ROUNDED SHOULDERS*

SPINAL DEVIATION — LORDOSIS

Lordosis is a physiological forward-concave curvature of the **spinal column**.

I have difficulty in standing up because **I am ashamed of what I am and I don't love myself**. I often experience submission to my father or to whatever represents authority for me, for I underestimate myself with respect to him, I feel inferior to him, I am not worthy of being his son. I feel overwhelmed by others, I have very little self-confidence and I am incapable of expressing my ideas and my opinions. I want to be free. I bow down despite myself, having the impression that I am limp and incapable of dealing with issues straightforwardly. Things are not going fast enough and the results are late in coming. I therefore tend to depreciate myself. I feel divided between being proactive and trusting myself, or listening only to what others have to say. I seek safety by holding on to my old ideas. Thus, I do not dare change the status quo so as to not upset anyone. I am boiling inside, and this anger is eating at me. I refuse the help of others; I thus have more difficulty in reaching my goals and I tend to fail more often.

I must **learn to love myself**. I accept↓♥ to **claim my place**, for everyone has a role to play in the Universe. I learn to **freely express my ideas and opinions** and I feel better with myself. Everything happens at the right time.

---

10. **Scheuermann's disease** is named after its discoverer, Olga **Scheuermann**, a Danish physician and radiologist who in 1921 described the characteristic lesions of apprentice clockmakers' kyphosis (now named *Juvenile kyphosis*)

I dare to stand up and I trust myself. I feel safe because my inner voice tells me what to do for my greater good.

SPINAL DEVIATION — SCOLIOSIS

A **scoliosis** is a lateral deviation of the **spinal column**.

When I am affected by a **scoliosis**, I have the impression of carrying a very heavy burden on my shoulders. As this exceeds any hope of accomplishment, I feel helpless and despairing. My responsibilities scare me, and I am indecisive in my orientation. My energy blocks, and the **scoliosis** is its physical manifestation. It often occurs in adolescence: as I am in search of an identity, too old to be a child and too young to be an adult, my life and my responsibilities seem enormous. I refuse this body and this life, I refuse to grow up. I will tend to compare myself to my brothers and sisters (especially if they are a twin) and my cousins. As I often have the impression that they are better than me, I will depreciate myself, which will express itself by a **scoliosis**. I compare myself negatively with others, and this attitude haunts me constantly. I am afraid of being judged. I feel constantly pushed. I feel that I must be the pillar of the family, to honor it and be its pride. This, however, is demanding a lot of my **spine**, which symbolically represents the ship's mast. I bend to the left or to the right in order to compare myself with everything that is beside me. I may move away from others to protect myself or to avoid blows. Deep inside me however, I need to get closer to others, but I don't dare take the first steps. I may feel lost, for I need reference points to define myself as an individual. They are usually personified by my father and mother or by the most influential people I mix with (such as a teacher or a babysitter for instance). If these reference persons do not suit me or have disappointed me, my **spinal column** (which does not feel **supported**) will twist sideways. I cannot rely on myself, for I feel too fragile. My spine is collapsing, like my inner world. I live according to others. I prefer to ***fade out*** and steer clear rather than take the risk of asserting myself. The **scoliosis** is related to a **desire to flee** a situation or someone. I check out what is happening in my life and is preventing me from feeling well.

I accept↓♥ to live in the present: one day at a time. I become **Aware** that I am in the school of life, living in harmony with what surrounds me. I rediscover joy, and each day I realize I am strong and able enough to take up the challenge! I fully take over my own life. I live for myself. I stop comparing myself with others, for we are all different and unique.

SPINE — DISPLACED DISC *See: DISC — HERNIATED DISC*

SPINE (in general) *See also: BACK (IN GENERAL)*

According to the classification used in the West, **33 vertebræ** are counted, beginning from the top, namely:

7 cervicals[11], rather thin,

12 dorsals[12], rather thick,

5 lumbars[13],

5 sacrals[14], fused and forming a triangle toward the bottom,

4 coccygeals, fused and atrophied.

The **spinal column**, like a construction pillar, represents support, protection and resistance. My spine therefore supports and protects me through all the situations of my life. It is my physical and inner pillar. I would collapse without it. My **spine** also symbolizes my most fundamental and spiritual energy. It represents my flexibility and my resistance when faced with the different events of my life. It gives me the freedom to be able to flexibly move and turn around in any desired directions. **Spinal deviations** (scoliosis, lordosis, etc.) are related to the deeper part of my whole energy system. During a blocking, physical pains appear. Feelings of powerlessness, too heavy a burden to carry, or an unsatisfied affective or emotional need, make me feel attacked in my solidity and my resiliency. I receive blows from behind. I have the impression that I am the pillar in my family, at work and in any situation or organization where I am involved. What would happen to others if I weren't there? Would everything collapse? The **spine** is related by the skeleton to all the different aspects of my being, through the central nervous system and the central blood distribution system. Each thought, feeling, situation, response and impression is imprinted in the **spine** as well as in the relevant body parts involved. I look at the affected region and I identify the cause of the blocking.

Whatever the reason, I accept↓♥ to remain open about the cause, and integration is more harmonious. I rebuild the new person I want to be.

SPITTING / COUGHING UP BLOOD *See: BLOOD DISORDERS*

SPLEEN

The **spleen** is located under the diaphragm in the upper left part of the abdomen. The main functions of this lymphoid organ, which plays a part in the immune system, are to control the quality of the red blood cells and to fight off infection by the production of antibodies.

Nostalgia, unfinished business, regrets and worries can dwell there. If my **spleen** is not functioning well, it may well be that I too will have difficulty in functioning well, mainly because I remain fixed on dark and negative ideas. I am obsessed by someone or something. This lowers my level of energy and I no longer feel like doing anything. I have the impression that I am a failure,

11. **Cervical**: Comes from the Latin *cervis,* which means 'neck'.
12. **Dorsal**: Comes from the Latin *dorsum*, which means 'back'.
13. **Lumbar**: Comes from the Latin *lumbus*, which means 'lower back'.
14. **Sacral:** This word refers to what is inviolable or demands great respect. In this case, it is the starting point of Kundalini energy, the spiritual energy that starts from the base of the **spine** and rises to the top of the head, leading to illumination.

that I have made a mess or a ***massacre*** of my life because I could not finish certain things, or I was unable to 'turn over a new leaf". I 'missed the train' and some good opportunities, and I resent myself, for I now believe I am incapable of succeeding in life. I thus tarnish my family history. I want to compensate by forgetting myself for my family or my friends, but I can no longer take it! I have created a situation from which I can no longer extricate myself. This will eventually lead to a **removal of the spleen**. This negativism is often related to my way of seeing myself as ugly, 'not OK'. No good, not up to snuff. I rather feel like sleeping and being passive. I feed on anger, and there is nothing very fun in my life. Someone or something is grinding on my nerves: it may be someone in my family whom I consider a failure or a moron. The difficulties I am facing with my **spleen** give me an indication about my fears concerning **blood**, for example not having enough **blood** or ***bleeding*** too much (during menstruations or transfusions). I may believe that my **blood** is 'no good', or so rare that I doubt my life could be saved if I sustained a major accident and needed a **blood** transfusion. **The fear of death is thus often in the background**. As the **spleen** controls the quality of the **blood**'s red cells, a badly functioning **spleen** may indicate a great inner injury that has yet to heal. It is like a bleeding wound. As **blood** represents the joy of living, I may have the impression that life is such a hard struggle that maybe I should back down and beat a retreat. I want to be able to find refuge far from reality, in a more spiritual world, unconnected to the earth; this may produce a **swelling of the spleen**. I confine myself in a rigid structure, which removes me from a feeling of freedom. This can take the physical form of ***thinness*** in my body. I put up a wall between me and my emotions and I thus wear a mask: I have the impression that this is a good way to defend myself against the outer world and avoid being **humiliated**.

Instead of being obsessed with negative ideas that I tend to exaggerate, I accept↓♥ to change these ideas by finding ways to have a good laugh. I take my life less dramatically, and I learn to laugh at myself and at certain situations. I learn to communicate my emotions as they arise in order to maintain balance and harmony throughout my body.

SPOTS (all over the body) *See: SKIN — SPOTS*

SPRAIN / TWIST *See: JOINTS — STRAIN / SPRAIN*

SQUINTING / CROSS-EYED *See: EYES — STRABISMUS [CONVERGENT]*

STATUS LYMPHATICUS

Lymphatism, or **status lumphaticus**, is characterized by anemic paleness, flabbiness of the tissues and thin skin.

I am lacking in strength and rigor. I avoid forcing myself, I do nothing, I show slackness, a lack of nerve and vitality. I find no motivation in life and

I feel useless. I allow others to invade my life because I have difficulty in defining my vital space and making people respect it.

My lack of self-acceptance↓♥ often originates from situations where I judged myself severely. **Lymphatism** shows me how I need to settle my differences with myself. It is a sign that I must take myself back in hand, start moving and get things moving, in order to make energy circulate and shake off this lethargy that leads me to do less and less and to sink ever deeper into negativism.

I accept↓♥ to regain my momentum, I choose to give joy to those who need it, through small gestures, which makes me feel more useful and more appreciated.

S.T.D. (sexually transmitted diseases) *See: VENEREAL DISEASES*

STERILITY

Sterility is defined as the incapacity for reproducing oneself.

It leads to feelings of powerlessness, despair, guilt and the impression that 'it' is unfair. The extreme stress experienced, or the pressure I put on myself to have a child, are strong enough to prevent the process from being set off. **Sterility** may indicate a rejection, an unconscious resistance to the idea of having a child, or a fear that the child will be handicapped or deformed or will die. It may also be that I desire a child solely to meet the expectations of the persons around me but that, deep down, I do not truly want it. I may also believe that this way, I will be able to hold on to my spouse. Because I am afraid of giving birth or of being unable to play my role as a parent (fear of the responsibility, of the financial problems) or not wanting my child to be made to experience the suffering that I went through, I provoke **sterility** because the idea of having a child becomes unconsciously ***inconceivable***. I may feel too immature for this sort of experience; I may still be too selfish. ***Fright*** takes hold of me. If I am a **woman**, I may also be afraid of re-living, through my pregnancy, the memories of moments when my mother was bearing me and that may have affected me. I may, even unconsciously, reject the image of my mother (the one who gave birth to me) or the relationship we had. If I am feeling a great inner emptiness, I may not be able to fill it, even with a child. **Male sterility** often occurs when a man perceives that being a father, and taking on that role, is too huge a responsibility. I may unconsciously not want to ***reproduce*** the same mistakes that I believe my parents made. It may unconsciously be a grudge match, not necessarily with my spouse, but with my family, which has always wanted to dictate my life. I must understand that the desire to have a child can be very strong, but so can the fear of having one, whether it is conscious or not; this is the difference that must be weighed in the balance for the pregnancy process to be set off or not. I may also be carrying a heritage of fears from my mother or my grandmother. It would be in my interest to check whether I have had experiences in the past, as a man or a woman, which could have made me develop certain sexual blocks.

Some psychotherapeutic or energy-based work may be quite appropriate in this case. Do I want a child just to fill a void, to give meaning to my life, or feel useful and important at last? Or on the contrary, do I feel I don't have enough to offer to 'deserve' giving birth to a child? I look at my life and wonder in what area of my life I can be very fertile or 'productive'. As the case may be, I may fill my need for having a child in some other area of my life. I then ask myself if I still truly feel like having a child, and if so, I accept↓♥ that my creativity will take the form of a pregnancy. I may also not have to go through the experience of being a parent. It is essential for me to question myself about the nature of my desire to have a child, and that I trust my inner self in my decision to give life or not.

Whatever happens, I accept↓♥ to fully live my life by giving myself permission to have rich experiences that move me closer to my divine being. I must fully acknowledge my worth. I live for myself with the values and priorities that are important to me and make me resonate with the whole Universe. I reject any thought of "not being good enough, of being inferior or bad". Life tells me to be more open to myself and to take care of myself. I must already be happy to start with, rather than expect the coming of a child to make me happy. I thus avoid making my happiness depend on someone else, for that is a heavy responsibility to bear. I let go and I ask life that, when the right moment has come, everything will unfold naturally. Meanwhile, I cultivate my creativity and my fertility in as many areas of my life as I wish. I create my life as the ***weaver*** creates a tapestry.

STERNUM

The **sternum** is a flat bone located at the anterior and median part of the thorax and joined with the first seven pairs of ribs and with the clavicles.

As it is in full view when I puff out my chest, it is related to my self-image and also to the one I project. If I reject who I am, if I always have the impression that what I do is never good enough, my **sternum** may **bend inward**. I feel ***mediocre***. I may tend to revolt easily, and I react by confronting people aggressively because I was injured in the past. I ***rear up*** like a horse in front of an obstacle. I may also have found myself in a situation where I was unable to say goodbye to a person, could not take her in my arms. I have lost this child-like innocence and spontaneity, and have become a gladiator using his sword to fight in this world that I find barren.

When my belly is prominent and more thrust out than my **sternum**, I find it difficult to accept↓♥ what I am, and I resist something. I am all round because I hide my emotions, I am unable to claim my place and I want to please everyone, I am too gentle in my words and unable to set my limits. I turn frustrations and situations against myself. I stop resisting what I am and life's events.

I choose to know and appreciate myself as I am. I accept↓♥ to fully take part in transforming my life, for I am its creator. I accept↓♥ to stand straight and to express myself confidently.

STIES / STYES *See also: BOILS / FURUNCLES / CARBUNCLES*

A **stye** is a small red and painful furuncle [15] located on the edge of an eyelid, at the base of an eyelash.

It manifests itself when I experience sadness or resentment toward something or someone that I see and that does not suit me. It may be that a person (it may be my spouse) has a different opinion from mine and does things differently, and that I perceive this as a 'taint'. I was cast aside or I think I acted badly but I would like to do things right and I want to repair my 'error'. I do not feel safe and I feel a lot of uncertainty. It is as though I was not in control of myself, and I need the strength of someone on whom I can rely because I feel too little. I may even hide behind someone else, which prevents me from creating by myself the life I desire. I become passive, and I close myself off from the different opportunities available to me. My life becomes empty and cold. The difference between conjunctivitis and a **stye** is that in the latter case, I find some 'ugliness' in the situation.

Instead of repressing my emotions, I accept↓♥ to express them, for they might well appear in the form of **styes**. It is by taking charge of my life and being part of it, by being in the 'ringside seat' that I can fully flourish.

STIFF NECK *See: NECK [STIFF]*

STIFFNESS (joint, muscle)

Muscular stiffness due to accumulated lactic acid involves an accumulation of rigid and blocked mental energy. I thus manifest rigid thought patterns and obstinacy, as well as a refusal or an inability to 'surrender'. I resist movement. It may also be in relation to authority, a situation or my own self. I congeal in a structure; I stiffen instead of riding the flow. I put my spontaneity aside and I resist life. I do not allow my intuition to express itself. I become intransigent. A **stiffness** limits some of my movements: did I feel I had too much freedom in a certain situation, or does someone want to curtail my freedom? I must check out my mental attitudes in relation to the body part affected by **stiffness**. If it is the **joints** that are **stiff**, in my limbs or in my spine, there is a deep resistance manifested by bone, showing a deep rigidity and a refusal to move forward.

I accept ♥ to become more open and flexible about the new directions that are open to me, in order to avoid taking a steep downward slide. Instead of resisting, I let things flow and I follow the rhythm of life and the seasons.

STIFFNESS (muscular)

Muscle stiffness, also called a **charley horse**, is a sensation of aching pain and muscle fatigue after an unusual exertion or in the initial phase of some viral

15. **Furuncle**: An acute infection of a pilosebaceous follicle.

infections (flu, hepatitis, etc.). The **stiffness** shows itself by a blocking of energy in the muscles.

It is related to the pain felt when a need (affective or emotional) has not been satisfied. Whereas the energy stored in my muscles generally expresses itself by a movement or a gesture, I unconsciously block this energy in the muscle. I am therefore in inner reaction (mental pain), and I express it physically by these bouts of **stiffness**. I feel beaten or oppressed by a person or a situation. The **stiffness** is located at different levels, and the **bone pains** indicate a very deep inner pain. I am affected by it down to the bottom of my being and my space.

I accept↓♥ to change my behavior and move in the right direction without being reactive. I accept↓♥ to be what I am, to live in the present instant, knowing that inside of me, life fills my most basic needs.

STITCH / PAIN (referred)

A **stitch in the side** is a pain that occurs after having made an exertion while walking fast or running. Or it is an intercostal pain due to intense physical agitation or exasperation. This pain rings an alarm: why am I going so fast? What is so urgent for me? I refuse to listen to my inner voice, and I force myself to do certain things in order to present a good image, to fit with the social norms regarding success. Is this irritation due to exasperation, dissatisfaction or disappointment? I push myself to the limit, whatever the consequences for my physical body. I listen only to my head and my insecurities. The **stitch** forces me to slow down. I learn to allow energy to circulate without getting impatient: I take the time to make a pause.

I accept↓♥ to become **Aware** that I also must slow down in my everyday life and take the time to live. I listen to my inner voice that knows what I need and what is good for me. I live at my own pace and my body relaxes and no longer needs to protest!

STOMACH (in general)

The **stomach** receives food and digests it to fill the different needs of my body in vitamins, proteins, etc.

Similarly, I nourish my brain with the situations and events of my life. Each **stomach** has its own way of functioning. Though the general form is the same, digestion can vary from one person to another. My **stomach** reflects the way I absorb and integrate my reality and **my capacity for digesting new ideas or new situations**. It can be compared to a barometer indicating my degree of openness and my way of reacting in life.

I accept↓♥ to welcome new ideas with openness and non-judgment.

STOMACH DISORDERS *See also: STOMACH — HEARTBURN*

The **ailments** affecting my **stomach** are related to 'everyday bread' issues, to the material and maternal side of my existence. I know the work carried out by my **stomach**, and I know it represents **my way of digesting, absorbing and integrating the events and situations of my life**. My **stomach** problems occur when my everyday reality is in conflict with my desires and needs. These conflicts usually take place in my family, friendship or work relations. I am experiencing serious anxieties. Certain things 'stay on my **stomach**' and I am astounded! My digestion is difficult with my thoughts as well as my emotions, for I tend to hold on to the past and I have difficulty in forgiving myself and others. If I do not ***communicate*** or if I hide things, my **stomach** reacts. If I have things to reproach myself with, or if I am not at peace with my **conscience**, **stomach ailments** appear. If I have **stomach cramps**, I ask myself about what situation in my life I am feeling such massive insecurity. I feel lost and I have resigned myself, believing this situation is inescapable. **Stomach pangs** are often related to a need for **Love**, 'emotional nourishment' and food. Food represents affection, security, reward and survival. If I feel an emptiness in my life, I want to fill it with food, especially in moments of separation, death, and loss or lack of money. Food can also help me artificially in 'freeing' myself of material or financial tensions. I feel a sort of **lack** of something indispensable for my survival. **Fermentation** derives from the fact that I do not want to face certain emotions that I experience about persons or situations. I push these emotions aside, but they still remain present, accumulate and 'ferment' as a result of my 'acid' attitude. I constantly brood over certain situations that I experienced and that I 'just can't digest'. I therefore tend to ruminate over past situations and re-experience the same attitudes and the same negative emotions, and I thereby avoid conflicts. Conflicts therefore stay on my **stomach**. It is very difficult for my **stomach** to digest incompletely experienced emotions. As my reality is in conflict with my dreams and my needs, this leads me to experience various emotions. I do not express my annoyances, I am irritated. **Anger** and **aggressiveness** are rumbling in me, but I repress them. And bang! Here come the **ulcer** and the **heartburn**. I have great fears, and my digestion is becoming laborious because my **stomach** is nervous and fragile. What is the situation in my life that I 'just can't digest'? It is usually something that happened recently. It may be a vexation in my family, my work environment, my social circle or my neighborhood and in which I was actively involved. I am feeling very worried, due in part to my poor self-confidence, which makes it difficult for me to accept↓♥ my emotions. A **sore stomach** will appear when I experience a vexation in the area of my personal finances or my work life. Certain situations are so repugnant and disgusting that my **stomach** refuses to digest them. What is the situation or the person that I am close to and that I wish to see disappear from my life? Or is it a part of me or of my way of living that I want to change because I am becoming **Aware** of the fact that I am too artificial and rigid? About what person or situation do I feel ***misunderstood***? Why am I being treated so ungratefully? I react to my reality in a negative and 'acid' manner, and I suffer from **indigestions** and **nausea**. My **digestion is very slow** if my **stomach** is tense and rigid, preventing changes from taking place in my life. I ask myself whether I am also slow and passive in my life, not stepping forward because of my insecurity. This **digestive discomfort** after meals (**dyspepsia**) denotes inactivity and indecision.

I become **Aware** that I must show more openness in life and I accept↓♥ that situations and events are there to make me grow. Acceptance↓♥ transforms them into experiences, and the pressure or tension disappears. I accept↓♥ to live in truth and candidness and thus make peace with my deeper emotions and be in harmony with my entourage. Forgiving and reconciliation are keys for my healing. I thus find within me a true sense of security and fullness.

STOMACH — AEROPHAGY

Aerophagy is the fact of involuntarily swallowing a quantity of air that enters the esophagus and the **stomach**. It is physiological at any age, but when this phenomenon is too frequent, it can provoke a dilation of the esophagus or the **stomach** (**aerogastria**).

I feel great nervousness, an inner tension. I have difficulty in managing and 'digesting' my life, especially on the material and financial side. I am becoming permanently worried. My anxieties govern my life. I feel threatened and saturated, and I can't absorb or integrate anything new. Do I need to breathe new air into my life? What am I trying to swallow all at once? I want to go too fast, and I take no time for myself, which increases my risk of experiencing failures. What is rushing me so in my work, in my relationships, in my life?

I accept↓♥ to take a step back in order to reclaim my vital space. I learn to breathe, to chew, to take the time to live, and I stop allowing others to control my existence. I learn to choose myself when it is necessary. By accepting↓♥ my inner strengths and accepting↓♥ to let them express themselves, I recover my sense of security and my balance.

STOMACH (cancer of the) *See: CANCER OF THE STOMACH*

STOMACH — GASTRITIS *See also: INFLAMMATION*

Gastritis is an acute or chronic inflammation of the **stomach**'s mucous lining, where the digestive process begins.

If there is an inflammation, there is some irritation and anger about something or someone that I can't digest. I don't understand that certain things do not go as I wish, or that certain persons do not act as I desire. I may feel I have been deceived, and am trapped in a situation or betrayed by the silence of a person. I am irritated by something that was absorbed by my digestive system, and the 'digested' reality disturbs me to the highest point. I feel insecure and I wonder what is in store for me. I sense that my world could collapse at any moment. I am like a guard dog, constantly on the lookout for danger.

I learn to accept↓♥ situations and others as they are, knowing that the only power I have is my power over myself. I change my expectations positively: I expect the best from life. I stop worrying and I soon enjoy each living moment.

STOMACH — HEARTBURN

As its name indicates, **heartburn** is the sign that something, a situation, an event or a person is **burning** me, **acidifying** me, making me **angry**. I find the situation irritating, unfair and sinister, and I feel helpless inside. I feel that it is these elements outside of me that control me. I am dominated, and I can't free myself of this hold, which makes anger and even rage rise up in me. When such a situation happens to me, I can ask myself: "What is burning me up or making me angry? What is it that I don't like and just can't digest[16]?" I have an 'acid' and bitter attitude toward life. It is also quite possible that I am unconsciously holding on to this anger, for I am afraid of asserting myself, of letting go and expressing my needs, my desires and my intentions with my **heart♥**. I am altogether unique, and the others are altogether different from me. I must therefore remain open and attentive to my own needs and accept↓♥ total responsibility for my acts, even if people are different from me. Stifling or repressing an emotion (anger, sorrow, rage) increases the acidity of the gastric gases, and thereby prevents me from swallowing anything else (for the burns manifest a form of **inner pressure** in the region of the **stomach**).

I accept↓♥ to see the links between my true feelings and my **heartburn**. I remain calm and observe my way of being and my reactions to the situations I experience and my attitude toward everyday events. By focusing my attention on my conviction that life is good and all my needs will be fulfilled in good time, my personal self-esteem increases and my next angers will be less intense. I take the time to appreciate each moment of my life, and my **stomach** feels better for it!

STOMACH (sore) *See also: INTESTINES, STOMACH (IN GENERAL)*

For a child as for an adult, a **sore stomach** indicates a feeling of abandonment and solitude. I am sensitive to an external event that affects me without my being able to express it. This makes revolt rise in me. **Sore stomachs** in a child are often a way to be taken care of. It is the refusal to communicate, the fear of not being listened to. I am anxious because I don't know what to do with all my possibilities. Did I make the right decisions? I want to be 'correct'. I am afraid of suffering and dying. I have the impression I am constantly under surveillance, and my level of stress is very high. I can try to talk to myself to reassure myself and give myself more self-confidence.

I furthermore accept↓♥ to communicate with my entourage by letting **Love** flow toward others. I trust life.

---

16. "**I just can't digest**": Here, the expression must be taken in the figurative sense. It could be someone about whom I say: *"Her, I just can't digest"*. (I am fed up with her, I can't stand her). It means that I do not esteem this person, or I resent her for some reason.

STOMACH (upset) / BILIOUSNESS *See also: INDIGESTION*

The **liver** metabolizes food, eliminates excess proteins, fats and sugars, and purifies the blood of its impurities. It is essential to life. It is known as the "seat of **anger** and **criticism**". The **liver** is also related to my behavior and represents my readiness to adjust to the events and circumstances of life. The negative emotions I feel (sorrow, hate, jealousy, envy, aggressiveness) hinder the proper functioning of the **liver**. My **liver** has a capacity for accumulating stress and inner tension. It is also in my **liver** that my bitter and irritating thoughts and feelings, still unexpressed or unresolved, are deposited. This is why, when I detoxify my **liver** by physiological means (with phytotherapy or otherwise) or energy-based ones, I then feel more calm and more in contact with myself. **Liver disorders** can even lead me to experience depression, which is perceived as a disappointment with myself. I may then experience sadness, weariness and a general slackening. I want to justify myself for my feeling of guilt and my disquiet. When my **liver** is congested, it affects the inner and spiritual levels of my conscience. There, I may lose my way and the direction I must take. The **liver** gives life, as well as it can keep going my fear of this very life.

I accept↓♥ to act so that it will give me life. I take responsibility for my thoughts and acts, and I consciously choose to focus my attention only on the positive. This leads me to have a fresh outlook on life. I thus show greater openness, and **Love** will flow more easily inside of me and all around me.

STRABISMUS / HETEROTROPIA *See: EYES — STRABISMUS (IN GENERAL)*

STRAIN *See: JOINTS — STRAIN / SPRAIN*

STRESS

Stress is an adaptive response to an event, a situation or a danger, real or imaginary. The capacity for adjusting depends on different factors: any situation that creates a greater demand on my organism leads me to experience **stress**, which changes into di**stress** if it is experienced to an extremely intense degree. The **stress** may be psychological (the pressure of my entourage), physical (a strong demand on my body related to work, sports, heat, cold, etc.), chemical or biochemical (the taking of medications, chemotherapy, hormonal change).

Stress in itself, in short, is less important than my reaction to it. It can be quite as positive, stimulating and creative as it can be threatening for my body. Depending on my reaction to events and to the underlying emotions, the stressful effect will be beneficial or noxious for me. It is important to see that even a happy event can make me experience high **stress**. Thus, I may win a million dollars at the lottery, which can have the effect of making me experience a depression because I feel I now have so many things to change in my life that I am afraid of not being able to do them. Will I keep my job with the people I esteem? Will my friends still be the same with me? Will I have to move? Will I be able to adjust to all these changes?

I accept↓♥ to look inside of me and question my reactions, my motives and my attitudes rather than put the blame on external situations. I learn to relax and consider the benefits of **stress**.

STRETCH MARKS / STRIA *See: SKIN — STRETCH MARKS / STRIA*

STUTTERING *See also: MOUTH, THROAT (IN GENERAL)*

Stuttering is the manifestation of an elocution disorder, a partial or severe difficulty in speaking, saying and expressing myself clearly (it may vary from a few random words to a regular disorder). It is related to the throat, the center of communication and self-expression.

My **stuttering** may originate from an affective or sexual block resulting from my childhood. This does not necessarily mean that I experienced inappropriate touching, but consciously or not, I may have registered a fear about my sexuality in relation to a person or an event. It is a form of **deep insecurity** originating from my childhood and related to the fear of a parent (the father or the mother), usually the person who represents authority, and which manifests itself in the presence of others. It is a sort of **repression**, an incapacity for adequately controlling my thoughts and my intense emotions and the failed attempt to control the expression of my speech, which is no longer spontaneous (this type of disorder can appear in early childhood when a child has been impeded in its right to cry: "*Don't cry!*"). It may also be a trauma experienced when I was inhibited or prevented from doing certain actions. I then transform this emotion into **stuttering**. I hesitate, I can't get to say clearly what I feel, I repress and deform my words for fear of rejection or out of anxiety. *If I clearly say what I feel, will my parents accept↓♥ it? Am I acceptable enough for them? Do I meet their expectations? Do they allow me to be what I am? Do my words exceed my thoughts?* Chances are high that one or both of my parents are very authoritarian and domineering and that I will not be allowed to 'carry the ***ball***'. I feel judged, controlled, criticized and even ridiculed enough for me to end up believing that my words are worth nothing. As a child, I may also have been either prevented from expressing myself or forced to speak when I didn't feel like it. Am I afraid of betraying someone by revealing a secret? What is the thing that must not be told? And if I dare to say it, how will it prove harmful to me? If I found myself in a situation where I was very frightened and was unable to scream, the stress I felt crystallized in my mouth and my words 'froze' and are no longer able to express themselves normally. If I grew up in an environment where the law of silence was golden, (the unsaid and the secret), this is a heavy burden, and I must always take some time before speaking, to make sure that I am not 'transgressing the law'. I then show all sorts of behavioral disorders, ranging from timidity to withdrawing into myself. I feel I am living in a prison where it is difficult to breathe. I am seeking my power, which I currently see only in others. The outer world is hostile, so how can I take my place in it while expressing myself freely? When I was very young, I may have experienced much confusion about speech or what language to use. For example, if more than one language was spoken at home and there was some competition about which one should predominate, I will have developed some insecurity about the words to be used, and this hesitation will show itself in the greater time delay that I leave between words. I may find it very difficult to express my feelings or my needs. I have the impression that I 'beg' for the attention or the approval of others.

The first step is to accept↓♥ to open my **heart♥** to my **thoughts**, **words** and **actions**, and mainly my **emotions** and **desires**. It is important to take my time and respect my own 'speed of being'. I respect myself as I am, with no judgment or criticism. I accept↓♥ to express my ideas, my joys, my sorrows and my fears. I am more and more engaged in acting and asserting myself and my desires. I can then begin to trust myself, to feel my emotions and feelings and to open up to the people I **love**. I thus recover an inner calm that enables me to express myself much more confidently. I will thus avoid the stammering, the rush of words of an overactive mind, or the holding back of certain words that have possibly fearful repercussions. I resume contact with my true nature, and I allow **Love** to flow in me. Inner peace sets in, and my acceptance↓♥ of my whole being thus leads others also to accept↓♥ me as I am.

SUBLINGUAL GLAND *See: GLANDS [SALIVARY]*

SUBLUXATION *See: LUXATION*

SUDDEN INFANT DEATH SYNDROME (SIDS) / CRIB DEATH

The **sudden infant death syndrome** is the brutal and unexpected death of a baby so far considered as being in good health. **Sleep apnea** is sometimes thought to be a cause. Though the baby presented symptoms, nothing portended such a quickly fatal outcome.

I, a baby, see this life before me as a burden. I am nothing, not good enough for my Dad and Mom. I do not desire to live, I prefer to go back, for I have become frightened by the mandate I gave myself. I have a huge sorrow, a great disappointment. Or I have come to live this experience of birth-death in order to evolve and make the people around me progress through letting go and detachment. My sobs are choking me. If I am the parent, I see how this baby is my mirror: is it possible that I too am destroying myself because I don't believe that I am up to it? Because I feel guilty and inferior? What is my own identity? Do I protect my vital space, or allow myself to be invaded by others?

I accept↓♥ right now to live my life for myself. I give myself unconditional **Love**. By being autonomous and strong, I regain courage and can give more to others, especially my children. I become **Aware** and I accept↓♥ that everything in life is lent to us: people, things and situations. I discover that nothing is immutable or permanent and everything is a life experience to grow and develop.

SUICIDE *See also: ANGUISH, ANXIETY, MELANCHOLY*

If I am thinking about **suicide**, I make the decision to destroy myself. I feel devoid of energy, and this idea is constantly haunting my thoughts. I become melancholy, solitary and full of bitterness. I can no longer initiate any outside contacts; I am living inside my bubble in which I allow nobody else because "no one understands me". My suffering is such that I no longer see the **Light**. It has become intolerable. **Suicide is related to escape**. I can ask myself, then, what I am trying to flee: my inner pain, my responsibilities, my inner emptiness, my lack of **Love**, etc.

If I consume drugs or alcohol and my diet is deficient in certain nutriments essential for the balance of my nervous system, I may be more prone to having **suicidal** ideas. I may also feel like committing **suicide** as a means to punish someone else; thus, they will then bear the guilt of not having loved me enough.

I accept↓♥ to trust and I close my eyes: the **Light** is in my **heart♥**. **I talk to someone about it, or I write down on paper the distress I experience in asking for help**.

SUNSTROKE / INSOLATION *See: ACCIDENT, BURNS, HEATSTROKE, SKIN (IN GENERAL)*

SURDIMUTISM *See: DEAF MUTE / DEAF AND DUMB*

SUPRARENAL / ADRENAL GLANDS *See: GLAND — CAPSULE [SUPRARENAL]*

SWALLOWING (difficulty in) *See: ESOPHAGUS*

SWELLING (in general)

Swelling usually appears when I experience an emotional resistance and repress my emotions. I accumulate these emotions because I feel powerless or do not know how to express them, to avoid hurting someone or simply hurting myself. **Swelling** can also be a means of protection, and I can ask myself: why do I feel the need to protect myself, and from whom or what? Am I making up illusions for myself about a situation? Illusions are related to water, and if I become **Aware** of the fact that this illusion is a wrong perception of a situation or a person, it will be in my interest to realistically question my values and my perception of things. I may also feel some persons are lying to me or hiding the truth from me.

I accept↓♥ to go and check out my perceptions so that the situations in my life will be clearer. I learn to express what I experience in order to free myself, and thus make these **swellings** disappear.

SWELLING / BLOATING (of the abdomen)

Swelling, or bloating, of the abdomen makes me become **Aware** that I am feeling frustration about my spouse, my children or my family. I sense that I am being lied to. I probably feel limited on the affective level or in the expression of my feelings toward some of the persons in my entourage.

I accept↓♥ that, by changing my way of seeing things and taking a more positive attitude, I will become **Aware** of the full abundance that is in my life, in all areas: affective, intellectual, emotional, material, etc.

SYNCOPE *See: BRAIN — SYNCOPE*

SYNDROME (acquired immune deficiency) / AIDS *See: AIDS*

SYNDROME[17] (Burnett's) *See: MILK-ALCALI SYNDROME*

SYNDROME (carpal tunnel) *See: WRIST – SYNDROME [CARPAL TUNNEL]*

SYNDROME (chronic fatigue) *See: CHRONIC FATIGUE SYNDROME*

SYNDROME (Cushing's) *See: CUSHING'S SYNDROME*

SYNDROME (Down's) *See: MONGOLISM / TRISOMY 21 / DOWN'S SYNDROME*

SYNDROME (Gélineau's) *See: NARCOLEPSY*

SYNDROME (Guillain-Barré's) / ACUTE POLYRADICULONEURITIS

See also: SYSTEM [IMMUNE]

Guillain-Barré's[18] **syndrome** is typified by inflammation and demyelination (loss of myelin[19]) in many nerve roots. It sometimes follows an infectious or viral disease or a vaccination, but most often, it appears to result from immune disorders. It is mainly located in the lower part of the body, but it can affect all the roots of the spinal and cranial nerves.

I am in a situation where I have the impression that I am being spied on; someone or something is going about disguised like a chameleon and wants to attack me. My nerves are constantly on edge, I stay on the alert, I trust nobody and I feel powerless because I don't really know my adversary, who in any case is supposed to protect me. He has a 'two-sided face', as I sometimes do, and it bothers me. I become hypersensitive to everything around me to avoid danger, and I feel powerless to react because I don't know where the attack will come from. I may resent myself for having done or said certain things, hence a feeling of guilt. I have the impression of having betrayed or of

17. **Syndrome**: A syndrome is not a disease in the proper sense, but a set of symptoms, the specific cause of which is unknown. In this case, it involves people who drink too much milk!

18. **Guillain** (Georges), **Barré** (Jean-Alexandre), **Strohl** (André): French physicians who in 1916 showed the characteristic anomaly of an increase of the proteins in the cerebrospinal fluid with a normal cell count in two soldiers with transitory generalized paralysis.

19. **Myelin**: It is a whitish substance that sheathes the nerve fibres making up the nerves of the cerebrospinal system (it is considered as the core of the nerves).

having been betrayed. I may discover information that will force me to 'bar' a person from my life.

A contact was cut off somewhere between me and a situation or someone. The loss of a good friend scares me, and I may react by having superficial relations with people to protect my sensitivity. This cutting off may also be from myself, for there is a conflict between my individuality and the **Soul** that I am: I lie to myself, I am in denial somehow.

I accept↓♥ to become **Aware** and understand how doubt and lies are present in my life, and from now on, I must live in Truth in every instant, whether with myself or with my entourage. This is how I can develop frank, deep and durable relations with others. I am thus naturally protected, and my life becomes increasingly calm and luminous.

SYNDROME (milk-alkali) *See: MILK — ALKALI SYNDROME*

SYNDROME (over-use) *See also: BACK DISORDERS, INFLAMMATION, TENDONS*

The **over-use syndrome** is a disease mainly found in musicians. It is characterized by inflammation in the tendons of the fingers, the wrist, the elbows and sometimes the shoulders or the neck. It can produce back pains. It is said that 'constraining positions' can cause up to 53 % of symphony orchestra musicians to suffer from back pains.

As a musician, I am often confined in tight spaces, enjoying a degree of comfort poorly suited to the job. It may be that the long hours of practice make me find the work heavy to endure when my shoulders are affected. The job insecurity and fierce competition in this milieu make me experience great fears, and I do not feel supported enough: that is where my shoulder pains come from.

I accept↓♥ to stay flexible and harmonize my mental and spiritual energy when my tendons are affected. Each body part sends me an appropriate message about what I am experiencing. Though it may seem to be related to my profession as a musician, there is no randomness to it. I identify the affected part in order to reach the level of **Awareness** that will help me feel better in what I do.

SYNDROME (premenstrual) *See: MENSTRUATION — PREMENSTRUAL SYNDROME*

SYNDROME (Severe Acute Respiratory) / (SARS) / ACUTE INTERSTITIAL PNEUMONITIS *See also: LUNGS — PNEUMONIA, RESPIRATION*

Severe acute respiratory syndrome (SARS), or **atypical pneumopathy**, is a severe pulmonary infection characterized by the sudden appearance of a fever exceeding 100.4° F (or 38° C) and by certain respiratory symptoms: coughing, shortness of breath and difficulty in breathing.

I am afraid, I am breathing badly, I am choking and feverish. My temperature rises when I am feeling trapped somewhere, in my couple, at work or elsewhere. I know I must reconsider my vital space, for the situation in which I am is stifling me. I am afraid of settling down and committing myself. I feel invaded from all sides by people who are poisoning my existence. It is becoming urgent for me to raise my **Consciousness** and free myself of these fears in order to fully come to terms with my existence. I question myself about my fears of commitment.

I accept↓♥ to consider situations where I may find 'my' place, or decide that it is time for me to disengage, to extract myself, to break off or to change something in my behavior. I learn to choose myself on the basis of my needs, and I become in harmony again by breathing fully.

SYNDROME (yellow nail) *See: NAIL — YELLOW NAIL SYNDROME*

SYPHILIS *See: VENEREAL DISEASES*

SYSTEM (immune) *See also: AIDS*

My organism's defense is provided by a **self-protection system**, which is essential to protect me from attacks originating from the outside world, such as bacteria, viruses, microscopic fungi and other potential problems. It recognizes foreign cells, pathogenous infectious agents[20] and the cells of another organism, which thus accounts for the rejection of grafts. Without the total and complete functioning of this **system**, death would ensue.

It is directly related to my emotional states, and a deep pain in my existence can dramatically reduce its strength. The **immune** cells initially develop in the bone marrow, and those that will become T cells are carried, once matured, to the thymus gland located near the **heart♥**. The T cells play a primordial role in identifying and eliminating foreign cells or substances that are not beneficial for the body. Of course, they must also be capable of recognizing what is good for the human body. They differentiate, discern, tolerate or reject, as needed, for the purpose of maintaining my body in the most perfect state of health possible. The **immune system** takes care of my reference system and therefore of who I am, my individuality or my personality. It guards my fortress (physical and emotional) and deploys its resistance when it must combat an enemy. The location of the thymus gland near the **heart♥** makes me become more **Aware** of the 'body-spirit' relation that exists. The **immune system** responds to my feelings and to all my thoughts, whether positive or negative. Thus, all thoughts of anger, bitterness, hate, resentment and self-destruction will tend to weaken my **immune system**. On the other hand, all thoughts of **Love**, harmony, beauty and inner peace will tend to reinforce my **immune system**. The thymus is the endocrine gland that is associated with the chakra (energy center) of the **heart♥**. Therefore, when my **immune system** is affected,

---

20. **Pathogenous**: Which can cause a disease.

my need for **Love** is also very great. My brain also is closely linked to my **immune system**, and certain states of mind can powerfully affect the functioning of my system. I become **Aware** that my **immune system** may be far busier curbing my own negative thoughts (therefore the internal enemy) than the attacks from outside (the external enemy). This system can become weakened if my first concern is to doubt the place and respect I award myself. This may originate from the uncertainty I experienced in my childhood toward one of my parents: I felt that the nest was in danger, sensed that a gale of madness was sweeping the house. I am in a dynamic of emotional self-destruction. Am I forgetting myself, letting myself pass after others, thus denying who I am and quelling my true needs? I ask myself: "What am I worth, and what can I provide for others in any case?" My life is filled with the requisite conditions for accomplishing things or simply for being happy. I easily give up before the obstacles that face me because I no longer have the desire to live. I no longer have any reasons for defending myself. As I am not capable of seeing what is good or bad for me, or of properly identifying myself to others without any judgment or self-criticism, my **immune system** can no longer protect me as much. It no longer even knows whether it should do its job, since I show no intense desire to live.

I accept↓♥ right now to identify the emotions I am experiencing, whatever they may be. I immediately make a habit of getting rid of the wastes that can prevent or diminish the effectiveness of my **immune system**: I take care of my feelings of sadness, solitude, abandonment, depreciation, etc., by discovering the message or the life lesson that a special situation in which I feel those emotions is leading me to learn. I thus restore the balance between my inner and outer lives, and my **immune system** is fully operational. I detach myself from the expectations and values of society and build my own preferences. I thus connect myself to my power of creation and healing that nourishes and reinforces my natural immunity. I discover my inner richness and I decide to choose myself: by learning to be well with myself, I am more able to enjoy a more enriching social life based on true values.

SYSTEM (locomotor) *See also: BONES*

The **locomotor system** is related to my mobility and my flexibility as well as to my inner openness and my outer openness. It comprises the bones, the muscles, the tendons and the ligaments. The framework that holds up my whole body is made up of bones. **These are what represent my moral principles, my structure, my honesty, my integrity, my stability**. When I become too rigid in my thoughts, my bones too become rigid and risk breaking more easily. **The extremities of my body and my muscles symbolize action and movement**. With my hands, I can grasp things and hold on to them. **My legs enable me to advance in life**. A difficulty in moving indicates that I am afraid of progressing. A lack of humility or a refusal to 'bend' or to admit my mistakes has the effect of making it difficult for me to bend my knees. My feet represent stability. I thus keep contact with the ground; I have 'both feet on the ground'. Each body part helps me to become **Aware** of my suppleness or my rigidity.

I accept↓♥ to listen to my body and feel free in my movements, for it is the guide of my inner state.

SYSTEM (lymphatic) *See also: GANGLION [LYMPHATIC]*

The **lymphatic system** is made up of the ganglions and vessels that transport the lymph to the bloodstream. It plays an important role in the functioning of the immune system. The **lymphatic system** is, in a sense, in parallel with the cardiovascular system. It is more directly related to the emotional and affective side of me, to the humors[21]. Whereas my nervous system is more directly related to the mental side of my energy-flowing or astral body, my **lymphatic system** is more directly related to the affective side of my energy-flowing or astral body.

Love is certainly the best way to keep the **lymphatic system** healthy and effective.

SYSTEM (nervous) *See also: NERVES (IN GENERAL)*

My **nervous system** is made up of nerves and centers that serve to coordinate and command the different parts of my body (emission), as well as to receive sensory, psychic and intellectual information.

In fact, my **nervous system** is more directly related to my thoughts in relation to my energy-flowing or mental body. It is the electrical connection system on the physical level that enables my thoughts to take action in this world. The **nervous system** is affected (**neuropathy**) when I overly favor my rational side to the detriment of my emotions and my intuition. Everything is thought out, analyzed, programmed and organized in my life, and I find it difficult to make room for spontaneity, pleasure, the joy of living and my emotions that I tend to repress. I come to experience many inner tensions and deal poorly with everyday situations. My "neurons are overheating".

I accept↓♥ to learn how to humanize my interpersonal interactions and relations in order to become fully conscious of the emotions that dwell in me. I can thus fully live my life in a balanced manner.

---

21. **Humours**: The organic tissue fluids of the human body.

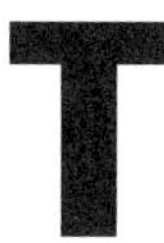

TACHYCARDIA *See: HEART♥ — CARDIAC ARRHYTHMIA*

TANTRUM *See also: HYSTERIA, NEUROSIS*

A **tantrum**, also called **self-centeredness**, is an inner surge of energy and vibrations that blocks, either at the level of speech because of an inability to communicate my point of view, or at the level of an activity, when I find it impossible to achieve or carry out an action.

At that point, the blocking becomes so strong and so great that I cannot release the energy harmoniously, and an **explosion occurs**. This leads me to say extreme words or carry out extreme gestures. These outbursts have their source in my attention, which is always attuned to my fears; I constantly fear that something negative will happen, but I do nothing to change the situation.

I accept↓♥ to stop and become **Aware**, while taking great breaths of air and relaxing deeply. I must accept↓♥ the situation and take the time to lower the pressure, while rebalancing my emotions.

TARTAR *See: TEETH — TOOTH AILMENTS*

TASTE DISORDERS *See also: NOSE, THROAT, TONGUE*

Ageusia is the total or partial (**hypogeusia**) loss of **taste**, often associated with a loss of smell.

Do I still feel like pursuing what I have undertaken? What do I need to change in the situation I am experiencing? I don't talk about it, but I feel that I am losing the expression of what I am. I may have the impression that I have to swallow a situation that I find disgusting: "Since I don't have the choice, it is better that I taste nothing!" It is a protective mechanism that enables me to escape unpleasant situations and also my deeper nature, my emotions. I protect myself from others but at the same time, I disconnect from myself, from my body and my feelings. I am no longer in contact with myself and the world around me. I diminish or 'neutralize' my sense of taste to protect myself.

I accept↓♥ to taste life, to allow myself new experiences in order to feel that I exist and let my radiance show. I trust my body and my deeper nature. I have the right to assert myself and say NO if a situation does not suit me. I respect myself more and more, and others will do as much for me!

TEAR DUCTS *See: CRYING*

TEARS *See: CRYING*

TEETH (in general)

The **teeth** symbolize **decisions**, the solid entranceway that enables me to take a full bite in life! Both inner and outer realities go through my **teeth**, which are one of the means I have to express myself wholly in this world. The **tooth** is one of the very hard auxiliary organs that represent the basic energy of my being, my integrity. The inner capacity for welcoming new ideas, **Love** and inner foods, as well as my balance and stability, manifest themselves by healthy and hard **teeth**.

The **teeth** are, in part, the mirror of a being. When food passes through my mouth, the mouth also transmits feelings that can affect my **teeth** in the more or less long term. A **tooth** is always affected first (even if it is, for example, a non-apparent cavity) and the related soft body organ is affected later on. Thus, **altered teeth** (decayed **teeth**, for example) indicate poor **self-assertion**, a reality unacceptable for me and the **fear of taking my place** in the world with the responsibilities this involves. My difficulty in acquiring my autonomy and my independence, in ***attaining*** what I desire, will take the form of ailments in my **teeth**. Even though I have difficulty in making certain beneficial decisions for myself, I must remain open to the available means that can enable me to overcome the most delicate situations. For many animals, their **teeth** represent the most effective means of self-protection and self-defense from external attacks. If I feel in danger and don't know quite how to react, my **teeth** will react.

My **teeth** also represent my will to move forward, to do things well, my capacity for giving life to my thoughts and my emotions. A deep conflict, guilt related to an emotional situation conveyed in words, or any other inner turmoil may manifest themselves by a reaction in the **teeth** and even in the **gums**. The **ailment** in a **tooth** or in the **gums** appears when I decide that the conflict will not be resolved and, consciously or not, I decide that "time will fix things". I want to limit the damage, and it is my **teeth** that will **decay**. Unresolved situations and poorly managed emotions 'decay' my **teeth**. I can therefore 'clench my **teeth**' to defend myself from an external attack in a situation that makes me strongly react. I close the door, resisting whatever wants to enter me or, on the contrary, whatever needs to come out of me. The **incisors** (the front **teeth**) represent the fact of having to decisively settle a choice between yes or no, between doing or not doing such and such an action, etc.

The **canines** are more related to the fact of being able to exercise a certain authority over the decisions I have to make. Somewhat like fangs, they symbolize my capacity or my duty to protect myself. They may be affected when I feel 'torn' by a decision to be made. I work relentlessly and yet, I have the impression that I will not be able to reach my goals. The **premolars** indicate how much I agree with my decisions. The **molars** represent my degree of satisfaction with the decisions I have made or that still remain for me to make. The **tooth enamel** will be affected when I have the impression that I don't have the right to 'bite' into a situation for moral reasons or because of the education

I received (I am too-well brought up to do any such thing). I may also sense that I am being 'used' by the people close to me because I have no barrier to defend me. The **dentin** will be affected if I think I am unable to 'bite' into a situation, doubting myself and my capacities. My everyday reality weighs heavily, and I want to escape it.

I accept↓♥ to remain open to **Love**, without fearing that I might lose the gratitude of others. When my **teeth** are healthy, I allow myself to smile more, and I thus open myself to nonverbal communication with others. I **love** myself as I am, with all my qualities. I must take care of my **teeth**; they 'dress up' my personality. They enable me to communicate clearly and precisely, being able to express my thoughts and my emotions with the appropriate words. **Teeth** do not wear masks! I remain myself, without judging myself and while remaining open to outside criticism. I transform my thoughts into true **Love**, and my **teeth** remain healthy.

TEETH — TOOTH AILMENTS

Dental problems are related to **decisions**, especially when I have **toothaches**. I **put off making decisions** because the consequences of these choices frighten me and make me feel insecure. It is associated with personal responsibility and with my capacity for making decisions-without fearing what may follow later on[1]. This indecision may derive from the fact that I don't have an overall view of a situation and thus can't draw any appropriate conclusions. My **teeth protrude** excessively when I am overly rushed in my decisions, when I want everything to go faster. I constantly make compromises for others to like me. If my **teeth** are slanted **backward**, I tend instead to apply the brakes and withdraw into myself. I have a **raging toothache**, and it may well be that **rage** has taken over in me because I resent myself for not being able to express what I want. I feel like 'baring my **teeth**', ***grumbling*** to take my place and show that I exist, or show off my power. I want to be listened to and respected. On the contrary, I 'shut my trap'. **In the root**, it shows the rage I feel over a situation where I am afraid of losing a member of my family.

Pain usually reappears in 'painful' situations where I must detach myself from a situation or a person. If I have not completely resolved a situation, the **pain** may remain even after the extraction of a **tooth**. The **pain** shows me that the anger I feel is useless and that I must stop putting pressure on myself because of the issue that the painful **tooth** represents. I become **Aware** that by communicating my needs and my desires, the **raging toothaches** will no longer have a reason to exist. When I am a child and **my teething is difficult**, I feel lost, not knowing what I can rely on. I feel anxious and uncertain. If on the contrary I have **no sensitivity**, it is my way of escaping unpleasant situations and turning a deaf ear to the messages that my body is sending me.

---

1. That is why so many people fear going to the dentist's. I often blame my fear of needles and shots to justify not going to the dentist's. But unconsciously, I know that working on my **teeth** will touch nasty emotions I want to flee. I often feel more emotional and febrile at the dentist's.

When there is **tartar on the teeth**, it is a form of internal aggression, an unresolved past reaction that is resurfacing. It may lead me to harden my positions about decisions I have to take or have already taken. I live for others instead of living according to my own aspirations and my personal will. **Tartar** becomes armor for my **teeth** to protect myself from external attacks. When I **break a tooth**, I am experiencing a confrontation with someone or something larger and more powerful than I, and I may stubbornly continue to fight for my ideas or what I believe in. I am rigid, always exceeding my capacities.

If my **baby teeth persist**, I am clinging to certain childish behaviors because I am afraid of growing up. If I **lose my teeth** prematurely, I have the impression that others are making the decisions in my place. I can't 'bite into life'. If I have reached the point of **losing my teeth**, for instance when I am getting on in age, it is as though my life no longer belongs to me, for others are making the decisions in my place. I can no longer 'bare my **teeth'**, and reluctantly forsake my creativity and my youth. If some of my **teeth have not developed**, it is difficult for me to be alive: I don't see how I can become independent, especially from my mother, and be able to express myself freely without fearing for the consequences. **Receding gums** are related to the fear of being discovered in an undisclosed secret. It wears me down over the years. I therefore lose myself and have no limits because, like a chameleon, I want too much to adjust to others so that they will like and accept↓♥ me. It would be time for me to delimit my vital space and free myself from this gnawing secret, to allow the energy to flow and bite into life.

I accept↓♥ to find a way to better structure my thinking and my ideas; it will thus be easier for me to take shrewd initiatives related to what I am currently experiencing and change my behaviors. I accept↓♥ to be **Aware** of what is going on in my life and to make sense of the determination that manages my Universe. I examine the side affected by **dental problems** and apply a suitable solution. If it is above, I think of intuition and instinct, whereas below, it is more a decision in the rational and logical domain, something physically needed.

TEETH — DENTURES / FALSE TEETH

A denture gives me the illusion of strong vitality. Indeed, similar to real **teeth**, it gives the impression of being real, of being as sincere as real **teeth**! Nothing is more false! As I want a clear answer, I go to the bottom of things. Am I capable of living my experiences with courage and sincerity, as with my real **teeth**? Am I determined to be what I truly am, to assert myself, to be wholehearted, to 'bite' into life? If the **denture injures me** (as following a so-called poor adjustment), I am still hurt, even unconsciously, by a parent who was monopolizing and demanding or who 'poisoned' my life (above, the father, my rational side, Yang; and below, the mother, my affective, intuitive side, Yin). It prevents me from becoming more autonomous.

I stop living according to others. I accept↓♥ to be myself, and by asserting myself I find satisfaction and happiness.

TEETH (grinding of) — BRUXISM *See also: AUTHORITARIANISM, JAW AILMENTS*

The **teeth** represent decisions and a certain form of aggressiveness. The **grinding of teeth**, also called **bruxism**, is therefore an **unconscious anger** that is surfacing, a **repressed rage** expressing itself, often at night.

I am very nervous inside, I hold back from saying or doing certain things. As I am unable to make clear and precise decisions, **grinding my teeth** is the **physical expression of my repressed sadness and aggressiveness** toward a situation that I find intolerable. Like a badly oiled door, the **grinding of teeth** throws **Light** on my fear of opening up to make decisions, and the sound of it expresses a form of inner moaning, feeling myself under the hold of an ***evil spell, bewitched***.

I speak in silence in order to release what I was unable to express in words during the day: all the things left unsaid, everything I buried inside. **Children** are very often affected by **bruxism**: it is from an early age that I learn the power games and the different authority relations that exist. If I am afraid of voicing my opinions, feeling 'too little' in front of my parents, my babysitter or my teachers, I **grind my teeth**.

Whatever my age, **bruxism** manifests my huge inner tension. I am facing a very great duality between my head and my **heart♥**, my reason and my passion, and the result is passivity.

I accept↓♥ to become **Aware** of this state without repressing it, and to express it as I currently experience it. I accept↓♥ my sensitivity and my surfacing emotions, and I realize that my uncertainties make me experience far more inner tension than just taking the needed initiatives. When I make a decision, I free myself and I feel more flourishing.

TEETH (root abscess) *See: TEETH — TOOTH [ROOT ABSCESS]*

TEETH (symbolism of)

N.B. I am always facing the person's right and left sides. Therefore:

On my left, I see the person's **right upper** (**teeth 11 to 18**) and **lower maxillaries** (**teeth 41 to 48**), which correspond to the left brain (the rational, concrete, material and analytic side).

On my right, I see the person's **left upper** (**teeth 21 to 28**) and **lower maxillaries** (**teeth 31 to 38**), which correspond to the right brain (affection, intuition, desire, sensitivity).

As the **teeth** are alive and follow a development process extending over several years, it is interesting to note that each one of them is related to a feeling or an emotion that, if it is poorly managed, will cause a weakness in that particular **tooth**.

If there is any **loss of teeth on the upper right side (teeth 11 to 18)**, I have difficulty in finding my place. The **left upper side (teeth 21 to 28)** indicates that I have difficulty in achieving my desire to be. The **lower right side (teeth 41 to 48)** refers to my difficulty in concretely building my life. The **lower left side (teeth 31 to 38)** indicates that I am not receiving the affective recognition I need from my family.

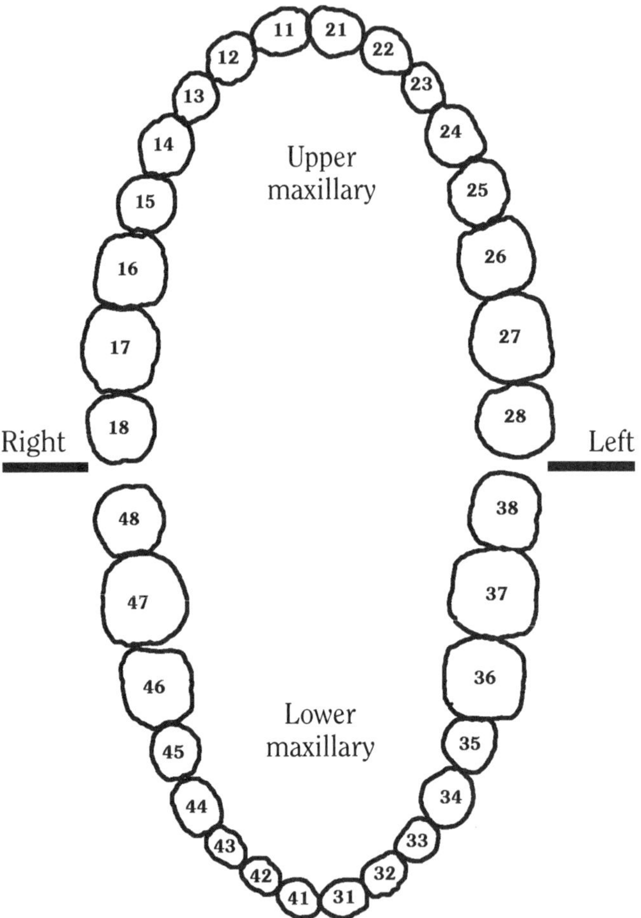

The **upper right central incisor (# 11)** corresponds to the father, the male part in humans, authority, God. The **upper left central incisor (# 21)** corresponds to the mother, the female part in humans. If a space is found between these two **teeth**, my female and male polarities are dissociated. If I am a woman, I constantly question my relationship with my spouse. If I am a man, I experience a duality toward women: I am attracted, but at the same time repelled by them. A **space between these two teeth** denotes my difficulty in forming a couple, outside of me as well as inside of me. If one of these **teeth** overlaps the other, the **overlapping tooth** represents the parent I perceive as the dominant one, and the **tooth** that is behind represents the parent I perceive as the dominated or self-effacing one.

The **lower central incisors** (**# 31 and #41**) refer to the place concretely occupied, namely in everyday life, by the mother or whoever represents her (**#31**) and the father (**#41**) or whoever represents him.

Just beside are the **lateral incisors** (**# 12, 22, 32, 42**). They are in direct relation with the central incisors. If I am having difficulty with one of my two parents or what they represent, lateral incisors will change positions, as my dynamic or my reactions to the male and female principles are called into question. These **teeth** will be **in front or will overlap the central incisors** if I want to be stronger than my parents, in front of them, independent, not subjected to authority. I want to dominate my parents or they will slip away of their own accord. The more forward they are, the earlier I wanted to distance myself from my parents. This situation prevails with my mother if the **left lateral incisor** (**#22**) **overlaps #21**, and it prevails with my father if it is the **right lateral incisor** (**#12**) **that overlaps # 11**. If the **lateral incisors** are **behind** the **central incisors**, I then take a submissive attitude toward one or the other or both parents, or I feel overprotected.

The **canine teeth** (**# 13, 23, 33, 43**) appear at puberty (around age 13–14), when sexual energy develops. They correspond to the great inner transformations I am experiencing. From my difficulties with my body and my incipient sexuality to my capacity for making choices, they will affect my **canines**. The **upper right canine** (**#13**) is related to changes that are visible or manifested outwardly, to projects and a view of the future, to duties and obligations that may lead me to not express myself. The **upper left canine** (**#23**) is related to inner changes and submission. For example, if I am having difficulty with the appearance of my menstruations, chances are that **#23** will be affected. The **lower left canine** (**#33**), being in front of **#23**, corresponds to inner changes that take effect outwardly, in my family. If I must endure everything in silence, **#23** will be affected. I tend to live like a slave and feel forced to serve others. The **lower right canine** (**#43**) represents my determination and the growth of my body. For example, if I stopped growing prematurely, it can be seen in **#43**.

The **first premolars** (**#14, 24, 34, 44**) represent who I am and what I want. If these **teeth** are extracted, as a child I will feel forced to melt into the crowd instead of standing out as a distinct individual. It is as though the collectivity were more important than the individual. I submit to an authority other than mine. The **upper right first premolar** (**#14**) shows how I express myself in society, with my inner qualities and richness. If I find it difficult to express my desires and take my place, this **tooth** will be displaced. The **upper left first premolar** (**#24**) is related to my sensitivity and my inner affective side. My poorly experienced desires and my unachieved childhood dreams involving these elements will bring difficulties with **#24**. The **lower left first premolar** (**#34**) indicates how I concretely express my will in my everyday life, especially on the affective level (and mainly concerning maternal **Love**), whereas the **lower right first premolar** (**#44**) is related to friendship and how I complete my projects. If I am markedly thwarted in conducting a project that I have set my **heart♥** on, **#44** will be affected.

The **second premolars (#15, 25, 35, 45)** are related to the desires I want to achieve and the betrayals (father, mother, in the couple, in friendship). My whole creativity is concerned here. If I can't express it, the latter will be affected. The **right second premolar (#15)** refers to what I want to develop outwardly. The fact of being unable to have children, for whatever reason, is an example of something I would like to create but has not materialized. The **left second premolar (#25)** contains my special abilities, whether or not I show who I truly am. It contains all of my past and present possibilities. The **lower left second premolar (#35)** is linked to my concrete relationship with my mother and how I am affected by her energies, how I feel free or stifled by her. The more I feel trapped and stifled by my mother, the more this **tooth** is **slanted inward**. The **lower right second premolar (#45)** refers to work and betrayal involving a friend. A difficulty in concretely organizing projects may also affect this **tooth**.

The **first molars (#16, 26, 36, 46)** appear at the age of 6 or 7 and they show how I take my place or not, and my need to be recognized by others. The **upper right first molar (#16)** is specifically related to the place I desire to take outwardly in society, whereas the **upper left first molar (#26)** is related to the place I desire to take and that enables me to outwardly express my sensitive and emotional side. The **lower left first molar (#36)** expresses whether I am well recognized affectively or not, especially by my parents. I may feel that I don't exist as I would like to, and **#36** reacts. The **lower right first molar (#46)** is very concretely related to work. The difficulty in materializing a project or in setting up a business will act on **#46**. It is related to the notion of desire, death and rebirth. If I came close to dying at a very early age, or if death was intensely present, whether the person died or not, **#46** will be affected.

The **second molars (#17, 27, 37, 47)** appear around the age of 12. They refer to my interactions with others and how I am perceived. The **upper right second molar (#17)** is related to everyday life and work. If my relations with others are conflicted, **#17** will react. The **upper left second molar (#27)** shows my inner relations with others at the level of my emotions. Unmet expectations involving the attitudes of others toward me will affect **# 27**. The **lower left second molar (#37)** also will react if, adding to a disappointment with a specific attitude, the person carries out a physical act that will amplify this disappointment. The **lower right second molar (#47)** is related to my relationships as such. Intense conflicted situations where words and acts have been produced will make **# 47** more vulnerable.

The **wisdom teeth (#18, 28, 38, 48)** appear around the age of 21, an age when I integrate my spiritual side. They represent the world in which I live, but also the spiritual world, my mission, my personal worth and the helping relationship. The latter can be reached through the mystic path, which is more oriented toward religion and its mysteries, or through esoteric knowledge. I have chosen the path of knowledge rather than the mystic path if my **wisdom teeth** are absent. If I have **wisdom teeth only on the upper maxillary**, I have difficulty in integrating my knowledge of the higher, invisible planes in my everyday life. When they are **only on the lower maxillary**, I put a lot of energy in my everyday actions to reintegrate the physical world. The **upper right wisdom tooth (#18)** refers to the strength I must develop to embody myself and integrate myself in the world at all levels. The **upper left wisdom tooth (#28)** corresponds to my fear of not integrating myself in the world. My poor self-esteem carries a fear of being rejected. The **lower right wisdom tooth (#38)** refers to my capacity for outwardly expressing my points of view and my emotions to the world around me, and the **lower left wisdom tooth (#48)** is influenced by my capacity for integrating and solidly anchoring myself in the physical world.

TEETH — TOOTH DECAY

Tooth decay is the manifestation of an extreme **inner pain.**

It manifests outwardly what is going on deep inside my person. **Something is gnawing at me** in the depths of my being. I can't quite express this pain gnawing at me, and inflammation appears. A **tooth** begins to soften and is often painful because of the nerve sensitivity present in the **tooth**. When the emotional tension has become too intense, it physically transforms itself into **decay in the tooth**, which corresponds exactly to what I am experiencing[2]. As each **tooth** represents a particular aspect of my personality and my life, the **decay** shows me that I am refusing or rejecting this particular aspect and that I am destroying myself. If I have this **tooth filled**, the emotions linked to it will stay imprisoned there until I become **Aware** of them. The structure of a **tooth** is the most rigid one in the human body. **Dental decay** concerns the 'mental' aspect. Is it **hate**, remorse or **resentment** toward someone, especially toward authority? I may 'bare my **teeth**' when I feel under attack. What is the actual cause of my pain? Knowing the initial reason will increase my chances of reversing this destructive process. I may resent myself for remaining silent and thus doing harm to myself. I may also have experienced a situation where I felt like 'biting' someone in a situation of self-defense but I didn't do it because "a well-brought-up child does not do such things". I often had **decayed teeth** as a child because I bore a grudge against someone. I received little affective nourishment (marks of affection, tenderness, sweets, etc.). I was laughed at and deeply hurt, to the core of my **teeth**! I may also be experiencing a family conflict where I have difficulty in accepting↓♥ what I receive from my entourage, and where I must filter this conflict with my **teeth** through the process of masticating. Indeed, my **teeth** enable me to filter and discriminate what enters my body and thus into my Universe in general. The more **cavities** I have, the more I cut myself off from myself and unconsciously move closer to death. For each **cavity** manifests a vital part of me that is dead or dying because a conflict I am experiencing remains unresolved. The pain will express itself through **decay** and may also generate other related physical ailments.

I accept↓♥ to stop looking for the physical cause (diet, sugar, etc.). Instead, I allow my thoughts to evolve and change my way of seeing the situations of

---

2. See the explanation for each **tooth** under: **Teeth (Symbolism of)**.

my life. I can ask myself: what is the emotional and rational 'food' (my thoughts) that no longer benefits me and that I would be better off replacing with healthier, better-balanced 'food'? I take life 'with a pinch of salt' and thus enable my **wisdom teeth** to develop and strengthen. It will be far more profitable for me!

TEETH — TOOTH (impacted wisdom) *See also: TEETH — SYMBOLISM OF TEETH*

Wisdom is a great quality. I have the good fortune to manifest it in this life. It enables me to open myself to the Universe and provides me with **solid bases** in everything I undertake.

Wisdom teeth symbolize this autonomy that I have been acquiring over the years. Thus, a **wisdom tooth** that refuses to come out and 'take its place' means I am still mentally refusing to claim all the space that is rightfully mine and trust myself. I keep inside what displeases me in myself so I can thereby please others.

I accept↓♥ to consciously claim my rightful place in order to nurture all the divine qualities essential to my development. I can thus create more solid bases for my life. I accept↓♥ to allow nature to follow its course and open my **consciousness** so I can grow and see the changes in me! They will be bountiful!

TEETH — TOOTH (root abscess)

As this **abscess** is found in the tissues enclosing the dental root, it shows my anger over a decision to be made. As the infection is located in the central hollow of the **tooth**, it indicates the annoyance I am feeling over a decision that is gnawing at me inside. It is like a small volcano erupting and allowing long-repressed negative emotions to burst out. I may feel intense inner pain about the affective nourishment I need and of which I feel deprived. If I am **affectively cut off**, especially from my mother or my children, and I store sorrow and disappointment while feeling guilty of what is happening, an **abscess** will appear. My deep roots are in question.

I accept↓♥ to make this decision as **lovingly** and congenially as possible, while taking into account the highest values that govern my life and respecting myself and others.

TENDINITIS *See: TENDON (IN GENERAL)*

TENDON (in general)

A **tendon** is the link between a muscle and the bone to which it is attached. It is made up of conjunctive tissue.

This tissue of soft consistency, therefore made up of mental energy that is joined to spiritual energy, has the effect of unifying expression and complete movement. It creates a direct link with my 'body-spirit'. My **tendons** represent how I can adjust to different situations in my life and how I advance by listening to my inner voice or not.

Supple **tendons** show my suppleness with myself and others. By contrast, the rigidity of my **tendons** reflects rigid tendencies. If my mental energy is stiff and rigid, I become inflexible. My soft tissue will thus sense this state, which then provokes its rigidity. When I am conflicted between what I think I should do and my inner voice telling me what I really want to do, I then feel a pain in the **tendons**. I tend to depreciate myself. My mental energy (**tendon**) decides on one direction, whereas my fundamental, deep and spiritual energy (**bones**), wishes to go in an opposite direction. Looking at which **tendon** is affected indicates to me what aspect of my life I depreciate.

For instance, if I have a **tendinitis in the wrist**, I must ask myself: "In what activity, requiring the use of my wrists and hands, do I feel that I am not good enough or that I could do better? What is making me so apprehensive? In what situation do I need to improve myself to achieve my goals in the future, although I feel powerless to do so?" I feel chained and incapable of reaching my goals. I need to be lent a helping hand. I **tend** to move toward my objectives, but am afraid of not getting there. I wonder how capable I am of merging the dualities of my life. If I am able, for example, to shift from my old ideas to my new ones, openly, knowing that I can totally rely on my inner authority, my **tendons** will be in good condition. If I am constantly foiled, if I live only according to others, my **tendons** will become fragile and will **tend** to tear. They will weaken if I too am feeling weak or not good enough. I may think that my actions are deemed to be worthless.

I accept↓♥ to see the importance of balancing my energies and advancing in life. I can trust my divine wisdom.

TENDON (Achilles' heel)

The **Achilles' heel tendon** connects the calf muscle to the heel bone. This most powerful **tendon** in the body can support up to 880 pounds (400 kilograms).

It enables my thoughts and my desires, physical as well as spiritual, to be achieved. It also serves to express any blocking in the movement of the ankle. For example, I may have a great desire for stability, but this is difficult to achieve because of a precarious financial situation.

The **Achilles' heel tendon** can support a lot: do I, too, feel that I am carrying such a heavy load? It can be strong and carry a heavy load if the inner base is solid, but if I feel nothingness inside of me, what can I lean on? Maybe I give too much importance to the 'container', to the outsides of things, but what about the 'content'? What are my priorities, my values? What is my life based on? Am I in contact with my divine essence, or am I dealing with mere appearances? Is there a break in my relations with others, especially my children or my parents? Do I always need to move, to go away, as if I can't remain in one place for too long, a little like a Gypsy? I become **Aware** that the **Achilles' heel tendon** works more when I am standing (vertical) than when I am lying down.

It becomes fragile if I find that it is impossible for me to rise. This may involve a desire for a promotion, a change in social rank, a desire to be part of a professional sports team, but obstacles prevent this from materializing.

I accept↓♥ to set things in motion to achieve my dreams and reach the goals I have set for myself. I ground my life on sure human values. I increase my inner strength by being myself.

TENIA / TAPEWORM *See: INTESTINES — TENIA*

TENNIS ELBOW *See: ELBOWS — EPICONDYLITIS*

TENSION (arterial) — HYPERTENSION (too high)

The image that evokes a person suffering from **hypertension** is the **pressure cooker**[3]. I am this person who accumulates unexpressed thoughts and emotions over long periods; I am often hypersensitive and control myself poorly. My anger and my annoyances for which I have not yet found any solutions are choked back, which makes me boil inside. I am confused. I may also tend to procrastinate and hold off the things I have to do or say, out of fear or for lack of self-confidence, and I come to experience intense nervous tension, for I make a mountain out of all that, and I don't know whether I will be able to carry out all my projects. I can also make up stories, amplify my problems, and my guilt will quickly increase the 'pressure'. My desire to control everything and resolve the situations of my life increases my pressure, which can become unbearable. I feel powerless, often because I no longer can, or want to, obey orders, especially at work. Having a deep fear of being rejected, I feel in danger and I stay on guard. I feel crushed and defenseless. I feel intense **tension** over an emotional or passionate situation, and it would be in my interest to diminish my level of stress. I have difficulty in feeling and receiving **Love** from others. I have closed myself against this **Love**, to no longer suffer; so I no longer want to give any or receive any. The **hypertension** I am experiencing may also have its source in my fear of death, whether it is conscious or not, and in my desire to get the most out of my life, for I want to achieve the many goals I have set for myself. It is the brain that commands the nervous tension, and the **heart♥** that sets the rhythm and heats the blood: together, they regulate the **tension**. Am I pressuring myself, or do I have the impression, instead, that this pressure comes from others? Am I denying any aspects of my personality that are desperately trying to emerge in full daylight? Do I feel ***suppressed***? I may feel in danger of expressing my true feelings, and this can lead to a depressive state. I must be the best, performing at the top of

---

3. **Pressure cooker**: A cooking pot with an airtight lid and a controlled steam escape mechanism, used to cook food under steam pressure.

my capacities. If I do not succeed as well physically as intellectually, the ***pressure*** and the **tension** will be enormous. I seek harmony in everything and I feel responsible for it, even when other persons are concerned. What a mandate I have given myself! As I tend to be hyperactive (which helps me to forget my worries), a good way to do it would be to put my priorities on the things to be done and give myself time to see what is going on inside of me and express all these emotions that are only asking to show themselves out in the open.

I accept↓♥ to learn how to gently 'let off steam' and to become **Aware** of the pressure I put on myself. I avoid the accumulation that will provoke an explosion. I learn to trust myself. I accept↓♥ to no longer need this pressure in order to feel alive. I accept↓♥ myself as I am, and I recognize that I am a unique being.

TENSION (arterial) — HYPOTENSION (too low)

Contrary to hypertension, **hypotension** is found in a person whose pressure is too low (however, a person can have a pressure that is below normal and yet feel quite fit. This pressure is therefore adequate for this person, as long as their quality of life is not affected by it).

If I am a person with **low pressure**, it may indicate that my desire for living is lacking. I have the impression that nothing is going right, that it is useless to make any efforts because I feel that it won't work anyway. I feel drained of energy and I can no longer bear the weight of events. I give in to discouragement and defeatism. My **heart♥** is no longer in it. I live as a victim, and I have the impression that my life resembles a dead end. I feel powerless about what I am asked to do in order to meet the norms set by society, which do not necessarily fit with my personal values. I am afraid I have to give up some of my dreams. **Hypotension** can lead to a loss of **Consciousness**. It is a sign that I want to flee my responsibilities, certain situations or certain persons, because facing them would lead me to take positions and actions that I may not feel like doing. I feel responsible for everyone around me, which is very heavy to bear. It may have started very early on in my life. I feel so weak, helpless and exhausted. I no longer feel like investing myself in life. The message my body is sending me is to trust myself and forge ahead. I choose to let myself be guided by my inner strength.

I accept↓♥ to take some time for myself. By recreating a state of serenity and discovering what I like, by resuming contact with what makes me passionate and by living each day with the simplicity of a child, I recover my joy in living. I leave their own responsibilities to others and only take care of my own. My **arterial tension** may stay low, but it will then be only a sign that I have reached a level of stress that is almost nil and that I am attuning my life to the flow of life itself.

TESTICLES (cancer of the) *See: CANCER OF THE TESTICLES*

TESTICLES (in general) *See also: PENIS AILMENTS*

The **male sexual glands** represent the male aspect. A problem in the **testicles**, commonly called 'my **family jewels**', is often related to fears, insecurity, the father image, or doubts concerning my manhood and my capacity to procreate. It may indicate a lack of acceptance↓♥ of my sexuality or my sexual preference. The fear of being judged on my performance may even lead to **impotence**. I feel weak and vulnerable. Why do I have to prove myself, in bed as well as in the family or at work? What do I have to prove? When I experience a tense situation, I sometimes have the impression of '**being held by the balls**', especially if my partner is a person of power. I become a ***witness*** and a spectator instead of being the main actor of my life. ***Commitment*** becomes a very dangerous thing that can even prove ***fatal*** for me. I may also feel curtailed in the action of my creativity, ***dispossessed*** of my talents. In the background, there is a fear of ***losing*** that is omnipresent. It may be someone from my family whom I **love**, but it can also be the fear of losing my identity, my time, my hopes, my memory. I then tend to feel guilty, disparaged or torn, often by a person of the opposite sex. I feel, or I am made to feel, like a 'little kid'. I retreat into my corner and hide behind a mask to avoid being hurt again. A **twist of the testicle**, which usually happens in childhood, represents how harshly, or even brutally, I discovered the false image I had of my father. In another case, I need to be ***attested***, my actions to be ***witnessed***, hence the appearance of a **cyst** or a **tumor**. I repress who I am so much that I become completely separated from my deeper forces. If there is an **inflammation of my testes** (**orchitis**), my frustration and my anger grow day by day, for I can no longer stand my emotional prison or the rejection of my spontaneity and my creativity. My incapacity in setting up certain projects burns me up. If there is a **failure of one or both testes to descend into the scrotum** (**cryptorchidism**), I probably had a childhood where scant words were exchanged with my father, often because he was very authoritarian and powerful. I feel stifled, and I feel great distrust toward others. If the **scrotum** is affected, I want to protect myself for I am afraid that something will happen to me, especially in my **testes**. I am in a conflict in which money is involved; so the saying: "Your moneybag or your life!" applies here. **Varicocele** indicates a fear of having children, for I myself have the impression that I did not have any parents, or that one of them was absent and I felt I was an orphan.

I accept↓♥ to explore my feelings about my virility and re-examine my understanding of the male principle.

TETANUS *See: MUSCLES — TETANUS*

TETANY

Tetany is characterized by seizures that make my muscles and nerves contract, mainly in the extremities. I feel my hands, my feet and all my muscles tensing.

This state originates from hyper-excitability and occurs during annoyances. In some cases, during severe seizures, my fingers squeeze shut and my thumb hides itself under my fingers by curling itself inside my hand, as if to isolate itself from the outside world. Maybe I too want to isolate myself and cut myself off from the world, maybe even with an unconscious desire to die, for I no longer feel like living or feel any joy in living. I react to a situation where I feel oppressed and hindered in my movements. I resent myself for not being able to express myself or to react in certain situations. I no longer can stand repressing my frustrations and my aggressiveness. I feel like 'tossing everything up in the air', but my fear of the consequences prevents me from acting it out.

I accept↓♥ to learn how to control myself. I eliminate negative thoughts and I minimize the effect of annoyances. By learning to express my emotions with words, I no longer need to do it with my body.

TETRAPLEGIA *See: PARALYSIS (IN GENERAL)*

THALAMUS

The **thalamus** has the form of two voluminous nuclei made of a gray substance, which are located on each side of the third ventricle of the anterior brain, and serve as relays for the sensory pathways.

A dysfunction in the **thalamus** indicates great questionings about myself, about who I am and how I am perceived. I am feeling a **distress** in my couple that I dare not admit. I may be inclined to deep despair. I may experience it toward myself or toward a loved one. I am afraid of being judged by others, afraid of being under-estimated or humiliated. I am often the first person however to judge myself and condemn myself. I tend to compare myself to others. In a sense, my affective side is dead. I am in a period of great changes: it is as though I were molting and shedding everything that could prevent me from moving ahead, but it scares me. I am in search of my true identity.

I learn to accept↓♥ myself as I am, and I realize that by being true with the people around me, I thus manifest far more **Love** and I maintain healthy and durable relationships.

THIGHS (in general) *See also: LEG(S) / (IN GENERAL) / AILMENTS*

The **thigh** contains the muscle group that represents the movement and strength for moving forward. **Strong** and **powerful thighs** indicate a well-grounded person with great energy reserves for their authority and their **spiritual development**. These natural 'reservoirs' also indicate one's state of mind. Thus, if I remain inactive for too long, I risk accumulating useless reserves. Either I want to do something but I cannot, or others want to force me to do things that do not suit me. I am afraid of taking my place, and I find that several situations in my youth, mainly experienced with my parents, were **unfair** and I have not accepted↓♥ them and feel very **resentful** about them. I may have been forced to separate from a person who was dear to me. **Lacking** something can be very frightening for me. Therefore, I make 'reserves'. I continue to pack these unconscious thoughts in my **thighs** and carry all this excess matter. I often have the impression that "It is too late" to say or do things. "I am toast!": a secret or an information that I wanted to keep for myself was found out. I feel anger, **resentment** and frustration because I have the impression that I have been working with no great success. By having **large, plump thighs** (very tightly pressed together), I unconsciously block the energy in this area and my sexuality risks changing, for energy remains 'stagnant' in the pelvis. I may have the impression that this way, I can be less easily reached and that I can hide my deepest emotions under this fat or these muscles. There may be a barricade of mental resistances that prevents me from fully expressing myself or finding my direction. It is time for me to free myself and let through this energy of **Love** that only wants to express itself.

I accept↓♥ to allow this energy to flow downward to my **thighs** and my legs that need it more, which helps me to root myself on earth, to be better grounded and thereby bring more balance between my spiritual and physical sides. This helps me make my blues go away. My body balances itself and I get rid of the accumulated resentment of my youth. Even though I sometimes have the impression that I am closed, I look at my material possessions and I accept↓♥ them for what they are in this world, namely servants of the Universe.

THIGHS (ailments of the) *See: LEGS — UPPER PART*

THIRST *See also: BLOOD — DIABETES, KIDNEYS — RENAL PROBLEMS, SUN STROKE*

Thirst is a natural phenomenon that contributes to balance substances such as salt or sugar, among others, in my cardiovascular system.

When my sensation of **thirst** is exaggerated (polydipsia), my thoughts are cloudy, my **heart♥** pounds wildly, I can no longer see clearly, my throat is dry and I am **thirsty**. Something is missing for me to be happy. Drinking! For a brief moment my **thirst** diminishes, but it very quickly returns because it involves my mind. I must therefore discover its cause: what is boring me in my life? Does my work seem boring? What thought or what fear is drying my mouth or my mind? Do I have the impression I am never quite satisfied in my life? Of what do I remain unquenched, what do I still feel the need for and never get enough of? Once I have found that, my seemingly unquenchable **thirst** will be controlled. Strong spices are known to intensify sexual desire. Properly used, this stimulant can enable me to eliminate **thirst**. On the other hand, an unsatisfactory sexual relation will have the effect of increasing **thirst**, adding to the feeling of loss. To fill this want, this desire to drink represents my need to live, for water represents life. On the other hand, when I drink very sparingly, am rarely **thirsty** and have too much saliva, I am too self-centered to see what is going on outside of 'my little world', and I do not open myself up enough to the outside world.

I accept↓♥ to open myself more to life and **Love** so I can find at last the situation that will 'quench my **thirst**'.

THROAT (in general) *See also: GLAND (THYROID) — (IN GENERAL)*

The **throat** contains the vocal cords (the larynx) and the pharynx. The thyroid gland is located just below the larynx. It enables me to express who I am and also to exchange with the people around me.

The **throat** is related to the laryngeal energy center, also called the **throat** chakra (the fifth chakra), the center of creativity, truth and affirmation. It also works in close collaboration with the sacral energy center or second chakra, the sexual energy center, sexuality being a way to communicate with another person. This energy center is important for self-assertion. It is also said: "Thought creates, speech manifests". Thus, through speech, I enable my thoughts to materialize in the physical world. Therefore, although negative thoughts can have repercussions on my health, negative words may have still more. This is also true on the positive side.

I accept↓♥ to have more to say positively, thus respecting my temple of flesh that shelters my divine element. The more I express the truth through this means of communication, the more I can harmoniously exchange with my environment.

THROAT DISORDERS *See also: THRUSH, TONSILS*

It is with my **throat** that I swallow my emotional experiences and my reality; it is where I take life in through respiration, water and food. It represents my power and my inner strength, because my capacity for expressing myself depends upon these two elements. It is also there that I release my feelings, from my **heart♥** to my voice. It is the two-way bridge between the head and the body, the spirit and the physical. If my **throat is sore**, I may feel guilty of having said certain words, or I may think I should have expressed something. It is as though I were punishing myself with pain. My rage and my anger want so much to express themselves, but I fear the reactions of others; I will therefore swallow my emotions that are putting my **throat** on fire. It may be time for me to say what I am experiencing, in order to release myself from it. My **throat** can also become **inflamed** if I repress rage, and this emotion then **rises in my throat**. If I do not say what I want to say or if there is a conflict in my self-expression, then my **throat** senses this repression. As the **throat** is the expression of self-affirmation, if I have difficulty in asserting myself and defending my point of view, I may want to compensate for that by becoming authoritarian toward myself or others, which limits my energy in that area. I prefer to hide things rather than take the risk of being ridiculed. I am very attached to the people around me and I easily allow myself to be affected by their words or gestures. An **infection in the throat by the streptococcus bacterium** is one of the most frequent forms of infection. It involves irritation and the holding in of energy. As the **throat** also represents conception and the acceptance↓♥ of life, if I have difficulties in my **throat**, I may be facing a deep conflict in the acceptance↓♥ of my existence. I seek my power within me, while denying it at the same time. I am also seeking my inner father. When having a **difficulty in swallowing** (**dysphagia**), I can ask myself what person or situation I have difficulty in swallowing, or what reality I feel compelled to swallow even if it does not suit me (for instance, it may be something that goes against my principles). I want to defy someone or something because I just can't allow this to pass! I may then try to cut myself off from my physical reality, maybe in hopes of escaping the obligation to assert who I am with my needs, and therefore the obligation to make changes in my life. In the case where food follows the 'wrong path' ('**swallowing the wrong way**[4]') because the epiglottis did not close as it should have, I ask myself in what area of my life I have the impression of 'going down the wrong path' and where I should re-examine my directions with respect to my priorities. I want to rush things and 'have control over the situation', for I feel in danger. If I **gulp things down whole**, I swallow everything from others and I have difficulty in forming my own opinion. I tend to be passive, waiting for others to do the work for me. If I have **mucosities in the throat**, I have accumulated too many negative words and emotions that ask only to be expressed. The **throat** chakra and the sexual chakra are more directly related. More precisely, the hypophysis stimulates the thyroid, which in turn transmits the messages to our genital organs. Both are related to creativity: the **throat** chakra concerns the creativity of my thoughts, while the sexual chakra concerns my creativity in matter. These two energy centers are also related to communication: through my voice, I communicate my thoughts, and through my sexuality, I physically communicate my feelings. Thus, if I have problems in the **throat**, it is good that I ask myself questions on what I have to express about myself, and I must go and check whether I am experiencing frustration with my sexuality.

I accept↓♥ that my happiness and freedom come from **my capacity to express myself in Truth**, thus increasingly approaching my divine essence. All the emotions I feel are positive and are here to help me in learning something about myself. I must release them to remove the tensions that might accumulate.

THROAT — *Laryngitis See also: APPENDIX III, HOARSENESS, INFLAMMATION*

Laryngitis is an inflammation of the larynx, accompanied by coughing and hoarseness. In children below age 5, it is called **pseudo croup** instead.

This infection is caused by a difficulty in expressing myself for fear of ridicule, very often toward authority. I can't express my own opinions and affirm what I have set my **heart♥** on. I submit to authority. This may be related to the fact of experiencing rejection from others and, if I assert myself, of being misunderstood by them. Losing my voice can also be a means to escape from a situation that would have required me to express myself. **I repress revolt, I**

4. **To swallow the wrong way**: This expression symbolizes the wrong path taken by food passing through the larynx and the trachea instead of the esophagus.

feel stifled, too many emotions have remained jumbled together. It may have followed the announcement of a great piece of news that amazed me and left me in open-mouthed astonishment[5]. When I remain silent instead of expressing myself, out of shame, fear or guilt, these feelings that I hide with my silence cause a blocking of energy that takes the form of **laryngitis**. A great resistance may then appear when those emotions try to express themselves later on. The larynx is inflamed and a high level of emotional energy is joined with the voice and self-expression. My creativity tries to find its own affirmation; it wants to be free to speak and skillfully voice its emotions. My powerlessness to express myself very quickly turns into anger against myself. I believe I am no longer safe if I refrain from speaking. However, I quickly realize how very frustrated I am because I can't make my opinion heard, I can't assert myself and I can therefore not exercise my authority in situations where it is necessary. I may therefore have fits of anger because this is 'just too much', but I then regret it. As my guilt is strong, I attract **laryngitis**; this way, I now have a 'good reason' for not speaking.

I must learn to say things and express my feelings, which will allow this energy to flow freely. If, with my current personality, I find it difficult to express myself by saying things, then I may express them in writing. As the larynx is related to the energy center of the **throat**, which is communication, I can communicate my feelings by writing them, even if I keep these writings for myself. This will enable me to communicate better with myself and enable me to clarify what I want to express.

THROAT — LARYNX *See also: APHONIA, CANCER OF THE LARYNX, HOARSENESS*

The **larynx** is the part of the upper airways located between the trachea and the pharynx.

It symbolizes my affirmation through speech and words, my will to express with authority what I experience and what I think. An **ailment in the larynx** generally occurs following an event that "took my breath away", where I was astonished and ***disconcerted***[6]. I was so frightened that "no sound could issue from my mouth". I was taken by surprise, and often I feel in danger, to the point that I have the impression my life is in peril. It may also concern something in my territory. It may follow that I wanted to scream or cry out for help but was unable to. It is important for me to retrace this event that probably occurred just before my **larynx** was affected by the disease. I can thus remove the trauma that was long 'hooked' to my **larynx** and allow it to heal. As the **larynx** is the essential organ of phonation, or the production of sounds, I must ask myself which of my emotions and states of feeling I want to express through my voice, but which I repress and keep for myself. I may have reached the point where I want to change my priorities and my life structures, and I fear the reactions of others. As my voice is unique, I examine how I accept↓♥

5. **To stay open-mouthed**: To have one's mouth open out of astonishment, stupor or admiration.

6. **Disconcerted**: Astounded, bewildered.

myself in what I am: am I comfortable in giving my own opinion, or do I wait for the opinions of others before voicing mine? Do I talk only about myself, or do I tend to talk about others and in their place? Do I allow my inner voice to speak? Do I tend to speak conditionally, or am I affirmative in my way of communicating? I want to get my message through, but am not succeeding. Am I refraining myself, or being forbidden to say things or even scream? Are there things I find difficult to ***swallow***?

I accept↓♥ right now to allow my **heart♥** to speak and quite simply express my emotions and opinions. My voice is becoming increasingly strong and solid and perfectly reflects my assurance and my self-confidence.

THROAT — PHARYNGITIS *See also: ANGINA, APPENDIX III, COLD*

Pharyngitis is far more commonly known by the expression a '**sore throat**'. All the emotions, feelings or energies that block my **throat** must enter through the nose or the mouth. Or again, they come from the depths of my inner being and they block in the **throat**. They are often emotions or situations that I ***swallow*** and find difficult to accept↓♥ and that involve a family member. It may be a situation where I want someone or something inaccessible and out of reach, that I cannot 'catch' and yet need in my life. I therefore 'smell' (nose) that all is not going well, or I am not absorbing (mouth) some of the energies that become available to me. It is sometimes the same emotions that have become amplified after a cold. These emotions affect me more deeply and closer inside of me than a simple cold. I also look at how my relationships with others are, and how dependent I can be upon them. I can be very easily influenced. I feel like shouting who I am, but my anxiety and uncertainties prevent me from doing so. I have such a strong impression of living in the background and not having the first place. I must therefore analyze these feelings that 'catch' and block in my **throat**, so I can accept↓♥ them and let them go.

I accept↓♥ to express myself and I reclaim power over my life because I assert who I am and what my needs are. I thus recover my autonomy. I accept↓♥ to give the same freedom to others, and my anger disappears and makes place for more understanding and calm in my life.

THROAT — PHARYNX *See also: POLYPS*

The **pharynx**, which corresponds to the **throat**, is a canal that goes from the back of the mouth down to the entrance of the esophagus.

If my **pharynx** is affected, I am regretting a choice that I made. I realize that I took the wrong direction or the wrong way. A passage is taking place from one situation to another (such as adolescence, a change of jobs, a separation, etc.), which I did not accept↓♥ or was not made at the right moment: I regret it but I can't turn back. I resent myself and I find it difficult to ***swallow***. I am disappointed; I am poisoning my own existence by brooding over the past. I may also lack something essential (some information for example) for implementing a project, and if it is impossible for me to find it in order to complete the project, I may develop a **cancer**. This leads me to depreciate myself and feel guilty.

I accept↓♥ to re-examine my priorities: what is really necessary for my happiness, and what is secondary or superfluous? I accept↓♥ that all the choices I have made so far have been the right ones and have enabled me to learn the life lessons I needed. I am always guided, and I listen to my inner voice that shows me the right way.

THROAT (sore) *See: THROAT — PHARYNGITIS*

THROAT (to have a frog in one's)

To **have a frog in my throat** manifests, quite despite myself, something that I desire to express but keep inside of me. Am I afraid of being ridiculed, criticized, rejected or misunderstood? Something is congesting and prickling my **throat**. This fear is clearly related to my sensitivity, consciously or unconsciously.

I accept↓♥ to trust myself and tell things as they are, while remaining true to myself; I will thus gain the respect of others and myself.

THROAT (to have a lump in one's)

I have a **lump in my throat** when I experience anxiety. I feel held in a stranglehold. I may also be lacking in self-confidence and doubting my capacities, especially in front of someone who intimidates me and represents some form of authority. I have the impression that my breath has been taken away. I prefer to subject myself to this rather than stand by my choices. I am paralyzed by anxiety, and social life frightens me. I have difficulty in taking position, and I question my beliefs. I may feel vulnerable, but I must trust in life.

I accept↓♥ to express myself freely and overcome my fears. I find inner peace for I am fully guided. I am the Ruler of my life!

THROMBOANGIITIS OBLITRANS *See: BUERGER'S DISEASE*

THROMBOSIS *See: BLOOD — THROMBOSIS*

THROMBOSIS (coronary) *See: HEART♥ — CORONARY THROMBOSIS*

THRUSH *See also: MOUTH / (IN GENERAL) / AILMENT, CANDIDA, THROAT / (IN GENERAL) / DISORDERS, INFECTIONS (IN GENERAL)*

Thrush, also called **oral candidiasis**, is a disease due to a yeast and is characterized by the presence of creamy white plaques caused by parasites on the oral and pharyngeal mucous membranes, namely in the mouth and the throat. This disease is very frequent **in children**.

It appears following the incessant screams and crying of my child who desires to receive caresses and physical contacts with us, her parents. If I put myself in the child's place, especially a baby's, I remember that I need the contact with my mother or my father to feel safe and out of danger, for I know that I am vulnerable. The only way I have to seek my parents' attention and have them take me in their arms is for me to scream and cry. It is the only way to 'gorge' myself (larynx!) on human warmth. As my parents can wrongly interpret these cries and believe that I am hungry, thirsty, cold, etc., I won't obtain what I need. And my **larynx**, the essential organ of phonation, being incapable of filling my need for physical contact, will trigger **thrush**. For the **thrush** to go away, my parents need to hug me in their arms as often as possible, caress me and make me feel secure. When **thrush** appears in me as an **adult**, it may have occurred following an infection in my lungs or my airways. My needs are then the same as those of the child mentioned above, with the difference that it is my inner child who needs to be given attention and made to feel safe. I feel a great affective emptiness and I am melancholy. The adult part of me can comfort this child in me and reassure it. Harmony will settle more steadily, which will allow health to resume its place. As an adult, I have difficulty in making my needs heard and I feel incapable of communicating what I feel. I want them to know what I need, I want them to be able to 'guess', and this is not how it happens; so I am then very frustrated and aggressive. Everything is blurred for me and I don't know in which direction to go. Making decisions is very difficult for me. I have the impression of remaining in place instead of developing. Yet, I know that I have all the necessary potential for implementing my projects.

I accept↓♥ to acknowledge my potential and put things forward in order to enact all this inner power in the physical world. I am now able to show all my gentleness and understanding, while daring to fully live my life.

THUMB *See: FINGERS — THUMB*

THUMB SUCKING

By **sucking my thumb**, I wish to thus recreate the sensation of well-being I felt when I was in my mother's womb. The **thumb** is sometimes replaced by the middle finger, which represents sensitivity. The warmth and moisture of my mouth give me security and the sense of being sheltered from the outside world.

By **sucking my thumb** or any other finger, I have the impression of thereby finding temporary satisfaction. I become **Aware** of how powerless and dependent I can feel in front of others. I am hungry to learn and to accomplish myself, and instead of filling my needful emptiness with food, I do it by **sucking my thumb**. I console myself by myself. I remain in my world. If I am a young child, with this gesture I express my fear of growing up into an adult. If my **fingers are pressed against my palate**, I need my father, his presence and his protection. If I place them **under my tongue**, behind the lower incisors, I rather need affection and a maternal presence. I must reinforce my feeling of inner safety while taking care of myself and enjoying myself.

I accept↓♥ to express what I feel and I make an effort to go toward others and ask for help if I need any. Instead of relying on my **thumb** to sustain me, I rely on my inner strengths and I accept↓♥ that I am constantly protected.

THYMUS *See: GLAND — THYMUS*

THYROID *See: GLAND THYROID (IN GENERAL)*

TIBIA *See: LEGS — LOWER PART*

TICS *See: BRAIN — TICS*

TIMIDITY

Timidity makes me bypass some marvelous things. I avoid people I don't know. For fear of being judged, I give up new things under the pretext that they are not for me. I give up and refuse to fight. I tend to seek security in the routine. I have little **Love** for myself and my poor self-esteem and low self-confidence prompt me to remain within a well-established framework where I do not feel hurt, rejected or misunderstood. This form of escape, due to my **timidity**, leads me to remain withdrawn. In some sense, it is quite possible that this may suit me, for I thereby protect myself from situations or persons that could injure me. I keep my communications to a minimum, with the persons from whom I sense no threat.

I accept↓♥ to make a habit of acting calmly and I give myself the opportunity to discover, every day, new things and new persons.

TINEA *See: HAIR — TINEA*

TINGLING / PRICKLING / PINS and NEEDLES

Tingling is a sensation of prickling on the surface of the body, which usually occurs spontaneously after a mechanical compression of a nerve or a blood vessel.

The location where the **tingling** takes place on my body indicates the temporary annoyance or irritation that I may be experiencing in relation to an aspect of my life.

I accept↓♥ to become **Aware** of it and I allow energy to flow freely.

TINNITUS *See: EARS — TINNITUS*

TOES

The **toes** represent the details of the future. They are a point of balance and enable me to perceive the ground, and therefore the world. If I feel insecure about that, **cramps** will appear, and if I experience guilt, I may **knock** my **toe**,

cut myself (if there is a loss of joy) or injure myself more severely (**broken** or **cracked toe**). A **cracked toe** (or a **benign sprain**) shows me that I want to change directions and make a decision, but I resist change because I am too attached to something, someone or a situation. I am tired of always having the responsibility for seeing to it that everything unfolds congenially. A **fracture** highlights my feeling of being in a dead end. My little routine makes me feel secure but at the same time, I need some change! I may be a little flighty and up in the clouds, like an ***artist*** who lives in his imaginary world. Consciously or not, I may want to omit some important details, and the fact of injuring myself will wake me up so that I will become more vigilant and attentive. Or I become overly concerned with the small details to be settled in the future, and this distracts me from more pressing issues. If I have difficulty in moving straight for the goal I have set for myself, or on the contrary if I want to rush things too fast, my **toes** will be affected. Rushing things often expresses itself by the fact that I bump one or several **toes**. If I do violence to myself in my thoughts, I will hurt myself just to remind myself of it. If someone **mashes my toes**, I am feeling increasingly jammed over a direction to be taken. The "vise is closing", I want to run away, but I know deep inside that this is not the solution. If I have a **bunion**, which is a deviation of the **big toe** toward the second **toe**, there is a very deep conflict involving my values. A **bunion** generally appears when experiencing a relationship with a partner or a parent whom I find very dominant. As I allow the other to make the decisions, I evade my responsibility for my own decisions. The expression "stick to your knitting" aptly conveys my feeling that some people around me are minding my business, which does not concern them, unless I am the one reproaching myself for indirectly minding other peoples' businesses. A **bunion** may disappear if I take charge of myself and take my responsibilities, thus enabling me to fully live my life. As the **toes** are the part of my body that move forward first, **toes turned downward** may indicate insecurity in moving forward, a desire to 'grip the ground' to avoid advancing. My **toes** are like hooks, and I therefore tend to remain in place. **Toes turned upward** indicate my tendency to live my life superficially and to elevate myself to the more abstract realities rather than to the earthly ones. **Crooked toes** indicate a great confusion in the direction to take and an absence of inner freedom and clarity, which makes me want to flee. A **hammer toe** indicates stress and a repugnance to move forward. It may also be the fear of an abstract or poorly structured way of being. To know the metaphysical meaning of each of my **toes**, I can refer to the meaning of each of my fingers, beginning with the thumb for the **big toe**, and ending with the little finger, the pinkie, for the **little toe**. I simply transpose the meanings of the fingers, which are the details of everyday life, to those of the **toes**, which are the details of the future. It is often the **big toe** that is affected by an ailment. It represents my ego, my convictions, my territory. When it is affected, I can ask myself if I am experiencing a conflict with my obligations, with the law or with the authority that my mother wields over me, whether this mother is real – **big toe of the right foot** – or symbolic – **big toe of the left foot**. I feel compelled to obey. If the **big toe overlaps the second toe of the foot**, do I feel that I am responsible or that I must provide for the needs of a little brother (or sister)? If the **big toe is under the next toe**, I may feel I am submitting to, or enduring, a big brother (or big sister). If it is **deviated toward the other toes (hallux valgus)**, I am feeling guilty for being happy. I withdraw into myself, I no longer have my place in this world. So many things are imposed on me that I want to run away, but I don't know which direction to take.

I accept↓♥ to remain open and flexible about the future. By trusting myself about my choices and the directions to be taken, my **toes** will be in great shape and free of any ailments. I move forward in life with conviction!

TONGUE *See also: TASTE DISORDERS*

The **tongue** is a muscular organ to which taste is related and it is appended to the digestive system.

If I want to express a thought orally, I need my **tongue**. If I '**bite my tongue**', I must ask myself if I resent myself for what I have just said and am feeling guilty. Do I know how to hold my **tongue**? Where does it hurt me for not saying things as I experience them, for not expressing my feelings because I am unable to find the right words? When I use expressions such as: "It is ***burning*** my **tongue**" or "You have the **gift of the gab**", it denotes a situation involving the 'said' and the 'unsaid' that may generate '**tongue**' **ailments** (**prickling**, a **burning sensation**). What am I burning to do or to say and that I am holding back from? My feeling of powerlessness makes me remain silent. I can keep for myself a family secret which, were it to be divulged, would risk making me feel shame. As I have the impression that I am not being listened to, I become completely indifferent to others. If I feel guilty for what I said, I **bite my tongue**. The French saying: « Se tourner la langue sept fois avant de parler » (literally: "to turn over one's **tongue** seven times before speaking", meaning: to think long and hard before speaking) illustrates this well. A **pain in the tongue** indicates something specific that I refuse to say and that stays on the "tip of my **tongue**". A **pimple on the tip of my tongue** shows me how I can repress my surges of passion, verbal as well as physical. It may be a painful memory that I want to express in order to free myself of it. If my **tongue** is **fissured**, I want to stop playing the 'good boy / good girl' and tell the whole world: "That's enough! Now listen to me!" I have had quite enough of feeling divided, caught in a duality between what I want to express and what I actually say. My **tongue is numb or swollen** when I want to taste more of life or when I feel disgust for a person, a thing or a situation. A **thick tongue** shows me how entangled I feel in my words, not knowing how to express myself. An **ulcer on the tip of my tongue** shows me that something I want to say is burning me. A withdrawal into myself or guilt about a pleasure offered to me will make my **tongue** react, for instance in a case of **glossitis (inflammation)**. I do not dare taste all the flavors of life. I only punish myself, and I live like a slave. **Mycosis** (**tongue covered with a whitish coating**) manifests the criticism and rage that are brewing inside of me and that I do not dare to express. I was hurt in the past, and that still pursues me; I prefer to stay alone with my pain.

I accept↓♥ right now to savor all the joys that are offered to me. I learn to state my opinion and make myself respected in my differences, and I enjoy life!

TONGUE (cancer of the) *See: CANCER OF THE TONGUE*

TONSILS — TONSILLITIS / AMYGDALITIS *See also: INFECTION, THROAT*

The **tonsils**, which mean '**almonds**', are part of my lymphatic system and therefore of my immune system, and are defined as filters that control everything that passes through the throat (which embodies creativity and communication).

They keep only what is good for me and reject what is harmful. When they are inflamed, I have **difficulty in swallowing** and I risk choking. I thus repress my emotions and stifle my creativity. There is a situation stifling me, through which I repress my feelings of **anger** and **frustration**. **Tonsillitis** or **amygdalitis** (**-itis = anger**) generally manifests itself when the reality I swallow brings **intense irritation**, to the point where my filters (the **tonsils**) cannot take on everything and become red with anger at what is going on and with the inner revolt I am feeling. It may be the fear of being unable to reach a goal that was set, or of not being able to achieve something important for me, for lack of time or opportunity. This leads me to cling excessively to someone. I sense that I am on the point of obtaining something dear to me (a job, a spouse, a car, etc.), but I fear it will escape me and I will have to do without it, or I may only get to enjoy it in part, which I find 'hard to swallow'. A very intense inner conflict is 'smothered' and goes unexpressed. It is a blocking, a closing of this channel of communication. I feel helpless, stuck, a prisoner. I feel like releasing a full-throated ***shout***! Do I feel there is a situation that I am 'swallowing the wrong way'? I am in rebellion, or even revolt, against a person close to me (family, school, work). It may involve friendship, as I suspect that I cannot really count on my friends. If I am a **child**, I often have **tonsillitis** because I am not yet **Aware** enough of what is going on, or I don't control events. I experience **frustration** related to what I must 'swallow' in life. I feel very vulnerable and I wonder how I can protect myself from everything that assails me. I feel under attack and I want to defend myself, but I have difficulty in expressing myself. How can I face everything that offers itself to me and make choices that are congruent with who I am? As a **child**, I have far less experience and resources than adults, so I am more likely to experience **tonsillitis**. I feel that my parents don't take enough care of me, that I don't benefit from their presence. As my **tonsils** represent the outward expression of my deeper essence, at whatever age, my **tonsils** react to my doubts and my despair, mostly when I rely more on others than on myself to accomplish and create things. I may desperately want to reunite my parents' couple. It seems that a child's dream is becoming increasingly inaccessible.

I accept↓♥ things as they are around me, and I take the time to calmly and serenely analyze the situations that disturb my life. It is possible and easy to teach this attitude to children who are ready for it. Let us note that the **removal of the tonsils** means accepting↓♥ to swallow reality without filtering or censoring (protecting) it in advance. It is a removal of protection. I must deal with this situation in a different way, more congenial to me. I must learn to discover myself and be myself and have full confidence in myself.

TOOTH AILMENTS *See: TEETH – TOOTH AILMENTS*

TOOTH (impacted wisdom) *See: TEETH — TOOTH [IMPACTED WISDOM]*

TOOTH (root abscess) *See: TEETH — TOOTH [ROOT ABSCESS]*

TOOTHACHE *See: TEETH — TOOTH AILMENTS*

TORPOR / TORPIDITY *See: NUMBNESS*

TORSION of the TESTICLE *See: TESTICLES (IN GENERAL)*

TORTICOLLIS *See: NECK — TORTICOLLIS / STIFF NECK*

TRACHEITIS *See: RESPIRATION — TRACHEITIS*

TRACHEOBRONCHITIS *See: BRONCHI — BRONCHITIS, RESPIRATION — TRACHEITIS*

TRAVEL SICKNESS *See also: ANXIETY, NAUSEA, SEA SICKNESS, VERTIGO*

Travel sickness occurs when I am experiencing a duality or a discrepancy between two different sources of information, which makes it difficult for me to adjust my bearings with respect to certain persons or situations. For example, what Mom and Dad are saying doesn't agree. My inner, imaginary world is quite different from reality, from the external world. I may feel well and in control of my car, but not of the people around me. I feel insecure and uncomfortable. It disturbs my set habits and I may have the impression that I am losing control over what is going on in my life. The unfamiliar – and indirectly, death – frightens me. I have the impression that I must put up with things and persons, as in my life. There is something I want to flee, because I want to have already reached my destination right away! The fact of feeling resentment will give me fits of nausea along the way. **Car sickness** often refers to a sensation of feeling caught, stuck, or choked. If I have difficulty in driving my car myself, I ask myself how I am 'driving' my own life: am I the one in charge, or am I allowing others to manage it because I am afraid of the authority and the responsibility inherent in making decisions? If I don't like someone else to be driving, am I capable of trusting others, or do I tend to want to control everything, believing it is the only way for me to feel safe? Sometimes my discomfort about a **means of transportation** may be related to a past experience that was traumatic for me or only unpleasant. When I put myself again in a similar situation, my body recalls the negative memory and reacts. For example, I may have received very bad news while travelling. I now unconsciously associate trips with bad news to come. I may invent all sorts of reasons to not put myself again in a similar situation, in case I receive bad news again. I then tend to place the blame for my sorrow on the **means of transportation** used to make that trip, and I have the impression that in the future a **train** or an **aircraft** for example will be signs of a bad spell that I must avoid at all costs to prevent myself from suffering.

I accept↓♥ to make peace with myself and become **Aware** that the means of **transportation** are safe; it is in myself that I must trust and build this sense of safety. I know I am fully guided and always in the right place at the right time. I must trust in the future and accept↓♥ to explore new experiences, knowing it will broaden me.

TREMORS / SHIVERING / TREMBLING *See also: Parkinson's disease*

Tremors affect especially the upper limbs of the body and mainly the hands.

They are irregular movements that often occur after excessive anger or after a fright or a physical weakness. It is a reaction of the nervous system. Feeling caught and helpless, my **muscles** tense and start to tremble. I am like an erupting volcano, with my aggressiveness rumbling in me. This **trembling** may also occur following news or information of which I refuse to consciously see the consequences; it is like lying to myself. There is then a conflict between my **conscious** part and my subconscious. This tension that forms between the two provokes involuntary **trembling** in one of the parts of my body (arms, face, legs, trunk). It may be following a question I asked myself for so many years and to which I know the answer, but the truthfulness of which I doubt or ***fear***. I am shaken inside, and this shows up as **tremors**. I vacillate, I can't make up my mind in some situations, and my body does the same. The energy I accumulated in my subconscious, by dint of wanting my answer, is released in the form of **tremors**. These reach the **epidermis** only when I face a difficult situation of separation.

I accept↓♥ to learn to take my place and relax, and I live one day at a time. I ***sing*** to life and happiness!

TRISMUS *See: MUSCLES — TRISMUS*

TRISOMY 21 *See: MONGOLISM*

TUBE (fallopian) INFECTION *See: SALPINGITIS*

TUBERCULOSIS *See also: LUNG DISEASES*

Tuberculosis is an infection by Koch's bacillus[7], often lodged in the lungs but also able, through the blood, to reach the kidneys, the urinary system, etc. The

7. **Koch** (Robert): German physician (1843–Baden-Baden). In 1882, he identified the **tuberculosis** bacillus. He listed the modes of transmission of this disease and invented a diagnostic method. In 1905, he received the Nobel Prize in Medicine for all of his discoveries.

main symptoms are repeated bronchitis, abnormal fatigue, prolonged fever and the coughing up of blood.

Each of them shows me that I feel anger and that my life is joyless. I have the impression of being left behind, abandoned, feeling myself at a loss with my family. I no longer have any breathing space. I hope to be able to keep the people I **love** all for myself. My selfishness makes me jealous of what others possess, and I feel a 'victim', resenting the rest of the world and seeking revenge on it. As the lungs are affected, **tuberculosis also reveals my fear of imminent death, which is very present and invades my thoughts**. This is why a new outbreak of **tuberculosis** follows wars; for, in many cases, I may have found myself in situations where bombs fell close to where I was, where the enemy could 'put me down' (kill me). In fact, I have found myself in several situations where I could have died. I may have been left for dead, or I or my parents thought I would die young at a specified age. Gentleness then is absent from my life. I forbid my inner being from manifesting itself. The hardness of life and its experiences has, in turn, made me hard too, with a taste for vengeance. I simply want to protect myself from danger. My struggle to survive makes me wear a mask of iron, with a stone wall around me. I feel oppressed, something is stifling my breath. I feel like renewing contact with this child in me whom I have pushed away for too long. I carry bitter memories of the events of my past. I isolate myself, thus preventing new ideas or attitudes from entering me. I no longer communicate with my body, whether in kisses or hugs or in sexual intercourse. I thus do not transmit my fear of death, and I feel I am protecting others. I can escape from my emotions in work. It is very important for me to become **Aware** of all my inner feelings and to discover the object of this fear of death.

I accept↓♥ that I am protected at all times. I dare to be more fearless and take more risks. I must overcome this fear of death and live the present moment, savoring each instant. I allow gentleness to take place in my life. I renew contact with my divine essence, and nobody can hurt me.

TUMOR (brain) *See: BRAIN [TUMOR IN]*

TUMOR (malignant) *See: CANCER (IN GENERAL)*

TUMORS *See also: CANCER (IN GENERAL), CYST*

A **tumor** is comparable to a shapeless mass of tissues that may be found in different locations in the body.

It generally takes form following an emotional shock. By keeping inside of me old injuries and negative thoughts from my past, they accumulate and form a mass that eventually becomes solid. I easily become attached to someone, and my lack of self-confidence leads me to experience jealousy, envy and disappointment in myself and others. I have an unlimited potential that is dormant in me. I feel deeply sad about a situation and I feel resigned because I tell myself that I have 'lost the game' and I let myself drift, wanting to end things with life. I experience it as a moral and emotional downfall, not knowing whether I can pick myself up again. I have too many emotions trapped inside, and my body can no longer stand it. I think that by dominating others, criticizing them and using some power over them, it will change something; but deep down, I know that is not the solution. A **benign tumor** becomes larger and **malignant** (**cancer**) when I become increasingly anxious and focus my attention more and more on the past events that are still gnawing at me inside. My emotions are strengthening and my injuries are raw. I become so negative that I am always on alert and expecting the worst. It is therefore a negative energy that is surrounding me and that eventually becomes stronger than me.

I accept↓♥ to become **Aware** that this mass is blocking the flow of some of my energy that needs to flow freely. It is important for me to be able to express the distress inside of me; I must take seriously this message my body is sending me. I make room for the present and express my feelings. If I refuse this, I will feel that a little inner voice is telling me: **you are dying**, little by little. I practice detachment and I learn to trust myself totally.

TURISTA / MONTEZUMA'S REVENGE *See: INTESTINES — DIARRHEA*

TWINS *See: BIRTH [HOW MY BIRTH TOOK PLACE]*

TYMPANISM

Tympanism is an increase in the sonority of the thorax or the abdomen. It can be detected by striking a zone of the body with the fingers: it 'resonates' as on a drum.

This state may be the sign that I am a very highly sensitive person and that I hold in my emotions instead of letting them go freely. I feel like a puppet that is used against its will. To protect myself from my sensitivity, I 'reason' with my emotions to have the impression I can exert control over them with my intellect.

I accept↓♥ to fully experience my emotions, for they are a rich source for discovering different facets of myself.

TYPHOID *See: SALMONELLOSIS*

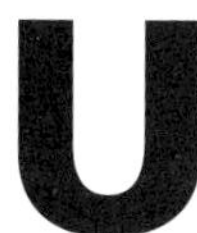

ULCER(S) (in general)

An **ulcer** is a loss of substance of the skin or of a mucous membrane, taking the form of a lesion that does not scar over and tends to spread and produce pus.[1.]

An **ulcer** can develop on the outer skin of the body (arms, legs, the cornea of the eye, etc.) or on the wall of an internal organ (stomach, intestine, mouth, etc.). An **ulcer** makes me become **Aware** that I am feeling great fears and insecurity. It indicates that an intense stress inhabits me and that **I feel worn down**, **distressed**, **devoured**: All that is burning me up from inside. The **ulcer** is the result of the fire of revolt, rancor and violent resentment. I have the impression of being tied to a ball and chain and I can't move forward as I would like to. I push myself to the limit, and I know I have reached a stage in my life where I must make some major changes, but I don't know quite how to go about it. My head is filled with thoughts and is overheating. My repressed aggressiveness leads me to meet people who are experiencing the same situation. Depending on the location on my body where my **ulcer** develops, it is possible for me to discover what is provoking this condition. If it is in my **mouth** for example, I can ask myself what it is that I have to say but am swallowing back. I cut myself off from my spontaneity of speech. **Stomach ulcers** show that there is something that I am digesting badly. I want to flee and get out of a situation. My anxiety makes me wear a mask, to be accepted↓♥ by others and thus find some safety. If it is in the **large intestine**, I am feeling stifled by this past that I refuse to let go. As a general rule, an **ulcer** indicates that I allow things or people to irritate me.

I accept↓♥ to let things flow and calm down. I rely on my own inner strength. I can extinguish the fire inside of me only by taming the emotions that inhabit me. By recovering my inner peace, the **ulcer** has no reason to exist.

ULCER (oral herpes) / CHANCRE *See: MOUTH DISEASE*

ULCER (peptic / gastric) of the DUODENUM[2] / STOMACH

Ulcers in the stomach can appear if I have low self-esteem. I want so much to please others that I am ready to swallow anything. I repress my emotions and my own desires by acting like this; I don't respect myself and I end up reproaching others for not respecting me. I feel eaten up inside, and I reach the point of dramatizing each event in my life. I am finding it increasingly difficult to **digest** all these bothers, concerns and uncertainties that make my

1. This superinfection is specific to cutaneous **ulcers** that have been neglected.
2. **Duodenum:** The initial part of the small intestine.

feeling of helplessness grow even larger. It is like an excess of irritants that transforms itself into an **ulcer**. This irritant may be a person or a situation I want to avoid seeing or facing, but this is impossible and it stays on my **stomach**! I wish I could expel this irritant from my vital space, from my 'territory'. I feel misunderstood, in part because I have difficulty in ***communicating*** my needs. As I want to please others at all costs, I prefer to chafe away in silence. As I have difficulty in asserting myself, the frustration grows in me until it becomes aggressiveness, which I must acknowledge and accept in order to better channel it. Otherwise, it could take on excessive proportions or even become a desire for vengeance. I tend to criticize myself severely and I can even reach the point of destroying myself. I worry a lot about one special aspect of my life: it may involve the affective side as much as the work-related side. This worry is 'eating me up inside'. It gives me knots in the **stomach**. All this torment makes me more fragile and vulnerable. If I have an **ulcer in the duodenum**, it refers especially to my fear of not meeting the expectations of all the persons who represent authority for me.

I accept↓♥ that my body is indicating that it is high time for me to discover the qualities that are in me, to appreciate myself at my true worth and to accept↓♥ my need for **Love**.

UMBILICAL HERNIA *See also: HERNIA*

An **umbilical hernia** can be a sign of my disappointment or my regret over having had to detach myself from the cozy and safe environment of my mother's womb. Now, I feel that I must manage alone, and I have efforts to make in order to reach the goals I have set for myself and that suddenly seem far less exciting.

I accept↓♥ the fact that I have all the necessary potential to reach my goals and that life supports me completely. By accepting↓♥ to serve unselfishly, I open my **heart♥** to the **Love** of others.

UMBILICUS

The **umbilicus** is the opening in the fetus' abdominal wall through which the umbilical cord passes. Shortly after birth it becomes a scar, which is then commonly named the **navel** or **umbilicus**.

A pain in this area means that I must open myself up more to others instead of remaining focused on myself. I may be '**cutting the umbilical cord'**, namely my dependence upon my mother or my family. When I was a fetus, it was through the **umbilicus** that I received all the nourishment essential for my growth and my survival. An **anomaly** or an **ailment** in this area can therefore also give me an indication about something I vitally need in my life and that I am not receiving, or on the contrary something that I would want to reject and evacuate because I have consumed or received it in excessive quantities and it may no longer be beneficial for me. I may have difficulty in detaching myself from my parents' influence and 'cutting the cord'. Everything that I carry around uselessly becomes a burden. I question my place within the clan, with the impression that I am not part of it. If I am a **baby with a red navel** and there is **inflammation**, this indicates that I am feeling much anger over my incapacity for experiencing things. I need to be close to Mother and at the same time I need some space. If I am the parent of this baby, I must see whether I too am experiencing the same thing, for the baby is very sensitive to what I am experiencing. The **umbilicus** is also considered by certain persons as an important energy center for openness, for there even exists a group called 'the **navel** adorers' who do meditation exercises on this part of the body that represents the opening of the passage of life when I was a fetus in my mother's womb.

I learn to accept↓♥ my ***eccentric*** side, to humbly recognize my qualities, thus not 'taking myself as the **navel** of the world' and enabling me to see all the beauty that exists in each being and each thing. I let go of any relation or situation that is no longer beneficial for me, and I allow new knowledge or new contacts to come to me, bringing with them a breeze of freshness and positive change in my life.

UPSET STOMACH / BILIOUSNESS *See: INDIGESTION*

UREMIA *See also: KIDNEYS [RENAL PROBLEMS]*

Uremia is the level of **urea** in the blood. **Urea** is a component of **urine**. This level can be abnormally high, due to renal failure; conversely, hepatic failure (of the liver) can be the cause of an abnormally low level.

The proteins are badly managed and I must ask myself: "What aspect of my life is not managed as I would want it to be?" I feel forced to leave everything behind me. I have the impression of losing everything. **Uremia** often appears when I feel uprooted from my native land, when I must go into exile on the other side of the ocean. I no longer know where I am in my life. What is truly good for me? I limit myself to doing certain things, sometimes with hardness and rigidity. It is not my **heart♥**, but my head, that is managing my life. I try to be the best, which complicates my relations with authority. **Urine** is related to my old emotions that need to be eliminated.

I accept↓♥ to put some order in what is disturbing my life and I remain open to new dispositions. I listen to my needs and my inner voice.

URETHRITIS *See also: APPENDIX III*

Urethritis is an inflammation of the canal conducting urine from the bladder neck to the external urethral orifice, the meatus.

This condition indicates that I reluctantly accept↓♥ to give way to a new situation and that I make place for aggressiveness. An unresolved situation with my mother can often generate **urethritis**. I have difficulty in delimiting my boundaries. I want to control the lives of others. I feel a lot of anger. I want to have the impression that I have my life under control, but I must become

Aware that it is an illusion, and that I must let go of certain things or persons. I can only have power over myself!

I accept↓♥ to allow new ideas to circulate more freely and to keep an open mind about my opinions, which can change, knowing that I am constantly evolving and changing.

URINE (urinary infections) / CYSTITIS *See also: BLADDER DISORDERS. INCONTINENCE [URINARY], INFECTIONS (IN GENERAL), LEUKORRHEA, VAGINA — VAGINITIS,*

Urine represents my old emotions that I no longer need and that I eliminate from my system. An inflammation of the bladder (**cystitis**) causes pain when I **urinate** (even in small quantities) and a constant desire to **urinate**. It is more frequent in young women, diabetics and pregnant women. As it is an **infection**, it means that this ailment is very often related to anger that I have accumulated. It may also be bitterness, resentment or exasperation that are boiling or burning in me and touching new aspects of myself or my personal relationships. As in a case of **vaginitis** (or **leukorrhea**), I may have a feeling of frustration over my sexual relations. As my **urinary** system and my reproductive system (vagina) are connected, the one will affect the other. It may be that my sexual relations are going admirably well and I don't understand why I was experiencing frustration. Precisely because everything is going quite well, I may ask myself: Why did I have to wait for so many years to succeed in having satisfying sexual relations? Unexpressed frustration and anger may originate from there. **Cystitis,** for example, may also occur following a separation. As I was incapable of expressing my negative emotions, fears and inner conflicts will surface about what is in store for me. Having great unfulfilled expectations, I blame the people around me for this void, and most of the time, my spouse suffers from it. I go from frustration to frustration because I leave to others the responsibility for my well-being. My inner rage is usually turned against persons of the opposite sex or my sexual partner. Do I feel imprisoned in a situation? Does someone have a hold over me? There follows a feeling of helplessness and the impression that my life is ruined.

It is therefore time for me to take myself in charge, and that I accept↓♥ responsibility for my life. I decide to move forward, I am reborn to myself, independently of my current and past relationships. I welcome myself gently. I allow my creativity to express itself. I live my life with my **heart♥** instead of constantly being in my head.

URTICARIA / HIVES / NETTLE-RASH *See: SKIN / URTICARIA / HIVES / NETTLE-RASH*

UTERUS (in general) *See also: CANCER OF THE CERVIX, FEMALE DISORDERS, PROLAPSE OF UTERUS*

The **uterus** symbolizes my status as a woman: **it is the core of my creativity**. It also represents the power to give birth, security and warmth. It is a refuge.

It is in this warm and safe sanctuary that nidation takes place. **Ovary** or **uterus** problems such as the **tilting** of the uterus indicate that it is time for me to develop my creativity, which will give me back the power to manage my life. It is in my interest to question myself about: "How do I feel as a woman? Do I feel guilty, ashamed or betrayed for having had children or not? Am I disappointed at not having the family I wished for, or disappointed at the child I will never have? Do I find it difficult to be a woman, a wife, a mother, a businesswoman, a lover?" Maybe I have the impression of regressing! This region touches my deepest, most secret feelings. Guilt, shame and solitude can gnaw at me inside. An unresolved bereavement can be the cause. These feelings will be more strongly present at the time of a hysterectomy: the despair of seeing that I am no longer a 'real woman', a 'fine ***lady***', that I am useless and undesirable, can even lead me to depression. I may feel myself less well **matched**, poorly suited to my spouse, and this makes me sad. I blame him for my misery, and this can induce an **inflammation of the uterus**: what I see in him constantly reminds me of what annoys me in myself, for he is my mirror. I reject my life and my own body. In this region of the pelvis, it is possible for me to give birth again, to awaken new aspects of my being; I can go forward in my quest for myself. If a disease develops in my **uterus**, such as a **tumor** for instance, I ask myself how I perceive the sexuality of others, and especially that of my children and grand-children. Do I have the impression that it is 'not OK', that it is 'unusual', that 'this is not done'? Do I feel that they are in any moral or physical danger? Do they risk injuring themselves? Is there something I find 'ugly' about my children or their lives as couples? Am I bothered about the role or the place that each member of the family is taking? Am I losing my 'little ones' because they are 'growing too fast' (I would like so much for them to remain small and safe)? I almost feel it as my duty to resume the role of a parent with my grand-children. My feeling of freedom is thus once again curtailed. It is as though a misfortune were threatening my family and my home. All these questionings may concern my real children or grand-children, or a nephew, a neighbor or a pupil whom I consider as such. I hold on to so many things from the past that it prevents my creativity from expressing itself. I turn down the child that I am and that I stored in a box in the belief that this is what I must do when I become an adult. Deep down, I want to move forward and accomplish things, but I am frustrated because something is preventing me from doing so. When there is **retention**, I become **Aware** of the state of fear in which I am. I am afraid of letting go. I worry, I cannot let 'my little one' go out into this new world, and I try to hold part of them back. I therefore lose blood, which is related to a loss of joy. "Am I losing the joy of having this child in me*? For soon they must face the world, and I am afraid for them"*.

I accept↓♥ to be reborn to myself.Instead of wanting to silence the customs that dictated my life, I accept↓♥ to integrate them into it harmoniously. I become **Aware** that I have no power over the lives of others and that everyone lives their own life in their own way. I have given my children the best education in the best possible way, and I can be proud of it! I accept↓♥ to allow the child in me to live, and who is **Love**, joy and hope.

UTERUS (cancer of the cervix) *See: CANCER OF THE UTERUS [CERVIX AND CORPUS]*

V

VAGINA (in general)

The **vagina** is the muscular membrane that is located between the vulva and the uterus in women.

The diseases that are related to the **vagina** often originate from my frustration over not being able to accomplish the act of carnal union, either because I do not morally permit it for myself or because I do not have the man with whom I could explore new experiences. "Am I satisfied with my present spouse?" If I am afraid of ***kisses*** and intimacy, either because of my principles that are very limiting with respect to sexuality, or because of past events where I felt guilty and ashamed because of what happened, I develop **ailments in my vagina**, notably **vaginal dryness**, as I unconsciously want to delay penetration. I push sexuality away, but for fear of losing my spouse, I give in to his advances and requests. By living in my head and my worries, I cut myself off from my body, my impulses and life in me. Pleasure is forbidden and full of guilt. I have locked myself into a 'physical and psychological corset'. I have the impression that I do not belong to anyone. Do I fully accept↓♥ my sexual impulses, even if this means that I feel subjugated and sometimes out of control? Was I ever the victim of a **denunciation**? Have I ever experienced a situation where my child was leaving and I had the impression it was like going off to war and he might never come back? I suffer from not having a partner, from not 'belonging to someone'. I experience it as a tragedy that has lasted too long. All these situations may cause a **vaginal prolapse** or associated disorders. I then feel powerless about myself and what is happening. This state usually involves a conflict or a rejection related to my sexuality and how I perceive myself.

I accept↓♥ to open myself up to **Love** in all its forms in order to fully flourish.

VAGINA — ITCHING (vaginal) *See: ITCHING [VAGINAL]*

VAGINAL DISCHARGE *See: LEUKORRHEA*

VAGINAL HERPES *See: HERPES [VAGINAL]*

VAGINAL SPASMS *See: SPASMS*

VAGINITIS *See also: CANDIDA, LEUKORRHEA, URINE [URINARY INFECTIONS]*

Vaginitis is an infection of the **vagina** (such as candidiasis or fungi) accompanied by nauseating odors.

In most cases, it shows that I feel frustration toward my sexual partner, or I am experiencing guilt. If I use sex to wield power or control over my spouse, it is possible that I will regularly experience problems of **vaginitis**. It may provide the ideal excuse for not making **Love**, and thus punish my spouse by depriving him of sex. My overly puritanical or moralizing side leads me to punish myself with **vaginitis**. The intimacy generated by a sexual relationship can trigger several feelings linked to memory or fear: the fear of feeling misunderstood, hurt again, or losing my partner who might feel trapped or possessed. Emitting unpleasant odors also enables me to release negative emotions, accumulated sorrows and anxieties, which are deeply buried in the vaginal tissue itself. The **vagina** is the place from where all my feelings involving sexuality emerge: if they are positive, I will experience sexual pleasure. On the contrary, an infection appears if I feel guilt, fear, shame, conflicts, confusion, as well as my memories of abusive experiences, or if I want to punish myself.

I accept↓♥ to be open to experiencing congenial sexuality. It is part of life and the happiness I am entitled to.

VARICELLA / CHICKENPOX *See: CHILDHOOD DISEASES — VARICELLA*

VARICOCELE *See: TESTICLES (IN GENERAL)*

VARICOSE VEINS *See: BLOOD — VARICOSE VEINS*

VEGETATIVE STATE (chronic) *See: BRAIN — CHRONIC VEGETATIVE STATE*

VEIN DISORDERS *See also: BLOOD — BLOOD CIRCULATION*

A **vein** is a blood vessel that returns blood from the organs back to the **heart**♥[1]. When the **veins** return from the lungs to the **heart**♥, they bring back purified 'red', oxygen-laden blood. When the **veins** return from the other organs to the **heart**♥, they bring back 'blue' blood, poorly oxygenated and laden with carbon monoxide, CO_2.

I have never had any **luck** in life! This is like saying that I was never able to find any joy in living. The blood flows in my **veins**; blood is life and the joy in living. I am constantly in contradiction with my inner voice and what I achieve in my life. I feel disappointed and outdated. I feel in a state of inertia, and no longer even see the beautiful things that happen to me. I am short of energy and I feel empty. I do not feel sustained by life or by my entourage and I see everything darkly. I am incapable of coming to terms with my life and I cannot return home. I want to get rid of my torments, but something is preventing me. My **coronary veins** are especially affected if I am afraid of losing someone or something I 'possess' and am reluctant to let go of. I experience it like a danger threatening my territory, namely my spouse, my home, my family, my work, my ideas. I am afraid of not belonging to anyone because I

---

1. Whereas an **artery** is a blood vessel that carries blood from the **heart**♥ to the organs.

am experiencing dependence: I suffer from indifference, mainly from my spouse. I feel neglected and abandoned. I give a lot, but I feel I am not receiving as much in return. I "no longer have any blood in my **veins**", I am lacking in energy and courage.

I accept↓♥ to allow joy to flow in me. I recognize the good moments, I learn to relax, and I find inner peace.

VEINS — VARICOSE VEINS *See: BLOOD — VARICOSE VEINS*

VENEREAL DISEASES *See also: CHANCRE, HERPES / (IN GENERAL) / GENITAL*

A **venereal disease** can suggest that a feeling of guilt subsists about my sexuality. Often my religious education portrayed sexuality as something dirty and impure. Feeling ***ashamed*** of my thoughts and actions, often betrayed by the other who 'transmitted the disease to me'; I believe I must punish myself by rejecting my genitals. I punish myself by destroying myself. Sexual energy is extremely important and powerful, it is an integral part of my genetic program for the survival of the species. Therefore a **venereal disease** involves an illness or an infection related to this energy. If I underestimate it, abuse it, or use it negatively or in a way that does not respect who I am or who others are, my body warns me by developing a **venereal disease**. Does my sexuality suit me and more importantly, do I feel well and flourishing with the person with whom I share my intimacy? Do I respect myself, or do I feel I am being abused? My non-acceptance of myself may even lead me to experience rejection and frustration, and feeling more in control over my impulses, I 'catch' a **venereal disease** that forces me to stay away from any sexual contact for some time. I may also attract this disease to myself to get revenge on my spouse when I feel that he has already abandoned me emotionally. I no longer venerate anything in him. In the case of **chlamydia**, I am afraid of the power, especially sexual, that could lead to abuse (to be abused, or to abuse others). I feel guilty when I feel my impulses. I am afraid, as much by what is inside of me as by what is around me. What is the frustration that is bothering me in my sexual life? Is my body expressing something that I would feel like telling my partner about? Do I have the impression that I am helpless in this situation? I feel bullied or dominated somewhere in this male or female aspect that is in me. I need to gain some distance in order to take stock of my relationship with the other, and it is my body that sets the limits that I do not dare express because I feel myself in a state of weakness. I feel like changing certain aspects of this relationship, and I feel incapable of claiming my place. I cannot find the words to say it, but it itches in me. **Gonorrhea**, also called **blennorrhagia**, shows me my irritation at seeing my incapacity for accomplishing things. I want to achieve great exploits, but I denigrate myself so much that I have no energy left to undertake anything at all. I am also disappointed in my partner. **Syphilis** shows me that I escape into a meaningless sexuality. It brings a certain shame on the family. I escape my true feelings and entertain relations with my partner where I seek power and want to be Number One. If I have a **venereal disease**, is there a link with a feeling of loss or a fear related to an affective abandonment? What is the passage (or the transition) I must achieve in order to recover my balance and my oneness? Is there an inner aspect of me that is fused with the other, which I had not noticed among my relationships and that does not suit me?

It is important for me to accept↓♥ that sexuality is a way to express my **Love** and my desire to join the other. I learn to see what is good for me and what no longer suits me. I accept↓♥ to contact my inner feelings so that my relationships will be true and healthy. I use my sexual power positively, in order to enable all my creative energies to flow in me. I choose to re-examine my position in my affective and sexual relationships. I allow new ideas to flow freely and I keep an open mind. I adjust my way of thinking and accept↓♥ that this experience is a means for me to grow and recover my affective balance.

VERTEBRÆ (fracture of) *See: BACK— FRACTURE OF VERTEBRÆ*

VERTIGO and DIZZINESS *See also: BLOOD — HYPOGLYCEMIA*

Vertigo is a cerebral disorder, an error of sensation, under the influence of which I believe that my own person or the surrounding objects are impelled by a rotary or oscillatory movement (**rotary vertigo**).

Having **spells of vertigo** or **dizziness** is **a way to escape** an event or a person whom I refuse to see or hear: though I am not satisfied, I stay in this pattern. I refuse to obey an external or inner authority or my inner voice. I may have the impression that a situation is developing too fast for me, and I am afraid of the changes it will bring in my life. Can I always be up to it? A new task or job position that I perceive as much more demanding will cause me to experience a 'psychological **vertigo**' that will transform itself into a physical **vertigo**. I am afraid of not being able to follow. Everything is moving, "It is going too fast!" I am losing my vital space and feeling compressed. It is as though I had no reference points to orient myself, and I may therefore have the impression that 'my father', or whoever represents authority, is absent or should be helping me more about the directions to be taken. I am also afraid of the future, I don't know very well what direction I should take and I find myself all alone with myself, in a void. It 'gives me **vertigo**'. I have difficulty in positioning myself. I prefer to shut up, and I flee. I would want to control everything going on inside of me as well as outside of me, but as that is impossible, I become unstable and anxious. In most cases, when I suffer from **vertigo** and **dizziness**, I may be suffering from hypoglycemia. There are forces over which I have no control, and this bothers me. I constantly seek the truth. I am affected by a lie concerning my genealogy: I have the impression that something is amiss, but I don't know what. I am not in contact with the earth; I am not 'touching land'. I am going in circles and I see no way out. There are also things that I cannot stand to hear. I live in my thoughts, daydreaming. I am experiencing uneasiness or a deep questioning about the position I hold in my family or in society. What is my position, and am I comfortable with it?

My spells of **vertigo** throw **Light** on the inner imbalance I am experiencing, often between my male and female sides. It may have appeared following an emotional shock. For example, the departure of someone I **love**: I minimized the impact of that event, preferring to turn a deaf ear. I thus have the impression that I can control my life, but I only achieve an external balance that is an illusion and very fragile.

I accept↓♥ to discover the joy of living, to enjoy small pleasures and to trust the future. This enables me to recover a feeling of inner balance, essential for me to heal.

VITILIGO *See: SKIN — VITILIGO*

VOCAL CORDS *See: CANCER OF THE LARYNX, THROAT — LARYNGITIS, VOICE — HOARSENESS*

VOICE (loss of) *See: APHONIA*

VOICE — HOARSENESS

When my tone of **voice** becomes dull, husky or rasping, then my **voice is hoarse** (it is also called **dysphonia**).

Hoarseness means that I am suffering from mental and physical exhaustion. Something is preventing my 'wheels' from turning without a snag. I am experiencing an emotional block, an intense emotion, and I am holding back my aggressiveness. As the throat is linked to the energy center of truth, communication and self-expression (the throat chakra), I feel caught by the truth, which I have difficulty in assimilating, and by my personal convictions. I live according to very precise and sometimes rigid structures. For instance, my view of work and the notion that "you have to work hard to make a success of your life" leads me to overwork, which manifests itself among other things by **hoarseness**. I use certain expedients or stimulants such as coffee, alcohol, cigarettes, etc., and when the effect wears off, the **hoarseness** appears. The fatigue I feel amplifies the worries and concerns that I did not want to look at. It is as though my **voice** were hesitating to produce sounds, for I am afraid of hitting a wall; I no longer know what to say because people find me a little crazy, 'cracked'.

I accept↓♥ the need to have some time off to give myself some rest and enough time to regenerate myself. Once I have rested, situations and events reassume their actual proportions, so I will be far more objective and lucid to make the decisions that are needed. I sing, and I thus free up the way to self-expression.

VOMITING *See: NAUSEA*

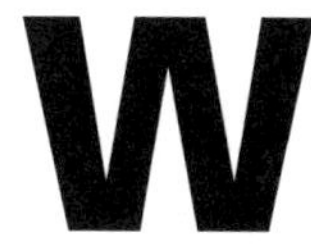

WALL / LINING

A **wall** is a part that circumscribes (limits) a cavity in the body or in a hollow organ (such as the bladder, the large intestine, the gallbladder, the small intestine, the stomach).

If it is affected, I must ask myself about what situation in my life I am feeling fragile. I have the impression that I do not have the power to change things. I feel limited in a role or a situation not of my choice. My words do not come out as I want them to; I do not feel I am 'the King', the master of my life. I thus live in submission, due to my poor self-esteem and the doubts that paralyze me. I feel separated, partitioned off, different from the others. I have difficulty in setting my limits and making myself respected in my needs. It is important to go and read the affected organ to find more information about what I am experiencing.

I accept↓♥ to renew contact with my needs and my emotions. I express them confidently while respecting myself and others. I am engaged in action and I thus take charge of my life again!

WARTS (in general) *See: SKIN — WARTS (IN GENERAL)*

WARTS (plantar) *See: FEET — WARTS [PLANTAR]*

WEAKNESS (state of) *See also: ASTHENIA, CHRONIC FATIGUE SYNDROME, FATIGUE (IN GENERAL)*

I find myself in a **state of weakness** when I feel a lack of strength in general. I may also have the sensation that I am about to lose **consciousness**.

I am hypersensitive and am experiencing annoyance or an intense emotion. I am **Aware** of what is going on, but I don't feel like being there and hearing what is going on. I feel the need to lie down to help me 'regain my senses'. This **weakness** may result from a situation that makes me feel very uncomfortable because I do not know very clearly how to situate myself. A member of my family is often involved. It is as though someone else had some control over this situation, whereas I can do nothing, which gives me an overpowering feeling of helplessness. Just thinking about it can trigger lassitude, bringing on a **state of weakness**, which is a way of escaping. It throws **Light** on my indifference to life, for I have lost interest in it. I follow a routine, whether at work or in my personal life, and I am tired of everything around me.

I accept↓♥ to face reality with strength and courage. I am **Aware** that I have the choice of taking 'my' place or letting others take 'the' place: it depends on me to do what needs to be done. I dare to express what I feel in order to reclaim my rightful place. I make the appropriate choices for my well-being and that of the people around me. I surround myself with **Light**, I let it envelop me with **Love**.

WEIGHT (excess) *See also: FAT*

The **excess fat** that my body puts between my inner being and my outer surroundings indicates that I unconsciously seek and want to isolate myself, either through my communication with the outer world or because there is an imprisoned emotion or feeling 'isolated' in me that I don't want to see. Through my **obesity**, I am seeking a **form of protection** that I continually accumulate in my inner thoughts. There is a gulf between me and the outer world. I want so much to **love** and approach the people I **love**, but I am so afraid! I thus camouflage my insecurities of being exposed or vulnerable, and thereby I want to avoid being hurt either by remarks, criticism or uncomfortable situations, notably those regarding my sexuality. If I experienced a traumatic situation involving sexuality (I may only have been frightened, or something may also have occurred physically), and if I am a **woman**, it may take the form of putting on weight in the thighs and hips, as though to 'protect' myself from an assault on the genital organs, whereas if I am a **man** I tend to have a well-rounded belly so that my genital organs will be less visible. It may also be any situation, even non-sexual, where I feel under attack. I can also interpret my excess weight as an indication of the fact that I want to possess everything. I entertain emotions such as selfishness and feelings that I refuse to let go of. I cling to the past. This can also be an imbalance, a way of revolting against my entourage, a reaction to gestures or situations that I no longer want to see or remember. Earthly nourishment also represents emotional nourishment. I will thus eat excessively to **fill an inner void**, the impression that I was ***abandoned***, or to compensate for the solitude or the isolation I am experiencing. I remain unconsciously in a relation of dependence, with a need for the other. I want to hide the shame and the **aggressiveness** I feel about a situation. Sometimes I prefer to ***run away*** and disappear in order to no longer suffer. I detest the '***imponderables***' in my life as well as all the things that are ***imposed*** on me. However, I feel the need to ***impose myself***, to assert myself or scare the others, who will then be more likely to go away and leave me in peace. I may experience great insecurities on an emotional as well as on a physical level, and unconsciously, I need to accumulate in order to avoid any 'shortages' or unmet needs that may arise. I want to 'have everything, just in case'. This lack of something may have been experienced in my childhood and may be connected to my mother, who was my direct link to nourishment and survival (breast feeding). If a **baby is overweight**, the mother has been feeding it a lot. It may develop a reflex of permanent demand, as though it could never be satiated. The mother has a desire, however unconscious, to remain in fusion with her baby, who will have difficulty later on in detaching itself from its mother. **Obesity** often develops after a great emotional shock or a major loss, when the void experienced becomes very ***hard to handle***. **I experience a great feeling of**

abandonment, an **inner void**. I often feel guilty over the departure or loss of a loved one. This ***abandonment*** may be experienced in relation to a person, but also to something non-physical such as the business that I had to ***abandon***, that I had to ***give up*** for personal reasons. I had to ***abdicate***, and that broke my **heart♥**. I had to ***abandon*** a project that was dear to me (to have a child for example), and I may consider myself as ***cowardly*** or as a loser. I also have the impression of losing control over a situation or a person. I am no longer connected to ***matter***. I have the impression that I 'carry no weight' in certain situations. I am seeking a goal in my life, and I want to accomplish 'something good'. I have difficulty in taking my place by using my words and my gestures. I therefore do it by taking up more space with my physical body. **I also depreciate myself regarding my physical appearance**: in my eyes, a small 'imperfection' or a few pounds gained will take on enormous proportions, and I then can't appreciate nor see my own physical qualities or attractiveness. Because I focus all my attention on what is 'awkward', my body reacts by adding more **weight** to show me how hard I am on myself and how self-destructive I am, even if it is only through negative thoughts. The sole fact of exercising or dieting will never be enough to lose weight, because I must first become consciously **Aware** of the real source of my **excess weight**, which results from a situation of **abandonment**. Whether I am a child or an adult, I become **conscious** of my self-rejection. I may **have the impression of feeling limited** with respect to different aspects of my life or to things I wish to achieve. This feeling of limitation makes my body expand and absorb a **weight** surplus. If I am a person who **accumulates thoughts, emotions or things**, my body also will 'accumulate', but in the form of fat. I must ask myself what benefits I derive from the fact of being **overweight**. What are the activities that I can thus avoid because they frighten me? Who are the persons from whom I remain distant? Do I have the impression that I have less control or less power in certain areas of my life, and do I feel it is just as well this way, because it means that I have less responsibilities and I can personally invest myself less? Another very important point to bear in mind is this: what danger threatens me if I reach my **ideal weight**? For example, a woman who, once she has lost some **weight**, will be more attractive in men's eyes and will be placed in situations where she will frequently have to say no to their advances. She may thus feel in danger of losing her freedom and her space, she will have to learn to assert herself, which can prove very difficult in certain cases. The fact of being attractive may also call up the 'nice body, but nothing in the head' stereotype, hence the fear of not being found intelligent. Therefore, if my brain has detected a danger linked to **weight** loss and having a good ***figure***, as soon as my body is in a situation where it is about to call upon its reserves of fat, an alarm signal will go off to neutralize this need. At that point, there will be a demand to absorb calories that will prevent my body from drawing on these reserves of fat. I may feel a significant lowering of energy, because all of my body's efforts are deployed in order to keep my weight stable or even to increase it if necessary. My body **resists**, just as I do in certain situations of my life. **Weight** is often related to the notion of strength. An **overweight** person is commonly called a 'stout person' or a 'large sized' person. Do I have the impression that I must be stout in order to survive or succeed in life? Must I be more physically imposing in order to be able to impose myself in my relations and make 'predators' flee? Is it my way of acting so that people will see me and easily spot me, because otherwise I would go unnoticed? Do I act as a 'counter-**weight**' in a situation that appears unfavorable for one of the parties? Or maybe I 'don't carry any **weight**' in a certain situation. If the reason for my **overweight** is due to a '**slow metabolism**', my insecurity is making me overly prudent, which prevents me from taking action.

I accept↓♥ to express my emotions, to recognize my value and all my possibilities. I now know that all the voids that I have the impression of experiencing in my life may be filled with **Love** and positive feelings toward myself. By accepting↓♥ myself and others, with the **Love** I surround myself with, I become free of this sadness and this need for protection.

WHITLOW / FELON

A **whitlow**, also called a **felon**, is the acute inflammation of a finger or, more rarely, of a toe.

If the **fingers** are affected, I have difficulty in proceeding through the details of everyday life, whereas the **toes** concern the details of the future. I am passive, indifferent and melancholy, and my action energy that needs to be externalized comes out through my fingers or my toes. «Do I feel like going toward others?» There is no doubt a deficiency in this respect. I need to get all these harmful repressed emotions and thoughts out of me, and go toward others and share. I want to release myself from my inner prison. I may even be keeping a secret that is now gnawing at me inside. I am now out of laughs and fun. Not being in contact with my inner self, I rely on others. It is as though I cannot manage my destiny. I allow my intimate space to be violated because I don't know my limits.

I accept↓♥ to decide right now what my territory is. I make contact with my power. I remove the bars from my prison. I am now free to create my life as I want it to be.

WORDS (spoken) *See also: APHONIA*

The **words** that I pronounce today create my future. There is a saying that "thought creates, and the verb (**speech**) manifests". Thus when I speak, I am already making my thoughts physically concrete, as though **speech** were material. If I have difficulty in **speaking** and choosing the words to express what I am experiencing, I can ask myself in what situation I was forced to either say nothing or tell a lie, and therefore to use words that did not respect my reality. For example, if I am a woman and I couldn't say that I was pregnant, then an enormous stress was registered from the fact of 'not saying', of hiding, of the unexpressed. After that, whenever any similar situations appear or whenever I sense that I am in a stressful situation, I have difficulty in **speaking**.

I feel inferior to others, and it is therefore difficult for me to express myself because I am afraid of not being up to dealing with the situation. I may want to play a role. The harmony or the disharmony in which I AM, or am living, will depend upon the quality of my **words** and my choices of **words**. If the song is melodious, if I speak from my heart♥, if cheerfulness, a positive outlook and encouragements issue from my mouth, I attract the sun. If my **words** convey but malicious gossip, a negative outlook, anger and destruction, then I attract gray clouds, thunderstorms and bad weather. **The choice is mine**!

I accept↓♥ to be true, quite simply.

WORMS (having) *See: INTESTINES / COLON / TENIA*

WORMS, PARASITES *See: FEET — MYCOSIS, HAIR — TINEA, INTESTINES / COLON (AILMENTS OF) / TENIA*

WOUND / SORE *See ACCIDENT*

WRINKLES

Wrinkles are cutaneous crevices. They can reflect expression or aging. There is a **rupture** of the elastic fibers of the dermis and an impairment of the rest of the conjunctive tissue.

Wrinkles appear when I experience an emotional shock, an upheaval or an inner suffering. These striations in my skin express and crystallize this suffering and pain gnawing at my skin. I may also be experiencing a **breakup** or an event where I must detach myself from a person, a situation or a material good. This makes me experience sorrow, despair, bewilderment and inner pain. If I worry constantly, which is often the case in my work, when I am troubled by doubts or do not feel up to facing the situation, these worries will impregnate my skin and form **wrinkles**. **Vertical wrinkles between the eyes** denote excessive tension, aggressiveness and impatience.

I accept↓♥ to let go of the past, I begin to sort out my life and my rigid psychological structures that slow me down in my progression. I learn to accept↓♥ that any event of my life is there to help me grow, and that it is through detachment that I manifest unconditional **Love**. My **wrinkles** will thus no longer have any reason to exist, and they may disappear. Wisdom brings the true youthfulness of the **heart♥**.

WRIST — SYNDROME (carpal tunnel)

Carpal tunnel syndrome is characterized by a sensation of numbness, tingling and sometimes even pain in the fingers. It mostly affects women in pregnancy or menopause, and occurs at night or on waking up in the morning.

It appears during great hormonal changes when I haven't sufficiently integrated my female side in its entirety. It usually appears at a point in my life when I feel I have been relegated to a secondary place, or when I no longer feel in my proper place. Previously I had the impression that I was the pillar that brought balance into my life and that of the persons close to me (it may be in my family, at work or in a social activity). Now that the attention is focused on someone else, I put pressure on myself in order to find new ways to get myself noticed. I do not know how to use my authority: I need to let go, but I refuse to relinquish control and "give the horse the reins". I tend to want to give orders. I feel remote from my spouse and am no longer in contact with my sexuality, which is nonexistent. I see few solutions and few roads to take; the "**tunnel** is very narrow". I feel pressed by life and compressed by my responsibilities, so it is more difficult to make decisions. The structures that I force myself to follow lead me to feel limited.

I accept↓♥ new things and the changes that appear in my life. The purpose of any situation or challenge that comes up in my life is to enable me to acquire or develop new strengths or qualities in order to achieve my full potential. It is essential that I handle this passage all alone, with who I am and with my physical and psychological changes. I accept↓♥ to take risks and discover different avenues that will give me huge personal satisfaction, for I will have overcome my fears! I choose to integrate what I am in my entirety, I free myself of what held me in chains and I am reborn to myself.

WRISTS *See also: JOINTS*

The **wrists** are the joints, the pivots that enable mobility, suppleness and flexibility in my hands and connect me to my forearms. They initiate the motions of my hands to execute any movement and thus to be engaged in action.

They manifest my will in action. If I act and move forward fluidly, my **wrists** will be strong and healthy. Rigidity in the **wrists** will therefore prevent me from dexterously grasping or choosing everything that life presents to me. There is thus an obstruction, a blocking or a refusal regarding the actions I should take. Any activities that require skill are affected by it. What advantage can I derive from the fact that I am now 'forced' to not perform certain movements, and therefore certain activities? The pressure I feel can be so great that I no longer know in which direction I should go. I am experiencing great indecisiveness. I want to reject my responsibilities for certain situations, I do not want to accept↓♥ or acknowledge the importance of my acts. **Pain in the wrists** can represent repressed energy concerning something that must be done, but that I hold back and do not carry out. It may also be something that happened in the past and weighs so heavily on me that I want to deny its existence. A **fracture** or a **sprain** indicates a deep conflict of expression with life and the way it uses me to carry out its work. The **fracture** calls me back to order and tells me to stop finding reasons to free myself of my responsibilities. I must stop blaming others for my own rigidity. An **ailment in my wrist** shows me how easily influenced I can be. I can resist new directions, new solutions or simply my own creativity. I feel ***chained*** and handcuffed in a situation or a relationship, and I am prevented from saying something. I must come to a halt and stop moving my hands.

I accept↓♥ to think about these pains in order to become **Aware** of the fact that I must release these energies with **Love** and trust, for their free flow enables me to act constructively through these actions. I trust myself, I am determined, and I maintain an openness that helps me to assess each situation. I thus remain at the level of **Love**, and everything I do is in harmony with my development. I grasp all the opportunities that life offers me.

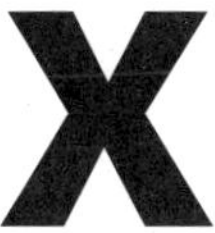

XANTHONYCHIA *See: NAILS — YELLOW NAIL SYNDROME*

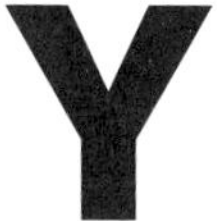

YELLOW NAIL SYNDROME *See: NAILS — YELLOW NAIL SYNDROME*

YAWNING

Yawning is a 'natural imitation reflex', more or less accepted↓♥ in polite society because of its conventions (I say 'natural', because so far there has been no medical therapy to treat it). I say **imitation** because it appears impulsively and unconsciously in a person who sees another person doing this action.

It is the sign for going to bed or taking a rest when I am fatigued or exhausted and I need to regenerate my strength. It is also a sign of dissatisfaction with food, because sometimes I will **yawn** if I haven't eaten enough or if my digestion is too slow. What is boring me, or what can't I digest in my life? I am bored to the point that I express it unconsciously, whether I am alone watching television or in the company of a person who doesn't suit me! "I want to be left alone!" Like a lion who is roaring, I show my dissatisfaction. I want to repel the enemy, I want to defend myself. Don't come too close to me!

Yawning is part of life, and I accept↓♥ it with **Love** and openness. It is important to just 'let be' this bodily expression that is still frowned upon by the educational principles of yesteryear! I let go of my resistances and I allow others to approach me and take care of me too.

Appendices

Appendix I

What Our Body Parts Stand For

THE HAIR	My strength.
THE SCALP	My faith in my divine side.
THE HEAD	My individuality.
THE EYES	My capacity for seeing.
THE EARS	My capacity for hearing.
THE NOSE	My capacity for smelling or sensing persons or situations.
THE LIPS	My upper lip is related to my female side and the lower lip, to my male side.
THE TEETH	My decisions, related to the female side above, related to the male side below.
THE NECK	My flexibility, my capacity for seeing several sides in the situations of life.
THE THROAT	The expression of verbal and nonverbal language, my creativity.
THE SHOULDERS	My capacity for bearing loads and responsibilities.
THE ARMS	My capacity for welcoming persons or life situations. They are extensions of the heart. They serve to carry out orders. They are related to what I do in life, such as my work.
THE ELBOWS	My flexibility in the changes of directions of my life.
THE FINGERS	The small details of everyday life.
THE THUMB	Related to worries or to my intellect or my hearing.
THE INDEX	Related to fears, to my personality (ego) or my sense of smell.
THE MIDDLE FINGER	Related to anger or to my sexuality or my vision.
THE RING FINGER	Related to sorrow or to my marriage or my sense of touch.
THE LITTLE FINGER	Related to pretention or to my family or my sense of taste.
THE HEART	My **Love**.
THE BLOOD	The joy that flows in my life.
THE BREASTS	My maternal side.
THE LUNGS	My need for space and autonomy. Related to my sense of living.

THE STOMACH	My capacity for digesting new ideas.
THE BACK	My support, my undergirding.
THE JOINTS	My flexibility, my capacity for bending myself to the different situations in my life.
THE SKIN	My interface between my inner and outer sides (balance).
THE BONES	The structure of laws and principles of the world in which I live.
THE UTERUS	My home.
THE INTESTINES	(Especially the large intestine, the colon): my capacity for releasing, for letting go what is useless to me, or for allowing events to flow in my life.
THE KIDNEYS	The seat of fear.
THE PANCREAS	The joy that is in me.
THE LIVER	The seat of criticism.
THE LEGS	My capacity for moving forward in life and embracing change and new experiences.
THE KNEES	My flexibility, my pride, my stubbornness.
THE ANKLES	My flexibility in the new directions of the future.
THE FEET	My direction (stamping in place). My understanding of myself and life (past, present, future).
THE TOES	The details of my future.

Brief Overview of Main Ailments and Diseases and Their Likely Meaning

List of the main ailments and diseases, with brief indications of their probable meanings.

Abcess	Often related to a difficulty in conveying something that irritates or annoys me. This difficulty will show itself in the form of an abcess.
Accident	Often related to fear or guilt.
Acne	Often related to poor self-esteem and a desire to hold people away from me for fear of being hurt.
AIDS	Often related to great disappointment and guilt regarding **Love** and sexuality.
Ailment, malaise	Often related to the fact of wanting to externalize an inner tension.
Alcoholism	Often related to the desire to escape my physical or affective responsibilities, to avoid being 'hurt again'.
Allergies	Often related to anger or frustration about a person or an event associated with the allergenic product. To whom or to what was I allergic when this situation occurred?
Alzheimer's disease	A disease often related to the desire to flee the realities of this world and to not want to take on any responsibilities.
Amputation	Often related to great guilt.
Anxiety, Anguishe	Often related to the feeling of being limited and restricted, with a very marked impression of smothering in a situation.
Anorexia	Often related to very low self-esteem and an unconscious desire to want to 'disappear'.
Appendicitis	Often related to anger because I feel in a dead end.
Arthritis	Often related to criticism of myself or of others.
Autism	Often related to escape because I have difficulty in dealing with the world around me.
Bleeding	Often related to a loss of joy (blood = joy).
Bulimia	Often related to the need to fill an inner affective void.
Burns, fever	Often related to my anger burning inside of me or against a person or an event.
Burnout	Often related to escape from an intense emotion experienced at work or in various occupations.
Cancer	Often related to a great fear or guilt, to the point of no longer wanting to live, even unconsciously.
Cellulitis	Often related to the fear of commitment and my tendency to cling to the emotions of the past.
Cholesterol	Often related to my joy in living that circulates with difficulty.
Cigarettes	Often related to an inner void that I want to fill.

Constipation	Often related to the fact of wanting to hold on to the persons or events of my life.
Cramps	Often related to tension in an action taken or to be taken.
Depression	Often related to the desire to remove pressure in my life. And so I have a 'de-pression'.
Diabetes	Often related to deep sadness that occurs following an event where I resented life.
Diarrhea	Often related to wanting to reject solutions or situations being offered to me to move ahead in life.
Dizziness Coma, Loss of consciousness,	Often related to a desire to flee a situation or a person, when I have the impression that things are going too fast.
Eczema	Often related to the fact of no longer having any contact with a loved one.
Fatigue	Often related to the fact that I scatter my energies and allow myself to be easily controlled by my fears, insecurities and worries.
Gangrene	Often related to resentment or fear about a situation involving the aspect of my life that is represented by the affected body part.
Gas	Often related to the fact that something or someone I cling to is no longer beneficial for me.
Heart	All heart-linked diseases are often related to a lack of **Love** for me, my loved ones or my environment.
Hypoglycemia	Often related to sadness resulting from my resistance to life's events.
Incontinence	Often related to a wish to control everything in my life.
Infarction	Often related to **Love**, which I must more fully accept↓♥ in order to receive it.
Infections	Often related to frustration over various aspects of my life.
Influenza	Often related to anger; I have taken a dislike to someone or something.
Insomnia	Often related to staying 'hooked' on a form of guilt.
Itching, Irritations	Often related to impatience, insecurity, or an annoyance with myself.
Joints, articulations	Often related to a lack of flexibility in life's situations.
Leukemia	Often related to no longer wanting to fight to obtain what represents **Love** in my life.
Lungs	Often the diseases involving the lungs are related to being able to take up my vital space, the 'air' I need to feel free and be able to live.
Mononucleosis	Often related to a great fear of facing a situation that would lead me to an affective commitment.
Multiple Sclerosis	Often related to having rigid thoughts about myself, about others and about life's situations.
Nausea	Often related to an aspect of my life that I want to reject because it disgusts me.

Numbness	Often related to a desire to become less sensitive to a person or a situation.
Pain	Often a form of self-punishment for a guilt feeling. May reflect a need for attention, or fear or anger.
Paralysis	Often related to escape, for a fear is paralyzing me.
Poisoning	I must ask: who or what is poisoning my existence?
Pressure (High)	Often related to long-standing worries or troubles.
Pressure (Low)	Often related to a form of discouragement.
Rheumatism	Often related to criticism, against myself or others.
Sciatic nerve	Often related to great insecurity about my basic needs: housing, food, money.
Scoliosis	Often related to my feeling so many responsibilities on my shoulders that I want to flee them.
Shingles Herpes zostra	Often related to great insecurity about the loss of the Love of someone or of a situation (e.g.: my work group) that brought me this Love.
Skin diseases	Often related to my feeling that I have no 'contact', physical or otherwise, to obtain the **Love** I need.
Smothering, Loss of breath	Often related to being overly criticized, held by the throat, lacking vital space and having difficulty in living what I want to live.
Snoring	Often related to old ideas, attitudes or material goods I cling to, which I would be better off to let go.
Stiffness (joint)	Often related to a lack of flexibility, stubbornness, resistance or rigidity, mainly with authority figures.
Strain, sprain	Often related to situations where I resist, worry, and need to increase my openness and flexibility.
Swelling, edema	Often related to feeling limited or afraid of being limited or stopped in what I want to do.
Tics	Often related to very great inner tension. Tics usually appear when I am experiencing pressure in dealing with authority.
Tinnitus	Often related to a need to listen to my inner needs and values.
Torticollis (Stiff neck)	Often related to one or more sides (aspects) of a situation that I avoid seeing or want to flee from.
Tumor, cyst	Often related to an emotional shock that solidifies.
Weight (excess)	Often related to accumulating things, ideas or emotions, a need to protect myself, feeling limited, experiencing an inner void.

Appendix III

Diseases with Names Ending in -itis

All diseases in **'itis'**are usually related to anger or frustration because they are related to inflammations. Here are a few examples:

Amygdal**itis**
Appendic**itis**
Arthr**itis**
Bronch**itis**
Burs**itis**
Col**itis**
Conjunctiv**itis**
Cyst**itis**
Diverticul**itis**
Epicondyl**itis**
Epiderm**itis**
Gastro-enter**itis**
Gingiv**itis**
Hepat**itis**
Ile**itis**

Appendix IV

Diseases with Names Ending in -osis

The diseases with names ending in **–OSIS,** such as arthr**osis,** cirrh**osis,** thromb**osis, etc.** are diseases that are non-inflammatory.
If I have one of these diseases, I am experiencing a situation in which either someone slows me down, or I am the one who applies the brakes because I **focus** my attention too much on my limits, whether external or internal. I do not **dare** to act, because I have an underlying fear. I am sensitive to the criticism of others, and experiencing such unpleasant situations leads me to be negative and sometimes even depressed.

I accept↓♥ to face my fears. **I DARE** to speak and undertake an action that will bring me greater freedom. I can thus create my life and achieve my dreams!

Acrokerat**osis**
Atheroscler**osis**
Arthr**osis**
Cirrh**osis**
Discarthr**osis**
Fibromat**osis**
Fibr**osis**
Kerat**osis**
Lord**osis**
Mediacol**osis**
Mononucle**osis**
Mucoviscid**osis**
Myc**osis**
Neur**osis**
Osteopor**osis**
Pedicul**osis**
Psych**osis**
Salmonell**osis**
Sarcoid**osis**
Scler**osis**
Scoli**osis**
Thromb**osis**
Tubercul**osis**

Appendix V

Principles of Healing

Here are some principles to help understand some of the mechanisms involved in the manifestation of diseases and healing. Each principle can be read individually or together along with the others listed below.

- Love is the true healer.

- Being 100% certain that I can heal will help the healing to happen.

- Illness is the brain's solution to lower the conscious or unconscious psychological stress.

- As soon as there is a solution, the conflict is eliminated, and the psychological overstress can be released.

- Stress results from the emotional conflict I experience and can trigger the disease.

- As diseases are programmable, consciously or unconsciously, they can also be de-programmed.

- Knowledge liberates and love helps with healing.

- The resolution of the conflict and the certainty of healing are important keys to complete healing.

- Diseases are the perfect brain solutions for reducing the psychological stress, and often are at the root of illnesses.

- Illness is a message of love to understand. I remain open to discover this message.

- The conflicts that are inside of me can cause an over stress.

- An illness is usually the biological transposition of a conscious or unconscious psychological conflict.

- Psychological stress is an internal conflict that I experience, either regarding a facet of myself, another person or a situation.

- An inner conflict results from a feeling of a lack of love at the heart ♥ level.

- All illness often comes from stress, conscious or unconscious.

- The Encyclopedia of Ailments and Diseases helps me to understand the emotions, thoughts or feelings I am experiencing that can have led me to manifest an illness.

- When I identify the emotion that is causing my stress, it shows me what I need to work on to eliminate it.

- It is important to keep my mind and heart ♥ open and to accept ↓♥ in my heart ♥ that I have something to understand through this illness (and not that I agree to be sick!)

- When I say THANK YOU in my heart ♥ to what is happening, I keep my heart ♥ open.

- I need to put the guilt aside!

- When I reintroduce love into a situation and heal, I find myself with more love, wisdom and freedom.

- **The Integration and Acceptance Technique** explained at the beginning of this encyclopedia helps accessing information through the heart ♥ allowing me to open the door for the healing process to take place.

- *The Encyclopedia of Ailments and Diseases* is a tool for understanding, investigation and transformation.

- Everything is possible! So, if I truly believe, I will seek and probably find a solution.

Love is the true healer

Index

✷ **Liver congestion**
See: Congestion

✷ **Liver — Hepatitis**

✷ **Locomotion**
See: System locomotor

✷ **Lordosis**
See: Spinal [deviation of] — Lordosis

✷ **Loss of appetite**
See: Appetite [loss of]

✷ **Low pressure**
See: Tension arterial— Hypotension [too low]

✷ **Lower back**
See: Back disorders — Lower back

✷ **LSD (consumption of)**
See: Drugs

✷ **Lumbago**
See: Back disorders- Lower back

✷ **Lumbalgia**
See: Back disorders — Lower back

✷ **Lung(s) (in general)**

✷ **Lung diseases**

✷ **Lungs (cancer of the)**
See: Cancer of the Lung

✷ **Lungs — Congestion**
See: Congestion

✷ **Lungs — Emphysema (pulmonary)**

✷ **Lungs — Legionnaires' disease**

✷ **Lungs — Pneumonia and Pleuresy**

✷ **Lupus (systemic lupus erythematosis [SLE])**
See: Skin — Lupus

✷ **Luxation / (Joint), Dislocation**

✷ **Lymph (lymphatic disorders)**

✷ **Lymphoma**
See: Hodgin's disease

✷ **Magic mushrooms (consumption of)**
See: Drugs

✷ **Malaise / Ailment**

✷ **Malaria / Paludism**

✷ **Male principle**

✷ **Malformation (in general) in the heart♥**

✷ **Mania**

✷ **Manic-depressive psychosis**
See: Psychosis

✷ **Marfan's syndrome**

✷ **Marijuana consumption**
See: Drugs

✷ **Masochism**
See: Sadomasochism

✷ **Mass / Lump / Swelling**
See: Hump / Lump

✷ **Mastication**
See: Mouth [in general]

✷ **Mastitis**
See: Breast — Mastitis

✷ **Mastoiditis**

✷ **Mastosis**
See: Breast disorders

✷ **Measles**
See: Childhood diseases

✷ **Medicine**

✷ **Melancholy**

✷ **Melanoma**
See: Skin — Melanoma [malignant]

✷ **Memory (failing)**

✷ **Ménière's disease — Labyrinthitis**

✷ **Meningitis**
See: Brain — Meningitis

✷ **Menisci**
See: Knee ailments

✷ **Meniscus**

✷ **Menopause disorders**

✷ **Menorrhagia**
See: Menstruation — Menorrhagia

✷ **Menses / Menstruation /**

Bibliography

ARNOLD, Roland, *La symbolique des maladies*, Éditions Dangles, 2000.

BALCH, James F., M.D., BALCH, Phyllis A., C.N.C., *Prescription for Nutritional Healing*, Avery publishing group inc., 1990.

BEERLANDT, Christiane, *La clef vers l'auto libération*, Édition Altima, 2000.

BOURBEAU, Lise, *Qui es-tu?*, Éditions Écoute ton Corps, 1988.

CAFFIN, Michèle, *Quand les dents se mettent à parler*, Éditeur Guy Trédaniel, 1994.

CHARPENTIER, Dr Gérard, *Les maladies et leurs émotions*, Editions de Mortagne, 2000.

COLIN, Docteur Antoine, *Dictionnaire des noms illustres en médecine*, Prodim, Édition-Librairie, Bruxelles, Belgique, 1994.

COLLECTIF, *Le nouveau petit Robert 2011*, Dictionnaires Le Robert, 2011.

DE SURANY, Marguerite, *Pour une Médecine de l'Âme*, Éditions Guy Trédaniel, 1987.

DE SURANY, Marguerite et JOURDAN, Jean-Claude, *Les deux inséparables: Crâne-Colonne*, union de l'âme et de l'esprit, Éditions Guy Trédaniel, 1990.

DRANSART, Dr Philippe, *La maladie cherche à me guérir*, Éditions Le mercure dauphinois, 1999.

DUHAIME, Bertrand, *L'humanité Métaphysique, A.U.M.*, Les ateliers universels de motivation.

DUNNE, Lavon J., *Nutrition Almanac (Third Edition)*, McGRAW-HILL, 1990.

DUPONT, Michel, *Dictionnaire historique des médecins dans et hors de la médecine*, Éditions Larousse, 1999.

FIAMMETTI, Roger, *Le langage émotionnel du corps*, Éditions Dervy, 2004.

FLÈCHE, Christian, *Décodage biologique des maladies*, Le souffle d'or, 2001.

HAY, Louise, *Heal your body*, Hay House, 1988.

HAY, Louise, *You can heal your life*, Hay House, 1990.

HAY, Louise, *How to love yourself*, Hay House, 1992.

KISTER, Pierre, *Dictionnaire encyclopédique alpha*, Éditions Grammont, Suisse, Lausanne, 1982.

LAROUSSE, *Larousse médical*, 2005.

MÜLLER, Brigitte et GÜNTHER, Hordt H., *A Complete Book of Reiki Healing*, Life rhythm, 1995.

ODOUL, Michel, *Dis-moi où tu as mal*, Éditions Dervy, 1999.

ODOUL, Michel Rémy, *Cheveux, parle-moi de moi*, Édition Dervy, 1997.

RAINVILLE, Claudia, *Métamédecine, la guérison à votre portée*, Éditions FRJ, 1995.

ROSSETTE, Alain, *Encyclopédie de décodage biologique en corrélation psycho cérébro-organique*, Éditions Holoconcept, 1999

SABBAH, Claude, *La biologie des êtres vivants décrite sous forme d'histoire naturelle*, notes de cours, séminaires 1, 2, 3, Holoconcept, 1997.

SHAPIRO, Debbie, *The Body mind workbook*, Element Books limited, 1990.

SHAPIRO, Debbie, *Your body speaks your mind*, Sounds True, 1998.

SHARAMON, Shalila & BAGINSKI, Bodo J., *REIKI, Universal Life Energy*, Guy Trédaniel, 1991.

VAN den bogaert, Eduard, *Le grand dictionnaire collégial de décodage biologique*, 2e édition, Rassemblé par et Réalisé par l'asbl Téligaté, Bruxelles, avril 2004.

VEREECK, Dre Estelle, *Dictionnaire de langage de vos dents*, Éditions Luigi Castelli, 2004.

About the Author

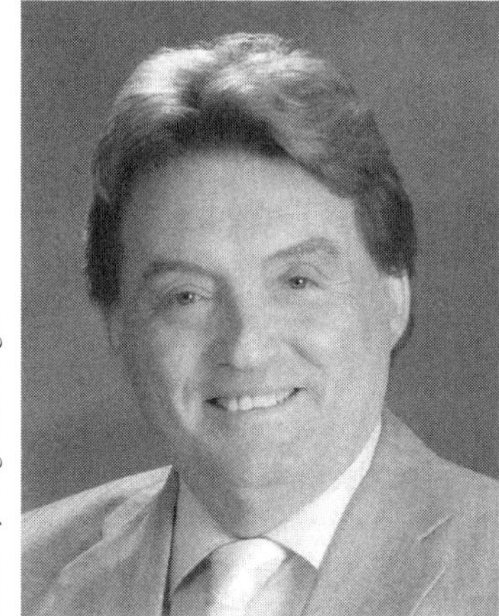

Photo by Serge Bourdages

Born in Montreal (Canada) in September 1950, Jacques Martel finished his training as an electrical engineer in 1977 at Laval University in Quebec City and became a regular member of the Order of Quebec Engineers. He later taught electricity and electronics for a government organization, the Canada Manpower Centre (CMC), and also worked as a trainer in private business.

He has always shown a keen interest for communication in all its forms. After completing his university studies, the electronic media attracted his attention, and in 1977 he undertook a training program at the Quebec College of Radio and Television Announcers (CART in French). Later on, for two years he took part as an anchorman and research assistant in more than 100 televised episodes on health and well-being that were shown on a private television network throughout the province of Quebec.

His desire to understand the "other side of things" led him on a spiritual quest that completely reoriented his life. In 1978 he undertook research on "Vitamin Therapy", also called the "Orthomolecular approach", following a holistic approach of being. His approach dovetailed with that of Canadian, American and European psychiatrists, researchers, chemists and biochemists in that field. It was in 1988 that he engaged in personal development training. This training touched such a chord that he became a leader of personal development workshops, an occupation that he then pursued full-time as a psychotherapist from as early as 1990.

Enriched by the truths he discovered, the communicator in him chose to share the fruits of his reflections with the greatest possible number of persons. Thus, the ATMA Growth Centre was born in 1990 and in 1996 it became ***ATMA Inc.,*** which grouped together **Les Éditions ATMA Internationales** (for books) and les **Productions ATMA Internationales** (for conferences, guided meditations and music on CDs). Jacques Martel is still the acting president.

Since 1990, he has continued to pursue his personal and professional training, which enabled him, over the years, to acquire a solid reputation in this field. It was in 1995 that he acquired his training as a Rebirther (a conscious breathing technique) at the Héléna Marcoux Centre.

His vast experience also enables him to intervene as a consultant with therapists and other health professionals.

In 1991, a writing project emerged in his life. Slowly but surely, the first French edition of the book ***The Complete Dictionary of Ailments and Diseases*** began to take form. The knowledge acquired during his training as an electrical engineer enabled him to learn how to travel from the tangible to the intangible and from practice to intuition; furthermore, his many workshops and conferences confirmed for him the close link between illnesses (ailments and diseases) and thoughts (feelings and emotions) as the sources of conflicts that can lead to the triggering of those illnesses. He was now quite ready to write his book, which finally appeared in its first edition in April 1998.

In 1993, he became a REIKI Master (a healing energy technique). From 1994 to 1998, he was the President of the Canadian and Quebec Association of REIKI Masters (ACQMR in French). In 2011, he was trained in "Reconnection" (another healing energy technique) and helped others to become reconnected so that they in turn could later be trained to become practitioners of this technique themselves. Since 04/04/04 (April 4, 2004), he has become more conscious of the Way that must be followed to further develop the means for moving toward physical, emotional, mental and spiritual healing.

Jacques Martel presents conferences, takes part in health and well-being fairs and leads workshops in Quebec. From 1988 to 2013, he led workshops in Europe and in the French D.O.M. (Overseas Territories), on Reunion Island, in French Polynesia and in Mauritius. He also, upon request, trains other therapists with his emotional healing technique, ITHT (the ***Integration Through the Heart Technique***), that he developed in recent years and which has given positive results to his clients. He also gives a training session entitled On the Road to Awakening, which helps those who wish to open themselves up in order to reach further levels of consciousness, safely and sincerely.

He also developed the ***Little Matchstick Figures Technique***, and the book introducing it was written by Lucie Bernier and Robert Lenghan: ***La Technique des Petits Bonshommes Allumettes*** (2015). It is a powerful and effective technique for becoming more keenly aware of our negative patterns and positively transforming them.

The interest stimulated among the general public and among therapists by the book ***The Complete Dictionary of Ailments and Diseases***, the first English edition of the present ***Encyclopedia of Ailments and Diseases***, demonstrates the relevance of such a work: it has been read so far by more than 1 million readers worldwide.

In addition to the second French edition (2007) of this book, Jacques Martel has published several other complementary books that are highly appreciated by people seeking healing and well-being. These other books include:

ATMA, the Power of Love (2005/2013)

The Power of the WORDS... that free me! (2011)

The 5 STEPS to achieve HEALING (2010)

Conscience, Amour et Guérison (Tomes I et II) (2016)
[Consciousness, Love and Healing (Tomes I and II)]

Le Pouvoir de l'ENGAGEMENT... ou comment agir en GAGNANT! (2014)
[The Power of COMMITMENT... or how to be a WINNER!]

ATMA et le Cercle de Guérison (2008/2013)
[ATMA and the Healing Circle]

Retour vers la Source (2011)
[Return to the Source]

Books co-authored with Jean-Jacques Robinet

LE POUVOIR DU REIKI, Énergie de Vie, Énergie de Guérison (2014)
[THE POWER OF REIKI, Life Energy, Healing Energy]

L'Oracle Indigo dévoilé (2018)

ATMA LE REIKI, Niveaux 1,2,3 et MAÎTRE Enseignant (2018)
[ATMA, REIKI, Levels 1,2,3 and Master Teacher]

Jacques Martel has also produced several conference CDs, guided meditation CDs and VIDEO capsules on different subjects involving health and well-being.

His Professional Career

1977	Diploma in Electrical Engineering, Laval University in Québec, Canada.
1977 - 1987	Member of the Quebec Order of Engineers.
1978 - 1988	Therapist in vitamin therapy (the orthomolecular approach).
1985 - 1986	Member of the Canadian Mental Health Association.
1987	Trained at the Quebec College of Radio and Television Announcers (CART in French).
1987 - 1990	Anchorman and program researcher for television programs on health and well-being (more than 100).
1990	Founding President of the ATMA Growth Centre.
1993	Trained as a REIKI Master.
1994 - 1998	President of the Canadian and Quebec Association of REIKI Masters (ACQMR in French).
1996	Diploma in Professional Rebirthing (a conscious breathing technique) at the Héléna Marcoux Institute.

1996 - 2002	Member of the Quebec Corporation of Alternative Medicine Practitioners (CPDMQ in French).
1998 - 2013	Personal development conferences and workshops in Europe (France, Switzerland, Belgium, French Polynesia, Réunion Island, Mauritius Island).
2011	Trained as a Practitioner of Reconnection© (Dr. Eric Pearl).

For more information about the author visit his website:
www.jacquesmartel.com

About the Co-author

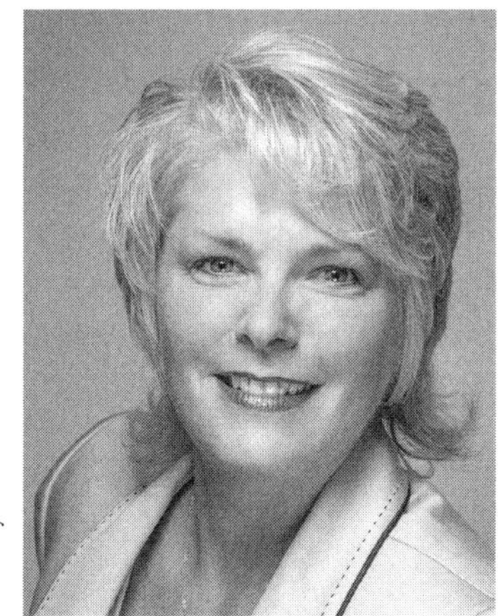

Photo by Don Ricker

Lucie Bernier is a psychotherapist, speaker and personal development workshop leader. She originates from Rivière-Ouelle, a municipality of Québec (Canada) located in the Lower Saint Lawrence River region. She completed her university training in Law and had a career as a flight attendant and a chief purser for 22 years with an international air carrier company.

In 1989 she undertook to engage in a process of working on her "Self". It was in 1993 that she became a REIKI Master (a natural healing technique applied by imposing the hands and using the universal neutral energy with no intention). She followed more than 2500 hours of personal and professional development workshops. She also acted as a workshop leader and/or assistant during the workshops given by Jacques Martel, mainly in Europe. She has also taught and given workshops and lectures in Québec, New Brunswick, Ontario, and in the United States.

From 1995 to 1998, she collaborated in the production of the first French edition of the book ***The Complete Dictionary of Ailments and Diseases***, now entitled ***The Encyclopedia of Ailments and Diseases***, and also took part in working out the second edition.

Discover the HU Chant

This mantra offers you exceptional opportunities to open your consciousness and raise your soul. It promotes peace, happiness and protection.

You can download the HU Chant here:

Or direct link:

https://soundcloud.com/jacques-martel-atma/le-chant-dunivers

You can download the "HU Chant" free of charge once you have signed up with SoundCloud.

Also of Interest from Findhorn Press

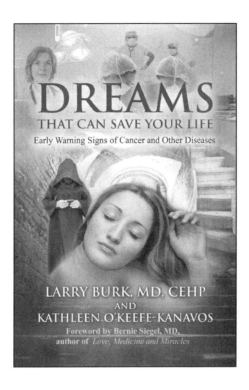

Dreams That Can Save Your Life

by Larry Burk, M.D., C.E.H.P.
and Kathleen O'Keefe-Kanavos

YOUR DREAMS CAN PROVIDE INNER GUIDANCE filled with life-saving information. Showcasing the important role of dreams and their power to detect and heal illness, Dr. Larry Burk and Kathleen O'Keefe-Kanavos, a three-time breast cancer survivor, share amazing medical research and true stories of physical and emotional healings triggered by dreams.

ISBN 978-1-84409-744-9

Also of Interest from Findhorn Press

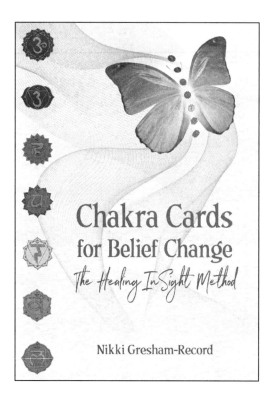

Chakra Cards for Belief Change

By Nikki Gresham-Record

A CARD DECK AND THERAPY TOOL in one, this boxed set offers 56 full-color cards to assist you in transforming your unhelpful beliefs and raising your vibration to begin creating the reality you desire. The cards feature high-vibration chakra images paired with powerful affirmations to help you clear the chakras and energetically realign your mindset.

ISBN 978-1-64411-040-9

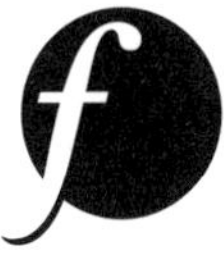

FINDHORN PRESS

Life-Changing Books

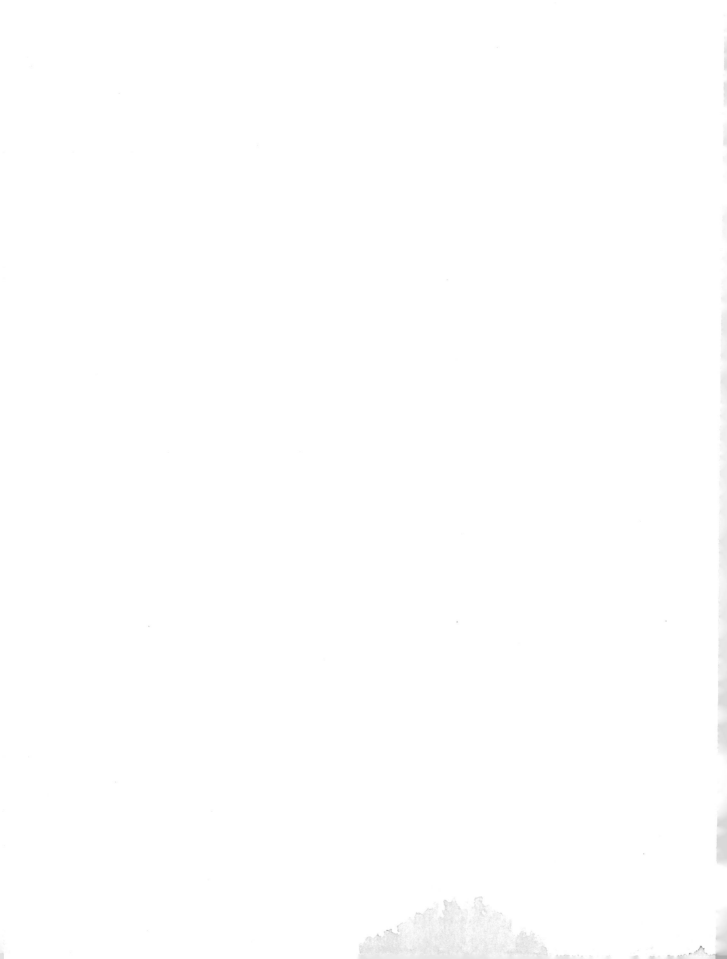